Genetics of Lactic Acid Bacteria

THE LACTIC ACID BACTERIA

Series Editor: Brian J. B. Wood

Strathclyde University
Glasgow, Scotland

Volume 3: *Genetics of Lactic Acid Bacteria*
Edited by Brian J. B. Wood and Philip J. Warner

Volume 2: *Genera of Lactic Acid Bacteria*
Edited by W. H. N. Holzapfel and Brian J. B. Wood

Volume 1: *Lactic Acid Bacteria in Health and Disease*
Edited by Brian J. B. Wood

Genetics of Lactic Acid Bacteria

Edited by

Brian J. B. Wood
Strathclyde University
Glasgow, Scotland

and

Philip J. Warner
Cranfield University at Silsoe
Bedfordshire, United Kingdom

Kluwer Academic / Plenum Publishers
New York, Boston, Dordrecht, London, Moscow

Library of Congress Cataloging-in-Publication Data

Wood, Brian, J. B.
Genetics of lactic acid bacteria/Brian J. B. Wood and Philip J. Warner.
p. cm. — (The lactic acid bacteria; v. 3)
Includes bibliographical references and index.
ISBN 0-306-47290-2
I. Lactic acid bacteria—Genetics. I. Warner, Philip J. II. Title. III. Series.

QR121.W66 2003
579.3′55—dc21

2003044722

ISBN: 0-306-47290-2

233 Spring Street, New York, New York 10013

http://www.wkap.nl/

10 9 8 7 6 5 4 3 2 1

A C.I.P. record for this book is available from the Library of Congress

Printed in the United States of America

Contributors List

1. **Girbe Buist**
Biologisch Centrum
University of Groningen
Kerklaan 30, 9751 NN Haren
The Netherlands

2. **Stéphane Chaillou**
Flore Lactique et Environnement Carné (FLEC)
INRA-CRJ, Domaine de Vilvert
78350 Jouy-en-Josas
France

3. **Luis M. Cintas**
Departemento de Nutrición y Bromotología III
Facultad de Veterinaria
Universidad Complutense de Madrid
28040-Madrid
Spain

4. **Willem M. de Vos**
Laboratory of Microbiology
Department of Biomolecular Sciences
Hesselink van Suchtelenweg 4
6703 CT Wageningen, The Netherlands
E-mail: willemdevos@algemeen.micr.wau.nl

5. **Gerald F. Fitzgerald**
Department of Microbiology and Food Science and Technology
The National Food Research Centre
University College
Cork, Ireland
E-mail: G.Fitzgerald@ucc.ie

6. **Michael J. Gasson**
Department of Genetics & Microbiology
Institute of Food Research

Norwich Research Park
Colney, Norwich
NR4 7UA, England
E-mail: mike.gasson@bbsrc.ac.uk

7. **Todd R. Klaenhammer**
Southeast Dairy Foods Research Center
Department of Food Science
Box 7624, North Carolina State University
Raleigh, NC 27695-7624, USA
E-mail: klaenhammer@ncsu.edu

8. **Michael Kleerebezem**
Wageningen Centre for Food Sciences
NIZO Food Research
P.O. Box 20, 6710 BA Ede
The Netherlands
E-mail: kleerebe@nizo.nl

9. **Jan Kok**
Biologisch Centrum
University of Groningen
Kerklaan 30, 9751 NN Haren
The Netherlands
E-mail: kokj@biol.rug.nl

10. **Oscar P. Kuipers**
Department of Genetics
University of Groningen
P.O. Box 14
9750 AA Haren
The Netherlands
E-mail: O.P.Kuipers@biol.rug.nl

11. **Aat Ledeboer**
Unilever Research Laboratorium
Oliver van Noortlaan 120
3133 AT Vlaardingen
The Netherlands

12. **Kees J. Leenhouts**
BioMaDe Technology
Nijenborgh 4, 9747 AG Groningen
The Netherlands
E-mail: c.j.leenhouts@chem.rug.nl

13. **Stephen McGrath**
National Food Biotechnology Centre
University College
Cork, Ireland

14. **Leo Meile**
Eidgenossische Technische Hochschule Zurich
Schmelzbergstrasse 9
ETH Zentrum
CH-8092 Zurich, Switzerland

15. **Annick Mercenier**
Nestlé Research Centre
P. O. Box 44
Vers-chez-les-Blanc
CH-1000 Lausanne 26
Switzerland
E-mail: annick.mercenier@rdls.nestle.com

16. **Ingolf F. Nes**
Laboratory of Microbial Gene Technology
Agricultural University of Norway
P.O. Box 5051
N-1432 Ås, Norway
E-mail: ingolf.nes@ikb.nlh.no

17. **Peter H. Pouwels**
TNO Prevention and Health
Post Box 2215
Leiden, The Netherlands
E-mail: p.pouwels@p.g.tno.nl

18. **Jane Rixon**
Institute of Bioscience and Biotechnology
Cranfield University at Silsoe
Silsoe, Bedfordshire
England, MK45 4DT

19. **Franziska Schwarz**
Eidgenossische Technische Hochschule Zurich
Schmelzbergstrasse 9
ETH Zentrum
CH-8092 Zurich, Switzerland

20. **Claire A. Shearman**
Department of Genetics & Microbiology
Institute of Food Research
Norwich Research Park
Colney, Norwich
NR4 7UA, UK

21. **Morten Skaugen**
Laboratory of Microbial Gene Technology
Agricultural University of Norway
N-1432 Ås, Norway

22. **Elizabeth Stanley**
National Food Biotechnology
University College
Cork, Ireland

23. **Michael Teuber**
Eidgenossische Technische Hochschule Zurich
Schmelzbergstrasse 9
ETH Zentrum
CH-8092 Zurich, Switzerland
E-mail: teuber@snickers.ethz.ch

24. **Douwe van Sinderen**
Department of Microbiology and Food Science and Technology
The National Food Research Centre
University College
Cork, Ireland

25. **Elaine E. Vaughan**
Laboratory of Microbiology
Department of Agrotechnology and Food Sciences
Wageningen University and Wageningen Centre for Food Sciences
Hesselink van Suchtelenweg 4
6703 CT Wageningen
The Netherlands
E-mail: elaine.vaughan@algemeen.micr.wau.nl

26. **C. Theo Verrips**
Unilever Research Laboratorium
Oliver van Noortlaan 120
3133 AT Vlaardingen
The Netherlands
E-mail: Theo.Verrips@unilever.com

27. **Shirley A. Walker**
Southeast Dairy Foods Research Center
Department of Food Science
Box 7624, North Carolina State University
Raleigh, NC 27695-7624, USA

28. **Philip J. Warner**
Institute of Bioscience and Biotechnology
Cranfield University at Silsoe
Silsoe, Bedfordshire
England, MR45 4DT
E-mail: P.J.Warner@cranfield.ac.uk

29. **Jerry M. Wells**
Microbial Genetics and Physiology
Institute of Food Research
Norwich Research Park
Norwich
England, NR4 7UA
E-mail: jerry.wells@bbsrc.ac.uk

30. **Brian J. B. Wood**
Bioscience Department
Royal College Building
University of Strathclyde
204 George St.
Glasgow
Scotland, 61 IXW
E-mail: b.j.b.wood@strath.ac.uk

Series Preface

The Lactic Acid Bacteria is planned as a series of volumes, and the interest shown in it to date justifies a cautious optimism that a series comprising at least five volumes will appear in the fullness of time. This being so, I feel that it is desirable to introduce the series by providing a little of the history of the events, which culminated in the decision to produce such a series. I also wish to indicate the boundaries of the group "The Lactic Acid Bacteria" (LAB) as I have defined them for the present purposes, and to outline my hopes for the future of the series.

Historical Background

I owe my interest in the LAB to the late Dr Cyril Rainbow, who introduced me to their fascinating world when he offered me a place with him to work on a Ph.D. on the carbohydrate metabolism of some lactic rods isolated from English beer breweries by himself and others, notably Dr Dora Kulka. I was given the topic of the preference exhibited by some of these isolates for maltose over glucose as a source of carbohydrate for growth, expressed in most cases as a more rapid growth on the disaccharide. One isolate, however, carried this to the extreme of growing on maltose alone. Eventually we showed that maltose was being metabolized by "direct fermentation" as the older texts called it. Specifically the bacteria were using phosphorolysis, which had first been demonstrated for maltose by Doudoroff and his associates in their work on a strain of *Neisseria meningitidis*.

I began work on food fermentations when I came to Strathclyde University, and I soon found myself involved again with the bacteria which I had not touched since completing my doctoral thesis. In 1973, J. G. Carr, C. V. Cutting, and G. C. Whiting organized the 4th Long Ashton Symposium *Lactic Acid Bacteria in Beverages and Food*, and from my participation arose a friendship with Geoff Carr, whom I had previously seen as a rather remote and awesome figure, but was in fact the most approachable and convivial of men, with whom I shared an enthusiasm for country pubs and cask-conditioned beers. The growing importance of the LAB (which had long been recognized as vital to several industries, notably dairying) was subsequently confirmed by the holding, on the 10th anniversary of the Long Ashton meeting, of the first of the Wageningen Conferences on the LAB. Discussions about the LAB, and the fact that they were significant enough to have entire conferences devoted to them, with Mr George Olley of Applied Science Publishers Ltd (who had proposed the idea which resulted in the production of *Microbiology of Fermented Foods*) generated the perception that there might be scope for a book on the LAB.

Subsequent discussions with Geoff Carr refined "a book" into "a multi-volume series". Rather slowly Geoff and I began to lay plans for such a series, generally in meetings convened in the delightful rural West of England pubs. Sadly, Geoff died before the plans reached fruition, but his thinking contributed much to my subsequent development of the ideas, which we hatched together, and I think that he would have approved of the form which the series is now taking. I also think that even he would have been amazed at how far knowledge, particularly in the genetics field, has advanced since that conference in Long Ashton. In every volume I have tried to achieve a multinational spread among the Authors, which would certainly have received his enthusiastic approval. I have also tried to achieve a direct and clear writing style through my directions to Authors and to my subsequent editing of the resulting manuscripts. Both Geoff and Cyril valued clarity in writing very highly and deplored the kind of scientific writing which seemed to have been generated under the delusion that proper science should demonstrate its importance by being as obscure as possible. In the intervening years, despite much talk about the need for increased clarity, the literary quality of such writing has, if anything deteriorated further, although with some notable exceptions. At the same time the continuing development of scientific effort in the developing countries makes it more important than ever that we communicate clearly in order to reach the workers for whom English is a second or even a third language.

The Lactic Acid Bacteria

Most of us think that we know what we mean when we use this expression. We tend to think of them as a reasonably coherent group, and this is convenient for a great many purposes. In fact, however, the LAB remind me of a cloud in the sky, which can look rather coherent and well-bounded when viewed from a distance, but that becomes more and more fuzzy and intangible the closer one approaches to it. The LAB are all Gram-positive; anaerobic, micro-aerophilic or aero-tolerant; catalase negative; rods or cocci; most importantly they all produce lactic acid as the sole, major, or an important product from the energy-yielding fermentation of sugars. It used to be thought that all LAB were nonsporing and nonmotile, although we now have the Sporolactobacilli and motile organisms within recognized groupings of LAB. *Listeria* species produce lactic acid as a major metabolic product, but I doubt if many people working with the LAB as normally understood, would wish to admit them to membership of the club. The LAB as a group had a "squeaky clean" image, with such adverse effects as have been reported being, in general, ascribed to unusual circumstances, such as abnormal immune status. This applied despite the Streptococci, as originally defined, including both beneficial and harmful organisms. Yet *Listeria* is closely related (according to modern classifications) to undoubted LAB, and *Streptococcus* as now defined seems to consist almost entirely of rather disagreeable organisms, so it seems a little irrational to admit one of these organisms and exclude the other. I can offer no real defence of my continuing decision to do so, despite the evidently logical argument to the contrary, other than the hoary old one of "accepted practice." After much discussion, and with due acknowledgment of the rapidly evolving situation which is leading to the establishment of several new genera, I choose to confine this series of books to the genera detailed in Volume II; *The Genera of Lactic Acid Bacteria*, plus a few which have become generally recognized since that was published. This must however recognize the right of individual contributors to the series to define the LAB in the manner which seems most appropriate to the story which they have to tell, and also acknowledge that the boundaries of the group have scope for development as the series of books progresses.

Future Plans for the Series

Production of the series to date has been strongly affected by the numerous changes of ownership which it has experienced as successive publishers have first taken it over, then divested themselves of it as their perceptions of their own future development have changed. This has been a most unsettling experience for everyone concerned. The present volume's production in particular has been set back very badly by these events. It is sincerely hoped that the series has now found a more permanent home, so that longer term plans can now be prepared with more confidence than has been possible recently.

Future plans will inevitably be modified in the light of experience gained as the series develops, not least the feedback from readers and the comments and suggestions of reviewers. At present a revision of *The Genera of LAB* is being actively considered, as the print run is exhausted and advances in the science make it inappropriate to simply reprint the present volume. Other obvious areas for coverage are (a) the physiology and biochemistry of the organisms; (b) their applications and uses. Both of these are potentially vast areas, requiring rigorous limitation to matters very particular to the LAB, multi-volume format, or some combination of the two. Readers' views on these matters, and on other areas appropriate for consideration as potential volumes in the series will be warmly welcomed.

It remains the intention that together these volumes will form a lasting primary source and, as the computer experts would say, "benchmark" against which future progress in our understanding of this diverse but important group of bacteria can be measured.

Brian J. B. Wood

Preface

Producing this book has been a long and arduous process, requiring great patience from our authors. We have never experienced book production beset with so many problems, and various authors have expressed entirely justified doubts as to the wisdom of continuing with an endeavor that began to look as if it would never achieve fruition. This was due to many factors, of which the changes in ownership were but one. The seriousness of these delays was compounded by the nature of the subject which it addresses. The speed at which knowledge advances is almost overwhelming in all areas, but the new methods and procedures, the sheer volume of information these generate, and the complexity of the subject, as well as the potential for applications in diverse commercial fields, make this a particularly complex volume to oversee and integrate. Additionally, one of the Editors (BJBW) freely admits that assimilating the arcane-seeming language of this burgeoning subject greatly taxes his remaining grey cells' capacity to harvest new information. Despite this, the exercise has been fascinating for us, and we believe that this experience will be shared by our readers. This new knowledge is already finding many applications, not only in the obvious ways, such as improving and stabilizing dairy organisms, but in such remarkable new areas as delivering drugs and vaccines, and in the expression of introduced genes and the export from cells of those genes' products. In any scientific area developing at the bewildering pace being experienced by this one, it is a truism that the book will be out of date before it leaves the Printer. Thus the best that we can hope for is that it will be a means whereby future progress can be judged. Obviously the individual worker will always be ahead of the textbook in her/his particular field of expertise, but a book like this will demonstrate the extent to which that person's knowledge overlaps with related areas, and sometimes with remarkably distant ones. We have a particular hope that the book will show workers in developing countries how understanding the genetics of the microbes which they are using can help in developing their safe application to solving local problems. We also hope that it will be seen as a positive contribution to the developing debate on the safe application of genetic control and manipulation to farming and commercial processes.

P. J. Warner
Brian J. B. Wood

Contents

Chapter 1

Introduction: Background, Relevant Genetic Techniques, and Terms 1
Jane E. Rixon and Philip J. Warner

Chapter 2

Plasmid Biology, Conjugation, and Transposition 25
Michael J. Gasson and Claire A. Shearman

Chapter 3

Comparative Genomics of Bacteriophage Infecting Lactic Acid Bacteria 45
Elizabeth Stanley, Stephen McGrath, Gerald F. Fitzgerald, and Douwe van Sinderen

Chapter 4

Genetics of the Metabolism of Lactose and Other Sugars 95
Elaine E. Vaughan, Michiel Kleerebezem, and Willem M. de Vos

Chapter 5

Regulation of Gene Expression in *Lactococcus lactis* 121
Oscar P. Kuipers and Kees J. Leenhouts

Chapter 6

Gene Expression in Lactobacilli 143
Peter H. Pouwels and Stéphane Chaillou

Chapter 7

Genetics of Proteolysis in *Lactococcus lactis* 189
Jan Kok and Girbe Buist

Chapter 8

Genetics of Bacteriocin Production in Lactic Acid Bacteria 225
Morten Skaugen, Luis M. Cintas, and Ingolf F. Nes

Chapter 9

Lactic Acid Bacteria as Mucosal Delivery Vehicles........................ 261
Jerry M. Wells and Annick Mercenier

Chapter 10

The Genetics of Phage Resistance in *Lactococus lactis*..................... 291
Shirley A. Walker and Todd R. Klaenhammer

Chapter 11

Antibiotic Resistance and Transfer in Lactic Acid Bacteria................. 317
Michael Teuber, Franziska Schwarz, and Leo Meile

Chapter 12

The Ratio between Benefits and Risk of Fermented Foods Produced by Genetically Modified Lactic Acid Bacteria 355
Theo Verrips and Aat Ledeboer

Glossary/Abbreviations 377

Index 379

1

Introduction

Background, Relevant Genetic Techniques, and Terms

Jane E. Rixon and Philip J. Warner

History and Background

It seems incredible now that 25 years ago we knew nothing of the molecular genetics of lactic acid bacteria (LAB). Whilst taxonomy had been to the fore in the early part of the last century, and the biochemistry of the organisms was established in its middle years, it was in the final quarter of the 20th century that we began to gain an insight into how the organisms function at the molecular level. This is well within the careers of many of those working in the field today and though it is an often-used phrase, in this case it is true that the pace of achievement has been nothing short of phenomenal.

Rather than give an overview of this dramatic progress, this book looks at the most important advances and states the state of knowledge at present. By and large, it takes a thematic approach, looking at the molecular dissection of the major activities of the LAB and of its importance to man. These include lactose metabolism, proteolysis, bacteriocin production, phage susceptibility and resistance, antibiotic resistance, etc. It also looks at some of the biology of the organisms themselves through chapters on, for example, gene expression and natural gene transfer systems. Whilst most major areas of study are covered, the breadth of the field and the rapid pace of progress in the field make it difficult to make this book completely comprehensive.

The LAB and their importance to man have been the subject of the two previous volumes in this series and the reader is referred to them for a more complete understanding of these topics. However, it may be appropriate here to remind the reader that we are discussing several genera of Gram-positive bacteria, including *Lactococcus, Leuconostoc, Pediococcus, Carnobacterium, Enterococcus, Streptococcus, Lactobacillus*, and

Jane E. Rixon and Philip J. Warner • Cranfield University at Silsoe, Silsoe, Bedfordshire, England, MK45 4DT; e-mail: p.j.warner@cranfield.ac.uk

Bifidobacterium. The DNA of the organisms is generally AT rich, being composed of only 34–40% GC.

But what has been the spur for advancing molecular studies? It is no-doubt true that studies of this type have been very fashionable but there have been two practical reasons why the work has gained extensive funding.

First, it has given us an understanding of how the organisms themselves control their metabolism. Knowledge of these control mechanisms imparts the ability to manipulate growth to optimize the industrial role of these bacteria. Second, the hope is that by direct manipulation of the genes themselves, we can enhance the traditional roles of LAB as well as making them fit for new ones, particularly in healthcare, for example, using LAB as live oral vaccines. At the time of writing the latter is the subject of some consumer resistance, particularly in the food sector, though there is less opposition to improvements in health gained through the use of genetically manipulated organisms (GMOs) and the LAB have every prospect of being important in this area.

The Lactic Acid Bacteria

The LAB are arguably the second only to yeast in importance in their services to mankind. They have been used worldwide in the generation of safe, storable, organoleptically pleasing foodstuffs for centuries. These foods include fermented milk products (such as cheese, yogurt, and kefir), bread and cereals (e.g., sourdough, ogi), beverages (malolactic fermentation in wines), vegetables (sauerkraut, silage, kimchi) and, particularly in the Far East, preserved and ensiled fish products. They came to the attention of microbiologists almost 100 years ago and, with recognition of their importance, have been studied almost continuously ever since. This book deals with the molecular dissection of the organisms at the levels of their proteins and nucleic acids, which is their molecular microbiology.

By its very nature this subject is specialist and thus it has developed a jargon all of its own. Many who are not in the field find this intimidating—as practicing scientists in the field we can state this was not an intention: the language has simply grown over the past quarter of a century as the field has developed. In this chapter we shall briefly describe some of the basics in order that readers may fully appreciate the following chapters of the book. For further general explanation there are a number of general texts available. The authors would recommend Lewin (1999).

Genetic Arrangement in the Lactic Acid Bacteria

Like other bacteria, the LAB have a single covalently closed circular piece of DNA, generally of the order of 10^9 base pairs in length, that forms the chromosome. This usually encodes all of the metabolic functions generally considered as essential to the organism and may also encode a number of nonessential functions to enable the organism to adapt to its environment.

In addition many bacteria also contain plasmids, autonomous DNA molecules, and transposon/insertion sequences, which add plasticity to the genome, as will be revealed later. We shall now look at these in a little more detail.

Plasmids of Lactic Acid Bacteria

Function

Plasmids are generally defined as circular double-stranded DNA molecules, capable of replication independent of the host genome. Plasmids have been identified in all genera of LAB and many strains are known to harbor multiple replicons. Although plasmids are usually dispensable to the host cell, some do carry genes that are essential for survival of the bacterium under particular environmental conditions. In the genus *Lactococcus*, plasmids have been associated with the production of bacteriocins, phage resistance, citrate utilization, sugar metabolism, proteolysis, and conjugative transfer (McKay, 1983; Dougherty et al., 1998; Akcelik, 1999). Besides their capacity to improve host survival and competitiveness, many of these plasmid-encoded traits are of significant industrial importance. With the exception of *Lactobacillus bulgaricus*, plasmids are also a common feature of *Lactobacillus*. However, while some of these plasmids have been linked to specific phenotypic traits such as *N*-acetyl-D-glucosamine production, carbohydrate metabolism, proteinase production, amino-acid metabolism, and bacteriocin production, most plasmids in *Lactobacillus* remain cryptic (Pouwels and Leer, 1993; Wang and Lee, 1997). Members of the genera *Pediococcus, Leuconostoc, Tetragenococcus, Oenococcus*, and *Streptococcus thermophilus* are also known to harbor extrachromosomal elements. In *Pediococcus*, plasmids have been shown to encode bacteriocins and are also associated with sugar metabolism (Gonzalez and Kunka, 1985). In the *Leuconostoc*, plasmids have been linked to lactose and citrate fermentation (Fantuzzi, 1991; Lin et al., 1991; Vaughan et al., 1995).

Replication

All plasmids replicate in a semi-conservative manner, one strand of the DNA molecule serving as a template for the synthesis of a complementary strand by DNA polymerase. As autonomous genetic elements, plasmids contain genes essential for their maintenance: genes controlling the initiation and control of replication. Nevertheless, the process of plasmid replication is still highly dependent on the host cell.

Plasmids replicate by one of two mechanisms: theta, or rolling circle replication (also known as sigma-replication) Both mechanisms are represented in LAB. During theta replication, the two strands of the DNA double helix separate at the origin of replication, and DNA synthesis proceeds in either one or both directions. Leading and lagging strand synthesis occurs simultaneously during θ-replication and is primed at closely located sites within the origin of replication. The plasmid molecule retains a circular conformation throughout the replicative process, and the DNA remains supercoiled ahead of the replication fork. On completion of the replication cycle, DNA gyrase nicks one of the circles to release a daughter plasmid molecule. The nicked plasmid is sealed and subsequently supercoiled.

Rolling circle or sigma replication (RCR) is initiated as the plasmid encoded replication protein (REP) nicks one strand of the DNA molecule at the double-stranded origin, *dso*, originally termed the positive origin of replication, ori(+) (te Riele et al., 1986). A new + strand of DNA is synthesized by DNA polymerase, displacing the original + strand and resulting in the formation of a single-stranded intermediate, which is released from the fully replicated molecule by REP as it recognizes a termination sequence within the origin of replication. Ligation of the ends of the displaced single-stranded DNA is catalyzed by

REP and single-stranded plasmid DNA molecules are finally converted to double stranded DNA molecules by host proteins. A large imperfect inverted repeat at the *sso* (single-stranded DNA origin) or minus origin, capable of forming a hairpin loop, is used to prime second strand synthesis. Further details can be found in Chapter 2 written by Gasson.

Broadly speaking, large plasmids of LAB belong to the pAMβ1/pIP501 or the pCI305/pWV02 family of replicons and replicate by the theta mode of replication, while the smaller plasmids belong to the pWV01/pSH71 family of plasmids and replicate via the mechanism of rolling circle replication (de Vos and Simons, 1994; de Vos et al., 1997).

Regardless of the mode of replication, the copy number of a plasmid is regulated such that a defined number are present in a given host under specific growth conditions. The mechanism by which this is achieved centers on a negative feedback loop to control the rate at which replication is initiated (Coutourier et al., 1988; Pouwels and Leer, 1993). Small countertranscript or antisense RNA molecules with complementarity to the 5′ end of a gene known as *repA* inhibit replication by transcription attenuation. Counter transcript RNA molecules may also inhibit replication by binding to the leader sequence of the *Rep* mRNA thereby preventing translation of and production of the REP protein required to initiate replication. The copy number of many LAB plasmids is controlled by an inhibitor target mechanism involving countertranscript RNA. The replication of other plasmids is thought to be controlled by the production of a repressor protein, which might act at the level of transcription to prevent the synthesis of *rep* RNA, or bind to the REP protein to suppress the initiation of replication (Coutourier et al., 1988; Del Solar and Espinosa, 1992).

Cloning Vectors

As commercially important microorganisms, much of the work on LAB has been driven by the desire to improve their potential for industrial applications. In the last 10–15 years, considerable effort has concentrated on the development of genetic techniques and molecular tools to allow us to develop a better understanding of these organisms at the molecular level. Much of this work has also opened up the possibility of strain improvement by genetic engineering, introducing or knocking-out specific genes, offering a more rational approach compared to the selection of spontaneous or induced mutants for particular traits. The introduction of heterologous DNA into any species of LAB requires, at the very least, (i) a suitable *cloning vector* in which the gene of interest can be inserted and subsequently amplified and maintained in the bacterial cell, and (ii) a means by which the vector and its insert can be introduced into the host cell. In many cases, the cloning vector will be a plasmid, although other nucleic acid molecules, such as the genome of a bacteriophage, can be used as an alternative.

With the exception of those designed for chromosomal integration, plasmid vectors must be able to replicate in their host cells. For this reason, all LAB vectors carry a Gram-positive replicon, and many are derived from endogenous plasmid species. The *Enterococcus faecalis* plasmid pAMβ1 (Clewell et al., 1974) was one of the first plasmids to be used as a cloning vector in LAB and, with a broad host-range, has formed the basis of a number of other cloning vehicles for use in lactococci and lactobacilli. Vectors exploiting native replicons include pWV01, pSH71 and their derivatives (of lactococcal origin) and those derived from the *Lb. hilgardii* plasmid pLAB1000 (Josson et al., 1990). Many of these plasmids are able to replicate in a variety of host species and are not limited to the strain from which they have originated.

Besides a functional origin of replication, plasmid vectors require one or more marker genes to allow bacteria that harbor them to be selected from those which do not. In addition they require one, or preferably more, unique restriction sites located within the marker gene(s) to facilitate the cloning of DNA fragments and subsequent identification of recombinants. A large number of the cloning vectors for use in *Escherichia coli* carry multiple restriction sites on a polylinker situated within the *lacZ'* gene encoding the α-peptide of the β-galactosidase enzyme. When introduced into an *E. coli* host capable of producing the complementary peptide, transformants can be identified by their ability to degrade the chromogenic lactose analogue: 5-bromo-4-chloro-3-indolyl-ß-D-galactopyranoside (X-gal), resulting in the formation of a blue product/colony. Insertional inactivation of the *lacZ'* gene means a functional β-galactosidase is not synthesized such that colonies appear white. This is often referred to as blue/white selection of recombinants.

The cloning sites in LAB plasmid vectors commonly reside within an antibiotic resistance gene. Since many strains of LAB are resistant to ampicillin, kanamycin, and tetracycline, but sensitive to erythromycin and chloramphenicol, genes conferring resistance to the latter are most frequently used as selectable markers. Despite their prevalence, antibiotic resistance genes are not necessarily the most appropriate markers for LAB vectors. The possibility of the genetic transfer of antibiotic resistance from genetically modified LAB to other microorganisms precludes the use of antibiotic resistance genes in strains engineered for release into open ecosystems. Several genes involved in carbohydrate utilization, have been used as selectable markers in place of drug resistance genes (Posno et al., 1991; Hashiba et al., 1992; MacCormick et al., 1995; Platteeuw et al., 1996). In addition, Klein et al. (1995) have suggested the use of peptidase genes as more suitable and safer genetic markers for *Lactobacillus* vectors and, more recently, several other food grade markers have been developed; these are discussed elsewhere in this book.

In general it is easier to clone DNA in *E. coli* than in species of LAB. Consequently, a number of bi-functional shuttle vectors containing two origins of replication, one for *E. coli* and one originating from a LAB, and at least two selectable markers, have been developed and used in *Lactobacillus, Lactococcus*, and *Leuconostoc* (de Vos and Simons, 1994; Mercenier et al., 1994). Shuttle vectors derived from cryptic lactococcal plasmids with a broad host range and capable of replicating in *E. coli* have also been described. Both types of vector allow DNA to be cloned in *E. coli*, amplified, and subsequently transferred to the Gram-positive host. Plasmid vectors for use in *Lactobacillus* and *Lactococcus* are discussed more specifically in several reviews (Pouwels and Leer, 1993; de Vos and Simons, 1994; Mercenier et al., 1994; Klaenhammer, 1995; Wang and Lee, 1997) and in other chapters of this book.

Plasmid Stability

If a genetically modified strain of LAB is to be of practical use, heterologous DNA introduced into the cell must be stably maintained in the absence of a selection pressure. Plasmid vectors that replicate by the θ mode, exhibit a high degree of stability in LAB. Those that replicate by rolling circle replication, however, are more prone to problems of both segregational and structural instability, resulting in loss of the plasmid over successive generations and the deletion or rearrangement of specific sequences, respectively.

During θ replication, plasmid multimers are converted to monomers by the action of a site-specific recombination system and the distribution of plasmid molecules between daughter cells is governed by a partitioning function. By contrast, the distribution of RCR plasmid molecules at cell division appears to be random (Novick, 1987) and this is thought to contribute to the poor segregational stability of vectors derived from such plasmids. Segregational instability of RCR plasmids has also been attributed to the inefficient conversion of single-stranded DNA molecules to double-stranded molecules in second strand synthesis (Shimizu-Kadota et al., 1991; Leer et al., 1992). The structural instability of RCR plasmids is frequently attributed to infidelity at various stages of the replicative process (Gruss and Ehrlich, 1989). The stability of lactococcal vectors is discussed in more detail by de Vos and Simons (1994) and the factors influencing the segregational and structural stability of *Lactobacillus* plasmids have been reviewed by Pouwels and Leer (1993) and Wang and Lee (1997).

Chromosomal Integration

In the absence of a selection pressure (i.e., the presence of the antibiotic to which the plasmid marker gene confers resistance), recombinant plasmids are frequently lost in successive generations as a result of segregational instability. To circumvent such problems, a number of methods have been employed to induce cloned genes to integrate into the bacterial chromosome where they are stably maintained. Integration can occur by one of several mechanisms including homologous recombination, site-specific recombination and illegitimate recombination, and integration vectors exploiting all three of these have been developed for the lactococci, streptococci, and lactobacilli. Integration vectors containing fragments of genomic DNA have been developed for *Lactococcus* and *Lactobacillus*. Integration is thought to occur by a Campbell-like mechanism involving a single crossover between the donor plasmid and recipient chromosome at homologous sequences (Campbell, 1962). Integration in this way is mediated by host recombination proteins and results in the insertion of DNA between two homologous flanking sequences. To stimulate integration, vectors of this type are derived from plasmids, which are either unable to replicate in the host cell (so-called suicide vectors) or exhibit a high degree of segregational instability (Leenhouts et al., 1989; Rixon et al., 1990; Bhowmik and Steele, 1993) and carry a small fragment of genomic DNA to provide a region of homology. Site-specific recombination was first described as the mechanism by which the *E. coli* bacteriophage lambda integrates and excises itself from the bacterial chromosome. Insertion of the phage into the host genome is catalyzed by a phage-encoded enzyme: integrase, which recognizes and binds to a specific attachment sequence on either or both the viral genome and the bacterial chromosome. The protein is then responsible for nicking and resealing the DNA molecules to promote recombination. Suicide site-specific integration vectors based on phage attachment sequences and integrase genes have been developed for *Lb. gasseri* (Raya et al., 1992; Fremaux et al., 1993), *Lb. plantarum* (Dupont et al., 1995), and *Lc. lactis* (Lillehaug et al., 1997; Brondsted and Hammer, 1999). Although integration vectors of the types described above have been used to stabilize heterologous genes in several species of LAB, the mechanism of insertion results in the co-integration of vector DNA. Insertion of the gene alone can be achieved by cloning it into the genomic insert of an integration vector to stimulate a double cross-over event resulting in replacement recombination. This method was adopted to mediate the integration of a number of genes into the chromosome of *Lactobacillus* (Fitzsimons et al., 1994; Hols et al., 1994; Lin et al., 1996).

Despite the apparent absence of homology or insertion sequences, a number of plasmids have been shown to integrate into the bacterial genome (Scheirlinck et al., 1989; Rixon et al., 1990; Bhowmik and Steele, 1993). Nonhomologous illegitimate recombination has been well documented in *Bacillus subtilis* (Hofemeister et al., 1983; Jannière and Ehrlich, 1987; Dempsey and Dubnau, 1989) and may be mediated by DNA gyrase or DNA topoisomerase (Marvo et al., 1983; Ikeda et al., 1984; Bashkirov et al., 1987) or stimulated by the creation of a recombinogenic structure during RCR or by exonuclease activity following the introduction of a nick (Dempsey and Dubnau, 1989). As a general rule, the unpredictability of illegitimate recombination renders it redundant as a method for gene stabilization.

Gene Transfer in Lactic Acid Bacteria

In nature, the transfer of genetic material between bacteria can occur by one of three mechanisms: conjugation, transduction, or transformation. These transfer systems have been adopted by molecular biologists for incorporation of heterologous DNA into microorganisms, including the LAB.

Conjugation

During the process of conjugation, genetic material is transferred from a donor to a recipient cell. Transfer is dependent on direct contact between the cells and controlled by a number of plasmid-borne genes. In Gram-negative bacteria, self-transmissible, or conjugative plasmids code for the synthesis and assembly of a sex pilus that binds to a protein in the outer membrane of the recipient cell to effect cell–cell contact. Other transfer or *tra* genes are responsible for plasmid replication and transfer. Replication is initiated at the origin of transfer, *oriT*. A nick is introduced into one strand of the DNA molecule and a single stranded copy of the plasmid generated by RCR. The single stranded molecule is subsequently transferred to the recipient cell where it is converted to a double stranded molecule by DNA polymerase and re-circularized. In addition to their own transfer, conjugative plasmids are capable of facilitating the transfer of certain nonconjugative plasmids. Cotransfer or mobilization is dependent on the presence of a specific *mob* recombination site involved in the formation of co-integrates of the two plasmids.

As a means of genetic exchange, conjugation is encountered less frequently among Gram-positive species of bacteria but has been described for several of the LAB, most notably the lactococci. In addition, some conjugative plasmids from other Gram-positive bacteria have been transferred into the organisms via conjugation. While the mechanism of conjugal transfer in Gram-positive bacteria is not fully understood, it is clear that sex pili are not involved in the formation of a conjugative bridge. Rather, cell aggregation appears to promote cell–cell contact prior to DNA transfer. Studies on conjugation in *Enterococcus faecalis* have shown that cell aggregation is mediated by a protein produced by donor cells in response to the secretion of small peptide "sex pheromones" by putative recipients. Lipoteichoic acid has been tentatively identified as the surface receptor for the aggregation clumping factor on both recipient and donor cells (Ehrenfeld et al., 1986). Conjugation in *Lactococcus* is similarly characterized by cell aggregation but not by the production of a sex pheromone. Although the precise mechanism has yet to be elucidated, the conjugal transfer of plasmid DNA in *Lc. lactis* sub-species is directed by the co-integration of a labile sex factor, which normally resides on the host chromosome (Gasson et al., 1995). More specific details of the molecular basis of conjugation in lactococci are given in Chapter 2 of this book.

In contrast to *Lactococcus*, native conjugation in the genus *Lactobacillus* has been reported only rarely (Chassy and Rokaw, 1981; Muriana and Klaenhammer, 1987). Furthermore, the conjugal transfer of heterologous plasmids to *Lactobacillus* species has been shown to be an inefficient process with frequencies typically ranging from 10^{-7} to 10^{-5} transconjugants per donor or recipient cell. Again, the mechanism of conjugal transfer in the lactobacilli is unclear, but work by Reniero et al. (1992) has provided evidence for the role of a proteinaceous aggregation-promoting factor in mediating a high frequency of transfer in *Lb. plantarum*. More recently, however, the cloning and sequencing of a gene encoding a protein that mediates autoaggregation in *Lb. reuteri* was found to exhibit a high degree of homology to ATP-dependent DEAD-box helicases (Roos et al., 1999). The significance of this finding is unclear at the present time.

Transduction

The exchange of genetic material by transduction is mediated by bacteriophage. Broadly speaking, bacteriophage can be classified into two distinct groups: virulent phage and temperate phage. Virulent phage exhibit a lytic lifecycle during which the host bacterium is converted into a phage-producing cell. Very briefly, after attachment to the bacterial cell wall, the viral particle penetrates the host cell and the phage genome passes into the cell cytoplasm. Bacterial RNA and DNA synthesis is shut down and the replication of viral DNA (or RNA) ensues. During morphogenesis, structural proteins synthesized by the phage are assembled and the phage genome is packaged to form new infective viral particles, which are released on lysis of the bacterial cell. In addition to a lytic cycle, temperate phage are also capable of a lysogenic cycle. On initiation of the lysogenic cycle, the phage genome integrates into the bacterial chromosome where it exists as a prophage until potentially lethal conditions stimulate the lytic cycle and the prophage is excised.

Transduction occurs when bacterial DNA is erroneously packaged into phage and transferred to a recipient phage-sensitive host. In generalized transduction, bacterial DNA fragments are randomly packaged into the viral capsid along with the phage genome. Specialized transduction, however, is mediated by temperate phage only, and occurs as a result of an inaccurate excision of prophage DNA from the host chromosome. In this case, bacterial DNA flanking the integration site is packaged into the viral capsid with the phage genome when lytic growth is induced.

Transduction is relatively common among the lactococci and gene transfer by virulent and, more frequently, temperate phage has been described. Much of the more recent work on *Lactococcus* bacteriophage is related to their importance in inducing cell lysis in commercial starter cultures to enhance the flavor development of matured cheeses. Transduction, as a mechanism for gene exchange in other LAB, however, has been reported only rarely.

Transformation

Transformation refers to the uptake of exogenous DNA by recipient cells from their surrounding environment. For certain species of bacteria (e.g., *Streptococcus mutans, Streptococcus pneumoniae, Streptococcus sanguis*) a state of natural competence for the active take up and processing of DNA, is induced by a specific cell density or certain environmental conditions. For a number of other bacteria, particularly Gram-negative species, artificial competence can be induced by a variety of physical or chemical treatments.

Many readers, of course, will be familiar with the use of $CaCl_2$/heat-shock treatment to induce artificial competence in *E. coli*. Transformation does not appear to constitute a means of genetic exchange in the LAB—neither natural nor chemically induced artificially competent cells have been described for this group of bacteria, although natural competence has been described for some species of *Streptococcus* that are not normally considered to be members of the LAB.

Transposition

Most bacteria have been found to contain integration sequences, which can move within the bacterial genome. When a selectable marker is located between two integration sequences, the resulting genetic element is known as a transposon. Many of the first transposons to be identified encoded antibiotic resistance. Tn917 represents a transposon of this type used extensively in lactic acid bacteria (Tomich et al., 1980; Perkins and Youngman, 1986) More recently they have been found to encode metabolic traits, such as the ability to utilize sucrose and produce the bacteriocin, nisin (Rauch and deVos, 1992). A number of self-transmissible transposons have also been reported; these are able to excise from the genetic material of one organism and transfer to that of another. Examples include Tn916 (Franke and Clewell, 1981), and a whole family of similar elements discovered since. Transposons and the phenomenon of transposition will be covered in more detail in a later chapter of this book.

Conjugation, Transduction, and Transformation as Genetic Tools

The systems of conjugation, transduction, and what may loosely be described as transformation have been exploited, to a greater or lesser extent, as genetic tools in the LAB, primarily, but not exclusively, for the introduction of heterologous DNA into cells. The introduction of the broad host-range plasmid: pAMβ1 into lactobacilli from streptococci was the first demonstration of conjugal transfer in the LAB (Gibson et al., 1979). By the late 1980s numerous groups had reported the intrageneric conjugal transfer of plasmid DNA in *Lactococcus* and *Lactobacillus*. Several groups have also reported the transfer of conjugative plasmids between different strains and even different genera of LAB and *Enterococcus faecalis* (Chassy and Rokaw, 1981; Vescovo et al., 1983; West and Warner, 1985; Shrago et al., 1986; Muriana and Klaenhammer, 1987; Benachour et al., 1996; Langella et al., 1996). Not all transconjugants, however, were able to act as donors in subsequent mating experiments. Probably more interesting than the straightforward transfer of conjugative plasmids from recipient to donor, a number of reports have described the co-mobilization of nonconjugative plasmids in lactococci and lactobacilli. Indeed, pAMβ1, pIP501, and their derivatives have been used to mobilize plasmids encoding antibiotic resistance, bacteriophage resistance, and proteinase production, among other traits, to and from *Lactococcus* and *Lactobacillus* strains (de Vos and Davies, 1984; Cheol and Stiles, 1990; Hayes et al., 1990a; Ahn et al., 1992; Thompson et al., 1999). The mobilization of nonconjugative plasmids is effected by the formation of a co-integrate with a conjugative plasmid. The analysis of transconjugants generated in the mobilization of proteinase plasmids by pAMβ1 identified a specific recombination site responsible for the formation of pAMβ1 :: proteinase fusion plasmids (Hayes et al., 1990b). Sub-cloning this sequence into a nonmobilizable *Lc. lactis–E. coli* shuttle vector subsequently resulted in the conjugal transfer of the plasmid by pAMβ1. Though not universal, one of the problems encountered in the co-mobilization of plasmids has been the failure of co-integrates to resolve in recipient cells (Shrago and Dobrogosz, 1988). In general the transfer of DNA to LAB by conjugation or co-mobilization occurs at relatively low frequencies (10^{-6}–10^{-8} transconjugants/ donor), and depends on the strain of both donor and recipient cells. Though Reniero et al. (1992) demonstrated the transfer of pAMβ1 to *Lb. plantarum* at frequencies of up to 10^{-2} transconjugants/donor, the high efficiency of conjugation was attributed to the production of a clumping factor promoting the aggregation of donor and recipient cells during the mating process. Despite the interest shown in conjugation as a mechanism for the transfer of heterologous DNA to LAB and its undoubted importance as a cloning strategy in early studies, in practice, the introduction of foreign DNA into many species of LAB is accomplished by electrotransformation.

Although transduction has been demonstrated in lactococci on numerous occasions (McKay et al., 1973; Gasson, 1990), its use as a means of genetic exchange has never been fully exploited. As an analytical tool, however, transduction has proven invaluable, and provided the first evidence that lactose metabolism in *Lc. lactis* subspecies *lactis* C2 was plasmid encoded (McKay et al., 1976). The exchange of genetic material by transduction has been described much less frequently for other genera of LAB. In fact, only one report of transduction in *Streptococcus thermophilus* has been published (Mercenier et al., 1988b). In the genus *Lactobacillus*, generalized transduction by a temperate phage was reported for *Lb. salivarius* (Tohyama et al., 1971) and plasmid transduction mediated by bacteriophage øadh demonstrated in *Lb. gasseri* ADH (formerly *Lb. acidophilus* ADH: Kleeman and Klaenhammer, 1982; Raya et al., 1989; Raya and Klaenhammer, 1992).

As alluded to previously, no LAB are known to express natural competence for the uptake of exogenous DNA and artificially induced competence has been demonstrated only in *Lc. lactis* where cells were mixed with DNA in the presence of polyethylene glycol (PEG; Sanders and Nicholson, 1987). The thick peptidoglycan layer characteristic of the Gram-positive cell wall, may explain the difficulties encountered in inducing competence in LAB. Partial or complete removal of the bacterial cell wall using muralytic enzymes (lysozyme and/or mutanolysin), has rendered many strains of *Lactococcus, Lactobacillus*, and *Strept. thermophilus* amenable to transformation or transfection, though reported frequencies are generally low (Lin and Savage, 1986; Simon et al., 1986; Chassy, 1987; Morelli et al., 1987; Cosby et al., 1988; Mercenier et al., 1988a), particularly for organisms other than *Lactococcus*. Protocols for LAB protoplast transformation are all based on that described for *Bacillus subtilis* (Chang and Cohen, 1979), which essentially, involves digestion of the bacterial cell wall, resuspension of the resultant protoplasts in an osmotically stable medium, the incubation of protoplasts with DNA in the presence of PEG, and finally the regeneration of recombinant cells. Success appears to depend upon a number of experimental parameters, which must be optimized for each strain. Composition of the growth medium has a profound effect on cell wall structure and therefore affects protoplast formation. The nature, source and purity of muramidase and composition of the incubation buffer for cell wall digestion are known to influence the efficiency of protoplast generation (Mercenier and Chassy, 1988). Prolonged incubation with lysozyme or mutanolysin has been shown to inhibit regeneration of the cell wall following transformation (Simon et al., 1986). The molecular weight and concentration of PEG, essential for protoplast transformation, growth phase of the recipient cells at harvest, the size of the transforming DNA, and the composition of the regeneration medium also influence the efficiency of DNA transfer and recovery of recombinants to a greater or lesser extent (Mercenier and Chassy, 1988). While on the subject of protoplasts, it would seem pertinent to mention protoplast fusion as a strategy for introducing genetic material in LAB. Plasmid DNA has been introduced into the species of *Lactobacillus* and *Lactococcus* by PEG induced protoplast fusion (Okamoto et al., 1983, 1985; Cocconcelli et al., 1986; Iwata et al., 1986). Protoplast fusion of *Lb. acidophilus* and *Lc. lactis* has also been achieved by exposing protoplasts to a DC current, though recombinants were recovered only where protoplasts were resuspended in sub-fusion concentrations of PEG (<20%), which presumably protects against cell lysis on the application of the electric current (Reed, 1987). Both intrageneric and intergeneric fusion has been reported but results are often difficult to reproduce and, like protoplast transformation, problems are frequently encountered in the regeneration of recombinant cells.

As previously stated, the LAB are an industrially important group of microorganisms and there is considerable interest in improving their potential as such by genetic engineering. However, the lack of an efficient method of gene transfer for many strains of LAB limited progress in this regard until Harlander (1987) showed that DNA could be introduced into intact cells of *Lc. lactis* by electroporation. Since then all genera of LAB have been transformed by electroporation and the technique has largely superseded other methods of gene transfer in the laboratory, favored for its relative simplicity and comparative reproducibility and efficiency. Transformation by electroporation involves the application of a brief, high voltage electrical pulse to a suspension of cells and DNA. Although the molecular mechanism of electrotransformation is not completely understood, the electrical pulse is thought to result in a rearrangement of phospholipids and proteins in the cell membrane to generate transient pores through which the DNA can pass into the cell (Benz and Zimmerman, 1981). Electroporation was initially used to effect the transfer of DNA into mammalian cells (Neumann et al., 1982) and scanning electron microscopy has been employed to examine the ultrastructure of red blood cell membranes and to investigate the dynamics of pore formation during electroporation (Chang, 1989; Chang and Reese, 1990; Chang, 1992). Observations suggested that pores were formed in the first few milliseconds after the application of the electrical pulse. Following a period of expansion, pore structures remained relatively stable until they started to re-seal. Despite decreasing in size with time, partially re-sealed pores had a long life-span and the diameter (20–120 nm) and duration of transient pores were deemed sufficient to allow large molecules such as DNA to diffuse through the membrane and into the cell. Electroporation has provided a convenient technique for the introduction of DNA into strains, which were previously untransformable or transformed only as protoplasts.

Numerous papers describing the transformation of LAB by electroporation have been published. In general, the method involves washing harvested cells several times in a low salt buffer (with or without sucrose) or distilled water, and resuspending them in ice cold low salt buffer, briefly incubating DNA and cells together on ice, before transferring the mixture to an electroporation cuvette and applying an electrical pulse of 5–10 kV/cm using a Gene Pulser apparatus. Shocked cells are usually held on ice for a short period before plating out onto selective media. Differences in the uptake of DNA by different strains of LAB have been noted by many groups. In addition, transformation frequencies (transformants/μg DNA) and efficiencies (transformants/surviving cells) appear to be influenced by culture conditions as well as many parameters of the electroporation protocol itself. Differences in the uptake of DNA by various strains of LAB may be related to differences in cell wall morphology. Growing cells in the presence of DL-threonine, glycine, or penicillin to weaken the cell wall has improved the transformation rate of *Lc. lactis* subsp. *cremoris* (Van der Lelie et al., 1988; Holo and Nes, 1989) and several *Lactobacillus* species (Aukrust and Nes, 1988; Hashiba et al., 1990; Wei et al., 1995; Thompson and Collins, 1996). The treatment of cells with lysozyme prior to electroporation similarly resulted in an increase in the transformation efficiency of *Lc. lactis* (Powell et al., 1988), *Lactobacillus* strains (Wei et al., 1995) and *Pediococcus acidilactici* (Kim et al., 1992). The effect of cell wall weakening agents, however, is not universal: the addition of glycine, threonine, and lysine to the culture medium had no effect on the transformation frequency of *Lb. sake* (Berthier et al., 1996).

A number of reports have suggested that bacterial cells may be more amenable to transformation by electroporation when harvested in early- or mid-log phase (Calvin and Hanawalt, 1988; Powell et al., 1988; Gaier et al., 1990; Natori et al., 1990). Others have demonstrated higher transformation frequencies for cells harvested in mid- to late-log or stationary phase (McIntyre and Harlander, 1989; Hashiba et al., 1990). In general, however, growth phase appears to have a minimal influence on transformation frequency or efficiency. Sanoja et al. (1999), however, found growing *Lb. manihotivorans* in the absence of air resulted in an increase in the transformation frequency.

With regard to the voltage applied to cells, higher field strengths are reported to generate higher transformation frequencies (Luchansky et al., 1988; Powell et al., 1988; David et al., 1989; Bringel and Hubert, 1990). Long pulses of high voltage, however, may result in cell death or damage. For many strains, a field strength of 4–6.25 kV/cm with a capacitance of 25 μF would be a good starting point in the development of a protocol for electrotransformation.

The composition of the cell/DNA suspension buffer can have a profound effect on transformation frequencies. The inclusion of sucrose as an osmoprotectant resulted in a 10-fold increase in the transformation frequency of *Leuconostoc mesenteroides* subsp. *cremoris* (Wyckoff et al., 1991), and *Lb. plantarum* (Thompson and Collins, 1996), though the addition of sucrose had no effect on the transformation frequency of *Lb. sake* (Berthier et al., 1996). While washing cells in a buffer containing magnesium chloride had a marked positive effect on the yield of *Lb. sake* transformants by reducing the amount of extracellular polysaccharide, adding NacCl to the actual electroporation buffer reduced transforma-tion frequencies 10-fold (Aukrust and Blom, 1992; Berthier et al., 1996). Substituting a phosphate-based electroporation buffer for 30% PEG-1000 resulted in a significant increase in the transformation frequency of *Lb. hilgardii* (Josson et al., 1989). The addition of PEG has similarly increased the efficiency of transformation of another species, *Lb. plantarum* (Rixon, J. E. and Gilbert, H. J., University of Newcastle, UK, unpublished) and *Lb. casei* (Natori et al., 1990). PEG has also been used to induce competence in *Lc. lactis* (Sanders and Nicholson, 1987) and to mediate the protoplast transformation of a number of LAB (Kondo and McKay, 1984; Morelli et al., 1987). However, the mechanism by which PEG is able to facilitate whole cell or protoplast transformation is largely unknown. Some evidence suggests that PEG may cause a certain degree of disruption in the cell wall or membrane so allowing the penetration of exogenous DNA (Sanders and Nicholson, 1987). PEG may also influence the uptake of DNA by inducing a conformational change in the DNA molecule (Bibb et al., 1978). Adding PEG to transformation mixtures has a pronounced effect on cell survival. Its potential to increase transformation frequencies may be a consequence of its ability to protect against cell lysis in high current fields (Reed, 1987). The positive effect of PEG on electrotransformation is not universal, however, and Berthier et al. (1996) found that the addition of PEG-3000 completely inhibited the uptake of DNA by *Lb. sake* by electroporation.

Increasing the DNA concentration in transformation mixtures resulted in an increase in both the number of transformants recovered and in the transformation frequency of *Lb. plantarum* (Rixon, J. E. and Gilbert, H. J., University of Newcastle, UK, unpublished). A positive correlation between DNA concentration and the yield of transformants has also been observed for many strains of LAB, though transformation frequencies are usually higher at lower DNA concentrations. In addition to concentration, the purity, conformation and size of DNA may influence the efficiency of transformation. Berthier et al. (1996) found small-scale DNA preparations less efficient than caesium chloride purified DNA, though Holo and Nes (1989) found purity to be less important. With respect to size, smaller plasmids are generally regarded as more efficient vectors for electrotransformation. However, Powell et al. (1988) were able to demonstrate a high frequency of transfer of the large plasmid pAMβ1 to *Lc. lactis* by electroporation and McIntyre and Harlander (1989) found no consistent correlation between plasmid size and the transformation frequency of *Lc. lactis* subsp. *lactis*. Linearized and ligated DNA has been used to transform LAB but, in general, supercoiled DNA is more efficient (Rixon Gilbert and Hazlewood, University of Newcastle unpublished; Berthier et al., 1996; Thompson et al., 1997).

Given the harshness of electroporation, it is not surprising that the recovery of transformants is greater if cells are incubated in nonselective liquid medium to allow recovery prior to plating out onto selective media. Interestingly, the addition of magnesium chloride to the liquid recovery medium further improved the transformation frequency of *Lb. sake* (Berthier et al., 1996) and *Lb. manihotivorans* (Sanoja et al., 1999). For *Lb. sake*, the increase in the number of transformants recovered was not related to improved cell survival. Berthier et al. (1996) have, therefore, suggested that magnesium chloride may facilitate plasmid maintenance in recipient cells, thus increasing the relative numbers of transformants in the surviving population rather than increasing recovery *per se*.

Numerous papers describing the electrotransformation of LAB have been published in the last 10 years. In writing this section, we have aimed to give a brief overview of electrotransformation as applied to LAB and highlight some of the most salient features of the technique. If optimizing a protocol for the transformation of a new strain, readers would be well advised to consult the literature in more detail.

Plasmid Incompatibility and Restriction–Modification

The successful introduction of heterologous DNA into any species of LAB is dependent on the host strain and plasmid vector employed. Certain strains of LAB appear to be recalcitrant to all methods of gene transfer in the laboratory. For a proportion of bacteria, the failure to recover recombinants might be attributable to problems of plasmid incompatibility or to the possession of an active restriction–modification system by the host bacterium.

Plasmids harboring an identical or similar replicon will compete with each other during replication and partitioning of daughter plasmids in cell division. Such plasmids are said to be incompatible and while one is usually stable, the other is segregationally unstable and ultimately lost from the bacterial population. In an attempt to avoid problems of incompatibility, several groups have tried using strains cured of their indigenous plasmids. However, this has not always resulted in improved transformation frequencies (Sanoja et al., 1999). As Cambourn et al. (1998) have pointed out, consideration of the plasmid status of recipient hosts and potential problems of incompatibility is particularly pertinent when attempting to modify industrial strains of LAB since the loss of a native plasmid might have a profound adverse effect on the industrial properties of the bacterium.

As a protective mechanism, many bacteria, including species of LAB, produce restriction endonucleases, which recognize and cleave foreign DNA at specific sequences. Native DNA is methylated to prevent cleavage but any incoming DNA not methylated at restriction sites will be degraded. The restriction–modification status of the host strain might, therefore, have a major influence on the recovery of recombinants. One further word of warning: the possession of a restriction–modification system may have some bearing on the future manipulation of DNA isolated from such strains since the methylation of DNA by hosts that possess a modification system might preclude its subsequent restriction by specific restriction endonucleases. Such considerations are particularly pertinent when using cloning vectors with a limited choice of cloning sites.

Gene Expression

Gene expression refers to the transcription of a gene and translation of the cognate messenger RNA to produce a protein. In bacteria, both transcription and translation are initiated at specific sequences upstream of the structural gene and the precise sequence and spacing of these signals has some influence on the expression level and amount of the encoded protein produced by the cell.

Transcription

The transcription of a gene is initiated by RNA polymerase, which binds to a specific sequence upstream of the coding region, known as the promoter. Prokaryotic RNA polymerases comprise five subunits: two identical α-subunits, one β-, one β'-, and one σ-subunit. The last mentioned binds reversibly to the catalytically active core RNA polymerase and is responsible for recognition of the promoter sequence (Helmann and Chamberlain, 1988). After transcription has been initiated, the σ-factor is released and the core enzyme elongates a mRNA chain (Travers and Burgess, 1969). The transcription of bacterial genes has been studied most extensively in *E. coli* and *Bacillus subtilis*. In *B. subtilis* the principal form of RNA polymerase contains a σ-subunit of 43 kDa known as σ^{43}. Alternative σ-factors exhibiting different promoter specificity can also interact with the core RNA polymerase but are usually associated with the expression of genes involved in the developmental processes or in the response of the bacterium to environmental stress (Losick and Pero, 1981; Doi and Wang, 1986). While cellular transcription in *E. coli* is predominantly controlled by the σ^{70}-RNA polymerase, at least two minor RNA polymerase holoenzymes have been identified and it is likely that alternative σ-factors are involved in gene expression in many species of bacteria. In 1993, Araya et al. cloned and characterized the gene for the major σ-factor in *Lc. lactis*. The encoded protein was 39 kDa in size and exhibited a high degree of similarity to the σ^{43} subunit from *B. subtilis*.

Analysis of the DNA sequence of promoters recognized by the principal form of RNA polymerase in *E. coli* shows two highly conserved hexanucleotides, located approximately -35 and -10 bp upstream of the transcriptional start site, known as the -35 region and the Pribnow box (or -10 region) respectively (Pribnow, 1975; Schaller et al., 1975;

Hawley and McClure, 1983). The spacing between these two hexamers is usually in the region of 15–19 bp such that the consensus sequence for *E. coli* promoters is TTGACA-N_{15-19}-TATAAT-N_{5-7}-transcriptional start. The AT-rich nature of the -10 hexamer is thought to be significant since the hydrogen bonding between A and T residues is weaker than that between G and C bases, which might facilitate melting of the DNA in this region and the formation of an open-promoter complex. It is generally believed that the degree of sequence conservation at the -10 and -35 regions is largely responsible for determining the strength of a particular promoter, and in this way, has a direct effect on the level of gene expression.

The alignment of both defined and undefined promoters from *Lactococcus* and *Lactobacillus* has revealed a consensus of TTGACA in the -35 region and TATAAT at the -10 region, analogous to the canonical -10 and -35 sequences of *E. coli* and *B. subtilis* promoters used by the major σ-factor dependent RNA polymerase (de Vos and Simons, 1994; Klaenhammer, 1995). In common with *B. subtilis* promoters, many *Lactococcus* and *Lactobacillus* promoters feature a TG doublet upstream of the -10 sequence. In addition to these specific sequences, *Lactococcus* and *Lactobacillus* promoters are typically rich in A and T residues in the spacer region between the two conserved hexanucleotides and in the region upstream of the -35 sequence. Since fewer have been sequenced, it is difficult to comment on the promoter structure in other species of LAB. However, the -35 and, particularly the -10 sequences reported are comparable to the consensus sequences exhibited by the vegetative promoters of *E. coli* and Gram-positive bacteria (Garmyn et al., 1995; Labarre et al., 1996; Jobin et al., 1997; Quirasco et al., 1999).

Sequences resembling *rho*-independent terminators have been observed in the 3′ non-coding region of the majority of *Lactococcus* and *Lactobacillus* genes sequences to date. Such termination sequences are characterized by a GC-rich region of dyad symmetry capable of forming a hair-pin loop, followed by a stretch of thymidine residues. The hair-pin loop is responsible for eliciting a pause by the RNA polymerase enzyme and ultimately leads to the termination of transcription. The series of uridine residues in the corresponding mRNA transcript is believed to facilitate dissociation of the mRNA from the template since RNA–DNA hybrids with rU–dA pairing are exceptionally unstable (Platt, 1986). Features of transcription initiation and termination signals in LAB genes will be discussed more specifically and in more detail in subsequent Chapters 6 and 7 by Pouwels and Kok.

Translation

The translation of mRNA in prokaryotes is initiated by the binding of the small subunit of a ribosome to a short sequence upstream of the translational start codon, known as the RBS or Shine–Dalgarno sequence. In *E. coli*, Shine–Dalgarno sequences generally conform to the consensus AGGA, which displays perfect complementarity to the 3′-terminus of 16S rRNA (Shine and Dalgarno, 1974). The ribosome-binding sequences of Gram-positive bacteria are often more extensive than those of *E. coli* and an analysis of Shine–Dalgarno sequences from *B. subtilis* has suggested that complementarity may extend to the extreme 3′-terminus of the 16S rRNA, which differs from that of *E. coli* (**A**UUCCUCC in *E. coli*; **UCU**UUCCUCC in *B. subtilis*) (Moran et al., 1982). The 3′-end of *Lc. lactis* 16S rRNA has the sequence 3′-CUUUCCUCC-5′ (Chiaruttini and Millet, 1993), but although all lactococcal translation initiation sites contain the sequence AGGA, their length and extent of complementarity to the 16S rRNA sequence is variable.

The 3′-end of 16S rRNA from a number of *Lactobacillus* species has been determined as 3′-CUUCUU-5′ (Martinez-Murcia and Collins, 1990a,b) and an analysis of sequences has shown that the majority of putative Shine–Dalgarno sequences in *Lactobacillus* species contain the highly conserved sequence AGGAGG (Pouwels and Leer, 1993). Many genes of LAB have been expressed in *E. coli* under the control of their endogenous promoters and Shine–Dalgarno sequences. The cloning of heterologous genes with their native transcription and translation initiation signals, however, has generally resulted in low levels of expression.

Heterologous Gene Expression in Lactic Acid Bacteria

Numerous genes from LAB have been cloned and expressed in *E. coli* under the control of their own transcription and translation initiation signals. The cloning of heterologous genes with their native promoter and Shine–Dalgarno sequences in LAB, however, has generally resulted in low levels of expression. Several reasons might account for this. First, members of the LAB appear to be more stringent in their utilization of promoter sequences. Indeed, using a library of synthetic promoters, Jensen and Hammer (1998) showed that modifying the −10 and −35 consensus sequences resulted in a decrease in promoter activity. A lack of fidelity to the −10 and −35 sequences, however, does not provide a sufficient explanation for the poor expression of heterologous genes in the LAB since endogenous promoters do not always display strict conformity to the canonical −10 and −35 sequences. In the early 1980s, Banner et al. (1983) showed that the AT-rich box upstream of the −35 region of the *spoVG* gene was essential for the efficient utilization of the promoter by *Bacillus subtilis* σ^{37}-RNA polymerase. Similar stretches of A and T residues are also a common feature of promoters, which are efficiently used by the σ^{43}-RNA polymerase of *B. subtilis* (Moran et al., 1982). More recently, the AT-rich region upstream of the −35 sequence of the *lac* promoter has been shown to enhance the efficiency of transcription initiation in *Lc. lactis*, although it had little effect on the efficiency of transcription in *E. coli* (van Rooijen et al., 1992). The evaluation of synthetic promoters further suggests that the length of the spacer region between the −35 and −10 regions is important in determining promoter strength in *Lc. lactis* (Jensen and Hammer, 1998). More specifically, Liu et al. (1997) showed that a TgTGt extension 5′ to the −10 consensus sequence of a promoter was a crucial determinant of promoter efficiency in *Lc. Lactis*.

In *Lactobacillus*, there is evidence to suggest that the sequence of the spacer region between the −10 and −35 consensus sequences might be important in determining promoter strength, and it is likely that efficient promoter utilization by lactobacilli depends on the interaction of RNA polymerase with multiple sequences within the promoter region. Recently, McCracken and Timms (1999) showed that the effect of modifying the sequence of the spacer region was dependent on both the strain of *Lactobacillus* and on context, that is, the specific sequence of the two consensus regions. This and other work, including that described by Platteeuw et al. (1994), which demonstrated significant differences in the ability of the same promoters to initiate transcription in *Lactococcus, Lactobacillus*, and *Leuconostoc* species, highlights the importance of using dedicated promoters in optimizing the expression of heterologous genes in different species of LAB.

An extended polypurine sequence with complementarity to the 3′-region of rRNA may be essential for the efficient translation of LAB mRNAs. Thus, the expression of foreign genes in LAB may be restricted at the level of translation by the inefficient binding of the ribosome to the Shine–Dalgarno sequence, particularly where genes are from a Gram-negative species. In addition, translation efficiency may be influenced by codon usage. While the assignment of a codon to a particular amino acid is universal, the preferred use of individual codons differs between taxonomic groups and it has been suggested that the degeneracy of the genetic code may be exploited to regulate gene expression (Grosjean and Fiers, 1982; Andersson and Kurland, 1990). Rare codons may modulate the expression of proteins synthesized at a low level by causing a pause in translation as a result of the relative paucity of appropriately charged tRNA molecules. Both *Lactococcus* and *Lactobacillus* species exhibit a bias in their utilization of codons (de Vos and Simons, 1994; Pouwels and Leer, 1993), and this will undoubtedly have some influence on the rate of translation and hence the overall expression level of heterologous genes.

Expression Vectors

Although problems arising as a result of differences in codon bias are difficult to negate, low levels of gene expression resulting from the use of sub-optimal promoter and/or ribosome-binding sequences can be overcome by the use of so-called expression vectors. These are specifically designed such that the gene of interest can be inserted into the vector and transcriptionally and translationally fused to more appropriate promoter and Shine–Dalgarno sequences. These regulatory sequences may originate from a characterized gene or may have been selected from the chromosome using a promoter–probe vector. Promoter–probe vectors carry a promoterless reporter gene that can only be expressed if DNA inserted upstream of the translational start codon carries a sequence, which will act as a promoter. Of course, there is no guarantee that the fragment of DNA cloned into the promoter probe vector constitutes a "true" promoter in its native host. Furthermore, if a promoter–probe vector is employed to isolate a promoter sequence in a host other than that for which it is intended to express the gene ultimately, there is no guarantee that the promoter will function as such in the desired strain. This is especially true if *E. coli* is used as the host organism since the species is particularly promiscuous in its use of promoter sequences. Fragments of DNA from LAB will frequently exhibit promoter activity in *E. coli* (i.e., act as a pseudopromoter) but fail to initiate transcription in the Gram-positive bacteria.

For many applications, the ability to control the production of recombinant proteins in LAB will be desirable. In bacteria, genes are regulated at both the level of transcription and at the level of translation through inducer and repressor systems, anti-terminators, RNA binding proteins, and binding of anti-sense RNA to mRNA species. Though gene regulation has been studied most extensively in *E. coli*, the last 5–10 years has seen a vast increase in knowledge regarding the regulation of gene expression in the LAB, and a number of expression systems responsive to environmental stimuli, inducers, or repressors have been described (recent reviews by de Vos et al., 1997; Kuipers et al., 1997; Djordjevic and Klaenhammer, 1998). More consideration is given to the control of gene expression and the development of regulated gene expression elsewhere in this volume.

Concluding Comment

This chapter has sought to introduce what follows and explain some of the underlying principles required to fully understand it. The reader will now enter all of the topics that have been well studied at the molecular level within the last few years and should emerge with a view as to the state of the art shortly after entry to a new millennium. We hope he/she enjoys being part of the adventure and emerges truly fascinated at what has been achieved.

References

Ahn, C., Collins-Thompson, D., Duncan, C., and Stiles, M. E. (1992). Mobilization and location of the genetic determinant of chloramphenicol resistance from *Lactobacillus plantarum* ca TC2R. *Plasmid* 27: 169–176.

Akcelik, M. (1999). The conjugal plasmid pLL10236 encodes lactose fermentation ability, restriction/modification activity, bacteriocin production and immunity in *Lactococcus lactis* subsp. *lactis* LL102. *Food Microbiology* 16: 487–494.

Andersson, S. G. E., and Kurland, C. G. (1990). Codon preferences in free-living microorganisms. *Microbiological Reviews* 54: 198–210.

Araya, T., Ishinashi, N., Shimamura, S., Tanaka, K., and Takahashi, H. (1993). Genetic and molecular analysis of the *rpoD* gene from *Lactococcus lactis*. *Bioscience Biotechnology & Biochemistry* 57: 88–92.

Aukrust, T., and Blom, H. (1992). Transformation of *Lactobacillus* strains used in meat and vegetable fermentations. *Food Research International* 25: 253–261.

Aukrust, T., and Nes, I. F. (1988). Transformation of *Lactobacillus plantarum* with the plasmid pTV1 by electroporation. *FEMS Microbiology Letters* 52: 127–132.

Banner, C. D. B., Moran, C. P., Jr., and Losick, R. (1983). Deletion analysis of a complex promoter for a developmentally regulated gene from *Bacillus subtilis*. *Journal of Molecular Biology* 168: 351–365.

Bashkirov, V. I., Khasanov, F. K., and Prozorov, A. A. (1987). Illegitimate recombination in *Bacillus subtilis*: nucleotide sequences at recombinant DNA junctions. *Molecular & General Genetics* 210: 578–580.

Benachour, A., Flahaut, S., Frere, J., and Novel, G. (1996). Plasmid transfer by electroporation and conjugation in *Tetragenococcus* and *Pediococcus* genera and evidence of plasmid-linked metabolic traits. *Current Microbiology* 32: 188–194.

Benz, R., and Zimmerman, U. (1981). The resealing process of lipid bilayers after reversible electrical breakdown. *Biochimica Biophysica Acta* 640: 169–178.

Berthier, F., Zagorec, M., Champomier-Vergès, M., Ehrlich, S. D., and Morel-Deville, F. (1996). Efficient transformation of *Lactobacillus sake* by electroporation. *Microbiology* 142: 1273–1279.

Bhowmik, T., and Steele, J. L. (1993). Development of an electroporation procedure for gene disruption in *Lactobacillus helveticus* CNRZ32. *Journal of General Microbiology* 139: 1433–1439.

Bibb, M. J., Ward, J. M., and Hopwood, D. A. (1978). Transformation of plasmid DNA into *Streptomyces* at high frequency. *Nature* 294: 398–400.

Bringel, F., and Hubert, J.-C. (1990). Optimized transformation by electroporation of *Lactobacillus plantarum* strains with plasmid vectors. *Applied Microbiology & Biotechnology* 33: 664–670.

Brondsted, L., and Hammer, L. (1999). Use of the integration elements encoded by the temperate lactococcal bacteriophage TP901-1 to obtain chromosomal single-copy transcriptional fusions in *Lactococcus lactis*. *Applied & Enviromental Microbiology* 65: 752–758.

Calvin, N. M., and Hanawalt, P. C. (1988). High-frequency transformation of bacterial cells by electroporation. *Journal of Bacteriology* 170: 2796–2801.

Cambourn, W. M., Tannock, G. W., Yu, P. L., Pearce, L. E., and Pillidge, J. (1998). Plasmids with homology to pFX3 and pCI3340 in starter lactococci and lactobacilli and electroporation of selected strains with these vectors. *International Dairy Journal* 8: 251–254.

Campbell, A. M. (1962). Episomes. *Advances in Genetics* 11: 101–145.

Chang, D. (1989). Cell poration and cell fusion using an oscillating electric field. *Biophysical Journal* 56: 641–652.

Chang, D. (1992). Structure and dynamics of electric field-induced membrane pores as revealed by rapid-freezing electron microscopy. In: D. Chang, B. M. Chassy, J. A. Saunders, and A. E. Sowers (Eds.), *Guide to electroporation and electrofusion* (pp. 9–27). London: Academic Press.

Chang, D. C., and Reese, T. S. (1990). Changes in membrane structure induced by electroporation as revealed by rapid freezing electron microscopy. *Biophysical Journal* 58:1–12.

Chang, S., and Cohen, S. N. (1979). High frequency transformation of *Bacillus subtilis* protoplasts by plasmid DNA. *Molecular & General Genetics* 168: 111–115.

Chassy, B. M. (1987). Prospects for the genetic manipulation of lactobacilli. *FEMS Microbiology Reviews* 46: 297–312.

Chassy, B. M., and Rokaw, E. (1981). Conjugal transfer of lactose plasmids in *Lactobacillus casei*. In: S. Levy, R. Clowes, and E. Koenig (Eds.), *Molecular biology, pathogenesis and ecology of bacterial plasmids* (p. 590). New York, USA: Plenum Press.

Cheol, A., and Stiles, M. E. (1990). Mobilization of plasmids mediating bacteriocin production using pAMβ1 in a lactic acid bacterium from meat. *FEMS Microbiology Reviews* 87: 6.

Chiaruttini, C., and Millet, M. (1993). Gene organization, primary structure and RNA processing analysis of a ribosomal RNA operon in *Lactococcus lactis*. *Journal of Molecular Biology* 230: 57–76.

Clewell, D. B., Yagi, Y., Dunny, G. M., and Schultz, S. K. (1974). Characterization of three deoxyribonucleic acid molecules in a strain of *Streptococcus faecalis*: Identification of a plasmid determining erythromycin resistance. *Journal of Bacteriology* 117: 283–289.

Cocconcelli, P. S., Morelli, L. Vescovo, M., and Bottazzi, V. (1986). Intergeneric protoplast fusion in lactic acid bacteria. *FEMS Microbiology Letters* 35: 211–214.

Cosby, W. M., Casas, I. A., and Dobrogosz, W. J. (1988). Formation, regeneration, and transfection of *Lactobacillus plantarum* protoplasts. *Applied & Environmental Microbiology* 54: 2599–2602.

Coutourier, M., Bex, F., Bergquist, P. L., and Maas, W. K. (1988). Identification and classification of bacterial plasmids. *Microbiological Reviews* 52: 375–395.

David, S., Simons, G., and de Vos, W. M. (1989). Plasmid transformation by electroporation of *Leuconostoc paramesenteroides* and its use in molecular cloning. *Applied & Environmental Microbiology* 55: 1483–1489.

de Vos, W. M., and Davies, F. L. (1984). Plasmid DNA in lactic streptococci: Bacteriophage resistance and proteinase plasmids in *Streptococcus cremoris* SK11. In: *Third European Congress on Biotechnology* (Vol. 3, pp. 201–205). Verlag Chemie Weisheim.

de Vos, W. M., Kleerebezem, M., and Kuipers, O. P. (1997). Expression systems for industrial Gram-positive bacteria with low guanine and cytosine content. *Current Opinion in Biotechnology* 8: 547–553.

de Vos, W. M., and Simons, G. F. M. (1994). Gene cloning and expression systems in lactococci. In: M. J. Gasson and W. M. de Vos (Eds.), *Genetics and Biotechnology of Lactic Acid Bacteria* (pp. 52–105). Glasgow: Blackie Academic & Professional.

Del Solar, G. H., and Espinosa, M. (1992). The copy number of plasmid pLS1 is regulated by two trans-acting plasmid products—the anti-sense RNAII and repressor protein, Rep A. *Molecular Microbiology* 6: 83–94.

Dempsey, L. A., and Dubnau, D. A. (1989). Identification of plasmid and *Bacillus subtilis* chromosomal recombination sites used for pE194 integration. *Journal of Bacteriology* 171: 2856–2865.

Djordjevic, G. M., and Klaenhammer, T. R. (1998). Inducible gene expression systems in *Lactococcus lactis*. *Molecular Biotechnology* 9: 127–139.

Doi, R. H., and Wang, L.-F. (1986). Multiple prokaryotic ribonucleic acid polymerase sigma factors. *Microbiological Reviews* 50: 227–243.

Dougherty, B. A., Hill, C., Weidman, J. F., Richardson, D. R., Venter, J. C., and Ross, R. P. (1998). Sequence and analysis of the 60 kb conjugative, bacteriocin-producing plasmid pMRC01 from *Lactococcus lactis* DPC3147. *Molecular Microbiology* 29: 1029–1038.

Dupont, L., Boizetbonhoure, B., Coddeville, M., Auvray, F., and Ritzenthaler, P. (1995). Characterization of genetic elements required for site-specific integration of *Lactobacillus delbrueckii* subsp. *bulgaricus* bacteriophage MV4 and construction of an integration-proficient vector for *Lactobacillus plantarum*. *Journal of Bacteriology* 177: 586–595.

Ehrenfeld, E. E., Kessler, R. E., and Clewell, D. B. (1986). Identification of pheromone-induced surface proteins in *Streptococcus faecalis* and evidence of a role for lipoteichoic acid in formation of mating aggregates. *Journal of Bacteriology* 168: 6–12.

Fantuzzi, L. (1991). Instability of lactose and citrate metabolism of *Leuconostoc* strains. *Biotechnology Letters* 13: 433–436.

Fitzsimons, A., Hols, P., Jore, J., Leer, R. J., O'Connell, M., and Delcour, J. (1994). Development of an amylolytic *Lactobacillus plantarum* silage strain expressing the *Lactobacillus amylovorus* α-amylase gene. *Applied & Environmental Microbiology* 60: 3529–3535.

Franke, A. E., and Clewell, D. B. (1981). Evidence for conjugal transfer of a *Streptococcus faecalis transposon (Tn 916)* from a chromosomal site in the absence of plasmid DNA. *Journal of Bacteriology* 145: 494–502.

Fremaux, C., de Antoni, G. L., Raya, R. R., and Klaenhammer, T. R. (1993). Genetic organization and sequence of the region encoding integrative functions from *Lactobacillus gasseri* temperate bacteriophage øadh. *Gene* 126: 61–66.

Gaier, W., Vogel, R. F., and Hammes, W. P. (1990). Genetic transformation of intact cells of *Lactobacillus curvatus* Lc2-c and *Lact. sake* Ls2 by electroporation. *Letters in Applied Microbiology* 11: 81–83.

Garmyn, D., Ferain, T., Bernard, N., Hols, P., Deplace, B., and Delcour, J. (1995). *Pediococcus acidilactici* LDHD gene—cloning, nucleotide sequence, and transcriptional analysis. *Journal of Bacteriology* 177: 3427–3437.

Gasson, M. J. (1990). *In vivo* genetic systems in lactic acid bacteria. *FEMS Microbiology Reviews* 87: 43–60.

Gasson, M. J., Gordon, J.-J., Pillidge, C. J., Eaton, T. J., Jury, K., and Shearman, C. A. (1995). Characterization and exploitation of conjugation in *Lactococcus lactis*. *International Dairy Journal* 5: 757–762.

Gibson, E. M., Chase, N. M., London, S. B., and London, J. (1979). Transfer of plasmid-mediated antibiotic resistance from streptococci to lactobacilli. *Journal of Bacteriology* 137: 614–619.

Gonzalez, C. F., and Kunka, B. S. (1985). Transfer of sucrose-fermenting ability and nisin production phenotype among lactic streptococci. *Applied & Environmental Microbiology* 49: 627–633.

Grosjean, H., and Fiers, W. (1982). Preferential codon usage in prokaryotic genes: the optimal codon-anticodon interaction energy and the selective codon usage in efficiently expressed genes. *Gene* 18: 199–209.

Gruss, A., and Ehrlich, D. (1989). The family of highly interrelated single-stranded deoxyribonucleic acid plasmids. *Microbiological Reviews* 53: 231–241.

Harlander, S. K. (1987). Transformation of *Streptococcus lactis* by electroporation. In: J. J. Ferretti and R. Curtis (Eds.), *Streptococcal genetics* (pp. 229–233). Washington, DC: American Society of Microbiology.

Hashiba, H., Takiguchi, R., Iskii, S., and Aoyama, K. (1990). Transformation of *Lactobacillus helveticus* subsp. *jugurti* with plasmid pLHR by electroporation. *Agricultural & Biological Chemistry* 54: 1537–1541.

Hashiba, H., Takiguchi, R., Jyoho, K., and Aoyama, K. (1992). Establishment of a host-vector system in *Lactobacillus helveticus* with β-galactosidase activity as a selection marker. *Bioscience Biotechnology & Biochemistry* 56: 190–194.

Hawley, D. K., and McClure, W. R. (1983). Compilation and analysis of *Escherichia coli* promoter sequences. *Nucleic Acid Research* 11: 2237–2255.

Hayes, F., Caplice, E., McSweeny, A., Fitzgerald, G. F., and Daly, C. (1990a). pAMβ1-associated mobilization of proteinase plasmids from *Lactococcus lactis* subsp. *lactis* UC317 and *L. lactis* subsp. *cremoris* UC205. *Applied & Environmental Microbiology* 56:195–201.

Hayes, F., Daly, C., and Fitzgerald, G. F. (1990b). High frequency, site specific recombination between lactococcal and pAMβ1 plasmid DNAs. *Journal of Bacteriology* 172: 3485–3489.

Helmann, J. D., and Chamberlain, M. J. (1988). Structure and function of bacterial sigma factors. *Annual Review of Biochemistry* 57: 839–872.

Hofemeister, J., Israeli-Reches, M., and Dubnau, D. (1983). Integration of plasmid pE194 at multiple sites on the *Bacillus subtilis* chromosome. *Molecular & General Genetics* 189: 58–68.

Holo, H., and Nes, I. F. (1989). High-frequency transformation, by electroporation, of *Lactococcus lactis* subsp. *cremoris* grown with glycine in osmotically stabilized media. *Applied & Environmental Microbiology* 55: 3119–3123.

Hols, P., Ferain, T., Garmyn, D., Bernard, N., and Delcour, J. (1994). Use of homologous expression-secretion signals & vector-free stable chromosomal integration in engineering of *Lactobacillus plantarum* for α-amylase & levanase expression. *Applied & Environmental Microbiology* 60: 1401–1413.

Ikeda, H., Kawasaki, I., and Gellert, M. (1984). Mechanism of illegitimate recombination: common sites for recombination & cleavage mediated by *Escherichia coli* DNA gyrase. *Molecular & General Genetics* 196: 546–549.

Iwata, M., Mada, M., and Ishiwa, H. (1986). Protoplast fusion of *Lactobacillus fermentum*. *Applied & Environmental Microbiology* 52: 392–393.

Jannière, L., and Ehrlich, S. D. (1987). Recombination between short repeated sequences is more frequent in plasmids than in the chromosome of *Bacillus subtilis*. *Molecular & General Genetics* 210: 116–121.

Jensen, P. R., and Hammer, K. (1998). The sequence of spacers between the consensus sequences modulates the strength of prokaryotic promoters. *Applied & Environmental Microbiology* 64: 82–87.

Jobin, M. P., Delmas, F., Garmyn, D., Divies, C., and Guzzo, J. (1997). Molecular characterization of the gene encoding an 18 kDa small heat shock protein associated with the membrane of *Leuconostoc oenos*. *Applied & Environmental Microbiology* 63: 609–614.

Josson, K., Scheirlinck, T., Michiels, F., Platteeuw, C., Stanssens, P., Joos, H., Dhaese, P., Zabeau, M., and Mahillon, J. (1989). Characterization of a Gram-positive broad-host-range plasmid isolated from *Lactobacillus hilgardii*. *Plasmid* 21: 9–20.

Josson, K., Soetaert, P., Michiels, F., Joos, H., and Mahillon, J. (1990). *Lactobacillus hilgardii* plasmid pLAB1000 consists of two functional cassettes commonly found in other Gram-positive organisms. *Journal of Bacteriology* 172: 3089–3099.

Kim, W. J., Ray, B., and Johnson, M. C. (1992). Plasmid transfers by conjugation and electroporation in *Pediococcus acidilactici*. *Journal of Applied Bacteriology* 72: 201–207.

Klaenhammer, T. R. (1995). Genetics of intestinal lactobacilli. *International Dairy Journal* 5: 1019–1058.
Kleeman, E. G., and Klaenhammer, T. R. (1982). Adherence of *Lactobacillus* species to human fetal intestinal cells. *Journal of Dairy Science* 65: 2063–2069.
Klein, J. R., Ulrich, C., Wegmann, U., Meyer-Barton, E., Plapp, R., and Henrich, B. (1995). Molecular tools for the genetic modification of dairy lactobacilli. *Systematic & Applied Microbiology* 18: 493–503.
Kondo, J. K., and McKay, L. L. (1984). Plasmid transformation of *Streptococcus lactis* protoplasts: Optimization and use in molecular cloning. *Applied & Environmental Microbiology* 48: 252–259.
Kuipers, O. P., de Ruyter, P. G. G. A., Kleerebezem, M., and de Vos, W. M. (1997). Controlled overproduction of proteins by lactic acid bacteria. *Trends in Biotechnology* 15: 135–140.
Labarre, C., Divies, C., and Guzzo, J. (1996). Genetic organization of the *mle* locus and identification of a *mleR*-like gene from *Leuconostoc oenos*. *Applied & Environmental Microbiology* 62: 4493–4498.
Langella, P., Zagorec, M. Ehrlich, S. D., and Morel-Deville, F. (1996). Intergeneric and intrageneric conjugal transfer of plasmids pAMβ1, pIL205 and pIP501 in *Lactobacillus sake*. *FEMS Microbiology Letters* 139: 51–56.
Leenhouts, K. J., Kok, J., and Venema, G. (1989). Campbell-like integration of heterologous plasmid DNA into the chromosome of *Lactococcus lactis* subsp. *lactis*. *Applied & Environmental Microbiology* 55: 394–400.
Leer, R. J., van Luijk, N., Posno, M., and Pouwels, P. H. (1992). Structural and functional analysis of two cryptic plasmids from *Lactobacillus pentosus* MD353 and *Lactobacillus plantarum* ATCC8014. *Molecular & General Genetics* 234: 265–274.
Lewin, B. (1997). *Genes VI*. Oxford University Press, ISBN 0-19-857778-8.
Lillehaug, D., Nes, I. F., and Birkel, N. K. (1997). A highly efficient and stable system for site-specific integration of genes and plasmids into the phage phi LC3 attachment site (attB) of the *Lactococcus lactis* chromosome. *Gene* 188: 129–136.
Lin, J. H.-C., and Savage, D. C. (1986). Genetic transformation of rifampicin resistance in *Lactobacillus acidophilus*. *Journal of General Microbiology* 132: 2107–2111.
Lin, J., Schmitt, P., and Davies, C. (1991). Characterization of a citrate-negative mutant *of Leuconostoc mesenteroides* spp. *mesenteroides*: Metabolic and plasmidic properties. *Applied Microbiology & Biotechnology* 34: 628–631.
Lin, M. Y., Harllander, S., and Savaiano, D. (1996). Construction of an integrative food-grade cloning vector for *Lactobacillus acidophilus*. *Applied Microbiology & Biotechnology* 45: 484–489.
Liu, C. Q., Harvey, M. L., and Dunn, N. W. (1997). Cloning of a gene encoding nisin resistance from *Lactococcus lactis* subsp. *lactis* M189 which is transcribed from an extended −10 promoter. *Journal of General Applied Microbiology* 43: 67–73.
Losick, R., and Pero, J. (1981). Cascades of sigma factors. *Cell* 25: 582–584.
Luchansky, J. B., Muriana, P. M., and Klaenhammer, T. R. (1988). Application of electroporation for transfer of plasmid DNA to *Lactobacillus, Lactococcus, Leuconostoc, Listeria, Pediococcus, Bacillus, Staphylococcus, Enterococcus* and *Propionibacterium*. *Molecular Microbiology* 2: 637–646.
MacCormick, C. A., Griffin, H. G., and Gasson, M. J. (1995). Construction of a food-grade host vector system for *Lactococcus lactis* based on the lactose operon. *FEMS Microbiology Letters* 127: 105–109.
Martinez-Murcia, A. J., and Collins, M. D. (1990a). Nucleotide sequence of 16S ribosomal RNA from *Lactobacillus viridescens* and *Lactobacillus confusus*. *Nucleic Acid Research* 18: 3402.
Martinez-Murcia, A. J., and Collins, M. D. (1990b). Nucleotide sequence of 16S ribosomal RNA from *Lactobacillus kandleri* and *Lactobacillus minor*. *Nucleic Acid Research* 18: 3401.
Marvo, S. L., King, S. R., and Jaskunas, S. R. (1983). Role of short regions of homology in intermolecular illegitimate recombination events. *Proceedings of the National Academy of Sciences USA* 80: 2452–2456.
McIntyre, D. A., and Harlander, S. K. (1989). Genetic transformation of intact *Lactococcus lactis* subsp. *lactis* by high voltage electroporation. *Applied & Environmental Microbiology* 55: 604–610.
McCracken, A., and Timms, P. (1999). Efficiency of transcription from promoter sequence variants in *Lactobacillus* is both strain and context dependent. *Journal of Bacteriology* 181: 6569–6572.
McKay, L. L. (1983). Functional properties of plasmids in lactic streptococci. *Antonie van Leeuwenhoek* 49: 259–274.
McKay, L. L., Baldwin, K. A., and Efstathiou, J. D. (1976). Transductional evidence for plasmid linkage of lactose metabolism in *Streptococcus lactis* C2. *Applied & Environmental Microbiology* 32: 45–52.
McKay, L. L., Cords, B. R., and Baldwin, K. A. (1973). Transduction of lactose metabolism in *Streptococcus lactis* C2. *Journal of Bacteriology* 115: 810–815.

Mercenier, A., and Chassy, B. M. (1988). Strategies for the development of bacterial transformation systems. *Biochimie* 70: 503–517.

Mercenier, A., Pouwels, P. H., and Chassy, B. M. (1994). Genetic engineering of lactobacilli, leuconostocs and *Streptococcus thermophilus*. In: M. J. Gasson and W. M. de Vos (Eds.), *Genetics and biotechnology of lactic acid bacteria* (pp. 252–293). Glasgow: Blackie Academic & Professional.

Mercenier, A., Robert, C., Romero, D. A., Costellino, I., Slos, P., and Lemoine, Y. (1988a). Development of an efficient sphaeroplast transformation procedure for *S. thermophilus*: the use of transfection to define a regeneration medium. *Biochimie* 70: 567–577.

Mercenier, A., Slos, P., Fallen, M., and Lecocq, J. P. (1988b). Plasmid transduction in *Streptococcus thermophilus*. *Molecular & General Genetics* 212: 386–389.

Moran, C. P., Jr., Johnson, W. C., and Losick, R. (1982). Close contacts between σ^{37}-RNA polymerase and a *Bacillus subtilis* chromosomal promoter. *Journal of Molecular Biology* 162: 709–713.

Morelli, L., Cocconcelli, P. S., Bottazzi, V., Damiani, G., Ferretti, L., and Sgaramella, V. (1987). *Lactobacillus* protoplast transformation. *Plasmid* 17: 73–75.

Muriana, P. M., and Klaenhammer, T. R. (1987). Conjugal transfer of plasmid-encoded determinants for bacteriocin production and immunity in *Lactobacillus acidophilus* 88. *Applied & Environmental Microbiology* 53: 553–560.

Natori, Y., Kano, Y., and Imamoto, F. (1990). Genetic transformation of *Lactobacillus casei* by electroporation. *Biochimie* 72: 265–269.

Neummann, E., Schaefer-Ridder, M., and Hofschneider, P. H. (1982). Gene transfer into mouse lyoma cells by electroporation in high electric fields. *EMBO Journal* 1: 841–845.

Novick, R. P. (1987). Plasmid incompatibility. *Microbiological Reviews* 51: 381–395.

Okamoto, T., Fujita, Y., and Irie, R. (1983). Fusion of protoplasts of *Streptococcus lactis*. *Agricultural & Biological Chemistry* 47: 2675–2676.

Okamoto, T., Fujita, Y., and Irie, R. (1985). Interspecific protoplast fusion between *Streptococcus cremoris* and *Streptococcus lactis*. *Agricultural & Biological Chemistry* 49: 1371–1376.

Perkins, J. B., and Youngman, P. J. (1986). A physical and functional analysis of Tn917, a *Streptococcus* transposon in the Tn3 family that functions in *Bacillus subtilis*. *Plasmid* 12: 119–138.

Platteeuw, C., Simons, S. G., and de Vos, W. M. (1994). Use of the *Escherichia coli* β–glucuronidase (*gusA*) gene as a reporter gene for analyzing promoters in lactic acid bacteria. *Applied & Environmental Microbiology* 60: 587–593.

Platteeuw, C., van Alen-Boerrigter, I., van Schalkwijk, S., and de Vos, W. M. (1996). Food-grade cloning and expression system for *Lactococcus lactis*. *Applied & Environmental Microbiology* 62: 1008–1013.

Platt, T. (1986). Transcription termination and the regulation of gene expression. *Annual Review of Biochemistry* 55: 339–372.

Posno, M., Heuvelmans, P. T. H. M., van Giezen, M. J. F., Lockman, B. C., Leer, R. J., and Pouwels, P. H. (1991). Complementation of the inability of *Lactobacillus* strains to utilize D-xylose with xylose catabolism-encoding of *Lactobacillus pentosus*. *Applied & Environmental Microbiology* 57: 2764–2766.

Pouwels, P. H., and Leer, R. J. (1993). Genetics of lactobacilli: Plasmids and gene expression. *Antonie van Leeuwenhoek* 64: 85–107.

Powell, I. B., Achen, M., Hillier, A. J., and Davidson, B. E. (1988). A simple and rapid method for genetic transformation of lactic streptococci by electroporation. *Applied & Environmental Microbiology* 54: 655–660.

Pribnow, D. (1975). Nucleotide sequence of an RNA polymerase binding site at an early T7 promoter. *Proceedings of the National Academy of Sciences USA* 72: 784–788.

Quirasco, M., Lopez-Munguia, A., Remaud-Simeon, M., Monsan, P., and Farres, A. (1999). Induction and transcription studies of the dextransucrase gene in *Leuconostoc mesenteroides* NRRL B-512F. *Applied & Environmental Microbiology* 65: 5504–5509.

Rauch, P. J. G., and de Vos, W. M. (1992). Characterization of the novel nisin-sucorse conjugative transposon, tn5276 and its insertion in *Lactococcus lactis*. *Journal of Bacteriology* 174: 1280–1287.

Raya, R. R., Fremaux, C., de Antoni, G. L., and Klaenhammer, T. R. (1992). Site-specific integration of the temperate bacteriophage øadh into the *Lactobacillus gasseri* chromosome and molecular characterisation of the phage (attP) and bacterial (attB) attachment sites. *Journal of Bacteriology* 174: 5584–5592.

Raya, R. R., and Klaenhammer, T. R. (1992). High-frequency plasmid transduction by *Lactobacillus gasseri* bacteriophage øadh. *Applied & Environmental Microbiology* 58: 187–193.

Raya, R. R., Kleeman, E. G., Luchansky, J. B., and Klaenhammer, T. R. (1989). Characterization of the temperate bacteriphage øadh and plasmid transduction in *Lactobacillus acidophilus* ADH. *Applied & Environmental Microbiology* 55: 2206–2213.

Reed, W. M. (1987). Protoplast fusion of *Lactobacillus acidophilus* and *Streptococcus lactis* via electric field or chemical induction. *Journal of General & Applied Microbiology* 33: 287–294.
Reneiro, R., Cocconcelli, P., Bottazzi, V., and Morelli, L. (1992). High frequency of conjugation in *Lactobacillus* is mediated by an aggregation-promoting factor. *Journal of General Applied Microbiology* 138: 763–768.
Rixon, J. E., Hazlewood, G. P., and Gilbert, H. J. (1990). Integration of an unstable plasmid into the chromosome of *Lactobacillus plantarum*. *FEMS Microbiology Letters* 71: 105–110.
Roos, S., Lindgren, S., and Jonsson, H. (1999). Autoaggregation of *Lactobacillus reuteri* is mediated by a putative DEAD-box helicase. *Molecular Microbiology* 32: 427–436.
Sanders, M. E., and Nicholson, M. A. (1987). A method for genetic transformation of non-protoplasted *Streptococcus lactis*. *Applied & Environmental Microbiology* 53: 1730–1736.
Sanoja, R. R., Morlon-Guyot, J., and Guyot, J. P. (1999). Electrotransformation of *Lactobacillus manihotivorans* LMG 18010(T) and 18011. *Journal of Applied Microbiology* 87: 99–107.
Schaller, H., Gray, C., and Hermann, K. (1975). Nucleotide sequence of an RNA polymerase binding site from the DNA bacteriophage fd. *Proceedings of the National Academy of Sciences USA* 72: 737–741.
Scheirlinck, T., Mahillon, J., Joos, H., Dhaese, P., and Michiels, F. (1989). Integration and expression of α-amylase and endoglucanase genes in the *Lactobacillus plantarum* chromosome. *Applied & Environmental Microbiology* 55: 2130–2137.
Shimizu-Kadota, M., Shibahara-Stone, H., and Ishiwa, H. (1991). Shuttle plasmid vectors for *Lactobacillus casei* and *Escherichia coli* with a minus origin. *Applied & Environmental Microbiology* 57: 3292–3300.
Shine, J., and Dalgarno, L. (1974). The 3′-terminal sequence of *Escherichia coli* 16S ribosomal RNA: Complementarity to nonsense triplets and ribosome binding sites. *Proceedings of the National Academy Sciences USA* 71: 1342–1346.
Shrago, A. W., Chassy, B. M., and Dobrogosz, W. J. (1986). Conjugal plasmid transfer (pAMβ1) *Lactobacillus plantarum*. *Applied & Environmental Microbiology* 52: 574–576.
Shrago, A. W., and Dobrogosz, W. J. (1988). Conjugal transfer of group B Streptococcal plasmids and co-mobilization of *Escherichia coli-Streptococcus* shuttle plasmids to *Lactobacillus plantarum*. *Applied & Environmental Microbiology* 54: 824–826.
Simon, D., Rouault, A., and Chopin, M.-C. (1986). High-efficiency transformation of *Streptococcus lactis* protoplasts by plasmid DNA. *Applied & Environmental Microbiology* 52: 394–395.
te Riele, H., Michel, B., and Ehrlich, S. D. (1986). Single-stranded plasmid DNA in *Bacillus subtilis* and *Staphylococcus aureus*. *Proceedings of the National Academy of Sciences USA* 83: 2541–2545.
Thompson, J. K., and Collins, M. A. (1996). Improvement in electroporation efficiency for *Lactobacillus plantarum* by the inclusion of high concentrations of glycine in the growth medium. *Journal of Microbiological Methods* 26: 73–79.
Thompson, J. K., McConville, K. J., McReynolds, C., and Collins, M. A. (1997). Electrotransformation of *Lactobacillus plantarum* using linearized plasmid DNA. *Letters in Applied Microbiology* 25: 419–425.
Thompson, J. K., McConville, K. J., McReynolds, C., and Collins, M. A. (1999). Potential of conjugal transfer as a strategy for the introduction of recombinant genetic material into strains of *Lactobacillus helveticus*. *Applied & Environmental Microbiology* 65: 1910–1914.
Tohyama, K., Sakurai, T., and Arai, H. (1971). Transduction by temperate phage PLS-1 in *Lactobacillus salivarius*. *Japanese Journal of Bacteriology* 26: 482–487.
Tomich, P. K., An, F. Y., and Clewell, D. B. (1980). Properties of erythromycin-inducible transposon, Tn917 in *Streptococcus faecalis*. *Journal of Bacteriology* 141: 1366–1374.
Travers, A. A., and Burgess, R. R. (1969). Cyclic re-use of the RNA polymerase sigma factor. *Nature* 222: 537–540.
Van der Lelie, D., van der Vossen, J. M. B. M., and Venema, G. (1988). Effect of plasmid incompatibility on DNA transfer to *Streptococcus cremoris*. *Applied & Environmental Microbiology* 54: 865–871.
Van Rooijen, R. J., Gasson, M. J., and de Vos, W. M. (1992). Characterization of the promoter of the *Lactococcus lactis* lactose operon: Contribution of flanking sequences and LacR repressor to its activity. *Journal of Bacteriology* 174: 2273–2280.
Vaughan, E. E., David, S., Harrington, A., Daly, C., Fitzgerald, G. F., and de Vos, W. M. (1995). Characterization of plasmid-encoded citrate permease (*citP*) genes from *Leuconostoc* species reveals high sequence conservation with the *Lactococcus lactis citP* gene. *Applied & Environmental Microbiology* 61: 3172–3176.
Vescovo, M., Bottazzi, V., and Gasson, M. J. (1983). Conjugal transfer of broad-host range plasmid pAMβ1 into enteric species of lactic acid bacteria. *Applied & Environmental Microbiology* 46: 753–755.
Wang, T.-T., and Lee, B. H. (1997). Plasmids in *Lactobacillus*. *Critical Reviews in Biotechnology* 17: 227–272.

Wei, M. Q., Rush, C. M., Norman, J. M., Hafner, L. M., Epping, R. J., and Timms, P. (1995). An improved method for the transformation of *Lactobacillus* strains using electroporation. *Journal of Microbiological Methods* 21: 97–109.

West, C. A., and Warner, P. J. (1985). Plasmid profiles and transfer of plasmid-encoded antibiotic resistance in *Lactobacillus plantarum. Applied & Environmental Microbiology* 50: 1319–1321.

Wyckoff, H. A., Sandine, W. E., and Kondo, J. K. (1991). Transformation of dairy *Leuconostoc* using plasmid vectors from *Bacillus, Escherichia*, and *Lactococcus* hosts. *Journal of Dairy Science* 74: 1454–1460.

2

Plasmid Biology, Conjugation, and Transposition

Michael J. Gasson and Claire A. Shearman

Introduction

The movement of genes between strains and species and the rearrangement of genetic material within the genome are critical factors in bacterial evolution. The importance of these processes to bacteria is matched by their value for the development of genetic tools with which to characterize and manipulate individual strains. In this regard, the lactic acid bacteria (LAB) are well endowed, possessing a rich complement of plasmids and transposable genetic elements. Natural processes for gene transfer are also of relevance to the safety evaluation of GM microorganisms. Given the potential of GM LAB for exploitation in food and health, understanding of these processes is important to the establishment of a scientific framework to support regulatory decision making. In this chapter some aspects of the biology of plasmids and transposable elements will be reviewed.

Plasmids

Plasmid-Encoded Traits

The lactococci were the first LAB to be subject to detailed molecular genetic analysis and much of the earliest work focused on their unusually large plasmid complements. These plasmids range in size from 2 to over 100 kb and they can be cryptic or encode traits of considerable relevance to the organisms' industrial use. The inherent segregational instability of plasmid DNA has been of value in the assignment of genetic traits to individual plasmid molecules by correlating trait curing with the loss of a specific plasmid. In addition, the phenomenon is important as a straightforward explanation for the frequently observed instability of industrially important properties of LAB. Thus, the chromosomal

Michael J. Gasson and Claire A. Shearman • Food Safety Science Division, Institute of Food Research, Norwich Research Park, Norwich, UK, NR4 7UA; e-mail: mike.gasson@bbsrc.ac.uk

integration of plasmid-encoded industrial traits by *in vivo* processes or recombinant DNA technology was one of the first targets for the biotechnological development of improved starter lactococci (McKay and Baldwin, 1978; Leenhouts et al., 1991b).

During the early genetic analysis of *Lactococcus lactis* it was difficult to gain molecular insight into individual plasmid-encoded traits due to the complexity and instability of the total plasmid complement. For this reason, strains cured of all plasmids were developed in order to provide clean backgrounds in which to study individual plasmid molecules. The two most widely used plasmid-free strains of *Lc. lactis* are MG1363 (Gasson, 1983) and IL1403 (Chopin et al.,1984).

A variety of interesting genetic traits have been found to be plasmid-encoded in the lactococci. These include genes for lactose catabolism (Kemplar and McKay, 1979a; McKay, 1983; Gasson, 1983, 1990), proteinase production (Kok, 1990), citrate uptake (Kemplar and McKay, 1979b; Hugenholtz, 1993), bacteriophage resistance (Forde and Fitzgerald, 1999), bacteriocin production (Klaenhammer, 1993), polysaccharide biosynthesis (Vedamuthu and Neville, 1986; Von Wright and Tynkkynen, 1987; Van Kranenburg et al., 1997), metal ion resistance (Liu et al., 1996; Leelawatcharamas et al., 1997; Khunajarakr et al., 1999), and antibiotic resistance (Teuber et al., 1999).

In other LAB, plasmids appear to be rather less abundant. However, a wide variety of cryptic plasmids have been found and some have been characterized in molecular detail including examples from *Streptococcus thermophilus* (Janzen et al., 1992; Solaiman and Somkuti, 1998), *Lactobacillus* (Bates and Gilbert, 1989; Pouwels and Leer, 1993; Kanatani et al., 1995; Cocconcelli et al., 1996; Oki et al., 1996; Sano et al., 1997; Wang and Lee, 1997; Aleshin et al., 1999; Lin and Chung, 1999; Thompson et al., 1999), *Leuconostoc* (Brito et al., 1996; Zuniga et al., 1996; Biet et al., 1999), *Pediococcus*, and *Tetragenococcus* (Benachour et al., 1995, 1997).

In addition, plasmids have been found to confer a variety of traits that include bacteriocin production (Klaenhammer, 1993), sugar catabolism (Pouwels and Leer, 1993; Benachour et al., 1996), heat stress response (Somkuti et al., 1998), and antibiotic resistance (Pouwels and Leer, 1993; Lin et al., 1996; Fons et al., 1997).

Vector Development

With the development of gene cloning methodology in the LAB, there was an interest in the development of plasmid vectors based on the naturally occurring replicons. Several vector series have been built using various small cryptic plasmids found in *Lc. lactis*. The first plasmids to be exploited in this way were pWV01 and pSH1 from *Lc. lactis* strains Wg2 and 712, respectively (Kok et al., 1984; Gasson and Anderson, 1985). These replicons were found to be unusually promiscuous, functioning in a wide variety of different genetic backgrounds that include both Gram-positive and Gram-negative species. For this reason, these vector derivatives have been exploited extensively in many different strains and species. The ability to replicate in *Escherichia coli* was of special value in providing instant shuttle vectors that facilitated convenient cloning stategies.

More recently other lactococcal plasmids have been exploited in a similar way, including pCI305 and pD125 from *Lc. lactis* strains UC317 and 5136, respectively (Hayes et al., 1990; Xu et al., 1991). In addition, naturally occurring plasmid replicons from other species of LAB have been exploited in the construction of gene cloning vectors (Pouwels and Leer, 1993; Klein et al., 1996; Wang and Lee, 1997; Solaiman and Somkuti, 1998; Aleshin et al., 2000; Biet et al., 1999; Lin and Chung, 1999).

Plasmid Replication by the Rolling Circle Mechanism

Several plasmids from the LAB have been sequenced in their entirety and in other cases the regions involved in DNA replication have been characterized following their isolation by cloning using replicon probe strategies. The availability of DNA sequence data and information on the minimal regions required for plasmid replication has provided valuable insight into the mechanisms by which plasmid DNA is replicated and segregated during bacterial growth and division.

This analysis has revealed that many plasmids, including both pWV01 and pSH71 from *Lc. lactis*, replicate by the rolling circle mechanism (DeVos, 1987; Leenhouts et al., 1991a). Indeed, it is now recognized that most of these plasmids belong to a very large family of small, promiscuous multicopy replicons that are found in many Gram-positive species and also in some Gram-negative hosts (Del Solar et al., 1993).

The rolling circle mode of replication has been reviewed in detail by Gruss and Ehrlich (1989) and Del Solar et al. (1993 and 1998). The most characteristic feature is the gene-ration of single-stranded DNA during plasmid replication. This phenomenon and the generation of high molecular weight multimers have been implicated as a cause of both segregational and structural instability. This has important consequences for the practical utility of gene cloning vectors based on plasmids such as pWV01 and pSH71 and these limitations were formally established in a comparative study featuring pWV01 and the enterococcal theta-replicating plasmid pAMβ1 (Kiewiet et al., 1993a,b).

Rolling circle replication depends on the involvement of three plasmid-encoded elements: a plus origin; a replication protein Rep; a minus origin. Replication proceeds via two distinct phases: first a single-stranded copy is made and second this is converted into double-stranded DNA. The Rep protein acts as an endonuclease and topoisomerase, it recognizes the origin sequence and introduces a nick to initiate replication. The plus DNA strand is displaced and a new plus strand is synthesized by 3′-OH extension from the nick. This process requires host cell functions that include DNA III, ssDNA-binding protein, and a helicase. Rep then recognizes a termination sequence that overlaps the origin sequence, producing a second nick to generate one fully replicated strand together with a single-stranded monomer of the displaced strand. The ends of the single-stranded DNA are ligated to form a circle and conversion to double-stranded DNA involves host factors that recognize a distinct minus or single-strand origin. Characteristically, the plus origin is located upstream or within the gene encoding Rep. Both the minus origin and the Rep protein exhibit sequence conservation across a large family of plasmids from diverse bacterial sources (Gruss and Ehrlich, 1989; Del Solar et al., 1998).

The efficiency with which the host converts single-stranded DNA into double-stranded DNA is governed by the ability of the host to act on the minus or single-strand origin. Poor efficiency in this reaction leads to the accumulation of single stranded DNA and this contributes to poor plasmid stability.

The large group of rolling circle replicons has been sub-divided into four distinct families on the basis of sequence homology in their plus origin region, which has been termed the leading strand initiation and control region (Del Solar et al., 1993). The lactococcal plasmids pWV01 and pFX2 and the *Lactobacillus* plasmid pLB4 are included in the very well characterized pLS1 family. A diagram of leading strand replication and its control in this plasmid family is shown in Figure 2.1. Key features are binding of the replication protein Rep to a conserved region of repeat sequences known as iterons, followed by the introduction of a nick at a distinct conserved site 5′-TACTACG/A-3′.

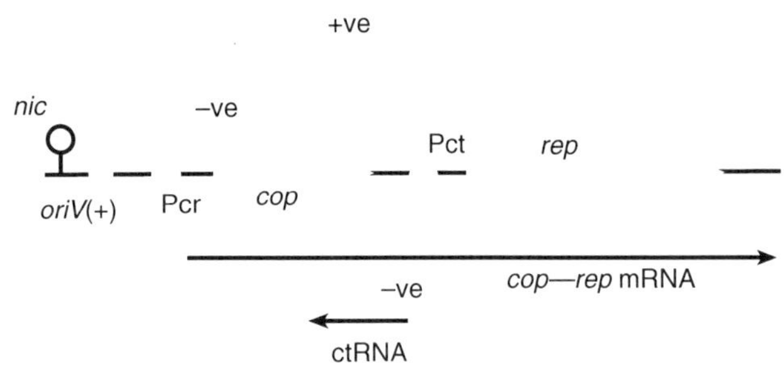

Figure 2.1. Model of leading strand replication in the pLS1 family of rolling circle-replicating plasmids based on Del Solar et al. (1993).

The availability of Rep protein is rate limiting and this is the target used by the cell to control plasmid replication and copy number. Transcription of *rep* is repressed by the binding of a small protein Cop to an operator site. Cop is encoded by DNA upstream of *rep* and the two proteins appear to be co-transcribed by a powerful promoter that is associated with the Cop-binding operator. From the DNA sequence data, the Cop proteins of pWV01 and pFX2 are predicted to be about 53 amino acids in size and that of pLB4, 52 amino acids. Cop proteins feature a helix-turn-helix motif typical of a DNA binding protein. In addition, control is exerted at the translational level by a countertranscript mRNA that inhibits Rep protein translation. Whilst much of this picture of replication control is based on generic data for the plasmid family, specific analysis of pFX2 has been reported recently (Grohmann et al., 1998).

The second part of rolling-circle plasmid replication, involving the conversion of single-stranded DNA into double-stranded DNA, uses a distinct origin of replication. In the case of pWV01, this single-strand origin has been characterized in some detail both *in vivo* and *in vitro* (Seegers et al., 1995). The region comprises 250 bp containing two inverted repeats both of which are required for full functionality.

The involvement of a trans-acting Rep protein in plasmid replication was exploited by Maugin et al. (1992) to generate a temperature sensitive derivative of the pWV01 replicon. This involved hydroxylamine mutagenesis to introduce several point mutations within the *repA* gene. This temperature sensitive replicon has been exploited in the development of valuable genetic tools based on the fact that plasmid replication be switched on and off by temperature shift. This has facilitated the development of suicide vectors that can be used to force chromosomal integration by homologous recombination or transposition.

Whilst many rolling circle replicons from the LAB are closely related to pWV01, the small cryptic lactococcal plasmid pWC1 has been shown to exhibit no homology to these molecules but rather to belong to a distinct group of which pC194 is the prototype. The distinct nature of the pWC1 replicon was shown by its compatibility with pWV01-family of replicons and, whilst it was maintained in several different Gram-positive species, it did not replicate in *E. coli* (Pillidge et al., 1996). The characteristics of several replicons isolated from *Lactobacillus* have been reviewed and these include further examples of pC194-like plasmids (Pouwels and Leer, 1993; Wang and Lee, 1997).

Plasmid Replication by the Theta Mechanism

In addition to rolling circle replication, some plasmids from LAB have been shown to use theta replication in which single-stranded DNA is not formed. One of the best characterized theta-replicating plasmids is pWV02, which like pWV01 was isolated from *Lc. lactis* Wg2 (Kiewiet et al., 1993b). The minimal replicon from this plasmid was identified and its DNA sequence provided further insight into its mode of replication. This involves a transacting replication protein RepB, 22 bp iteron sequences that are repeated three and a half times and, further upstream, another direct repeat of 10 bp located in an AT-rich region. Overall this structure resembles that found in iteron-containing theta replicons that have been characterized in *E. coli*. In contrast to the rolling circle replicons, plasmid pWV02 exhibited a narrow host range, and this feature is common to other theta replicons from LAB.

Several other theta plasmid replicons from lactococci have been characterized including pCI305 (Hayes et al., 1990), pUCL22 (Frere et al., 1995), pCI2000 (Kearney et al., 2000), pND324 (Duan et al., 1999), and those of the lactose plasmid pSK11L (Horng et al., 1991), the citrate plasmid pSL2 (Jahns et al., 1991), the cadmium resistance plasmid pND302 (Liu et al., 1997) and the bacteriophage resistance plasmids pCIS3 (Seegers et al., 2000), and pJW5633 (Gravesen et al., 1995). In addition, Seegers et al. (1994) demonstrated that several different plasmids maintained in a single lactococcal strain had related theta replicons.

Theta-replicating plasmids have been characterized in other species of LAB including, pUCL287 from *Tetragenococcus halophila* (Benachour et al., 1995, 1997), pMD136 from *Pediococcus pentosaceus* (Kantor et al., 1997), and pLA106 from *Lactobacillus acidophilus* (Sano et al., 1997).

Whilst most theta replicons from the LAB appear related, there are exceptions. Kearney et al. (2000) studied the replicon of plasmid pCI2000 and showed that it was a theta replicon unrelated to the pWV02 group. Plasmid pCI2000 belonged to a new family of which pLS32 from *Bacillus* is the prototype. These replicons do not possess an AT-rich region associated with their origin of replication and have iteron sequences within the coding sequence of the replication protein. In addition to characterizing the mode of pCI2000 DNA replication, these authors discovered a gene encoding a paritioning protein related to those found on some Gram-negative plasmids was discovered. The trans-acting gene was essential for stable plasmid inheritance and provided the first example of an active partition mechanism in Gram-positive bacteria.

The greater stability of theta replicons has been recognized as an advantage for use in gene cloning vectors for the LAB.

Conjugation

Heterologous Transmissible Plasmids

The transfer of genetic material by conjugation in the LAB involves both homologous systems and the exploitation of transmissible plasmids that have been introduced from heterologous species. With respect to the latter, the very widespread exploitation of pAMβ1 and pIP501 in the LAB has been reviewed extensively (e.g., Gasson, 1990; Gasson and Fitzgerald, 1994). These plasmids transfer readily between strains of most Gram-positive species and they have been exploited to mobilize several traits encoded by resident plasmids. Examples include proteinase production, bacteriophage resistance, lactose catabolism, polysaccharide production and antibiotic resistance (Gasson and Fitzgerald, 1994).

Specifically designed plasmid vectors have been used to take advantage of conjugal mobilization by the wide host range plasmids pAMβ1 and pIP501. In this way gene cloning can be undertaken in a transformation proficient strain prior to conjugal delivery into a desired host that may be recalcitrant to transformation or inefficient. Examples include the vectors pVA838 and pSA3 (Romero et al., 1987). Langella et al. (1993) investigated mobilization by pIP501 in *Lc. lactis* and defined a *mob* region that acted as a *recA*-dependent recombination hot spot to facilitate co-integrate formation.

The development of a conjugal delivery system that allows direct transfer from *E. coli* into *Lc. lactis* and other Gram-positive species was described by Trieu-Cout et al. (1987). This involved the exploitation of a conjugation transfer origin derived from the Gram-negative P group plasmid pRK2, together with replicons from both pAMβ1 and pBR322 and an antibiotic resistance marker that was selectable in both Gram-positive and Gram-negative hosts. Whilst this approach has been used in several species, especially where transformation methods are inefficient, its promise for the LAB has not been taken up to any great extent.

Transmissible Plasmids in the Lactic Acid Bacteria

In keeping with the presence of large plasmid complements, indigenous conjugation has been observed frequently in the lactococci. Examples of plasmid encoded traits that have been transferred by conjugation include production of bacteriocins (McKay et al., 1980; Scherwitz et al., 1983; Coakley et al., 1997), proteinases (Kok, 1990), and polysaccharides (Van Kranenburg et al., 1997), bacteriophage resistance (Klaenhammer and Fitzgerald, 1994; Garvey et al., 1995; O'Sullivan et al., 1998), and catabolism of lactose (Snook and McKay, 1981; Gasson, 1990) and raffinose (Kelly et al., 1998). Despite the widespread occurrence of conjugation, few systems have been characterized in any great detail. The major exception is the transfer system associated with the chromosomally located sex factor found in the *Lc. lactis* 712-C2-ML3 family of strains.

The Lactococcal Sex Factor

The earliest examples of plasmid transfer by conjugation in *Lc. lactis* involved the lactose plasmids that were present in strains ML3 and 712 (Gasson and Davies, 1980; McKay et al., 1980). It is now established that these strains, together with C2, are very closely related, although they have acquired a variety of differences during their maintenance in separate parts of the world (Davies et al., 1981). Lactose plasmid transfer from *Lc. lactis* ML3 or 712 donor strains is inefficient but transconjugants can acquire a radically improved transfer ability that is associated with the formation of a lactose plasmid co-integrate with a distinct sex factor. In the case of *Lc. lactis* ML3, this sex factor has been defined as a 48 kb plasmid pRS01, whereas in the case of *Lc. lactis* 712 and its plasmid free derivative MG1363 it has been shown to be a larger chromosomally integrated element (Walsh and McKay, 1981; Anderson and McKay, 1984; Gasson et al., 1992). Despite the isolation of pRS01 as plasmid DNA, strains harboring this element also carry a homologous chromosomally integrated molecule. The pRS01 element is largely homologous to the *Lc. lactis* 712 chromosomal sex factor and it is possible that this molecule exists in a state flux between chromosomal integration and an excised form as a covalently closed circular (CCC) DNA molecule. It is conceivable that under such circumstances it may not rely on efficient self replication for its maintenance in the cell. Indeed, CCC DNA has been isolated from *Lc. lactis* MG1363 at a copy number below one suggesting that it is not maintained solely by plasmid replication. Despite these differences in interpretation of its plasmid status, most of the observations on conjugal transfer are common for both pRS01 and the *Lc. lactis* 712 sex factor. Isolates of the related strain *Lc. lactis* C2 from different laboratories vary with respect to the presence of the sex factor DNA and those lacking the element cannot generate high frequency transferring derivatives of their lactose plasmid (Gasson et al., 1992).

The process of co-integrate formation between the sex factor and the lactose plasmid involves insertion sequence (IS)-mediated transposition events. These are controlled by IS*S1S* and IS*S1T* elements that have been identified on the lactose plasmid (Anderson and McKay, 1984; Gasson et al., 1992). Co-integration is independent of the host cell's generalized recombination system and results in the duplication of the IS element at the junctions between the two co-integrated molecules. The integration events involve specific sites on the lactose plasmid that are defined by the location of the IS element and random sites on the sex factor. This latter point is of considerable importance as the precise integration point will influence subsequent transfer properties if genes involved in conjugation are interrupted or their expression altered. One of the most striking consequences of co-integrate formation was the appearance in some strains of a constitutive cell aggregation phenotype and this property is assumed to represent a key stage in cell to cell contact formation. Indeed, there are obvious parallels with the role of aggregation substance encoded by the transfer systems of sex pheromone plasmids from *Enterococcus faecalis* (Godon et al., 1994).

In recent years, the transfer system associated with pRS01 and the *Lc. lactis* sex factor has been characterized in considerable detail. In the former case, advantage was taken of the plasmid co-integration process to map regions of pRS01 that were involved in conjugation. For this, use was made of pTRK28, a relatively small and high copy number plasmid that carried IS*S1S*. In this way four distinct regions of pRS01 involved in conjugation were mapped and characterized (Mills et al., 1994).

In the case of the *Lc. lactis* sex factor a chromosome walking strategy was used to clone the integrated element, including its junctions with the *Lc. lactis* MG1363 chromosome. The entire DNA sequence of this element has been determined, leading to the definition of genes involved in conjugation. A summary of the structure of the sex factor is given in Figure 2.2.

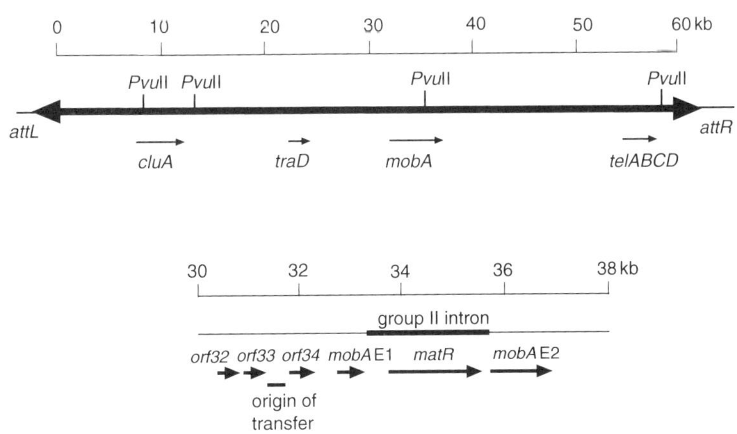

Figure 2.2. Genetic map of the *Lc. lactis* MG1363 sex factor shown in its chromosomally integrated state.

The gene responsible for cell aggregation is *cluA* (Godon et al., 1994). It encodes a cell surface presented protein of 1243 amino acids with a molecular size of 135 kDa. It has a 43 amino-terminal leader involved in its secretion from the cell and a cell surface-associated carboxy-terminus. The latter consists of a cell wall associated region followed by a classical cell membrane anchor as has been defined in cell surface-associated proteins from Gram-positive bacteria. This starts with a short region of positively charged residues followed by 30 hydrophobic amino acids and the conserved heptapeptide sequence LPXTGE. The amino acid sequence of CluA exhibits regions of homology with two distinct classes of bacterial surface protein: the Asc10 and Asa1 aggregation proteins involved in the conjugal transfer of *Enterococcus faecalis* sex pheromone plasmids and the Ssp5 and SpaP oral streptococcal proteins involved in binding to salivary glycoprotein. Inactivation of *cluA* results in a severe reduction in conjugal transfer ability. The role of CluA in promoting cell to cell contact was established by the upsteam integration of a *dnaK* promoter, which led to the appearance of a constitutive cell aggregation phenotype. More recently *cluA* has been cloned on an expression vector under the control of the lactococcal *nisA* promoter, which results in nisin inducible cell aggregation.

Another gene was found to encode a protein with homology to TraD from the *E. coli* sex factor F (Jalajakumari and Manning, 1989) and VirD4 from *Agrobacterium tumefaciens* Ti plasmids (Lessl et al., 1992). In both cases this protein is thought to play a role in the active transport of the transferred DNA strand into the recipient cell and it seems likely that this is the function of the homologous lactococcal protein (Frost et al., 1994).

Detailed characterization of the region involved in DNA transfer has been achieved both in pRS01 and the *Lc. lactis* sex factor. This includes the gene encoding the conjugation specific mobilization protein and the origin of transfer.

The mobilization protein gene, named *mobA* in *Lc. lactis* MG1363 and *ltrB* in pRS01, is remarkable in that it is interrupted by a complete and active group II intron (Shearman et al., 1996; Mills et al., 1996). At the time of its discovery this was a most unusual finding as the presence of introns in prokaryotes was not well established. The lactococcal intron provided the first evidence for a functional intron within a biologically active bacterial gene. A genetic map of this region is included in Figure 2.2. The sequence analysis of this region revealed an open reading frame encoding a protein with significant homology to the maturase of a mitochondrial group II intron. This gene, *matR* (*ltrA* in pRS01), was preceded by a ribosome binding site and it was not fused to an upstream gene. The open reading frame included a series of conserved reverse transcriptase domains and a possible zinc finger, features that are characteristic of other intron maturases. The intron maturase provides the essential catalytic activities involved in intron excision. The transfer gene *mobA* (*ltrB* in pRS01) was separated into two exons by the presence of a complete intron sequence. RT-PCR of this region produced an amplified cDNA that was 2.49 kb smaller than predicted from the genomic sequence, demonstrating that the intron was efficiently excised from the *mobA* mRNA. Sequencing of the cDNA revealed the splice site that was located in a conserved region of the mobilization protein. Inactivation of the *mobA* exons or the intron maturase severely inhibited conjugation, suggesting that the mobilization protein was an essential component of the conjugation process and that intron splicing was an active feature of conjugation gene expression. The intron mRNA sequence was modeled to form a well conserved structure consisting of six helical domains around a central wheel (Figure 2.3). The existence of an active self-splicing group II intron in a functional bacterial gene is a unique observation that has opened up new possibilities for the study of these genetic elements (Dunny 1999).

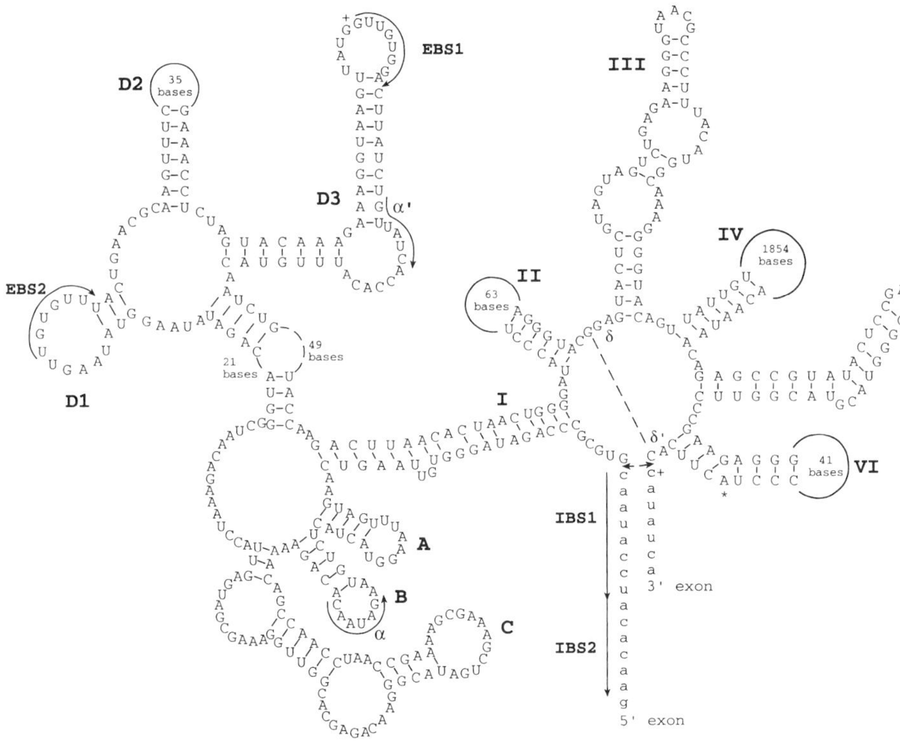

Figure 2.3. Group II intron found in the mobilization gene mobA of the *Lc. lactis* MG1363 sex factor.

One of the most interesting aspects of group II introns is their ability to transfer themselves to new sites within the genome. This can involve homing, in which the intron moves to the same site in an intronless version of its target gene. In addition and at a lower frequency, it can move to a distinct genomic site. The homing process has been very well studied in yeast mitochondria (Lambowitz and Belfort, 1993; Belfort and Perlman, 1995). The availability of an active intron in a bacterial system provides a unique opportunity to study intron mobility in a rather more manipulable genetic background. Mills et al. (1997) assayed homing in *Lc. lactis* using agarose gel electrophoresis of plasmid DNA from strains transformed with both an intron donor plasmid and an intron-free target plasmid. The homing process was found to take place efficiently, exhibiting target specificity that was equally efficient for either the complete target gene or a smaller 250 bp region across the splice site. Homing was independent of the host's generalized recombination system. Recently, Matsuura et al. (1997) described the functionality of the lactococcal intron both *in vitro* and in an heterologous *E. coli* host. In addition, an in depth analysis of homing was reported by Cousineau et al. (1998).

The region of DNA upstream of gene *mobA* (*ltrB* in pRS01) has been shown to contain the origin of transfer *oriT* where a single-strand nick is introduced to initiate transfer replication. The *oriT* was located by the use of a mobilization assay in which sex factor DNA was cloned on an otherwise nonmobilizable vector. The ability of this vector to be mobilized when other transfer functions, including the mobilization protein, were supplied *in trans* depended on the presence of the *oriT* sequence. The region had a series of inverted repeat and direct repeat structures that are characteristic of other bacterial origins of transfer (Mills et al., 1998).

DNA sequence data across the junctions between the integrated sex factor and the chromosome of *Lc. lactis* MGI363 has been determined. In addition, the chromosomal integration site of a sex factor cured derivative and the integration site of the sex factor in its excised state have been sequenced. This data revealed details of the integration/excision process that is characteristic of this genetic element. Both the sex factor and the chromosome have a unique homologous 24 bp sequence that controls integration and excision. When the sex factor is integrated within the chromosome this 24 bp sequence is duplicated at the junctions. PCR analysis suggested that the sex factor is maintained in a state of flux between its integrated and excised states. Furthermore, this integration and excision process was unaffected by the introduction of a *recA* mutation, suggesting that it was independent of the host's generalized recombination system. These observations are reminiscent of the site specific integration and excision processses associated with temperate bacteriophages such as *E. coli* phage lambda. Examination of the sex factor DNA sequence has not revealed the presence of a recombinase enzyme gene that might be responsible for the site specific recombination process and thus this may be undertaken by a host enzyme encoded by the lactococcal chromosome. Figure 2.4 shows the sequences involved in the site specific recombination process associated with sex factor integration and excision.

In order to investigate transfer of the sex factor as a discrete genetic element, it was marked by the integration of a selectable tetracycline resistance gene. This allowed its very high frequency of transfer between all tested strains to *Lc. lactis* to be established. Furthermore, a series of physically mapped chromosomal markers was used to demonstrate that the sex factor was able to mobilize the bacterial chromosome in a unidirectional and polarized manner that is reminiscent of Hfr transfer in *E. coli*. This phenomenon has been used in the authors' laboratory as a convenient method for the combination of chromosomal mutations in *Lc. lactis*. The fact that the sex factor can transfer at high frequency to a chromosomal integration site that appears to be present in all strains of *Lc. lactis* suggests that this genetic element has considerable potential for use as a vector for the stable and nondisruptive introduction of genetic material into industrial strains of this species.

```
1:
ACAGGTTAATAAAACCGTGGGAATAT AATCTTATTTATACCTAGAATATG CAAAAAAAGCGTAATAACGGTATTT

2:
CTTTAGTATTTAGTCTATAATAGAAC AATCTTATTTATACCTAGAATATG GCTGGGCGTTTCTACCTCGTACCGT

3:
CTTTAGTATTTAGTCTATAATAGAAC AATCTTATTTATACCTAGAATATG CAAAAAAAGCGTAATAACGGTATTT

4:
ACAGGTTAATAAAACCGTGGGAATAT AATCTTATTTATACCTAGAATATG GCTGGGCGTTTCTACCTCGTACCGT
```

DNA sequences at integration/excision sites are shown for:

1—the sex factor in its excised plasmid-like state;
2—the chromosome of a sex factor-free strain;
3—the left junction between chromosomally-integrated sex factor and the bacterial chromosome;
4—the right junction between chromosomally-integrated sex factor and the bacterial chromosome.

The conserved 24 bp region involved in site-directed integration/excision has no underline whereas sex factor DNA flanking this 24 bp sequence has a solid underline ______ and chromosomal DNA flanking this 24 bp sequence has a broken underline ....

Figure 2.4. Sites involved in the chromosomal interation and excision of the *Lc. lactis* MG1363 sex factor.

Transposable Genetic Elements

Conjugative Transposons

As well as conjugation associated with plasmids, both indigenous and heterologous conjugative transposons have featured in the genetics of LAB. With respect to the former, Tn*916* has been used widely, and with respect to the latter, transposons encoding sucrose catabolism and nisin biosynthesis genes have been characterized in some detail. In addition, an integrative conjugative element, ICE*St1*, has been described in *Streptococcus thermophilus*, which undergoes site specific integration within a gene encoding fructose-1,6-biphosphate aldolase (Burrus et al., 2000).

The transposon Tn*916* and the related element Tn*919* have been delivered to a variety of different LAB species by conjugation and shown to generate insertional inactivation mutants (Gasson and Fitzgerald, 1994). Examples in *Lc. lactis* include genes for maltose catabolism, citrate utilization, and the malolactic fermentation (Renault and Heslot, 1987; Hill et al., 1991). In some strains, the insertion specificity of Tn*916* appears to be nonrandom. More detailed analysis of the transposition process suggests that this may reflect the fact that its excision can be impaired in some background strains. The use of these strains as donors for conjugal delivery and transposon mutagenesis results in retention of the original integration site and the transposon is probably transferred passively by a distinct conjugation process. In the case of *Lc. lactis* MG1363, this appears to be the chromosomally located sex factor described above (Bringel et al., 1992; Gasson and Fitzgerald, 1994). The use of Tn*916* as a genetic tool in the LAB is relatively limited and more effective use has been made of Tn*917* as is described below.

The conjugal transfer of linked genes for sucrose catabolism and the biosynthesis of nisin was observed long before the nature of the genetic element that encodes the genes was discovered (Gasson, 1984). The combination of linked trait curing and transmissibility suggested that a plasmid was involved but it is now conclusively established that the genes are carried on a chromosomally located conjugative transposon. The first characterized elements were Tn*5301* and Tn*5276* (Horn et al., 1991; Rauch and deVos, 1992). Pulsed field gel electrophoresis was used to show that the transposon was approximately 70 kb in size and that when transferred into the *Lc. lactis* MG1363 background it appeared to integrate with site and orientation specificity at one of two chromosomal locations. DNA sequence determination of the chromosomal junctions with the transposon suggested integration into a specific target site. The DNA sequence 3′-TTTTTG-5′ was duplicated at the boundaries between transposon and chromosomal DNA. Analysis of the target for transposition in different strains revealed sequence conservation of 18 out of 25 bases, reinforcing the view that transposition was site-specific. Further data, including the discovery of *int* and *xis* genes near one end of Tn*5276* and the detection of a circular intermediate, suggested that the mechanism of transposition resembles that of the well characterized transposons Tn*916*, Tn*554*, and Tn*1545* (Gasson and Fitzgerald, 1994; Rauch and deVos, 1994).

Several attempts have been made to transfer transposons encoding sucrose fermentation and nisin biosynthesis genes from *Lactococcus* into heterologous species. Evidence for low frequency transfer to *Lactobacillus* and *Enterococcus* has been presented but in these cases no biosynthesis of nisin was detected (Broadbent et al., 1995; Gasson and Hill, unpublished data). Additional traits, including a bacteriophage resistance phenotype and production of N^5-(carboxyethyl) ornithine synthase have been shown to be encoded by some sucrose–nisin transposons (Gonzalez and Kunka, 1985; Murphy et al., 1988; Donkershoot and Thompson, 1990).

Exploitation of Transposon Tn*917*

The enterococcal transposon Tn*917*, which is not self-transmissible by conjugation, has been used extensively as a genetic tool in the LAB. This transposon has been developed for use in various Gram-positive bacteria, notably in *Bacillus* and sophisticated derivatives designed to integrate reporter genes have been designed. The potential for Tn*917* in the LAB is well demonstrated by the work of Israelson and Hansen (1993) who showed that the temperature sensitive replicon of the delivery vector pE194ts functioned in *Lc. lactis*. Random transposition was demonstrated and the transposon was used to integrate a promoterless β-galactosidase gene into the chromosome in order to detect environmentally regulated genes.

Insertion Sequences

A wide variety of insertion sequences has been discovered and characterized in the LAB. These elements are often present in large numbers within the genome. Some examples of IS elements found in the LAB are listed in Table 2.1. IS elements have been shown to be involved in a variety of *in vivo* DNA rearrangements and they have been used in the development of powerful genetic tools.

The involvement of ISS*1S* and ISS*1T* in the formation of lactose plasmid :: sex factor co-integrates was described above. In some cases IS elements are known to provide promoters that control the expression of adjacent genes. Transposition of IS*905* was shown to be responsible for switching on nisin gene expression during the construction of a system for the production of variant nisin molecules (Dodd et al., 1994). Spontaneous inactivation of a gene encoding an abortive infection system was shown to be the result of insertional inactivation following transposition of IS*1076* (Huang et al., 1991).

IS elements have been used to effect the integration of DNA into the chromosome. The iso-ISS*1* element IS*946* was cloned onto a suicide vector and shown to effect random integration of the plasmid into the genome of *Lc. lactis* (Romero and Klaenhammer, 1992). A similar result was achieved using the distinct IS element IS*981* (Polzin and McKay, 1992) and Le Bourgeois et al. (1992) exploited IS-promoted random integration to introduce additional sites for rare cutting restriction endonucleases during their physical mapping of lactococcal chromosomes.

Conclusion

The analysis of plasmids and transposable genetic elements in LAB has advanced significantly in recent years. A variety of valuable genetic tools have been developed and these support both GM technology and the use of conventional genetics for the manipulation of individual strains. Whilst plasmids have interest and significance in their own right, the development of methods to exploit the bacterial chromosome are especially important. A notable development is the use of temperature sensitive plasmid vectors and transposons to facilitate both directed and random chromosome integration. In addition the discovery of a genetic element that facilitates both high frequency conjugation and site-directed chromosomal integration in all lactococcal strains is notable. The fact that this genetic element can mobilize chromosomal genes opens up possibilities for strain development by the combination of individual mutations and the future construction of hybrid strains.

Table 2.1. Insertion Sequences from LAB

IS Element	Size (bp)	Inverted Repeats (bp)	Target Duplication (bp)	Transposase (a.a.)	Homology	Known Distribution	Known Iso-Elements	Accession Number	Reference
IS*L1*	1256	40	3	274	IS2/IS*3*	*Lactobacillus casei*	H	X02734	Shimizu-Kadota et al. (1985)
IS*S1*	808	18	8	226	IS*26*	*Lactococcus* *Enterococcus* *Streptococcus thermophilus*	IS*S1S* IS*S1T* IS*S1S*A IS*S1S*B IS*S1S*C IS*S1N* IS*S1W* IS*S1R* IS946	M18290 M18291 M18292 M18293 M18294 M37395 M37396	Polzin and Shimizu-Kadota (1987) Haandrikman et al. (1990) Romero and Klaenhammer (1990)
IS*904*	1241	39	4	253	IS2/IS*3* IS*600*	*Lactococcus*	IS*1068* IS*1076*	M27276 X52273	Dodd et al. (1990) Rauch et al. (1990)
IS*905*	1313	28	8	392	IS*256*	*Lactococcus*		L20851	Dodd et al. (1992)
IS*981*	1222	40	5	280	IS2/IS*3* IS*51* IS*150* IS*600* IS*629* IS*861* IS*904* IS*L1*	*Lactococcus* *Streptococcus thermophilus* *Lactobacillus bulgaricus*		M33933 L32790	Polzin and McKay (1991) Guedon et al. (1995)
IS*982*	1003	18		295	IS*256*	*Lactococcus* *Enterococcus*	 ISEfm1	L34754	Yu et al. (1995)
IS*1062*	1062	24	3	320	IS*1252* IS*6770*	*Enterococcus*		X96976	Hirt et al. (1996)

(continued)

Table 2.1. ***(continued)***

IS Element	Size (bp)	Inverted Repeats (bp)	Target Duplication (bp)	Transposase (a.a.)	Homology	Known Distribution	Known Iso-Elements	Accession Number	Reference
IS*1070*	1027	28	2 or 4	305	IS*30* IS*4351* IS*1086* IS*1161* IS*AS2*	*Leuconostoc*		U17353	Vaughan and de Vos (1995)
IS*1076*	1296	39	3		IS*3* IS*904*	*Lactococcus*	IS*1076R* IS*1076L*		Novel et al. (1988)
IS*1165*	1553	39	3 or 8	412		*Leuconostoc* *Pediococcus* *Lactobacillus*		X62617	Johansen and Kibenich (1992)
IS*1191*	1313	28	8	391	IS*1201* IS*256*	*Streptococcus thermophilus* *Lactococcus* *Lactobacillus bulgaricus*		L32789	Guedon et al. (1995)
IS*1194*	1200	16		332	IS*5*	*Streptococcus thermophilus* *Lactococcus*		Y13626	Bourgoin et al. (1998)
IS*1201*	1387	24	8	369	IS*256*	*Lactobacillus helveticus*			Tailliez et al. (1994)
IS*1223*	1493	25	5	OrfA 177 OrfB 313 translational fusion	IS*3* IS*150* IS*600*	*Lactobacillus johnsonii*		U09558	Walker and Klaenhammer (1994)
IS*1297*	1039	18		226	IS*S1*	*Leuconostoc*		U59101	Ward et al. (1996)
IS*1675*		26		440		*Lactococcus*		U91581	Dufour et al. (2000)
					IS*30*	*Pediococcus pentosaceus*		Z32771	Leenhouts et al. (1994)

In addition, the molecular characterization of plasmid replication, transposition, and conjugation has advanced rapidly in recent years. Overall, the natural processes of gene transfer and rearrangement in LAB are reasonably well-characterized providing insight into the evolution of these bacteria and a range of tools for their biotechnological development.

References

Aleshin, V. V., Semenova, E. V., Tarakanov, B. V., and Livshits, V. A. (2000). A family of shuttle vectors for lactic acid bacteria and other gram-positive bacteria based on the plasmid pLF1311 replicon. *Microbiology* 69: 63–67.

Aleshin, V. V., Semenova, E. V., Doroshenko, V. G., Jomantas, Y. V., Tarakanov, B. V., and Livshits, V. A. (1999). The broad host range plasmid pLF1311 from *Lactobacillus fermentum* VKM1311. *FEMS Microbiology Letters* 178: 47–53.

Anderson, D. G., and McKay, L. L. (1984). Genetic and physical characterisation of recombinant plasmids associated with cell aggregation and high frequency conjugal transfer in *Streptococcus lactis* ML3. *Journal of Bacteriology* 158: 954–962.

Bates, E. M., and Gilbert, H. (1989). Characterisation of a cryptic plasmid from *Lactobacillus plantarum*. *Gene* 85: 253–258.

Belfort, M., and Perlman, P. S. (1995). Mechanisms of intron mobility. *Journal of Biological Chemistry* 270: 30237–30240.

Benachour, A., Frere, J., and Novel, G. (1995). pUCL287 plasmid from *Tetragenococcus halophila (Pediococcus halophila)* ATCC 33315 represents a new theta-type replicon family of lactic acid bacteria. *FEMS Microbiology Letters* 128: 167–176.

Benachour, A., Flahaut, S., Frere, J., and Novel, G. (1996). Plasmid transfer by electroporation and conjugation in *Tetragenococcus* and *Pediococcus* genera and evidence of plasmid-linked metabolic traits. *Current Microbiology* 32: 188–194.

Benachour, A., Frere, J., Flahaut, S., Novel, G., and Auffray, Y. (1997). Molecular analysis of the theta-replicating plasmid pUCL287 from *Tetragenococcus (Pediococcus) halophilus* ATCC33315. *Molecular and General Genetics* 255: 504–513.

Biet, F., Cenatiempo, Y., and Fremaux, C. (1999). Characterisation of pFR18, a small cryptic plasmid from *Leuconostoc mesenteroides* FR52, and its use as a food grade vector. *FEMS Microbiology Letters* 179: 375–383.

Bourgoin, F., Guedon, G., and Decaris, B. (1998). Characterization of a novel insertion sequence, IS1194, in *Streptococcus thermophilus* CNRZ368. Direct DNA sequence submission Accession number Y13626.

Bringel, F., Van Alstine, G. L., and Scott, J. R. (1992). Transfer of Tn*916* between *Lactococcus lactis* subsp. *lactis* strains is nontranspositional: Evidence for a chromosomal fertility factor in strain MG1363. *Journal of Bacteriology* 174: 5840–5847.

Brito, L., Vieira, G., Santos, M. A., and Paveia, H. (1996). Nucleotide sequence analysis of pOg32, a cryptic plasmid from *Leuconostoc*. *Plasmid* 36: 49–54.

Broadbent, J. R., Sandine, W. E., and Kondo, J. K. (1995). Characteristics of Tn5307 exchange and intergeneric transfer of genes associated with nisin production. *Applied Microbiology and Biotechnology* 44: 139–146.

Burrus, V., Roussel, Y., Decaris, B., and Guedon, G. (2000). Characterisation of a novel integrative element, ICE*St1*, in the lactic acid bacterium *Streptococcus thermophilus*. *Applied and Environmental Microbiology* 66: 1749–1753.

Chopin, M. C., Chopin, A., Rouault, A., and Simon, D. (1984). Two plasmid-determined restriction and modification systems in *Streptococcus lactis*. *Plasmid* 11: 260–263.

Coakley, M., Fitzgerald, G. F., and Ross, R. P. (1997). Application and evaluation of the phage resistance- and bacteriocin-encoding plasmid Pmrc01 for the improvement of dairy starter cultures. *Applied and Environmental Microbiology* 63: 1434–1440.

Cocconcelli, P. S., Elli, M., Riboli, B., and Morelli, L. (1996). Genetic analysis of the replication region of the *Lactobacillus* plasmid vector pPSC22. *Research in Microbiology* 147: 619–624.

Cousineau, B., Smith, D., Lawrence-Cavanagh, S., Mueller, J. E., Yang, J., Mills, D., Manias, D., Dunny, G., Lambowitz, A. A., and Belfort, M. (1998). Retrohoming of a bacterial group II intron: Mobility via complete reverse splicing and rehoming via full reverse splicing. *Cell* 94: 451–462.

Davies., F. L., Underwood, H. M., and Gasson, M. J. (1981). The value of plasmid profiles for strain identification in lactic streptococci and the relationship between *Streptococcus lactis* 712, ML3 and C2. *Journal of Applied Bacteriology* 51: 325–338.

Dodd, H. M., Horn, N., and Gasson, M. J. (1990). Analysis of the genetic determinant for production of the peptide antibiotic nisin. *Journal of General Microbiology* 136: 555–566.

Dodd, H. M., Horn, N., Hao, Z., and Gasson, M. J. (1992). A lactococcal expression system for engineering nisins. *Applied and Environmental Microbiology* 58: 3683–3693.

Dodd, H. M., Horn, N., and Gasson, M. J. (1994). Characterization of IS*905*, a new multicopy insertion sequence identified in lactococci. *Journal of Bacteriology* 176: 3393–3396.

Donkershoot, J. A., and Thompson, J. (1990). Simultaneous loss of N5-(carboxyethyl) ornithine synthase, nisin production and sucrose fermenting ability by *Lactococcus lactis* K1. *Journal of Bacteriology* 172: 4122–4126.

Duan, K., Liu, C.-Q., Liu, Y.-J., Ren, J., and Dunn, N. W. (1999). Nucleotide sequence and thermostability of pND324, a 3.6 kb plasmid from *Lactococcus lactis*. *Applied Microbiology and Biotechnology* 53: 36–42.

Dufour, A., Rince, A., Uguen, P., and Le Pennec, J. P. (2000). IS1675, a novel lactococcal insertion element, forms a transposon-like structure including the lacticin 481 lantibiotic operon. *Journal of Bacteriology* 182: 5600–5605.

Dunny, G. M., and McKay, L. L. (1999). Group II introns and expression of conjugative transfer functions in lactic acid bacteria. *Antonie van Leeuwenhoek* 76: 77–88.

Fons, M., Hege, T., Ladire, M. Raibaud, P., Ducluzeau, R., and Maguin, E. (1997). Isolation and characterisation of a plasmid from *Lactobacillus fermentum* conferring erythromycin resistance. *Plasmid* 37: 199–203.

Forde, A., and Fitzgerald, G. F. (1999). Bacteriophage defense systems in lactic acid bacteria. *Antonie van Leeuwenhoek* 76: 139–155.

Frere, J., Herreman, C., Boutibonnes, P., Novel, M., and Novel, G. (1995). Segregational stability and copy number of the theta-type replicon *Rep22* in *Lactococcus*. *Current Microbiology* 30: 33–37.

Frost, L. S., Ippen-Ihler, K., and Skurray, R. A. (1994). Analysis of the sequence and gene products of the transfer region of the F sex factor. *Microbiology Reviews* 58: 162–210.

Garvey, P. D., Van Sinderen, D. P., Twomey, C., Hill, C., and Fitzgerald, G. F. (1995). Molecular genetics of bacteriophage and natural phage defense systems in the genus *Lactococcus*. *International Dairy Journal* 5: 905–947.

Gasson, M. J. (1983). Plasmid complements of *Streptococcus lactis* NCDO712 and other lactic streptococci after protoplast-induced curing. *Journal of Bacteriology* 154: 1–9.

Gasson, M. J. (1984). Transfer of sucrose fermenting ability, nisin resistance and nisin production into *Streptococcus lactis* 712. *FEMS Microbiology Letters* 21: 7–10.

Gasson, M. J. (1990). *In vivo* genetic systems in lactic acid bacteria. *FEMS Microbiology Reviews* 87: 43–60.

Gasson, M. J., and Anderson, P. H. (1985). High copy number plasmid vectors for use in lactic streptococci. *FEMS Microbiology Letters* 30: 193–196.

Gasson, M. J., and Davies, F. L. (1980). High frequency conjugation associated with *Streptococcus lactis* donor cell aggregation. *Journal of Bacteriology* 143: 1260–1264.

Gasson, M. J., and Fitzgerald, G. F. (1994). Gene transfer systems and transposition. In: M. J. Gasson and W. M. de Vos (Eds.), *Genetics and biotechnology of lactic acid bacteria* (pp. 1–52). London: W. M. Blackie Academic & Professional.

Gasson, M. J., Swindell, S. R., Maeda, S., and Dodd, H. M. (1992). Molecular rearrangement of lactose plasmid DNA asociated with high-frequency transfer and cell aggregation in *Lactococcus lactis*. *Molecular Microbiology* 6: 3213–3223.

Godon, J.-J., Jury, K., Shearman, C. A., and Gasson, M. J. (1994). The *Lactococcus lactis* sex factor aggregation gene *cluA*. *Molecular Microbiology* 12: 655–663.

Gonzalez, C. F., and Kunka, B. S. (1985). Transfer of sucrose fermenting ability and nisin production phenotype among lactic streptococci. *Applied and Environmental Microbiology* 49: 627–633.

Gravesen, A., Josephsen, J., Von Wright, A., and Vogensen, F. (1995). Characterisation of the replicon from the lactococcal theta-replicating plasmid pJW563. *Plasmid* 34: 105–118.

Grohmann, E., Moscoso, M., Zechner, E. L., del Solar, G., and Espinosa, M. (1998). *In vivo* definition of the functional origin of leading strand replication on the lactococcal plasmid pFX2. *Molecular and General Genetics* 260: 38–47.

Gruss, A., and Ehrlich, S. D. (1989). The family of highly integrated single-stranded deoxyribonucleic acid plasmids. *Microbiological Reviews* 53: 231–241.

Guedon, G., Bourgoin, F., Pebay, M., Roussel, Y., Colmin, C., Simonet J. M., and Decaris B. (1995). Characterization and distribution of two insertion sequences IS*1191* and iso-IS*981*, in *Streptococcus* *thermophilus*: does intergenetic transfer of insertion sequences occur in lactic acid bacteria co-cultures? *Molecular Microbiology* 16: 69–78.

Haandrikman, A. J., C. Van Leeuwen, J. Kok, P. Vos, W. M. de Vos and G. Venema (1990). "Insertion elements on lactococcal proteinase plasmids." *Applied and Environmental Microbiology* 56: 1890–1896.

Hayes, F., Daly, C., and Fitzgerald, G. F. (1990). Identification of the minimal replicon of *Lactococcus lactis* subsp. *lactis* UC317 plasmid pCI305. *Applied and Environmental Microbiology* 56: 202–209.

Hill, C., Daly, C., and Fitzgerald, G. F. (1991). Isolation of chromosomal mutants of *Lactococcus lactis* subsp. *lactis* biovar *diacetylactis* 18–16 after introduction of Tn*919*. *FEMS Microbiology Letters* 81: 135–140.

Hirt, H., R. Wirth and A. Muscholl (1996). "Comparative analysis of 18 sex pheromone plasmids from *Enterococcus facaelis*: detection of a new insertion element on pAD1and implications for the evolution of this plasmid family." *Molecular and General Genetics* 252: 640–647.

Horn, N., Swindell, S., Dodd, H. M., and Gasson, M. J. (1991). Nisin biosynthesis genes are encoded by a novel conjugative transposon. *Molecular and General Genetics* 228: 129–135.

Horng, J. S., Polzin, K. M., and McKay, L. L. (1991). Replication and temperature-sensitive maintainance functions of lactose plasmid pSK11L from *Lactococcus lactis* subsp. *lactis*. *Journal of Bacteriology* 173: 7573–7581.

Huang, D. C., Novel, M., and Novel, G. (1991). A transposon-like element on the lactose plasmid of *Lactococcus lactis* subsp. *lactis* 2270. *FEMS Microbiology Letters* 77: 101–106.

Hugenholtz, J. (1993). Citrate metabolism in lactic acid bacteria. *FEMS Microbiology Letters* 12: 165–178.

Israelson, H., and Hansen, E. B. (1993). Insertion of transposon Tn*917* derivatives into the *Lactococcus lactis* subsp. *lactis* chromosome. *Applied and Environmental Microbiology* 59: 21–26.

Jalajakumari, M. B., and Manning, P. A. (1989). Nucleotide sequence of the *traD* region of the *E. coli* F sex factor. *Gene* 81: 195–202.

Jahns, A., Schafer, A., Geis, A., and Teuber, M. (1991). Identification, cloning and sequencing of the replication region of *Lactococcus lactis* subsp. *lactis* biovar *diacetylactis* Bu2 citrate plasmid pSL2. *FEMS Microbiology Letters* 80: 253–258.

Janzen, T., Kleinschmidt, J., Neve, H., and Geis, A. (1992). Sequencing and characterisation of pST1, a cryptic plasmid from *Streptococcus thermophilus*. *FEMS Microbiology Letters* 95: 175–180.

Johansen, E. and A. Kibenich (1992). "Isolation and characterization of IS*1165*, an insertion sequence of *Leuconostoc mesentaroides* subsp. *cremoris* and other lactic acid bacteria." *Plasmid* 27: 200–206.

Kanatani, K., Tahara, T., Oshimura, M., Sano, K., and Umezawa, C. (1995). Identification of the replication region of *Lactobacillus acidophilus* plasmid pLA103. *FEMS Microbiology Letters* 133: 127–130.

Kantor, A., Montville, T. J., Mett, A., and Shapira, R. (1997). Molecular characterisation of the replicon of the *Pediococcus pentosaceus* 43200 pediocin A plasmid pMD136. *FEMS Microbiology Letters* 151: 237–244.

Kearney, K., Fitzgerald, G. F., and Segers, J. F. M. L. (2000). Identification and characterisation of an active plasmid partition mechanism for the novel *Lactococcus lactis* plasmid pCI2000. *Journal of Bacteriology* 182: 30–37

Kelly, W. J., Davey, G. P., and Ward, L. J. H. (1998). Conjugative transfer of raffinose metabolism in *Lactococcus lactis*. *FEMS Miocrobiology Letters* 167: 145–149.

Kemplar, G. M., and McKay, L. L. (1979a). Genetic evidence for plasmid-linked lactose metabolism in *Streptococcus lactis* subsp *diacetylactis* strains. *Applied and Environmental Microbiology* 37: 1041–1043.

Kemplar, G. M., and McKay, L. L. (1979b). Characterisation of plasmid deoxyribonucleic acid in *Streptococcus lactis* ssp. *diacetylactis*: evidence for plasmid-linked citrate utilization. *Applied and Environmental Microbiology* 37: 316–323.

Khunajarakr, N., Liu, C.-Q., Charoenchai, P., and Dunn, N. (1999). A plasmid-encoded two-component regulatory system involved in copper-inducible transcription in *Lactococcus lactis*. *Gene* 229: 229–235.

Kiewiet, R., Kok, J., Seegers, J. F. M., Venema, G., and Bron, S. (1993a). The mode of replication is a major factor in segregational plasmid instability in *Lactococcus lactis*. *Applied and Environmental Microbiology* 59: 358–364.

Kiewiet, R., Bron, S., De Jonge, K., Venema, G., and Seegers, J. F. M. L. (1993b). Theta replication of the lactococcal plasmid pWV02. *Molecular Microbiology* 10: 319–327.

Klaenhammer, T. R. (1993). Genetics of bacteriocins produced by lactic acid bacteria. *FEMS Microbiology Reviews* 12: 39–86.

Klaenhammer, T. R., and Fitzgerald, G. F. (1994). Bacteriophage and bacteriophage resistance. In: M. J. Gasson and W. M. de Vos (Eds.), *Genetics and biotechnology of lactic acid bacteria* (pp. 106–168). London: W. M. Blackie Academic & Professional.

Klein, J. R., Ulrich, C., Wegmann, U., Meyer-Barton, E., Plapp, R., and Henrich, B. (1996). Molecular tools for the genetic modification of dairy lactobacilli. *Systematic and Applied Microbiology* 18: 493–503.

Kok, J., Van der Vossen, J. M. B. M., and Venema, G. (1984). Construction of plasmid cloning vectors for lactic streptococci which also replicate in *Bacillus subtilis* and *Escherichia coli*. *Applied and Environmental Microbiology* 48: 726–731.

Kok, J. (1990). Genetics of the proteolytic system of lactic acid bacteria. *FEMS Microbiology Reviews* 87: 15–42.

Lambowitz, A. M., and Belfort, M. (1993). Introns as mobile genetic elements. *Annual Review of Biochemistry* 62: 587–622.

Langella, P., Le Loir, Y., Ehrlich, S. D., and Gruss, A. (1993). Efficient plasmid mobilisation by pIP501 in *Lactococcus lactis* subsp. *lactis*. *Journal of Bacteriology* 175: 5806–5813.

Le Bourgeois, P., Lautier, M., Mata, M., and Ritzenthaler, P. (1992). New tools for the physical and genetic mapping of *Lactococcus* strains. *Gene* 111: 109–114.

Leelawatcharamas, V., Chia, L. G., Charoenchai, P., Kunajar, N., Liu, C.-Q., and Dunn, N. (1997). Plasmid-encoded copper resistance in *Lactococcus lactis*. *Biotechnology Letters* 19: 639–643.

Leenhouts, K. J., Bolhuis, A., Kok, J., and Venema, G. (1994). The sucrose and raffinose operons of Pediococcus pentosaceus PPE1.0 Direct DNA sequence submission Accession number Z32771.

Leenhouts, K. J., Gietema, J., Kok, J., and Venema, G. (1991b). Chromosomal stabilisation of the proteinase genes in *Lactococcus lactis*. *Applied and Environmental Microbiology* 57: 2568–2575.

Leenhouts, K. J., Tolner, B., Bron, S., Kok, J., Venema, G., and Seegers, J. F. M. L. (1991a). Nucleotide sequence and characterisation of the broad-host-range lactococcal plasmid pWV01. *Plasmid* 26: 55–66.

Lessl, M., Pansegrau, W., and Lanka, E. (1992). Relationships of DNA-transfer-factors-systems: Essential transfer factors of plasmids RP4, Ti and F share common sequences. *Nucleic Acids Research* 20: 6099–6100.

Lin, C. F., and Chung, T. C. (1999). Cloning of erythromycin resistance determinants and replication origins from indigenous plasmids of *Lactobacillus reuteri* for potential use in construction of cloning vectors. *Plasmid* 42: 31–41.

Lin, C. F., Fung, Z. F., Wu, C. L., and Chung, T. C. (1996). Molecular characterisation of a plasmid-borne (pTC82) chloramphenicol resistance determinant (cat-TC) from *Lactobacillus reuteri* G4. *Plasmid* 36: 116–124.

Liu, C.-Q., Leelawatcharamas, V., Harvey, M. L., and Dunn, N. W. (1996). Cloning vectors for lactococci based on a plasmid encoding resistance to cadmium. *Current Microbiology* 33: 35–39.

Liu, C.-Q., Khunajakr, N., Chia, L. G., Deng, Y.-M., Charoenchai, P., and Dunn, N. W. (1997). Genetic analysis of regions involved in replication and cadmium resistance of the plasmid pND302 from *Lactococcus lactis*. *Plasmid* 38: 79–90.

Matsuura, M., Saldanha, R., Ma, H., Wank, H., Yang, J., Mohr, G., Cavanagh, S., Dunny, G. M., Belfort, M., and Lambowitz, A. M. (1997). A bacterial group II intron encoding reverse transcriptase, maturase and DNA endonuclease activities: Biochemical demonstration of maturase activity and insertion of new genetic information within the intron. *Genes Development* 11: 3333–3345.

Maugin, E., Duwat, P., Hege, T., Ehrlich, D., and Gruss, A. (1992). New thermosensitive plasmid for Gram-positive bacteria. *Journal of Bacteriology* 174: 5633–5638.

McKay, L. L. (1983). Functional properties of plasmids in lactic streptococci. *Antonie van Leeuwenhoek* 49: 259–274.

McKay, L. L., Baldwin, K. A., and Walsh, P. M. (1980). Conjugal transfer of genetic information in group N streptococci. *Applied and Environmental Microbiology* 40: 84–91.

McKay, L. L., and Baldwin, K. A. (1978). Stabilization of lactose metabolism in *Streptococcus lactis* C2. *Applied and Environmental Microbiology* 36: 360–367.

Mills, D. A., Choi, C. K., Dunny, G. M., and McKay, L. L. (1994). Genetic analysis of regions of the *Lactococcus lactis* subsp. *lactis* plasmid pRS01 involved in conjugative transfer. *Applied and Environmental Microbiology* 60: 4413–4420.

Mills, D. A., McKay, L. L., and Dunny, G. M. (1996). Splicing of a group II intron involved in the conjugative transfer of pRS01 in lactococci. *Journal of Bacteriology* 178: 3531–3538.

Mills, D. A., Manias, D. A., McKay, L. L., and Dunny, G. M. (1997). Homing of a Group II intron from *Lactococcus lactis* subsp. *lactis* ML3. *Journal of Bacteriology* 179: 6107–6111.

Mills, D. A., Phister, T. G., Dunny, G. M., and McKay, L. L. (1998). An origin of transfer (*oriT*) of the conjugative element pRS01 from *Lactococcus lactis* subsp. *lactis* ML3. *Applied and Environmental Microbiology* 64: 1541–1544.

Murphy, M. C., Steele, J. L., Daly, C. C., and McKay, L. L. (1988). Concomitant conjugal transfer of reduced-bacteriophage-sensitivity mechanisms with lactose- and sucrose-fermenting ability in lactic streptococci. *Applied and Environmental Microbiology* 54: 1951–1956.

Novel, M., Huang, D. C., and Novel, G. (1988). Transposition of the *Streptococcus lactis* ssp. *lactis* Z270 lactose plasmid to pVA797: demonstration of an insertion sequence and its relationship to an inverted repeat sequence isolated by self-annealing. *Biochimie* 70: 543.

Oki, M., Kakikawa, M., Taketo, A., and Kodaira, K. (1996). Genome structure of a *Lactobacillus* plasmid pNMO belonging to the rolling-circle type replicon. *Journal of General and Applied Microbiology* 42: 271–283.

O'Sullivan, D., Coffey, A., Fitzgerald, G. F., Hill, C., and Ross, R. P. (1998). Design of a phage-insensitive lactococcal dairy starter via sequential transfer of naturally occurring conjugative plasmids. *Applied and Environmental Microbiology* 64: 4618–4622.

Pillidge, C. J., Cambourn, W. M., and Pearce, L. E. (1996). Nucleotide sequence and analysis of pWC1, a pC194-type rolling circle replicon in *Lactococcus lactis*. *Plasmid* 35: 131–140.

Polzin, K. M., and McKay, L. L. (1991). Identification, DNA sequence and distribution of IS*981*, a new high-copy number insertion sequence in lactococci. *Applied and Environmental Microbiology* 57: 734.

Polzin, K. M., and McKay, L. L. (1992). Development of a lactococcal integration vector by using IS*981* and a temperature sensitive lactococcal replication region. *Applied and Environmental Microbiology* 58: 476–484.

Polzin, K. M., and Shimizu-Kadota, M. (1987). Identification of a new insertion element, similar to gram-negative IS*26*, on the lactose plasmid of *Streptococcus lactis*ML3. *Journal of Bacteriology* 169: 5481–5488.

Pouwels, P. H., and Leer, R. J. (1993). Genetics of lactobacilli: Plasmids and gene expression. *Antonie van Leeuwenhoek* 64: 85–107.

Rauch, P. J. G., Beerhuyzen, M. M., and de Vos, W. M. (1990). Nucleotide sequence of IS*904* from *Lactococcus lactis* subsp. *lactis*NILO R5. *Nucleic Acids Research* 18: 4253.

Rauch, P. J. G., and de Vos, W. M. (1992). Characterisation of the novel nisin-sucrose conjugative transposon Tn*5276* and its insertion in *Lactococcus lactis*. *Journal of Bacteriology* 174: 1280–1287.

Rauch, P. J. G., and de Vos, W. M. (1994). Identification and characterisation of genes involved in excision of the *Lactococcus lactis* conjugative transposon Tn*5276*. *Journal of Bacteriology* 176: 2165–2171.

Renault, P. P., and Heslot, H. (1987). Selection of *Streptococcus lactis* mutants defective in malolactic fermentation. *Applied and Environmental Microbiology* 53: 320–324.

Romero, D. A., and Klaenhammer, T. R. (1990). Characterization of insertion sequence IS*946*, an iso-ISS*1* element, isolated from the conjugative lactococcal plasmid pTR2030. *Journal of Bacteriology* 172: 4151.

Romero, A., and Klaenhammer, T. R. (1992). IS946-mediated integration of heterologous DNA into the genome of *Lactococcus lactis* subsp. *lactis*. *Applied and Environmental Microbiology* 58: 699–702.

Romero, A., Slos, P., Castellina, R. L., and Mercenier, A. (1987). Conjugative mobilization as an alternative vector delivery system for lactic streptococci. *Applied and Environmental Microbiology* 53: 2405–2413.

Sano, K., Otani, M., Okada, Y., Kawamura, R., Umesaki, M., Ohi, Y., Umezawa, C., and Kanatani, K. (1997). Identification of the replication region of the *Lactobacillus acidophilus* plasmid pLA106. *FEMS Microbiology Letters* 148: 223–226.

Scherwitz, K. M., Baldwin, K. A., and McKay, L. L. (1983). Plasmid linkage of a bacteriocin-like substance in *Streptococcus lactis* subsp. *diacetylactis* strain WM4: Transferability to *Streptococcus lactis*. *Applied and Environmental Microbiology* 45: 1506–1512.

Seegers, J. F. M. L., Bron, S., Franke, C. M., Venema, G., and Kiewiet, R. (1994). The majority of lactococcal plasmids carry a highly related replicon. *Microbiology* 140: 1291–1300.

Seegers, J. F. M. L., Zhao, A. C., Meijer, W. J. J., Khan, S. A., Venema, G., and Bron, S. (1995). Structural and functional analysis of the single-strand origin of replication from the lactococcal plasmid pWV01. *Molecular and General Genetics* 249: 43–50.

Seegers, J. F., Van Sinderen, D., and Fitzgerald, G. F. (2000). Molecular characterization of the lactococcal plasmid pCIS3: Natural stacking of specificity subunits of a type I restriction/modification system in a single lactococcal strain. *Microbiology* 146: 435–443.

Shearman, C. A., Godon, J.-J., and Gasson, M. J. (1996). Splicing of a group II intron in a functional transfer gene of *Lactococcus lactis*. *Molecular Microbiology* 21: 45–53.

Shimizu-Kadota, M., Kiraki, M., Hirokawa, H., and Tsuchida, N. (1985). ISL*1*: a new transposable element in *Lactobacillys casei*. *Molecular and General Genetics* 200: 193.

Snook, R. J., and McKay, L. L. (1981). Conjugal transfer of lactose fermenting ability among *Streptococcus cremoris* and *Streptococcus lactis* strains. *Applied and Environmental Microbiology* 42: 904–911.

Solaiman, D. K. Y., and Somkuti, G. A. (1998). Characterisation of a novel *Streptococcus thermophilus* rolling circle plasmid used for vector construction. *Applied Microbiology and Biotechnology* 50: 174–180.

del Solar, G., Giraldo, R., Ruiz-Echevarria, M. J., Espinosa, M., and Diaz-Orejas, R. (1998). Replication and control of circular bacterial plasmids. *Microbiology and Molecular Biology Reviews* 62: 434–464.

del Solar, G., Moscoso, M., and Espinosa, M. (1993) Rolling circle-replicating plasmids from Gram-positive and Gram-negative bacteria: a wall falls. *Molecular Microbiology* 8: 789–796.

Somkuti, G. A., Solaiman, D. K. Y., and Steinberg, D. H. (1998). Structural and functional properties of the hsp16. 4-bearing plasmid pER341 in *Streptococcus thermophilus*. *Plasmid* 40: 61–72.

Tailliez, P., Ehrlich, S. D., and Chopin, M. C. (1994). Characterization of IS*1201*, an insertion sequence isolated from *Lactobacillus helveticus*. *Gene* 145: 75–79.

Teuber, M., Meile, L., and Schwarz, F. (1999). Acquired antibiotic resistance in lactic acid bacteria from food. *Antonie van Leeuwenhoek* 76: 115–137.

Thompson, J. K., Foley, S., McConville, K. J., Nicholson, C., Collins, M. A., and Pridmore, R. D. (1999). Complete sequence of plasmid pLH1 from *Lactobacillus helveticus* ATCC15009: analysis reveals the presence of regions homologous to other native plasmids from the host strain. *Plasmid* 42: 221–235.

Trieu-Cout, P., Carlier, C., Martin, P., and Courvalin, P. (1987). Plasmid transfer by conjugation from *Escherichia coli* to Gram-positive bacteria. *FEMS Microbiology Letters* 48: 289–294.

Van Kranenburg, R., Marugg, J., Van Swam, I. I., Willem, N. J., and de Vos, W. M. (1997). Molecular characterization of plasmid-encoded *eps* gene cluster essential for exopolysaccharide biosynthesis in *Lactococcus lactis*. *Molecular Microbiology* 24: 387–397.

Van Kranenburg, R., and de Vos, W. M. (1998). Characterisation of multiple regions involved in replication and mobilization of plasmid pNZ4000 in *Lactococcus lactis*. *Journal of Bacteriology* 180: 5285–5290.

Vaughan, E. E., and de Vos, W. M. (1995). Identification and characterization of the insertion element IS*1070* from *Leuconostoc lactis* NZ6009. *Gene* 155: 95–100.

Vedamuthu, E. R., and Neville, J. M. (1986). Involvement of a plasmid in production of ropiness (mucoidness) in milk cultures by *Streptococcus cremoris* MS. *Applied and Environmental Microbiology* 51: 677–682.

Von Wright, A., and Tynkkynen, S. (1987). Construction of *Streptococcus lactis* ssp. *lactis* strains with a single plasmid associated with mucoid phenotype. *Applied and Environmental Microbiology* 53: 1385–1386.

de Vos, W. (1987). Gene cloning and expression in lactic streptococci. *FEMS Microbiology Reviews* 46: 281–295.

Walker, D. C., and Klaenhammer, T. R. (1994). Isolation of a novel IS3 group insertion element and construction of an integration vector for *Lactobacillus* spp. *Journal of Bacteriology* 176: 5330.

Walsh, P. M., and McKay, L. L. (1981). Recombinant plasmid associated with cell aggregation and high-frequency conjugation in *Streptococcus lactis*. *Journal of Bacteriology* 146: 937–944.

Wang, T. T., and Lee, B. H. (1997). Plasmids in *Lactobacillus*. *Critical Reviews in Biotechnology* 43: 143–148.

Ward, L. J. H., Brown, J. C. S., and Davey, G. P. (1996). Identification and sequence analysis of IS*1297*, an ISS1-like sequence in a *Leuconostoc* strain. *Gene* 174: 259–263.

Xu, F., Pearce, L. E., and Yu, P.-L. (1991). Construction of a family of lactococcal vectors for gene cloning and translational fusion. *FEMS Microbiology Letters* 77: 55–60.

Yu, W., Mierau, I., Mars, A., Johnson, E., Dunny, G. and McKay, L. L. (1995). Novel Insertion Sequence-like Element IS*982* in Lactococci. *Plasmid* 33: 218–225.

Zuniga, M., Pardo, I., and Ferrer, S. (1996). Nucleotide sequence of plasmid p4028, a cryptic plasmid from *Leuconostoc oenos*. *Plasmid* 36: 67–74.

3

Comparative Genomics of Bacteriophage Infecting Lactic Acid Bacteria

Elizabeth Stanley, Stephen Mc Grath,
Gerald F. Fitzgerald, and Douwe van Sinderen

Introduction

Lactic acid bacteria (LAB) are Gram-positive, acid tolerant rods, or cocci, which produce lactic acid as the major end product of fermentation (Axelsson, 1993). This group comprises the genera *Lactococcus, Lactobacillus, Leuconostoc, Streptococcus, Pediococcus*, and *Carnobacterium*, many of which play important roles in the food fermentation industry (McKay and Baldwin, 1990). LAB are used as starter cultures for the production of a wide range of fermented dairy foods (i.e., cheeses, yogurts, and fermented milks) as well as a diversity of other products such as fermented meats, sour dough bread, and silage (Mercenier et al., 1994). In addition to their capacity to rapidly acidify the fermentable food product, thereby inhibiting growth of pathogens and spoilage microorganisms, their metabolic activities are also responsible for the development of a range of flavor and texture characteristics of the food.

Bacteriophage (phage) are obligate intracellular, bacterial parasites that are found ubiquitously in nature. Phages infecting LAB are of considerable economic importance because they represent one of the main causes of fermentation failure. The dairy industry has implemented a number of technological strategies to alleviate the problem of phage infection including air filtration, separation of bulk starter tanks from the production area, direct vat inoculation, the use of closed vats, rotation of starter strains, and the application of phage-resistant starter cultures (Neve, 1996). However, these measures have not

Elizabeth Stanley, Stephen Mc Grath, and Gerald F. Fitzgerald • National Food Biotechnology, University College, Cork, Ireland **Gerald F. Fitzgerald and Douwe van Sinderen** • Department of Microbiology, University College, Cork, Ireland **Gerald F. Fitzgerald** • Food Science and Technology, University College, Cork, Ireland; e-mail: g.fitzgerald@ucc.ie

eliminated phage as a serious problem in industrial practice. As an alternative strategy a significant amount of research has been aimed at understanding phage–host interactions as well as phage biology in the expectation that a fundamental understanding of the LAB phages may assist in providing an efficient and long-term solution to phage infection. Due to these investigations, a significant body of knowledge is now available on the primary genome structure and organization of many phages infecting LAB thus giving an insight into their evolutionary history while at the same time providing the information for the development of "intelligent" phage resistance strategies. This review will summarize the accumulated information available on LAB phage biology and genomics.

General Properties of LAB Bacteriophage

Phage were first identified by Twort (1915) and two years later by d'Hérelle (1917) who coined the name "bacteriophage." The first report of bacteriophage infecting lactococcal starter cultures was made by Whitehead and Cox (1935), who identified these agents as a major threat to dairy fermentations. Primary classification of bacteriophage is based on morphology (Bradley, 1967). Bacteriophages with contractile tails are classified as morphotype A; those with long non-contractile tails as morphotype B; and those exhibiting short non-contractile tails as morphotype C. In addition, morphotypes 1–3 describe differences in the phage heads morphology (small isometric headed, prolate, and large prolate headed phage representing morphotypes 1, 2, and 3, respectively). Ackerman and DuBow (1987) subsequently differentiated bacteriophages into a number of families and reclassified and renamed Bradleys groups A–C as *Myoviridae, Siphoviridae*, and *Podoviridae*, respectively.

All LAB bacteriophages studied to date are composed of a proteinaceous head and tail, and contain a single molecule of double stranded DNA that has a % G + C content similar to that of its host. Consequently, G + C values may range from 37% in the case of lactococcal bacteriophages to 48% for phages infecting *Lactobacillus* (Klaenhammer and Fitzgerald, 1994). Genome sizes are usually within the range of 18–55 kb (Jarvis et al., 1991) but they have also been reported to be much longer (Prévots et al., 1990; Moineau et al., 1992). The genomes of LAB bacteriophages appear to be quite compact with few non-coding DNA regions (e.g., Schouler et al., 1994; Lubbers et al., 1995; Van Sinderen et al., 1996; Kodaia et al., 1997; Stanley et al., 1997).

Overview of the Life Cycle of Bacteriophage

Bacteriophages can be divided into two groups based on their life cycles. "Virulent" or "lytic" phages are only capable of one method of propagation. Briefly, at the beginning of the infection a lytic phage adsorb to a specific receptor site on the LAB host cell, using the distal end of their tails. Electron microscopic studies of lactococcal phages have shown that they can bind either uniformly over the cell or in small groups (5–30 phages) at evenly distributed spots (Budde-Niekiel and Teuber, 1987). The linear phage genomic DNA is then injected into the cytoplasm of the cell. Following DNA injection, phage replication takes place and subsequent assembly of mature phage progeny, the latter event being coupled to DNA packaging. The final stage of the lytic life cycle involves the release of the progeny phage from the infected cells in a process that involves the activity of two different types of phage-encoded proteins. The first has a lytic activity, which is involved in the degradation of the cell wall, while the second is a facilitative protein, which disrupts

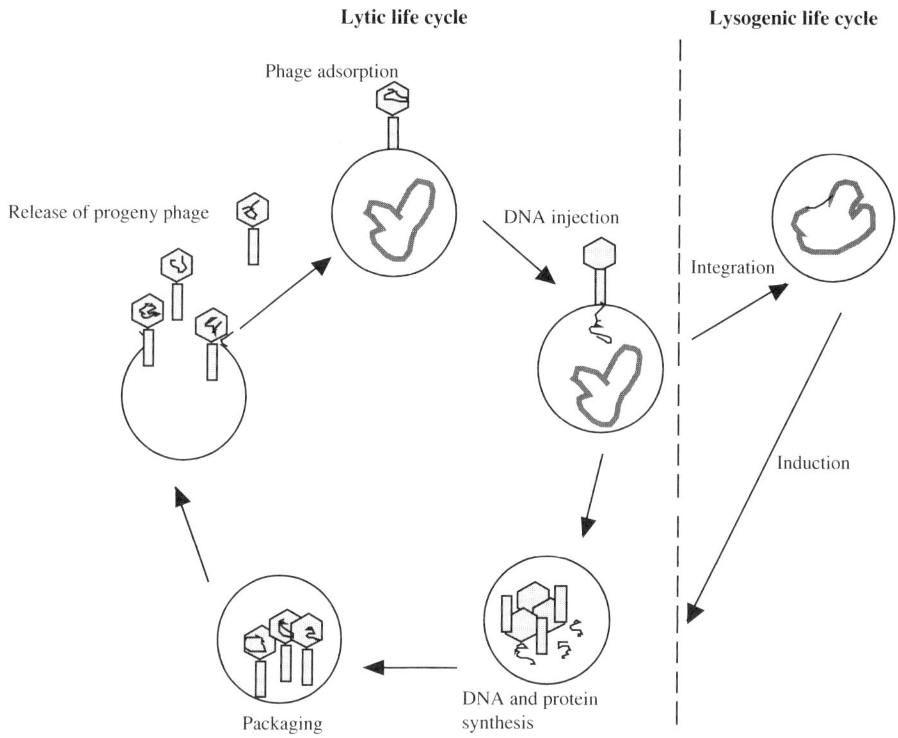

Figure 3.1. The life cycle of a lytic and a lysogenic bacteriophage (adapted from Nauta [1997]). See text for details.

the cell membrane thereby allowing the lytic enzyme to gain access to the wall (see below for more detail). The progeny phage are then released into the environment where the lytic cycle can be repeated (Figure 3.1). For a comprehensive review see Young (1992).

The "lysogenic" or "temperate" bacteriophages are more versatile because in addition to the lytic pathway, they can enter into a life cycle, which does not result in the death of the host. This alternative course is known as the lysogenic life cycle and involves the integration of the phage DNA into the chromosome of the host where it is then referred to as a prophage. The integration event involves site specific recombination between short homologous DNA sequences or attachment sites on the host (the *attB* site) and phage genomes (the *attP* site). Once integrated into the bacterial genome, the prophage can remain in this state indefinitely, a situation which is mediated by a phage-encoded repressor protein. Alternatively, prophage induction (i.e., relief of repression) may take place resulting in excision of the prophage and initiation of the lytic cycle (Figure 3.1). Lysogeny is discussed in more detail below.

Classification of Bacteriophages Infecting Lactic Acid Bacteria

Much of the research on LAB bacteriophages has been directed towards the development of a coherent classification scheme, which ideally should reflect relationships between phages in terms of their evolutionary origin. Early classification schemes relied on morphological and serological properties as well as phage–host interactions and protein content. In recent years, classification schemes could apply additional parameters, which include genetic comparisons of phage through DNA homology studies and sequence analysis. These classification methods are discussed below.

Morphology

Due to the relative ease with which it can be determined, the initial step in bacteriophage classification usually involves characterizing morphological properties. All *S. thermophilus* bacteriophages analyzed to date (Deane et al., 1953; Accolas and Spillman, 1979; Reinbold et al., 1982; Krush et al., 1987; Larbi et al., 1990; Carminati and Giraffa, 1992; Fayard et al., 1993; Brüssow et al., 1994a; Le Marrec et al., 1997; Stanley et al., 1997) belong to the *Siphoviridae* family corresponding to group B1 as defined by Bradley (1967). The main characteristics of these phages are a small isometric head (50–90 nm in diameter) and a relatively long striated non-contractile tail (100–360 nm).

Although some *Podoviridae* lactococcal phages have been reported, most bacteriophages infecting *Lactococcus* species belong to the *Siphoviridae* family and exhibit either small isometric heads (i.e., morphotype B1 as defined by Ackermann and DuBow [1987]) or prolate heads (morphotype B2), with phages of morphotype B1 being the more common (Klaenhammer and Fitzgerald, 1994).

Bacteriophages infecting *Lactobacillus* are generally members of the *Siphoviridae* family displaying small isometric heads although some prolate headed *Lactobacillus* bacteriophages have been reported (Tohyama et al., 1972; Séchaud et al., 1988; Forsman, 1993). Bacteriophages infecting *Lb. helveticus* were found to possess isometric heads with contractile tails of variable length, a feature that was taken as a basis for classification (Séchaud et al., 1992).

Bacteria belonging to the *Leuconostoc* genus are heterofermentative coccoid LAB and are often used as a minor component of mixed strain cultures in the food industry (Davidson et al., 1996). *Leuconostoc oenus*, reclassified as *Oenococcus oeni* (Dicks et al., 1995), is used in the malolactic fermentation of wine. Few *Leuconostoc* phages have been reported but this may be due to difficulties in phage detection because of the slow growth characteristics of this bacterial species. The *Leuconostoc* phages that have been described display long non-contractile tails and isometric heads, which places them in the *Siphoviridae* family, subgroup B1 (Arendt et al., 1991; Arendt and Hammes, 1992; Boizet et al., 1992; Poblet-Icart et al., 1998).

Host Range

Classification of bacteriophages of LAB based on host range has been described in numerous studies and is particularly relevant to the users of LAB cultures in food (especially dairy) fermentation processes. However, groupings based on host range analyses rarely converge with schemes based on other classification criteria. For example, Mata and Ritzenthaler (1988) reported that a certain group of *S. thermophilus* bacteriophage exhibited very similar host ranges despite limited DNA homology. Conversely, other phage displaying very similar restriction profiles exhibited a completely different lytic spectrum. Similar observations were made for bacteriophages infecting *L. lactis* by Relano et al. (1987). Host range appears, therefore, to be of poor taxonomic value when classifying LAB bacteriophages.

Serology

Several attempts have been made to classify *S. thermophilus* and lactococcal bacteriophages on the basis of their serological properties (Kivi et al., 1987; Mata and Ritzenthaler, 1988; Jarvis, 1989; Brüssow et al., 1994a). However, a serious drawback of this method is that it is based on differences in antigenic properties exposed at the external structure of the virion and is, therefore, indicative of the expression of only a small part of the genome.

Structural Protein Profiles

Protein profile analysis has been commonly employed to classify *S. thermophilus* bacteriophages and as a classification method it correlates well with other schemes. However, it must be remembered that proteins with identical molecular weights are not necessarily closely related and classification by this method should be supported by genetic information. To date, three different types of protein profiles have been described for *S. thermophilus* phages. Kivi et al. (1987) described phages in which four major proteins with molecular masses of approximately 63, 49, 42, and 11 kDa were identified. All other reports describe phages with either two major structural proteins with molecular masses of approximately 31 and 27 kDa or three major structural proteins with molecular masses of approximately 40, 24, and 15 kDa (Neve et al., 1989; Prévots et al., 1989; Benbadis et al., 1990; Fayard et al., 1993; Le Marrec et al., 1997; Stanley et al., 1997). The availability of sequence data has resulted in the identification of the genes encoding each of the major structural proteins from øO1205 (Stanley et al., 1997) and the two major structural proteins from ø7201 (Le Marrec et al., 1997; Proux et al., 2002). Le Marrec et al. (1997) demonstrated that the genomes of *S. thermophilus* bacteriophages, which contain three major structural proteins, displayed homology to the genes encoding the three major structural protein from øO1205. Similarly, the genes encoding the two major structural proteins of ø7201 exhibited DNA homology to genomic DNA of all tested *S. thermophilus* bacteriophages, which also displayed a protein profile of two major structural proteins (Le Marrec et al., 1997; Proux et al., 2002). Interestingly, Le Marrec et al. (1997) noted that the bacteriophages containing three major structural proteins packaged their DNA using a *pac* site while the packaging mechanism of the phages with two major structural proteins employed a *cos* site. Therefore, a correlation appears to exist between the possession of a particular set of structural proteins and the method of packaging employed by *S. thermophilus* phages.

The structural composition of lactococcal bacteriophages has also been analyzed. Generally, one to three major structural proteins are detected, in addition to a number of minor structural proteins (e.g., Kim and Batt, 1991b; Arendt et al., 1994; Lubbers et al., 1995; Johnsen et al., 1996; Van Sinderen et al., 1996). Phages of different morphotypes tend to have different protein profiles (Neve, 1996).

Similar to what is observed in *S. thermophilus* phages, Forsman and Alatossava (1991) reported that three of four *Lb. delbrueckii* subsp. *lactis* bacteriophages examined packaged their DNA utilizing a *pac* site and were found to contain major structural proteins of 34 and 19 kDa in addition to a number of minor proteins. Conversely, the fourth phage utilized a *cos* site and possessed two major structural proteins of 30 kDa and 28 kDa in addition to a number of minor proteins. Antisera from one of the *pac* phages cross reacted with almost all of the structural proteins from the other two *pac* phages indicating that their proteins are quite similar. In contrast, only three structural proteins from the *cos* phage (including the larger of its major structural proteins) reacted with the antiserum.

Oe. oeni phages have also been classified on the basis of their structural composition. Arendt and Hammes (1992) noted that ten *Oe. oeni* bacteriophages isolated from wine could be divided into three groups based on this criterion. Group 1 phages contained two major structural proteins of 35.5 and 28.5 kDa, group 2 contained three major structural proteins of 37, 34.5, and 27 kDa, while group 3 phages contained structural proteins of 41.5, 39.5, and 15 kDa. Boizet et al. (1992) examined eight *Oe. oeni* phages (none of which was common to the study of Arendt and Hammes [1992]) seven of which contained a *cos* site and shared common proteins of 26 and 34 kDa. All of these phages belonged to the same homology group. Interestingly, the *pac* phage (which contained a major protein of 45 kDa) did not hybridize to any of the *cos* phages.

DNA Homology

Classification of LAB phages based on DNA homology has the advantage of evaluating the entire phage genome as opposed to a specific portion, which may encode, for example, the structural genes. *S. thermophilus* phage genomes have been analyzed by Southern hybridization and dot blot assays (Neve et al., 1989; Prévots et al., 1989; Benbadis et al., 1990; Fayard et al., 1993; Brüssow et al., 1994a,b; Le Marrec et al., 1997) and results indicate that these phages belong to a single homology group. The degree of homology between the phage does vary however and, as a consequence, the identification of two (Prévot et al., 1989; Benbadis et al., 1990), three (Neve et al., 1989), or four (Fayard et al., 1993) subgroups has been made.

Lactococcal bacteriophages are now routinely classified according to DNA relatedness as determined by hybridization analysis in combination with their morphological characteristics. On the basis of these data Jarvis et al. (1991) have defined 12 genetically distinct phage species (Table 3.1). The majority of lactococcal phage encountered in the dairy industry were found to be members of the (a) lytic, small isometric headed 936 species, (b) the small isometric-headed P335 species, which include both lytic and lysogenic phage, or (c) the lytic, prolate headed c2 species. In Australia, New Zealand, the

Table 3.1 Lactococcal Phage Species, Type Phage and Members (Adapted from Jarvis et al., 1991)[a]

Family	Morphotype Species	Phage Type	Phage	Members
Siphoviridae	B1	936	P008	P008, F4-1, sk1, bIL41, bil170, bIL66, øUS3
	B1	P335	P335	øLC3, r1t, Tuc2009, TP901-1, ø31, ø50
	B1	P107	P107	
	B1	1483	1483	
	B1	P087	P087	
	B1	1358	1358	
	B1	BK5-T	BK5-T	BK5-T
	B1	949	949	
	B2	c2	c6A	c2, bIL67, øvML3, ø197, P001
Podoviridae	C2	P034	P034	
	C3	KSY1	KSY1	

[a]For clarity, only those members mentioned in the text are included. The phage species Rzh was omitted as this phage is no longer available.

United States, and Europe the majority of phage tend to be small isometric headed phage (Daly et al., 1996), while members of the c2 phage type appear to be the most common phage isolated in Canada (Moineau et al., 1992).

Bacteriophages of *Lb. delbrueckii* have also been classified on the basis of DNA homology. Four different homology groups have been defined (Mata et al., 1986; Lahbib-Mansais et al., 1988; Séchaud et al., 1988; Forsman and Alatossava, 1991; Forsman, 1993) with most of the phages belonging to one specific group designated "a." This group contains both lytic and lysogenic phage and two of the most thoroughly studied *Lb. delbrueckii* phages, mv4 (lysogenic) and LL-H (lytic), belong to this homology group (Mata et al., 1986).

Lahbib-Mansias et al. (1988) studied five phages of *Lb. helveticus* and found that they all appeared to belong to a single DNA homology group, which was distinct from the groups of *Lb. delbrueckii* phages.

Arendt et al. (1991) isolated five lysogenic *Oe. oeni* bacteriophages and showed that they all belong to the same homology group. However, Boizet et al. (1992) detected two homology groups among the eight *Oe. oeni* phages they studied.

The relative ease with which specific genomic regions and even entire bacteriophage genomes may nowadays be sequenced is giving researchers cause to re-evaluate the taxonomic relationships between bacteriophages. Brüssow and coworkers have performed several interesting comparative analyses of LAB bacteriophage genomes (Lucchini et al., 1998; Desiere et al., 1999; Lucchini et al., 1999a,b; Foley et al., 2000; Brüssow and Desiere, 2001; Brüssow and Hendrix, 2002). Using analysis based not only on DNA sequence similarity, but also on genome organization, it was proposed that two new genera of *Siphoviridae* corresponding to Sfi21-like and Sfi11-like phage be recognized (Brüssow and Desiere, 2001). Labrie and Moineau (2002) have performed a comparative analysis of a number of phages infecting *L. lactis*. In this study they compared the entire genome sequence of øBK5-T, a phage that has been designated to represent a distinct species, to the genome sequences of six P335-type phages. They found that, in certain cases, BK5-T displayed greater levels of DNA sequence identity with members of P335 phage group than was noted between certain members within the same group. This finding led them to propose that BK5-T be included in the P335 species, thereby reducing the number of LAB phage species from 12 to 11. Further comparisons and bioinformatic analyses of phage genome sequences will undoubtedly shed new light on the heredity of phages, which in turn will lead to reliable taxonomic assessment of phage species.

General Phage Biology

Genetic Switch

Substantial knowledge on the molecular biology of bacteriophages infecting LAB has been generated directly through experimental approaches, and via comparative analysis of sequences available on a large number of LAB bacteriophages. The next section will introduce general phage biology, sections of which are based primarily on *Escherichia coli* bacteriophage systems.

The "lysogenic-lytic decision" or genetic switch is well understood in the *E. coli* phage lambda (for a review see Ptashne, 1986). More recently, several regulatory regions involved in lysogeny of LAB bacteriophages have been described and investigated in considerable detail (e.g., Boyce et al., 1995a; Nauta et al., 1996; Ladero et al., 1998; García et al., 1999; Ladero et al., 1999; Madsen et al., 1999; Blatny et al., 2001).

These data have uncovered interesting analogies between lambda and lysogenic LAB phages with respect to the mechanism by which the genetic switch operates. Therefore, the genetic switch of lambda is briefly reviewed here.

Upon lambda infection of an *E. coli* cell, divergent transcription of the early genes *N* and *cro* is initiated from the two main promoters P_L and P_R (Figure 3.2). The N protein is an anti-terminator protein, which allows RNA polymerase to continue transcription through regions that would otherwise cause transcriptional termination. Consequently, genes encoding three regulators *cII, cIII*, and *Q*, in addition to genes, which allow DNA replication and site-specific recombination will be transcribed. *cIII* protects *cII* against degradation by host encoded proteins, and a high concentration of *cII* is essential for ensuring synthesis of the repressor, *cI*, from the promoter P_{RE} (*P*romoter for *r*epressor *e*stablishment) as well as the integrase protein from P_I. *cI* binds to two operators, O_L and O_R, and when bound to these operators transcription from P_L and P_R is blocked. As a result all phage genes except for *cI* are switched off and lysogeny is established. *cI* is essential for maintenance of the lysogenic life cycle and once lysogeny is established transcription of *cI* switches from P_{RE} to P_{RM} (*P*romoter for *r*epressor *m*aintenance).

Cro is a regulatory protein required for the development of the lytic life cycle. It binds to the two operators, O_L and O_R, thereby preventing the synthesis of the repressor *cI*. The anti-terminator protein Q then makes the expression of the late genes from $P_{R'}$ possible.

Therefore, both *cI* and Cro can bind to O_L and O_R, but with different affinities causing opposing effects on the activity of the relevant promoters. The operators regulate the activity from the two promoters P_L and P_R, and consist of imperfect symmetrical binding sites. The differences in the sequence of the operators form the basis for the affinity differences between *cI* and Cro binding to these sites. The choice between lysogenisation and lytic infection is determined by the relative concentrations of Cro and *cI*, which, in turn, is dependent on a number of environmental factors. For example, lysogenisation tends to occur in starving cells, while the lytic cycle is predominant in cells growing in a rich medium. The prophage can be induced to enter into the lytic life cycle by the activity of DNA damaging agents such as mitomycin C or UV irradiation, which induces the SOS response of the host cell. If the SOS response is sufficiently strong phage repressor is rapidly inactivated by RecA-induced autocleavage and as a consequence expression of the *cro* gene is switched on. This results in the simultaneous expression of the *int* and *xis* genes encoding the integrase and excisionase proteins, respectively, both of which are required for excision of the prophage from the host chromosome (Ptashne, 1986).

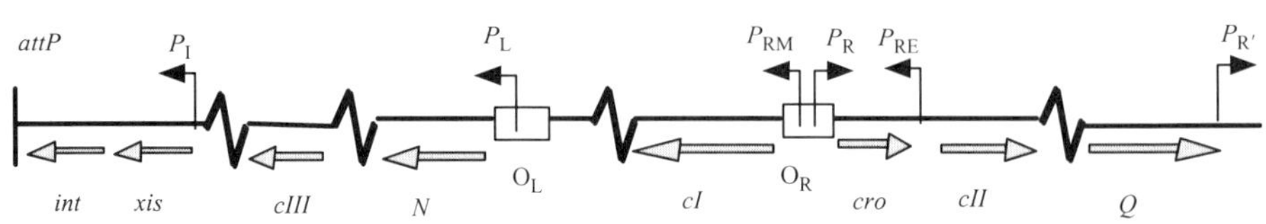

Figure 3.2. Gene organization of the regulatory region of lambda. O_L and O_R, leftward and rightward operators; P_L and P_R, leftward and rightward promoters; P_{RM}, promoter for repressor maintenance; P_{RE}, promoter for repressor establishment; $P_{R'}$, late promoter; P_I, promoter responsible for *int* transcription. Filled arrows show the direction and relative position of genes, with their name given beneath them.

Site-Specific Integration

Many phages use site-specific recombination between a phage attachment site (usually called *attP*) and a bacterial attachment site (usually referred to as *attB*) to allow integration of the phage genome into the bacterial chromosome in accordance with the model describing the integration of lambda (Gottesman and Weisberg, 1971). This results in the production of two hybrid sites, *attL* and *attR*, which flank the integrated phage chromosome. The integrative recombination is catalysed by a site-specific recombinase, which is specified by a gene located directly adjacent to the attachment site sequence. Genes encoding tRNAs are frequently used as sites for bacteriophage insertion (although a notable exception is lambda (e.g., Reiter et al., 1989; Hauser and Scocca, 1990; Campbell, 1992; Stanley et al., 1997). It has been proposed that tRNA-encoding genes are favored because the presence of a portion of a tRNA gene may increase the potential for the formation of stem-loop structures in the integrase mRNA thereby stabilizing the message, or alternatively, the structures may play a role in transcription (McShan et al., 1997). Furthermore, tRNAs are very conserved sequences and consequently are unlikely to undergo sequence changes, which would result in the host becoming resistant to lysogeny. The *Lb. delbrueckii* subsp. *bulgaricus* phage mv4 integrates into a $tRNA^{Ser}$ gene, and Auvary et al. (1997) applied this knowledge to construct an integration vector, which was able to integrate into the chromosome of a wide range of bacterial hosts based on the integrative elements of mv4. The region within which the attachment site is located is often AT rich (Landy and Ross, 1977; Raya et al., 1992; Lillehaug and Birkeland, 1993; Christiansen et al., 1994). Because regions of high AT-content tend to be more susceptible to strand opening this may facilitate the integration of phage DNA into the host chromosome (Weisberg and Landy, 1983).

Replication

Although a significant amount of sequence data is available for LAB bacteriophages, no model has yet been described for a general mechanism of LAB phage replication. However, due to the apparent similarities between some LAB phage-encoded proteins with replication proteins from *E. coli* and lambdoid phages a brief overview of replication of *E. coli* and lambda will be outlined below.

Replication of *E. coli* chromosomal DNA is initiated when 20–30 copies of the DnaA protein bind to the origin of replication (*ori*), thus causing opening of the double stranded DNA helix in an ATP-dependent reaction. The parental duplex must then be unwound and Okazaki fragments synthesised (for reviews see Kornberg and Baker, 1992; Marians, 1992). A complex of two enzymes (known as a primosome), composed of the helicase (DnaB), which is responsible for unwinding the DNA, and the primase (DnaG), which delivers short RNA primers to the lagging DNA strand, complete the replication initiation reaction. DnaC is responsible for guiding the helicase to the origin of replication, while single stranded binding proteins (SSB) function to maintain the single stranded state of the opened double stranded DNA template.

Replication of lambda requires two phage-encoded proteins, gpO and gpP. These initiate bi-directional replication from an origin located within *O*. gpO is an analogue of the *E. coli* DnaA protein whose function is to bind to the repeated regions of *ori* and as a consequence, destabilize the AT-rich sequence to allow replication initiation. The N-terminal end of gpO binds to *ori* while the C-terminal end binds gpP (Furth and Wickner, 1983) which in turn establishes an interaction with the host-encoded DnaB helicase (Zylicz et al., 1987). Initially replication proceeds via the theta-mode, but at some point will switch to rolling circle replication to generate concatemeric, double stranded DNA (Campbell, 1994).

Packaging of Phage DNA

Phage DNA replication results in the accumulation of DNA concatemers which must be cut and packaged into the (pro)-capsid before mature progeny phage can be released. In LAB bacteriophages, cutting and subsequent packaging may occur through one of two mechanisms, although it has been suggested that some phage use a combination of both methods (Van Sinderen et al., 1996). In phage using the headful mechanism of DNA packaging, the concatemeric DNA is cut initially at a specific sequence known as a *pac* site. Each subsequent cut occurs when the prohead has reached its maximum filling capacity of DNA, which is more than one unit length of the genome, resulting in circularly permuted molecules with terminal redundancy. Alternatively, the concatemeric DNA may be cut at a specific sequence known as a *cos* site resulting in self-complementary single stranded termini (cohesive ends). Bacteriophages of Gram-positive bacteria that utilize a *cos* site tend to produce 3′ overhangs (Perrin et al., 1997). Results of *in vitro* experiments have indicated that a combination of proteins, namely the terminase complex, the portal protein, and the expanded major protein are essential for DNA translocation in double-stranded DNA phage (Roa and Black, 1985; Guo et al., 1986; Hamada et al., 1986). Black (1989) has provided a comprehensive overview of DNA packaging in double stranded DNA phages, briefly; packaging of the phage genomic DNA is initiated when the terminase binds to a specific *pac* or *cos* site. The terminase is composed of two subunits—the small subunit, which binds and hydrolyzes ATP, is assumed to bind to the phage DNA, while the large subunit appears to attach to the prohead and may be involved in cutting the concatemeric phage molecules (Black, 1989). The portal protein is a structural component of the phage and is responsible for forming the entrance to the phage head (Dube et al., 1993). In addition, it is involved in conjunction with the terminase in initiating DNA packaging, in DNA translocation, and in determining the amount of DNA to be packaged in phage utilizing the headful cutting mechanism (Black, 1989). The expanded major capsid protein assists in translocating the DNA by the hydrolysis of ATP.

Analysis of the nucleotide sequences surrounding *cos* regions of numerous phages has revealed the presence of several structural features thought to be essential for binding of the phage terminases (Lillehaug et al., 1991; Chandry et al., 1994; Nakashima et al., 1994; García et al., 1997). High % G + C contents of *cos* regions have been reported (Lillehaug et al., 1991; García et al., 1997; Perrin et al., 1997) and these may reflect the necessity for stable base pairing of the *cos* region once the phage genome has entered the cell (García et al., 1997). For a more in depth discussion of packaging of double stranded phage DNA, the comprehensive review by Black (1989) should be examined.

Protein Composition

In lambda, once replication of the phage genome is initiated, synthesis of the bacteriophage structural proteins begins to form proheads and loose tails. The concatemeric DNA is cut at the *cos* site by the terminase complex and pumped into the prohead. The DNA is then cut at the next *cos* site and once the prohead is filled, it expands and other phage structural proteins are added to form a mature head to which the tails are finally attached. The genes encoding head proteins are clustered together and are located in a specific region of the genome, followed by the genes encoding tail proteins. Furthermore, the last gene of the head cluster encodes a product, which is located at the head–tail junction and this protein interacts with the protein encoded by the first gene of the tail cluster (Campbell, 1994). Recent sequence data suggests that this organization also appears to be present in LAB bacteriophages (see below).

Bacteriophage Lysis

The final step of the lytic life cycle is the release of the progeny phage from the infected bacterial cell. This is achieved by the combined activity of two types of phage encoded proteins, that is, lysins and holins, which represent the lysis cassette of the bacteriophage. The function of the lysin is to solubilize the bacterial cell wall, which ultimately leads to cell lysis and the subsequent release of the mature phage (for reviews on bacteriophage lysis, see Young, 1992; Gasson, 1996). Three classes of lytic activity have been recognized based on the peptidoglycan bond which they hydrolyze (Rodgers et al., 1980): (a) glycosidases, which hydrolyze the glycosidic linkage between the amino sugars of the peptidoglycan, and which include endo *N*-acetylglucosaminidases (or glucosaminidases) and endo *N*-acetylmuramidases (muramidases or lysozymes); (b) *N*-acetylmuramoyl-L-alanine amidases (amidases), which hydrolyze the *N*-acetylmuramoyl-L-amide linkage between the glycan strand and the cross-linking peptide, and (c) endopeptidases, which break the peptide chain of the peptidoglycan. García et al. (1990) have proposed a modular design for lysins based on sequence analysis and biochemical characterization of host cell autolysin and phage encoded lysins of *S. pneumoniae*. The premise of the lysin modular design is that the N-terminal region of the lysin determines the lytic activity of the protein while the C-terminal domain is involved in substrate binding of the enzyme to the cell wall (Figure 3.3). Atypical start codons have been reported for the lysins of a number of prolate headed lactococcal and *Oe. oeni* phages (Geis, 1992; Schouler et al., 1994; Shearman et al., 1994; Lubbers et al., 1995; Gindreau and Lonvaud-Funel, 1999; Parreira et al., 1999), and it has been speculated that these may act as a control mechanism to sprevent premature lysis of the host (Parreira et al., 1999).

Lysins generally do not contain a signal sequence and require holin proteins to cross the cell cyctoplasm. Holins are small membrane-associated proteins that cause nonspecific lesions in the cytoplasmic membrane thus allowing the lysin a passage to the cell wall (Bläsi and Young, 1996). Although there is little primary sequence relatedness between holins (Young and Bläsi, 1995) they can be recognized on the basis of their extremely hydrophilic and charge-rich C-terminus, two membrane-spanning regions separated by a β-turn linker region and a hydrophilic N-terminus (Figure 3.3). Although a methionine

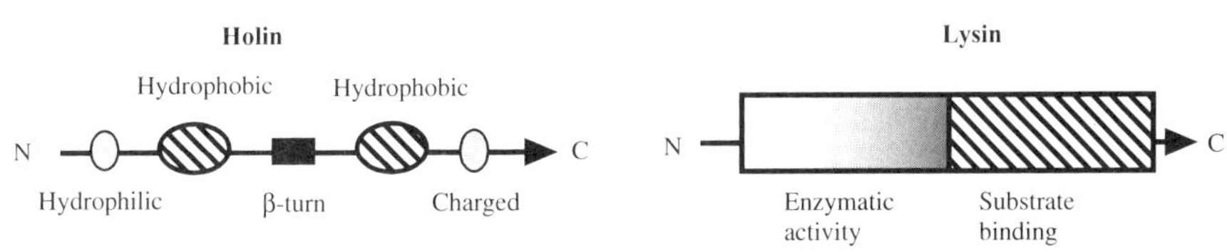

Figure 3.3. Schematic representation of the holin and lysin proteins, which are involved in bacteriophage lysis (adapted from Garvey et al., 1995).

dual start motif has been described for quite a number of holins, it is not a characteristic feature of most holins (Bläsi and Young, 1996). The dual-start motif is thought to allow the synthesis of two products of slightly different lengths, one of which acts as the inhibitor of the other, and this configuration is believed to be crucial for accurate timing of the lysis event (Young, 1992; Young and Bläsi, 1995; Graschopf and Bläsi, 1999). Young and Bläsi (1995) have described three distinct groups of holins. Type I holins are at least 87 amino acids in length and contain three or more membrane-spanning regions. Type II holins are less than 78 residues in length and contain two membrane-spanning regions. The holin of T4 t has been classified as a separate, type III, holin since it does not possess any structural or sequence similarity to the other two holin types.

Biology of Bacteriophage Infecting Lactic Acid Bacteria

With the advent of modern molecular biological and large-scale sequencing techniques, tremendous strides have been made into gaining a thorough understanding of the structural and functional organization of LAB phage genomes. At the time of writing, the entire sequence of thirteen bacteriophages infecting various LAB species are available in the databases (Table 3.2). In addition, substantial sequence information is available for a further 12 LAB bacteriophages (Table 3.2).

The genomes of all well studied bacteriophages are organized in such a way that functionally related genes are arranged in clusters and these clusters form modules (Botstein, 1980; Campbell, 1994). This also appears to be the case for bacteriophages of LAB. A module can be defined as a group of adjacent genes encoding proteins, which carry out a specific biological function. It has been speculated (Botstein, 1980) that bacteriophage evolve through the exchange of interchangeable genetic modules. Casjens and Hendrix (1974) postulated that the conserved gene order minimizes the number of unproductive interactions that arise by recombination between phages having partially homologous chromosomes. This functional organization is conserved among phage species (Casjens et al., 1992) and Figure 3.4 depicts schematic representations of the genomes of sk1 (a 936 phage), c2 (a prolate headed lactococcal phage), and P335 lactococcal phages. It is interesting to note that the modular organization of the completely sequenced *S. thermophilus* phages øO1205, ø7201, DT1 Sfi19, and Sfi21 and the *Lactobacillus* phages LL-H, øadh and øg1e appears to be similar to that of the P335 lactococcal phages.

Prolate Headed Phage

The two sequenced prolate headed phages of *L. lactis*, bIL67 (Schouler et al., 1994) and c2 (Lubbers et al., 1995), display a very similar genetic organization (Figure 3.4). The genomes of both phages are divided into two divergently oriented clusters consisting of the "early" and "late" transcribed regions. The divergent clusters are separated by the assumed origin of replication and both package their DNA utilizing a *cos* site. They have a relatively small genome with the complete sequence of bIL67 being 22,195 bp, compared to 22,163 bp of that of c2.

c2 and bIL67 share about 80% overall nucleotide sequence identity (Lubbers et al., 1995). However, this is not evenly distributed along the entire genome, with some regions sharing more than 90% identity and others less than 40% (Lubbers et al., 1995). The early region of c2 encompasses approximately 7 kb of DNA, which harbours 22 putative ORFs.

Table 3.2. List of LAB Bacteriophages for which the Genome Has Been Completely Sequenced

Phage	cos/pac Site	Size/bp	Small Isometric/ Prolate Headed, Lytic/Temperate	Number of Putative ORFs	Reference
Lactococcus					
bIL67	cos	22,195	Prolate, lytic	37	Schouler et al. (1994)
c2	cos	22,163	Prolate, lytic	39	Lubbers et al. (1995)
sk1	cos	28,451	SI[a], lytic (936)	54	Chandry et al. (1997)
biL170	cos	31,754	SI, lytic (936)	64	Crutz-le Coq et al. (2002)
r1-t	cos	33,350	SI, temperate (P335)	50	Van Sinderen et al. (1996)
Tuc2009	pac	38,347	SI, temperate (P335)	56	Van Sinderen et al. unpublished results
ul36	pac	36,798	SI, temperate (P335)	59	Labrie and Moineau (2002)
BK5-T	cos	40,003	SI, temperate (BK5-T)	63	Mahanivong et al. (2001)
TP901-1	pac	36,667	SI, temperate (P335)	56	Brondsted et al. (2001) Johnsen et al. (1996) Madsen and Hammer (1998) Walker et al. (1998)
Lactobacillus					
LL-H *(Lb. delbrueckii)*	pac	34,657	SI, lytic	52	Mikkonen et al. (1996b) Mikkonen and Alatossava (1994)
øg1e *(Lb. plantarum)*	pac	42,259	SI, temperate	62	Kodaira et al. (1997)
øadh *(Lb. gasseri)*	cos	43,785	SI, temperate	62	Altermann et al. (1999)
S. thermophilus					
øO1205	pac	43,075	SI, temperate	57	Stanley et al. (1997)
ø7201	cos	35,466	SI, lytic	44	Proux et al. (2002)
DT1	cos	34,820	SI, lytic	46	Tremblay and Moineau (1999)
Sfi19	cos	37,392	SI, lytic	44	Desiere et al. (1998)
Sfi21	cos	40,739	SI, temperate	53	Desiere et al. (1998)
Sfi11	pac	39,807	SI, lytic	53	Lucchini et al. (1998)

[a] SI: small isometric.

Similarity-derived functions have been assigned to some of these and they include a DNA polymerase, a recombination protein, a sigma factor protein and a transcription regulator protein (Jarvis, 1995a,b; Lubbers et al., 1995). The late region spans around 16 kb and 17 ORFs have been identified in this section of the genome. N-terminal sequence analysis identified three major structural and eight minor structural proteins (many of which appear to be post-translationally processed) (Lubbers et al., 1995). In addition, two putative holins and a lysin were identified (Jarvis, 1995a,b; Lubbers et al., 1995).

Similarly, the early region of bIL67 harbors 21 ORFs spanning approximately 7 kb while the late region consists of about 15 kb of DNA and contains 16 putative ORFs. A holin, terminase subunit, minor tail subunit, lysin, DNA polymerase, and a protein involved in recombination were tentatively identified on the genome (Schouler et al., 1994).

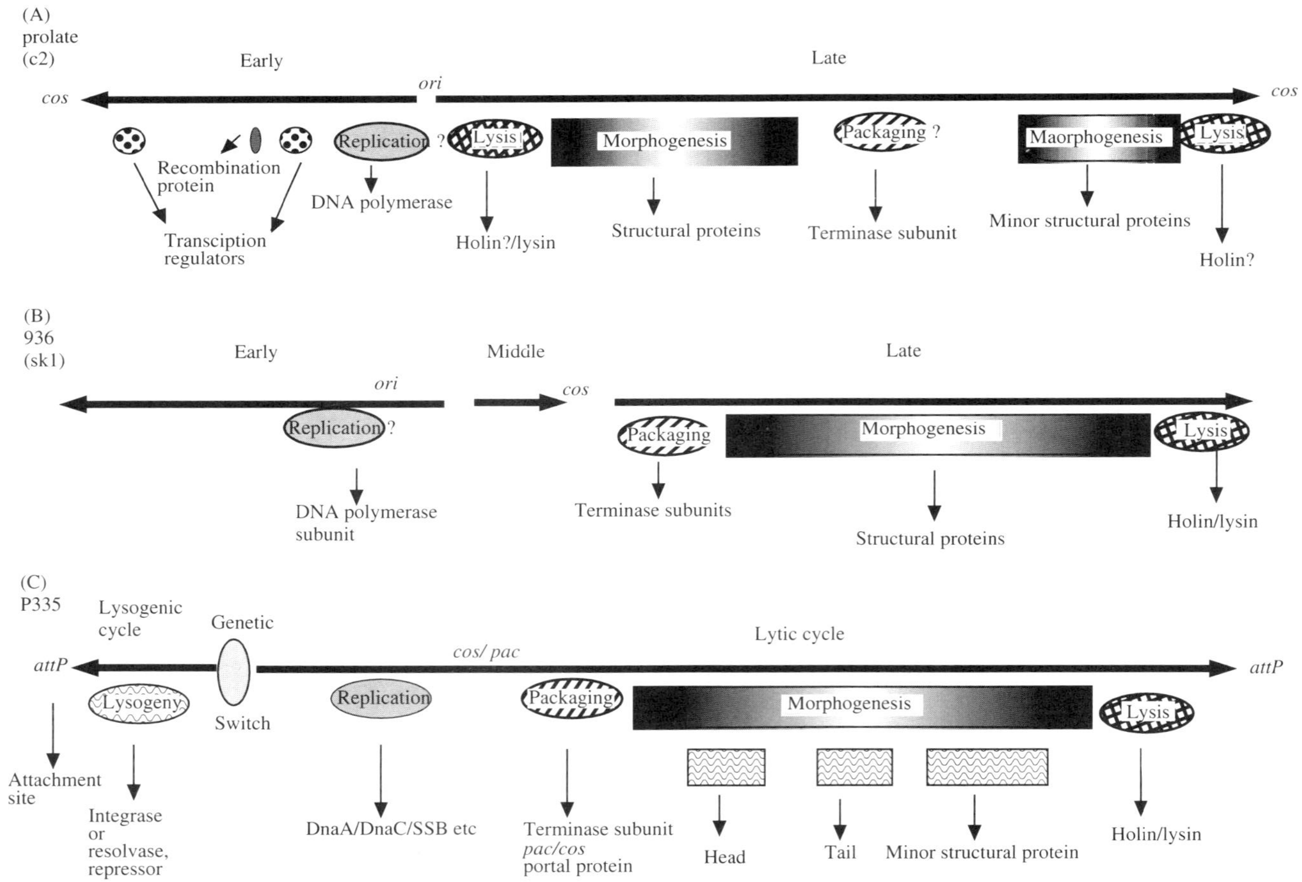

Figure 3.4. Schematic representation of the genomic arrangments of the lactococcal phage groups (A) prolate headed, (B) small isometric headed (936), and (C) small isometric headed (P335). Putative or proved functions are indicated. For a more detailed description, see text.

Small Isometric Headed Phage

All remaining LAB phages for which the entire genome sequence has been determined possess small isometric heads. They include five *S. thermophilus* phages, three *Lactobacillus* phages and four lactococcal phages (Table 3.2). Of the four completely sequenced small isometric headed lactococcal phages, sk1 is a member of the 936 species, while r1t, Tuc2009, and ul36 are P335 phages (see below). Analysis of the genome of *L. lactis* IL1403 revealed the presence of six prophages (Chopin et al., 2001). Bioinformatic analysis of these prophage sequences revealed that the three of the six encoded bacteriophages belong to the already described P335 group of temperate phages, whereas the remaining three are most probably satellites relying on helper phage(s) for multiplication (Chopin et al., 2001).

Three consecutive phases of transcription (early, middle, and late) were apparent for the 936 phage, sk1 (Chandry et al., 1997) (Figure 3.4). The remaining sequenced phages, which include phage of the lactococcal P335 species, in addition to bacteriophage infecting *S. thermophilus* and *Lactobacillus*, all share a very similar genetic organization. The genomes of the lysogenic phages are arranged in two divergent clusters separated on one side by the attachment site and on the other by an intergenic region involved in the genetic switch (Figure 3.4). The genome of the lytic *S. thermophilus, Lactobacillus*, and lactococcal P335 phages is, for the most part, transcribed in one direction.

936 Phage

The first complete 936-type phage genome sequence available was that of øsk1 (Chandry et al., 1997). Several of its 54 putative ORFs show sequence similarity to both the small isometric and prolate headed morphotypes. From a transcriptional point of view the genome is organized into three segments, represented by the early (30 ORFs), middle (4 ORFs) and late (20 ORFs) transcribed regions. These three regions are separated from each other by intergenic regions containing the *cos* site (middle and late), a transcription terminator (late and early) and divergent promoters (early and middle).

The early region consists of ORFs thought to specify replication functions (the DNA polymerase subunits). The middle region is composed of four small ORFs just upstream of the *cos* site. No function has been assigned to these ORFs. The late region of the genome putatively encodes various structural proteins, proteins involved in DNA packaging, and the lysis functions of the phage (Chandry et al., 1997).

The complete genome sequence of bIL170 has recently been published (Crutz-le Coq et al., 2002). Analysis of the putative structural protein genes gpl12 (putative fibre) and gpl20 (putative base plate protein) revealed that the deduced protein products are related by at least one of their domains to a number of multi-domain proteins encoded by a number of lactococcal and streptococcal phages. It was proposed that these proteins form a complex multi-component system involved in host range determination. Comparison of the bIL170 genome to that of sk1 showed that insertion/deletion events of one or two ORF's was the main source of divergence in the early gene clusters. It was proposed that such an event resulted in the replacement of a direct repeat-containing genomic fragment in bIL170, which thereby acquired a distinct origin of replication (Crutz-le Coq et al., 2002).

Partial sequence information is available for other 936-type phages including F4-1 (Chung et al., 1991; Kim and Batt, 1991b), bIL41 (Parreira et al., 1996), and bIL66 (Bidnenko et al., 1995). Sequence comparisons indicate that these 936-type phages are very closely related. For example, over 2 kb of the genome of sk1 (including most of the middle region) shows 84.9% identity to the middle expressed region of bIL66 (Chandry et al., 1997). Also, a 10.2 kb segment from the late region of bIL41 has been sequenced (Parreira et al., 1996) and this DNA fragment displays between 69% and 98% identity to the corresponding segment from sk1 (Chandry et al., 1997).

P335 Phage

Members of the P335 phage species are small, isometric-headed phages with genomes ranging from 30 to 42 Kb. The P335 species is heterogenous, having phages utilizing both *cos* and *pac* sites for DNA packaging, being the only lactococcal phage species containing both virulent and temperate members. The first complete P335 phage genome sequence published was that of r1t (Van Sinderen et al., 1996). r1t is a temperate phage and its genome is arranged in two divergent clusters of three and 47 ORFs. This appears to be a life cycle-specific orientation, that is, the orientation of the ORFs believed to be involved in the lysogenic life cycle is opposite to the remaining ORFs, which are associated with the lytic life cycle. It appears therefore that the r1t genome is arranged, such that all of the ORFs involved in the lytic life cycle are grouped in one large cluster. These clusters appear to be composed of a number of functional modules which are organized in a way that apparently reflects the chronological order of the life cycle itself, that is, those ORFs required for replication are transcribed first followed by modules involved in DNA packaging, morphogenesis and, finally, cell lysis (Figure 3.4). All other temperate P335-type phage whose genomes have been sequenced to date appear to exhibit this type of gene organization. The most recent complete P335 phage genome available that of ul36, also represents the first virulent P335 member to be completely sequenced (Labrie and Moineau, 2002). Interestingly, the genome of this lytic phage appears to be arranged into two divergent clusters of 6 and 53 ORF's. The cluster of 6 ORF's represents a cryptic lysogeny module containing genes, the deduced protein products of which display similarities to phage integrases, repressors, and cro proteins. Similarly an incomplete lysogeny module was identified in another lytic P335 phage, ø31 (Madsen et al., 2001). These observations indicate that virulent P335-type phage are derived from temperate phage.

S. thermophilus *Phage*

The five completely sequenced *S. thermophilus* phages appear to have a genetic arrangement very similar to that of the P335 species of lactococcal phage, that is, they have a modular arrangement made up of replication, packaging, morphogenesis, and cell lysis components. In fact it has been speculated that øO1205 is closely related to the P335 group of lactococcal phages (Stanley et al., 1997). Sequence comparisons of *S. thermophilus* phages revealed a substantial amount of homology between them (Bruttin et al., 1997a; Desiere et al., 1998; Lucchini et al., 1998; Neve et al., 1998; Desiere et al., 1999; Lucchini et al., 1999b; Desiere et al., 2002; Proux et al., 2002).

Lactobacillus *Phage*

The genomes of the *Lactobacillus* phage øgle (Kodaira et al., 1997), øadh (Altermann et al., 1999), and LL-H (Mikkonen et al., 1996b) have been completely sequenced and similar to the genomes of the P335 group of lactococcal bacteriophage, the putative ORFs identified on the genome of these phages are clustered into a number of functional modules. Interestingly, although LL-H is a lytic phage, remnants of an integrase and an attachment site (similar to that of mv4 [Auvray et al., 1997]) can be discerned, indicative of a direct evolutionary relationship between these two *Lb. delbrueckii* phages (Mikkonen et al., 1996a). Furthermore, the genes encoding some of the structural proteins of these two phages were also shown to be highly conserved (Vasala et al., 1993).

Comparative Genomics of LAB Bacteriophage

The emergence of genome sequence information has provided the substrate for comparative analysis of LAB phages. In some cases, high sequence similarity is observed between the genes, although these phages have been isolated from a number of different species. Furthermore, all appear to have a compact genome organization and contain very little non-coding DNA.

Lysogeny Module

Lysogeny appears to be widespread among *Lactobacillus* (Kiliç et al., 1996; Séchaud et al., 1988), *Lactococcus* (Huggins and Sandine, 1977; Jarvis, 1989; Davidson et al., 1990), and *Oe. oeni* (Arendt et al., 1991; Poblet-Icart et al., 1998). In contrast, lysogeny does not appear to be prevalent in *S. thermophilus*. However, while frequencies as low as 1.5% have been reported, incidences as high as 40% have also been described in literature (Smaczny and Krämer, 1984; Carminati and Giraffa, 1992; Fayard et al., 1993; Brüssow et al., 1994a; Brüssow and Bruttin, 1995; Le Marrec et al., 1997).

The assumed lysogeny module consists of a number of genes whose products establish and maintain lysogeny in the host. In this review, the genes encoding the integrase, two elements of the genetic switch, that is the repressor and Cro-like protein and the genes located between the integrase and Cro-like protein genes will be discussed as elements that are assumed to be part of the lysogeny module, without excluding the involvement of other genes. The entire sequence of this module has been determined in a number of LAB bacteriophages, for a recent review see Desiere et al. (2002).

When comparing the lysogeny module of LAB temperate bacteriophages, an overall similarity with respect to the relative position and orientation of the genes encoding the integrase, repressor and Cro-homologue is apparent. However, there are considerable differences in the number and size of the ORFs located between the integrase and repressor genes (Figure 3.5).

Site-Specific Integration

To date, two classes of integration systems have been identified in lactococcal phages. The most prominent class is that described in the lactococcal phages BK5-T (Boyce et al., 1995b), øLC3 (Lillehaug and Birkeland, 1993; Lillehaug et al., 1997), Tuc2009 (Van de Guchte et al., 1994b), and r1t (Van Sinderen et al., 1996). The integrase from these phages (and many other LAB phages) belong to the Int family of site-specific recombinases. For a recent review on the organization and function of the active site of the integrase family of recombinases see Grainge and Jayaram (1999). The putative integrase gene is almost identical in BK5-T, øLC3, Tuc2009, and r1t (Boyce et al., 1995b; Van Sinderen et al., 1996) and they all share a common 9 bp attachment site core sequence (5′ TTCTTCATG 3′). The near identity of the DNA region encoding the integrase and attachment site of

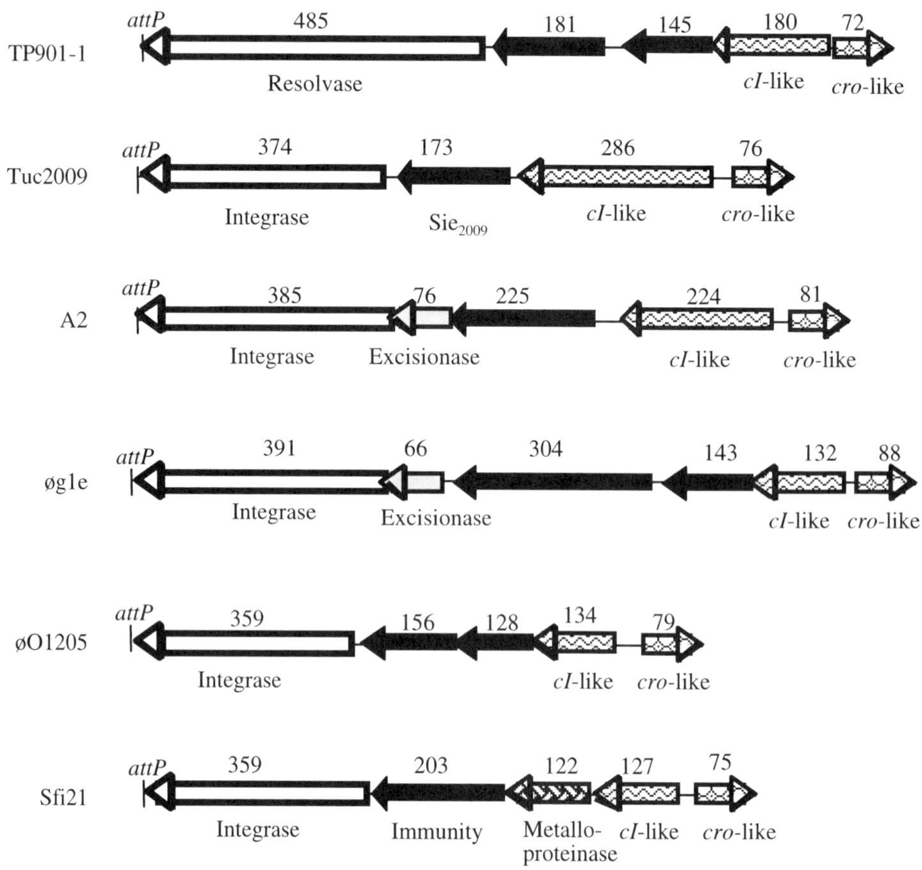

Figure 3.5. Schematic representation of lysogeny modules from LAB bacteriophages. Putative or proven functions are depicted below each of the proteins and the number of amino acids they contain is indicated above the protein. The direction of the arrow indicates the assumed direction of transcription.

these phages suggests that an essentially identical integration system may be employed by all (Van Sinderen et al., 1996). Identical sequences also surround the *attP* core in these phages and a number of inverted and direct repeats have been identified in this region, which may be important in the binding of the integrase (Boyce et al., 1995b). Under the current classification scheme BK5-T is placed in a homology group different to that of øLC3, Tuc2009, and r1t (Jarvis et al., 1991) (Table 3.1), and therefore it would appear surprising that the sequence of each of these four lactococcal phages is almost identical over this region of their genomes. However, Labrie and Moineau (2002) recently reported a comparative analysis of six complete P335-like phage genomes in which they demonstrate a genetic relationship between P335 phages and the phage-type of the BK5-T species. This finding led them to propose that phage BK5-T should be included within the P335 species. øLC3 and r1t were shown to integrate into an ORF for which no function could be identified (Lillehaug and Birkeland, 1993; Van Sinderen et al., 1996) (Table 3.3).

The P335 phage TP901-1 utilizes an integrative system, which has proven to be quite different from other LAB temperate phages (Christiansen et al., 1996). This system

Table 3.3. LAB Phage Integration

Phage	Size of Core Sequence	Integration Site	Reference
L. lactis phage			
øLC3	9 bp	Gene of unknown function	Lillehaug and Birkeland (1993) Lillehaug et al. (1997)
r1t	9 bp	Gene of unknown function	Van Sinderen et al. (1996)
Tuc2009	9 bp	Gene of unknown function	Van de Guchte et al. (1994b)
BK5-T	9 bp	Gene of unknown function	Boyce, et al. (1995b)
TP901-1	5 bp	Fimbriae precursor	Christiansen et al. (1994) Christiansen et al. (1996)
Lactobacillus phage			
øadh	16 bp	Not determined	Raya et al. (1992)
mv4	17 bp	$tRNA^{Ser}$	Dupont et al. (1995)
øg1e	24 bp	Not determined	Kakikawa et al. (1997)
A2	19 bp	$tRNA^{Leu}$	Alvarez et al. (1998)
S. thermophilus phage			
øO1205	40 bp	$tRNA^{Arg}$	Stanley et al. (1997)
TP-J34	40 bp	$tRNA^{Arg}$	Neve et al. (1998)
Sfi21	40 bp	$tRNA^{Arg}$	Bruttin et al. (1997a,b) Lucchini et al. (1999)
Oe. oeni phage			
ø10MC	15 bp	$tRNA^{Leu}$	Gindreau et al. (1997)

was shown to include (a) a gene encoding a protein showing similarity to site-specific recombinases of the resolvase family, (b) an *attP* containing region, and (c) an additional 425 bp sequence presumably containing the promoter for the resolvase-like protein, all of which were shown to be necessary for integration of TP901-1 into the chromosome of its host (Christiansen et al., 1996). Furthermore, recent work has shown that a fragment containing 56 bp of the *attP* containing region is sufficient for the site-specific integration of a non-replicating plasmid into the chromosome of *L. lactis* subsp. *cremoris* when the resolvase gene is supplied *in trans* (Brondsted and Hammer, 1999). Subsequent analysis revealed that a 43 bp *attB* region was found to be the smallest fragment able to participate fully in recombination, whereas *in vitro* studies showed that the TP901-1 integrase binds to this 43 bp *attB* fragment, the 56 bp *attP*, and a larger *attP* fragment with equal affinity (Breuner et al., 2001). Mutational analysis of the 5 bp common core region (TCAAT) showed that the TC dinucleotide is essential for recombination, but not for binding of the integrase, whereas none of the last three bases are important for recombination. When a number of *attL* sites, obtained by recombination between an *attB* site containing a mutation in this TC dinucleotide and a wild-type *attP* site, were sequenced, a mix of sites with the wild-type or the mutated sequence was obtained. These results are consistent with the hypothesis that the TC dinucleotide constitutes the TP901-1 overlap region. A 2 bp overlap region has been observed in recombination reactions catalyzed by all other members of the resolvase/invertase family tested so far. By selecting for *attB* sites with a decreased ability to participate in recombination, two bases located outside the core region of *attB* were shown to be involved in the *in vitro* binding of the TP901-1 integrase (Breuner et al., 2001).

The resolvase-like protein shares no similarity to members of the Int family of site specific recombinases, but instead is assumed to be a member of a subfamily of resolvases. This subsection differs from other members of the overall family in that they are more than twice their size. The core attachment site of TP901-1 does not show homology to any other identified core site and the phage integrates into an ORF which displays homology to a number of genes encoding precursors of fimbriae and secretion pathway proteins from different bacteria (Christiansen et al., 1994) (Table 3.3).

The integration system of each of three lysogenic *S. thermophilus* phages ø01205 (Stanley et al., 1997), Sfi21 (Bruttin et al., 1997a,b; Lucchini et al., 1999c), and TP-J34 (Neve et al., 1998) has also been identified (Table 3.3) and the integrases of these phages belong to the Int family of site-specific recombinases. All share an identical 40 bp core sequence which overlaps the 11 terminal bp of a $tRNA^{Arg}$ gene and all of these integrases exhibit up to 99% identity to each other (Neve et al., 1998; Stanley et al., 1999).

The integrases from the *Lactobacillus* bacteriophages øadh (Fremaux et al., 1993; Altermann et al., 1999), mv4 (Dupont et al., 1995), øgle (Kodaira et al., 1997), and A2 (Alvarez et al., 1998) are also members of the Int family of site-specific recombinases. The core sequence and integration site have also been determined for a number of these phages (Table 3.3). The integrase protein of øg1e was overexpressed and purified and was shown to bind specifically to the *attP* region (Yasukawa et al., 1997).

Analysis of a DNA fragment containing the *attP* region and the putative *int* gene from the *Oe. oeni* phage fOg44 (Parreira et al., 1999) and comparison with the corresponding sequence from another *Oe. oeni* phage, ø10MC (Gindreau et al., 1997), revealed significant sequence similarities. The *attP* of fOg44 is located between a putative excisionase and the integrase. However, no functional analysis of this putative excisionase has been reported (Parreira et al., 1999).

Lysogenic/Lytic Switch

The essential genetic elements necessary for the control of the lysis–lysogeny decision have been identified in a number of LAB bacteriophages. In lambda the Cro protein is a small protein (66 aa) containing a helix-turn-helix motif and is the first protein of the lytic cycle to be transcribed (Ptashne, 1986). Putative Cro-like proteins from many LAB bacteriophages have been identified based on their relative position on the genome in addition to their (small) size and the presence of a helix-turn-helix motif.

In this way putative Cro-like proteins were identified in several phages infecting LAB. For a discussion on this topic see Lucchini et al. (1999c). Only occasionally do these putative Cro-like proteins exhibit similarity to each other. Interestingly, genes encoding a Cro-like protein as well as putative operator-like sequences have been identified on the lytic *S. thermophilus* phages DT1 (Tremblay and Moineau, 1999) and Sfi19 (Lucchini et al., 1999b), which suggests that lytic phages, in some cases, have evolved from a lysogenic ancestor.

Two classes of LAB bacteriophage repressors are apparent (Table 3.4). Class I repressors are proteins with a size of between 220 to 300 amino acids, and two distinct domains can be discerned within these proteins. The N-terminal domain, consisting of approximately 100 amino acids, contains a helix-turn-helix motif, which is assumed to be necessary for the specific binding of repressor to its target DNA substrate (the operators). The C-terminal domain, analogous to the lambda repressor, is believed to be involved in oligomerization (co-operative binding of repressor proteins), and possesses a conserved

Table 3.4. LAB Phage Repressor Classification

Phage	Size of Repressor (aa)	Helix-Turn-Helix Motif	Ala/Gly Motif	Class
BK5-T	297	Yes	Yes	I
r1t	278	Yes	Yes	I
Tuc2009	286	Yes	Yes	I
A2	224	Yes	Yes	I
øg1e	132	Yes	No	II
øadh	108	Yes	No	II
øO1205	134	Yes	No	II
Sfi21	127	Yes	No	II
TP-J34	121	Yes	No	II
TP901-1	180	Not apparent	No	II

Ala/Gly motif required for RecA-mediated cleavage of the hinge region between the N- and C-terminal domains (Little, 1993). The second class of LAB phage repressors consists of considerably smaller proteins and although a helix-turn-helix motif can usually be discerned, members of this class do not contain an apparent RecA-mediated cleavage site. Despite the absence of such a Ala/Gly motif, induction of phages which possess these repressors does take place following the onset of the SOS response, for example, after addition of mitomycin C, indicating the involvement of RecA. However, the exact mechanism of how this is accomplished has not yet been elucidated. Class I repressors appear to be most prevalent among lactococcal phages, but have also been identified in bacteriophages infecting *Lactobacillus*, while Class II repressors seem to be typical for *S. thermophilus* phages, although they have also been found in *Lactobacillus* and lactococcal phages (Table 3.4).

Class I Repressors. The regulatory region of the temperate lactococcal phage r1t was the first to be examined in some detail. It encompasses two divergently orientated genes *rro* (*r*epressor of *r*-*o*ne) and *tec* (the *t*opological *e*quivalent of *c*ro). A helix-turn-helix motif was identified in the N-terminal domain of Rro while the C-terminal domain contains the conserved alanine/glycine amino acids thought to be essential for RecA-mediated autocleavage. The intergenic region between *tec* and *rro* contains two divergently oriented promoters (P_1 and P_2) and two almost identical 21 bp direct repeats with internal dyad symmetry (O_2 and O_3). A third putative operator site was identified within the coding region of *tec* (Nauta et al., 1996). Gel mobility studies revealed that Rro binds to the three operators. Co-operative binding of the repressor at the distantly separated operator sites is thought to occur through protein–protein contacts holding together a loop of intervening DNA (Matthews, 1992; Schleif, 1992). The function of P_1 is to establish lysogeny while P_2 is the transcriptional start for the expression of genes during the lytic phase (Nauta et al., 1996).

The putative repressor from Tuc2009 was identified on the basis of similarity searches (Van de Guchte et al., 1994a). Interestingly, high sequence similarity is observed between the C-terminal domains of the repressor from r1t and Tuc2009, while the N-terminal domains exhibit little if any sequence similarity (Nauta et al., 1996). This suggests that both repressors recognize different DNA sequences (i.e., operators).

ORF297 of the lactococcal phage BK5-T was identified as the repressor-encoding gene based on sequence similarities. ORF297 and ORF63 are arranged divergently to each other and the intergenic region between these two genes contains three operators and two divergently orientated promoters (Boyce et al., 1995a). By analogy to other phages, Boyce et al. (1995a) proposed that the DNA encompassing ORF297, ORF63, and its intervening DNA constitute the genetic switch region of BK5-T. The repressors from BK5-T, r1t, and Tuc2009 share high overall identity. This similarity however, is mainly concentrated at the C-terminal end (99% identity), with poor similarity being observed at the N-terminal domain (Boyce et al., 1995a)

Recently, the functional activity of the repressor from the *Lactobacillus* phage A2 was examined (García et al., 1999). Three operators (O_1–O_3) of 20 bp displaying partial symmetry were identified, as well as, the divergent promoters P_L and P_R. P_L transcribes Cro and Ant (anti-repressor) ORFs while P_R governs the expression of the genes encoding the repressor and site-specific integration machinery. In addition, the repressor was shown to suppress transcription of early lytic genes and to stimulate its own expression (García et al., 1999).

Class II Repressors. Although local similarity is found between the repressor from TP901-1 and the previously described Class I repressors there are also considerable differences between them (i.e., no RecA-mediated autocleavage site can be discerned and the repressor from TP901-1 is smaller than Class I repressors). In spite of these differences, functional analysis has shown that this repressor is capable of conferring immunity to infection by TP901-1 when present in the indicator strain (cited by Madsen and Hammer, 1998). Two divergent promoters p(R) and p(L) were identified in the intergenic region between the genes encoding the putative Cro and repressor proteins (Madsen and Hammer, 1998). The putative repressor was found to be necessary for repression of both promoters (Madsen et al., 1999). Furthermore, the presence of the putative Cro was found to be able to inhibit repression of the lytic promoter p(L) by the repressor. The results presented suggested that the relative amounts of the two proteins, repressor and Cro determine the decision between lytic or lysogenic life cycle after phage infection and that a protein complex consisting of repressor and Cro may constitute a new type of genetic switch in bacteriophages (Madsen et al., 1999).

To date, apart from comparative analyses, a detailed biochemical study has not been reported on the switch region of a lysogenic phage infecting *S. thermophilus*. The protein product of ORF4 from øO1205 shows weak similarity to the N-terminal (DNA binding) domain of the repressor of the lambdoid phage HK022 and a potential helix-turn-helix motif was identified (Stanley et al., 1997). It also exhibits high identity to the putative repressor from TP901-1 (Madsen and Hammer, 1998) with the similarity being most apparent in the N-terminal region. The putative repressor from øO1205 also shares some similarity (which is distributed equally over the entire protein) to the cI-like repressors from the *S. thermophilus* phages Sfi21 and TPJ-34. The repressors from Sfi21 and TPJ-34 show high identity to each other at the DNA level and homology is especially high at the 3′ end of the repressor encoding gene (Neve et al., 1998). Both show weak similarity to the repressor form Tuc2009. The typical RecA-mediated cleavage site is not apparent in the putative repressor of the three *S. thermophilus* phages.

The putative repressor protein from the *Lactobacillus* phage øadh displays similarities to the *B. subtilis* phage repressor from ø105. Similarity to the helix-turn-helix motif found in the repressors from Tuc2009 and r1t was also observed. However, no consensus RecA-mediated cleavage site could be discerned. In spite of this, functional analysis of this repressor demonstrated that it conferred immunity to øadh infection (Engel et al., 1998). The putative repressor from the *Lactobacillus* phage øg1e shows some similarities to lambda cI (Kakikawa et al., 1998). Three putative promoters were identified in the intergenic region between the cro-like and repressor-like proteins, but only two are expected to play a role in the lytic/lysogenic switch (Kakikawa et al., 1998). Five operator-like structures consisting of GATAC-boxes (boxes 2–6) were also identified in this region. A sixth copy (box 7) was located within the coding sequence of a protein directly downstream of the gene encoding the cI-like repressor and a seventh copy (box 1) was located within the gene encoding the Cro-like protein (Kodaira et al., 1997). Kakikawa et al. (1998) demonstrated that the repressor, in dimeric form, binds specifically to a DNA region (boxes 2–6) containing the GATAC-boxes. Subsequent analysis revealed that the Cro-like protein, which also binds as a dimer has a stronger affinity for two of the operator sequences than the repressor and that the relative concentrations of repressor-Cro molecules present in the cell determines which of the divergent promoters will be expressed (Kakikawa et al., 2000a,b).

Superinfection Exclusion

Temperate bacteriophages may express so-called superinfection-exclusion (Sie) functions that differ from immunity/repression systems in that they do not play a role in maintaining the lysogenic state and are not specific for homo-immune phages. These systems have been well characterized in phages infecting Gram-negative species, such as the Rex system encoded by the λ prophage, and the *sieA* and *sieB* systems encoded by P22 (Susskind et al., 1971; Matz et al., 1982). A Sie function, encoded by sie_{2009}, has recently been described in the temperate lactococcal phage Tuc2009 (McGrath et al., 2002a). The Sie_{2009} protein is associated with the host cell membrane and was demonstrated to provide a phage resistance phenotype against a number of phages of the 936 species, whilst having little or no effect on infection of phages belonging to the P335 and c2 groups. Evidence was presented to support the hypothesis that the Sie2009 protein prevents DNA injection by 936-type phage. Two additional prophage-encoded Sie systems were also identified, one on the chromosome of *L. lactis* IL409 and the other on the chromosome of *L. lactis* F7/2 (McGrath et al., 2002a). Bruttin et al. (1997a) have identified a gene (designated ORF203), which is positioned between the integrase and repressor-encoding genes on the lysogeny module of the temperate *S. thermophilus* phage Sfi21. It was found that when supplied on a plasmid vector, ORF203 confers a phage-resistant phenotype against twelve *S. thermophilus* bacteriophages. However, the mechanism by which the protein product of ORF203 confers this phenotype remains to be elucidated.

Replication

Replication Functions Identified in Lactococcal Phage

Sequencing of the prolate-headed, lactococcal phage c2 genome identified three ORFs (ORFe5, ORFe6 and ORFe7), which showed high sequence similarity to the three corresponding ORFs from bIL67 (ORF3, ORF4, and ORF5) (Lubbers et al., 1995). ORF3 contains five domains typically found in DNA polymerases and it was speculated that ORF3, ORF4, and ORF5 are subunits of a DNA dependent DNA polymerase enzyme (Schouler et al., 1994). The origin of replication of c2 has been identified (Lubbers et al., 1995; Waterfield et al., 1996) in the 611 bp intergenic region located between the divergently transcribed early and late regions of the phage genome (Lubbers et al., 1995).

In a subsequent study, 2-D gel electrophoresis was employed to determine the specific method of phage DNA replication utilized by c2 (Callanan et al., 2001). Results showed that c2 replicates via a theta mechanism and that DNA replication is in fact initiated within the *ori* sequence. This region is almost completely identical to the equivalent regions from the related phages bIL67 (Schouler et al., 1994) and ø197 (Schouler et al., 1992). Similar to other origins of replication, it is AT-rich and contains a number of repeated segments (Waterfield et al., 1996). When cloned on a non-replicative plasmid the origin was shown to be capable of mediating replication of the plasmid in *L. lactis*. These results suggested to the authors that phage-encoded proteins are not required for this type of DNA replication (Waterfield et al., 1996) despite the presumed presence of a putative DNA polymerase subunits, as mentioned above (Lubbers et al., 1995).

The small isometric-headed phage sk1 belongs to the lactococcal 936 family. Possible functions could be ascribed only to two of the 30 sk1 early region ORFs. Both ORF43 and ORF44 from sk1 show similarity to ORFe5 from c2 and ORF3 from bIL67. It was speculated therefore, that ORF43 and ORF44 encode subunits of a DNA polymerase (Chandry et al., 1997). Furthermore, the origin of replication from sk1 was localized to an 800 bp DNA fragment located just downstream of the intergenic region between the early and middle region of the phage genome (Chandry et al., 1997).

McGrath et al. (1999) have localized the putative origin of replication of the lactococcal bacteriophage Tuc2009 on a 160 bp segment of DNA, designated ori_{2009}. It is rich in direct repeats and is positioned within the ORF encoding the putative replisome organizer, Rep_{2009}. Furthermore, three additional ORFs were implicated in replication-associated functions based on similarity searches and included a putative single stranded binding protein, a type II methyltransferase and a topoisomerase I (McGrath et al., 1999). The putative topoisomerase I was identified based on its high similarity to the product of ORF11 from TP901-1 which in turn shows a low degree of similarity to topoisomerase I from two *Mycoplasma* species (Madsen and Hammer, 1998). In a further study the protein product of ORF17 from Tuc2009 was also shown to be an important component of the replication apparatus (McGrath et al., 2001). The protein specified by this gene was putatively identified as a helicase loader and homologues were identified in three other P335-type lactococcal phages. In fact, Southern hybridization analysis revealed that these three phages shared a high degree of homology to a number of genes contained on the Tuc2009 replication module (McGrath et al., 2001). The product of ORF12 from TP901-1 shows similarity to various single stranded binding proteins (Madsen and Hammer, 1998) including that from SPP1 (G36P) (Pedré et al., 1994). ORF11 and ORF12 from r1t are thought to play a role in the replication of this phage (Van Sinderen et al., 1996). The product of ORF12 shows similarity to *E. coli* DnaC, while the product of ORF11 shows significant similarity to G38P from the *B. subtilis* phage SPP1, which has been shown to act as a replisome organizer by binding to direct repeated sequences which make up the *ori* (Pedré et al., 1994).It is therefore believed to be a functional analogue of the *E. coli* DnaA protein and the lambda O protein (Furth and Wickner, 1983; Fuller et al., 1984). In a recent article it has been shown that the protein specified by ORF11 of r1t, Pro11, specifically interacts with a region containing four 6 bp direct repeats and it was proposed that this interaction may account for the torsion strain required for strand opening at the origin of replication (Zúñiga et al., 2002). Interestingly, the (putative) origins of replication of r1t (Van Sinderen et al., 1996), Tuc2009 (McGrath et al., 1999), lambda (Furth and Wickner, 1983), *E. coli* (Fuller et al., 1984), and SPP1(Pedré et al., 1994; Missich et al., 1997) are located within the coding regions of their respective replisome organizers. ORF14 of r1t has recently been identified as a RusA protein, which is responsible for resolving Holliday junction intermediates formed during DNA replication, recombination and repair (Sharples et al., 2002). ORF's highly homologous to ORF14 of r1t are present on the chromosomes of other lactococcal phages including ul36, Tuc2009, bil285, and BK5-T (Labrie and Moineau, 2002).

Replication Functions Identified in S. thermophilus *Phage*

The putative replication module of the *S. thermophilus* phage øO1205 has been identified and consists of at least 5.1 kb of DNA encoding a putative ATP/GTP binding protein (ORF9), a putative helicase (ORF10), and a putative primase (ORF13) (Stanley et al., 1997). Furthermore, the putative ATP/GTP binding protein shows very high similarity to a protein of unknown function in BK5-T (Boyce et al., 1995b); ORF10 and ORF11 show significant similarity to a conserved region found in lactococcal phages (Kim and Batt, 1991a; Kim et al., 1992) and ORF13 shows significant similarity to the putative primase from the cryptic plasmid pWS58 from *Lb. delbrueckii* subsp. *lactis* (accession number, Z50864). In addition, a 250 bp noncoding region, which is believed to constitute the origin of replication (*ori*), has also been described. High levels of homology were observed between this region and the highly conserved 5.1 kb replication region of a large number of other *S. thermophilus* phages (Desiere et al., 1997), which include Sfi21 and Sfi19 (Lucchini et al., 1999a). Foley et al. (1998) have shown that the Sfi21 *ori* acts as an origin of replication and requires phage-encoded proteins. In addition, these authors demonstrated that the putative origin of replication of Sfi21, when cloned on a vector in a *S. thermophilus* host is capable of conferring a phage-resistance phenotype against a large number of *S. thermophilus* phages (see below).

The replication module of the lytic *S. thermophilus* phage ø7201 contains ORFs whose products are significantly similar to the *E. coli* DnaA, DnaC, and SSB proteins. Interestingly, the replication module of ø7201 appears to employ two functional *ori*'s (Stanley et al., 2000). The replication modules of ø7201 and øO1205 are markedly different and Stanley et al. (2000) have classified *S. thermophilus* phages into two groups on the basis of their replication module. Members of group I employ an *ori* homologous to that of ø1205, while members of group II possess an *ori* homologous to at least one of the two identified for ø7201.

Replication Functions Identified in Lactobacillus *Phage*

The protein specified by ORF299 from the *Lactobacillus* bacteriophage LL-H shows similarity to G38P from SPP1 and it is therefore thought to encode the replisome organiser (Mikkonen et al., 1996b). However, unlike the situation found in other phages described above, the putative origin of replication is not located within the gene, but is separated from it by 18 kb. Mikkonen and Alatossava (1994) assigned the position of the origin of replication of LL-H to a 278 bp noncoding region located within the section of the phage genome encoding many of the structural proteins of this phage. This region is AT-rich and surrounded by eight copies of an 8 bp sequence present as both direct and inverted repeats. A putative ORF encoding a single stranded binding protein was also identified (Mikkonen et al., 1996b).

A putative DnaB-helicase was identified in the *Lactobacillus* phage øg1e on the basis of the presence of a number of conserved motifs found in helicases (Kodaira et al., 1997).

A putative helicase and nucleic acid polymerase have been identified in øadh on the basis of homology comparisons (Altermann et al., 1999). Furthermore, a potential replication origin was identified in a noncoding region of the genome. Interestingly, this region was found to be functional as a replicon in *Lb. gasseri* and *L. lactis*.

Replication module genes from phages infecting *L. lactis, S. thermophilus*, and *Lactobacillus* species coding for many different functions have been identified and the list is growing as new phage sequences become available. For reviews see amongst others: Forde and Fitzgerald (1999); Brüssow and Desiere (2001) and Brüssow (2001).

Packaging

cos-*Site Containing Phage*

Lactococcal Phage. The majority of lactococcal phage genomes appear to possess cohesive ends (Klaenhammer and Fitzgerald, 1994). The presence of cohesive termini can be demonstrated by comparing heated and non-heated restriction enzyme digests of phage DNA.

Perrin et al. (1997) compared the *cos* intergenic region of *L. lactis* bacteiophages of the c2 family and they noted a GC-rich region close to the *cos* site of all members. In addition, a four base pair indirect repeat TCAN-NACT has been found to be located close to *cos* in all sequenced *L. lactis* bacteriophages. The authors speculated that this repeat region determines terminase specificity. The *cos* site of the prolate-headed phage P001 is located in the intergenic region between the early and late regions, and it has a 3′ single stranded overhang of 12 nucleotides (cited by Schouler et al., 1994). This sequence was also identified in the intergenic region between the divergently transcribed early and late genes of bIL67 (Schouler et al., 1994) and the authors concluded that it was the corresponding *cos* site of this phage. ORF32 from bIL67 was the only identified ORF which specified a protein with recognizable DNA and ATP binding motifs typically found in terminase proteins and led the authors to suggest that this ORF specified a subunit of a phage terminase (Schouler et al., 1994).

The *cos* site of the lactococcal 936 bacteriophage bIL41 is located within the intergenic region between the middle and late transcribed genes (Parreira et al., 1996). Similarly, the *cos* site of the closely related phage sk1 was localized directly upstream of the terminase subunits, in the intergenic region between the middle and late regions of the genome (Chandry et al., 1997). Parreira et al. (1996) compared the sequence surrounding the *cos* site of bIL41 to the sequence of the 936 phages bIL66, P008 and sk1. It was concluded that the main structural features, which are assumed to play a role in the packaging of sk1 (Chandry et al., 1994), are conserved in these four phages.

The P335-type bacteriophage øLC3 possesses a *cos* site with a 13 nucleotide 3′ overhang (Lillehaug et al., 1991). Plasmids carrying this *cos* site could be transduced into its host with high frequency which demonstrated that *cos* plays an important role as a recognition signal for the packaging machinery (Birkeland and Holo, 1993). r1t possesses a *cos* site with a 13 nucleotide 3′ overhang (Van Sinderen et al., 1996), which is identical to the *cos* site in øLC3. The *cos* site of r1t is located just upstream of various packaging and structural components of the phage. Sequencing of r1t indicated that a significant portion of its packaged genomes contains ends which extend beyond the *cos* site, which suggested that packaging of the genome is accomplished by a combination of headful and unit length packaging mechanism (Van Sinderen et al., 1996).

S. thermophilus *Phage.* Le Marrec et al. (1997) have used the packaging mechanism of a number of *S. thermophilus* phages as a means of classification and identified two distinct groups. They noted a strict correlation between the method of DNA packaging utilized and the number of major structural proteins possessed by the phage. Examination of their phage collection revealed that all *pac* phages contained three major structural proteins while *cos* containing phages possessed just two.

The *cos* site of the lytic *S. thermophilus* phage ø7201 has been identified (Stanley et al., 1999, unpublished results). It consists of a 17 nucleotide sequence with a 3′ overhang. In addition, and similar to the situation in r1t (Van Sinderen et al., 1996), a significant portion of the packaged ø7201 genomes appear to possess termini which apparently extend much further than the *cos* site. In order to provide a possible explanation for these extended termini, Van Sinderen et al. (1996) proposed that the r1t genome was packaged by a combination of unit-length packaging utilizing the *cos* site and a headful mechanism which terminates when the prophage head is full (for a review see Black, 1989). It is conceivable that packaging of the ø7201 genome occurs in a similar manner. The *cos* site of ø7201 is located directly upstream of the putative small subunit of the terminase. DNA data base searches indicated that sequences homologous to the ø7201 *cos* site and surrounding region could be found in a number of *S. thermophilus* plasmids which may represent a mechanism to allow enhanced plasmid dissemination to other hosts by transduction. The temperate phage Sfi21 also possesses a *cos* site that consists of a 15 nucleotide sequence with a 3′ overhang. Furthermore, the *cos* site demonstrates 2-fold hyphenated rotational symmetry (Desiere et al., 1999). Putative terminase subunits were also identified. A putative terminase subunit in addition to the *cos* site were also identified in DT1 (Tremblay and Moineau, 1999). The packaging region of the three *cos*-site containing *S. thermophilus* phages show very high sequence similarity to each other and their *cos* sites are almost identical.

Lactobacillus *Phage.* The sequence of the *Lb. casei* bacteriophage A2 revealed a *cos* site with a 13 nucleotide 3′ overhang (García et al., 1997). A putative small subunit of the terminase was also identified in A2. As expected it possesses both helix-turn-helix and NTP-binding motifs and was shown to bind to a segment of DNA containing the *cos* site which was located directly downstream of this ORF. The *cos* site of the *Lactobacillus* phage PL-1 shows sequence homology to that of A2, but consists of 14 nucleotides (Nakashima et al., 1994). The *cos* site of øadh was also determined and found to consist of 12 bp with a 3′ overhang (Altermann et al., 1999).

pac-Site Containing Phage

Lactococcal Phage. The lactococcal phages ø50 (Alatossava and Klaenhammer, 1991), Tuc2009 (Arendt et al., 1994), and TP901-1 (Christiansen et al., 1994) have been shown to utilize a pac site to package their genomic DNA. The direction of packaging of Tuc2009 was determined to be an orientation opposite to that of the expected direction of transcription of the identified ORFs in the lytic module (Arendt et al., 1994).

S. thermophilus *Phage.* The *S. thermophilus* phages øTP-J34 (Neve et al., 1998), Sfi11 (Lucchini et al., 1998), and øO1205 (Stanley et al., 1997) were all reported to contain *pac* sites. The location of *pac* of øO1205 was determined to be located within the coding region of ORF25, which specifies a putative small subunit of the terminase. A similar position for *pac* has been observed for other phages, for example the *Salmonella* P22 phage (Black, 1989) and the *Bacillus* phage SPP1 (Chai et al., 1992). The direction of packaging was deduced to be the same as the orientation of this ORF (Stanley et al., 1997). In addition, the protein specified by ORF27 from øO1205 exhibited significant similarity to the portal protein from SPP1 (Chai et al., 1992).

Lactobacillus *Phage.* Forsman and Alatossava (1991) examined the genome of four *Lactobacillus* bacteriophage isolated from cheese processing plants in Finland. Three of these (LL-H, LL-K, and LL-S) packaged their DNA using a *pac* site, while the fourth, LL-Ku employed a *cos* site. A gene, *terL*, was identified in the øLL-H genome whose deduced protein product shows significant similarity to the large subunit of the *B. subtilis* phage SPP1 terminase. Interestingly, a 837 bp intron was discovered which interrupted this gene. The protein specified by the gene upstream of *terL* shows similarity to the small subunit of the *B. subtilis* phage SPP1 terminase (Mikkonen and Alatossava, 1995).

Protein Composition

Analysis of denatured LAB phage particles by SDS–PAGE and examination of the resulting protein profiles has frequently been used as a method of classification. Virion protein profiles have been described for several LAB bacteriophages and a number of the genes encoding these structural proteins have been sequenced.

Lactococcal Phage

P335 Phage. Three major and a number of minor structural proteins were identified in the *pac*-containing lactococcal phage Tuc2009, which belongs to the P335 phage group (Arendt et al., 1994). The genes *mp1* and *mp2* were identified on the phage genome and were shown to be separated by 9 kb (Arendt et al., 1994). MP4 has an estimated molecular mass of 32 kDa and is proposed to represent the major capsid protein.

A number of gel-purified protein products from the *pac*-containing lactococcal phage TP901-1 were used to obtain specific antibodies by affinity purification from polyclonal serum. These antibodies localized the major head (MHP) and tail (MTP) proteins in addition to components of the baseplate and neck passage structure (Johnsen et al., 1995). The DNA sequence encoding *mtp* was 91.1% identical to *mp2* from Tuc2009 and consequently it was assumed that the proteins encoded by these two genes have a similar function (Johnsen et al., 1996).

SDS–PAGE electrophoresis indicated that the lactococcal phage r1t consists of at least 11 protein bands. Five of these were N-terminally sequenced, including two protein bands of 190 and 160 kDa, which, interestingly, are larger than the predicted coding capacity of any of the ORFs identified on the r1t genome. N-terminal sequence analyses determined that these large proteins were in fact encoded by ORF31, the product of which had a molecular mass of just 32.2 kDa (Van Sinderen et al., 1996). It was proposed that the large protein bands represent covalently cross-linked pentameric and hexameric forms of the protein product of ORF31, a situation which was also observed for the head shell proteins of the mycobacteriophage L5 (Hatfull and Sarkis, 1993). It was therefore concluded that ORF31 represented the coding region for the major head protein. ORF37 of r1t was shown to specify the major tail protein while ORF27 and ORF45 were also found to encode structural proteins (Van Sinderen et al., 1996). ORF27 is located directly downstream of the *cos* site of r1t. Interestingly, ORF27 shows 98.3% overall identity to its (topological) homologue from the temperate lactococcal phage øLC3 (Van Sinderen et al., 1996) which was shown to contain one major structural protein and eight minor structural proteins (Lillehaug et al., 1991).

Prolate Headed Phage. At least 11 different proteins can be distinguished on a SDS- polyacrylamide gel of c2 phage particles, five of which are proteins with the same N-terminal amino acid sequence (Lubbers et al., 1995). These proteins are all encoded by the *l5* gene and it is believed that they may represent covalently linked multimers of the *l5* product. Using immunogold electron microscopy, two of these five proteins were identified as head proteins (Lubbers et al., 1995). Immunogold electron microscopy also identified the major tail protein (encoded by the *l7* gene) and a protein located at the tip of the tail (encoded by the *l10* gene). Homologues of the *l10* gene were also identified on the related phages bIL67 (Schouler et al., 1994) and ø197 (Schouler et al., 1992). Interestingly, a calcium-binding domain can be recognized in the protein encoded by *l10*, which may play a role in phage adsorption.

936 Phage. Western analysis indicated that a 7.6 kb *Hind*III/*EcoR*I fragment of the 936-type phage F4-1 encoded a number of structural proteins. These include the two minor structural proteins, P43 and P35, which are encoded by a single ORF and the major capsid protein, MCP (Kim and Batt, 1991b). Based on sequence homology to F4-1 a number of genes specifying structural proteins have been identified in the genomes of the related phages bIL41 (Parreira et al., 1996) and sk1 (Chandry et al., 1997). Chandry et al. (1997) predicted that the sk1 homologue of MCP from F4-1 is in fact a major tail protein suggesting the possibility that the F4-1 structural protein is localized in the tail.

S. thermophilus *Phage*

S. thermophilus bacteriophages have been classified into two groups on the basis of the observation that a particular packaging module, responsible for either *pac* or *cos* site-directed packaging, is associated with a specific set of structural proteins (Le Marrec et al., 1997). SDS–PAGE electrophoresis of *pac*-containing *S. thermophilus* øO1205 phage particles allowed the identification of three major and several minor structural proteins. N-terminal amino acid sequencing of the three major proteins indicated that they were encoded by ORF30, ORF31, and ORF37 (Stanley et al., 1997). Comparison of the sequence of the structural region of the two *pac* phages øO1205 and Sfi11, indicated that they were highly similar over a DNA segment spanning more than 20 kb (Lucchini et al., 1998; Proux et al., 2002). The first 7.5 kb of this segment of DNA encodes not only the three major structural proteins, but also a presumed portal protein and a number of proteins to which no function could be assigned (Lucchini et al., 1998; Proux et al., 2002). No similarity to *cos* containing phages was detected over this 7.5 kb region. Analysis of the sequence of øO1205 and Sfi11 indicates that these phages display remarkable similarities to a number of small isometric headed lactococcal phages belonging to the P335 species. The conserved gene order and sequence similarity between seven consecutive ORFs from øO1205 (ORF33 through ORF39) and Sfi11 (ORF113 through ORF105) with a gene cluster from the lactococcal TP901-1 is especially interesting and suggests a close evolutionary relationship between these phages (Stanley et al., 1997; Lucchini et al., 1998). A number of genes were identified in Sfi11, which were tentatively assumed to encode minor structural proteins (Lucchini et al., 1998). The DNA encompassing these ORFs exhibit very high homology to the *pac* phage øO1205, but also display considerable homology to the *cos* phages Sfi21 and Sfi19.

SDS–PAGE of the *S. thermophilus cos* phage ø7201 revealed the presence of two major structural proteins with molecular masses of 32 and 26 kDa. The gene encoding the smaller of these was identified (Le Marrec et al., 1997). N-terminal sequence analysis of the large major structural protein indicated that it is encoded by ORF26 and that the primary gene product of this ORF undergoes post-translational proteolysis in which the first 104 amino acids are removed to generate the mature phage protein (Stanley et al., 1999, unpublished results). Desiere et al. (1999) also speculated that the first 104 amino acids of the major structural protein of Sfi21, which is almost identical to the ORF26 encoded product, are removed. Putative proteins encoded by the highly homologous morphogenesis module from all these *cos-* phages also display similarity to proteins from various other lactic acid bacteriophages including the *Lactobacillus* phage LL-H, the lactococcal phage BK5-T. Most strikingly, high similarity was also detected to several adjacent ORFs of the *Oe. oeni* phage L10 (Stanley et al., 1999, unpublished results).

ORF18 of the lytic *S. thermophilus* phage DT1 was identified as a putative anti-receptor gene (Dupleiss and Moineau, 2001). Homologous genes were identified in six additional phages and a comparative analysis performed. Three distinct domains were identified in the deduced protein products. The N-terminal domain was conserved in all seven phages, the middle domain was found to be variable, whereas the C-terminal was found to contain both conserved and variable regions. Chimeric DT1 phages were constructed containing anti-receptor proteins with domains from different phages and it was found that host specificity was determined by the second variable region in the C-terminal (Dupleiss and Moineau, 2001).

Lactobacillus *Phage*

The *Lb. delbrueckii* phage LL-H is composed of at least seven structural proteins (Trautwetter et al., 1986). The major capsid protein (GP34) and major tail protein (GP19) have been identified (Trautwetter et al., 1986) and the amino acid sequence of the major capsid protein from the closely related *Lb. delbrueckii* phage mv4 displays a high degree of similarity to the capsid protein from LL-H (Vasala et al., 1993). Interestingly, the genes surrounding *gp34* are very similar at both the sequence and organizational levels in these two phages (Vasala et al., 1993). Subsequently, N-terminal sequence analyses identified the gene encoding a minor structural protein and an additional three genes encoding putative minor structural proteins were also identified in LL-H (Mikkonen and Alatossava, 1994). The *Lactobacillus* phage øg1e contains four major structural proteins with estimated molecular masses of 64, 43, 29, and 26 kDa (Kakikawa et al., 1996). The genes encoding the structural proteins were cloned and the sequence obtained from the N-terminal sequencing of the proteins matched the deduced amino acid sequence derived from the nucleotide sequence. The phage also contains more than 16 minor structural proteins. The genome sequence of øg1e (Kodaira et al., 1997) identified 12 consecutive ORFs showing similarity (29–49%) to ORFs encoding capsid proteins of the *Lactobacillus* phages LL-H and mv4 (Mikkonen and Alatossava, 1994). Two capsid protein genes were identified on the genome of øadh (Altermann et al., 1999) and interestingly, similar to what is observed in the *S. thermophilus* phages Sfi21 and ø7201, the larger of these proteins appears to be post-translationally processed.

Bacteriophage Lysis

The lytic systems of many phages infecting LAB have been characterized at a molecular level (see below) (Table 3.5). Holins are generally located directly upstream of the lysin

Table 3.5. Holins and Lysins of Bacteriophages of Lactic Acid Bacteria

	Holin		Lysin			
Phage	Size (aa)	Dual Start Motif	Size (aa)	Assumed Enzymatic Activity	Position Relative to Holin	Reference
L. lactis						
øvML3	71	Yes	226	Muramidase	Holin gene located within lysin gene	Shearman et al. (1994)
c2	161 (L2)	No	226	Muramidase	Downstream	Ward et al. (1993)
	96 (L17)	No			Removed	Lubbers et al. (1995)
bIL67	97	Yes	226	Muramidase	Removed	Schouler et al. (1994)
P001	N/A	N/A	226	Muramidase	N/A	Geis (1992)
sk1	117 (orf19)	Yes	246	Amidase	Downstream	Chandry et al. (1997)
	160 (orf53)	No			Removed	
øUS3	66	No	258	Amidase	Downstream	Platteeuw and de Vos (1992)
øLC3	88	No	429	Muramidase	Downstream	Birkeland (1994)
Tuc2009	88	No	428	Muramidase	Downstream	Arendt et al. (1994)
r1t	75	No	270	Amidase	Downstream	Van Sinderen et al. (1996)
S. thermophilus						
øO1205	141 (orf49)	No	281	Amidase	Downstream	Stanley et al. (1997)
	80 (orf50)	No			Downstream	Sheehan et al. (1999)
Sfi11	141 (orf141)	No	288	Amidase	Downstream	Lucchini et al. (1998)
	87 (orf87)	No			Downstream	

(*continued*)

Table 3.5. ***(continued)***

Phage	Holin Size (aa)	Holin Dual Start Motif	Lysin Size (aa)	Lysin Assumed Enzymatic Activity	Lysin Position Relative to Holin	Reference
Sfi19	141 (orf141)	No	289	Amidase	Downstream	Desiere et al. (1998)
	87 (orf87)	No			Downstream	
Sfi21	141 (orf141)	No	288	Amidase	Downstream	Bruttin et al. (1997a)
	87 (orf87)	No			Downstream	
DT1	80	No	200	Amidase	Downstream	Tremblay and Moineau (1999)
Lactobacillus						
øadh	114	No	317	Muramidase	Downstream	Henrich et al. (1995)
øg1e	142	No	422	Muramidase	Downstream	Oki et al. (1996)
PL1	N/A	N/A	N/A	Muramidase	N/A	Watanabe et al. (1984)
mv1	N/A	N/A	195	Muramidase	N/A	Boizet et al. (1990)
LL-H	107	No	297	Muramidase	Downstream	Vasala et al. (1995)
Oe. oeni						
fOg44	117	No	432	Muramidase	Downstream	Parreira et al. (1999)
ø10MC	163	No	432	Muramidase	Upstream	Gindreau and Lonvaud-Funel (1999)

N/A: Information not available.

gene, but exceptions to this rule appear to occur. For example, the predicted holin and lysin genes of the prolate headed phage bIL67 are separated by 12.6 kb (Schouler et al., 1994).

Holins of LAB Phage

Lactococcal Phage. The first putative holin to be identified from a bacteriophage infecting a member of the LAB was from the prolate headed phage øvML3 (Shearman et al., 1994). Interestingly, the gene encoding this presumptive holin was identified within the lysin-encoding sequence, a feature, which was considered to reflect the small size and compact nature of the phage genome. This putative holin consists of 71 amino acids, contains a potential dual start motif, a hydrophobic N-terminus, and a charged C-terminus. Putative holins have also been identified in the prolate headed phages c2 (Lubbers et al., 1995) and bIL67 (Schouler et al., 1994). Two possible holin-encoding genes were identified in c2. The first, l2, was located immediately upstream of the putative lysin gene, while the second, *l17*, was located almost 14 kb downstream of l2. Both exhibit the secondary structural motifs characteristic of holins. ORF37 from bIL67 is the analogue of *l17* (Lubbers et al., 1995) and, based on its secondary structure, Schouler et al. (1994) have suggested that it specifies a holin. In addition, the C-terminal portion of the product encoded by ORF37 display significant similarity to the characterized holin of the *B. subtilis* bacteriophage ø29 (Schouler et al., 1994).

ORF19 from the 936 phage sk1 displays many of the secondary structural features common to holins and following cloning and expression, Chandry et al.(1997) confirmed that its gene product has the functional properties of a holin. ORF19 is located directly upstream of the putative lysin and a region of the protein exhibits 97% identity to the putative holin from the 936 phage øUS3 (Platteeuw and De Vos, 1992). Interestingly, *orf53*, located in the middle region of sk1, exhibited 44% sequence identity to *l2* of the prolate headed phage c2, believed to encode one of its possible holins (see above).

Putative holins have also been identified for the P335 phages øLC3 (Birkeland, 1994), Tuc2009 (Arendt et al., 1994), and r1t (Van Sinderen et al., 1996). The putative holin gene of øLC3, *lysA*, is located upstream of the lysin gene, *lysB*, and has two transmembrane domains. LysA displays more than 42% identity to ORF2 from the *S. pneumoniae* phage EJ-1 which is located upstream of its phage lysin gene and contains characteristics common to holins (Díaz et al., 1992). LysA was shown to assist Lys-B mediated lysis when expressed in *E. coli* (Birkeland, 1994). The putative holin of Tuc2009 also shows high similarity to ORF2 from the *S. pneumoniae* phage EJ-1 (Arendt et al., 1994). ORF48 is thought to encode the holin of r1t. Analysis of the predicted protein product of ORF48 revealed that it contains the structural features necessary to define it as a holin (Van Sinderen et al., 1996).

S. thermophilus *Phage.* The *S. thermophilus* phages øO1205 (Stanley et al., 1997; Sheehan et al., 1999), Sfi11 (Lucchini et al., 1998), øSfi21 (Bruttin et al., 1997a), and Sfi19 (Desiere et al., 1998) all contain a very homologous lysis cassette consisting of two holin genes (*lyt49* and *lyt50* in øO1205) followed by a gene encoding a lysin (*lyt51* in øO1205). In contrast, the *S. thermophilus* phage DT1 (Tremblay and Moineau, 1999) appears to contain just one holin, exhibiting high identity to the holin directly upstream of the lysin of the other *S. thermophilus* phages. Expression of either *lyt49* or *lyt50* of øO1205 in *E. coli* was shown to cause cell death and leakage of the intracellular enzyme isocitrate dehydrogenase into the growth medium without apparent lysis of the cell (Sheehan et al., 1999). *lyt49* exhibits extensive homology to the gene encoding the holin of the streptococcal phage

Cp-1 (Martín et al., 1996), while *lyt50* exhibited significant homology to the holin gene of the staphylococcal phage phi11 (Weerakoon and Jayaswal, 1995) and the lactococcal phages Tuc2009 (Arendt et al., 1994) and øLC3 (Birkeland, 1994). It was speculated that the two adjacent holins may constitute a holin/antiholin system, where the antiholin acts as an inhibitor of the holin to ensure accurate timing of the release of the lysin (Sheehan et al., 1999).

Lactobacillus *Phage.* The holins from the *Lb. gasseri* phage øadh (Henrich et al., 1995; Altermann et al., 1999) and the *Lb. plantarum* phage øg1e (Oki et al., 1996) are located immediately upstream of their respective lysin genes. The holin from øadh does not display similarity to any proteins in the available sequence data bases, but does possess the structural features common to holins. Furthermore, it was shown to complement an *E. coli* bacteriophage lambda mutant in the *S* gene, which encodes a holin (Henrich et al., 1995). The holin from øg1e shares sequence similarity with the holin from øLC3 in addition to possessing the structural features common to holins.

Oe. oeni *Phage.* Putative holins have been identified in the two *Oe. oeni* phages, fOg44 (Parreira et al., 1999) and ø10MC (Gindreau and Lonvaud-Funel, 1999). Surprisingly, the putative holin of ø10MC is located immediately downstream of the putative lysin rather than in the usual upstream location.

Lysins of LAB Phage

The genes encoding a large number of LAB phage lysins have been identified (Table 3.5) and the deduced protein products of many of these genes have been characterized at both a molecular and biochemical level.

Lactococcal *Phage.* The gene encoding the lysin of øvML3 was the first lactococcal phage gene to be cloned and sequenced and it was initially reported to encode a protein of 187 amino acids with a molecular mass of 21 kDa (Shearman et al., 1989). However, subsequent experiments corrected a number of sequencing errors leading to the finding that the protein actually contained 226 amino acids and had a molecular mass of 25.2 kDa (Shearman et al., 1994). Oram and Reiter (1965) had previously characterized this lysin as a muramidase and described the conditions for its optimum enzymatic activity. The lysin showed significant similarity with protein 15 (a lysin) from the *B. subtilis* phages PZA and ø29. Interestingly, an isoleucine specifying codon (AUA) represents the start codon of the øvML3 lysin gene. Gene *13* encodes the lysin of c2 and this protein exhibits 94% amino acid identity with the lysin of bIL67 (Schouler et al., 1994). The gene *12*, located directly upstream of the gene encoding the lysin of c2 is considered a likely candidate to encode the holin.

The putative lysin of phages øUS3 (Platteeuw and de Vos, 1992) and sk1, which both belong to the 936 phage group, show 77% identity to each other (Chandry et al., 1997). Unlike the putative lysins from prolate headed lactococcal phages, data base searches indicate that the lysins from both øUS3 and sk1 show similarity to amidases. The lytic spectrum of the lysin from øUS3 was found to include all but one of the 35 strains of *L. lactis* tested, but it showed no activity against *Leuconostoc* and *Lactobacillus* strains (Platteeuw and de Vos, 1992). The lytic function of the putative lysin from sk1 was conclusively demonstrated when it was shown that simultaneous expression of the putative lysin and holin in *E. coli* caused cell lysis (Chandry et al., 1997). The N-terminal domain (i.e., enzymatic activity domain) of the putative lysin from the temperate phage øLC3 displays high similarity to the muramidases from the *S. pneumoniae* phages Cp-1, Cp-7, and Cp-9 as well as the *Lactobacillus* phages mv1 and mv4 (Birkeland, 1994). The lysin was expressed in *E. coli*, but required simultaneous expression of the holin to allow access of the lysin to the cell wall. An almost identical lysin gene has been characterized from the temperate phage Tuc2009 (Arendt et al., 1994; Sheehan et al., 1996). When this gene was overexpressed in *E. coli* it was found to be active against cell walls of a *L. lactis* subsp. cremoris strain. In addition, an active chimeric enzyme was constructed by fusing the region encoding the N-terminal section of the lysin from Tuc2009 with the C-terminal domain of the major pneumococcal autolysin. This fusion protein was shown to be capable of degrading pneumococcal cell walls (Sheehan et al., 1996). Sequencing of the entire genome of r1t identified an ORF whose deduced protein product contained an N-terminal domain which shows similarity to a family of chromosomally and phage-encoded cell wall lytic enzymes which are known to have amidase activity (Van Sinderen et al., 1996). In addition, the C-terminal section of the protein, which is assumed to be involved in cell wall recognition, shows significant sequence similarity to the C-terminal region of the lysins from the lactococcal prolate headed phages c2, bIL67, and vML3.

S. thermophilus *Phage.* The genomes of *S. thermophilus* phages are highly conserved and putative lysis cassettes have been identified in a number of these. All show high sequence identity to each other. The putative lysins from øO1205 (Stanley et al., 1997; Sheehan et al., 1999), øSfi19 (Lucchini et al., 1998), and øSfi11 (Lucchini et al., 1998) are between 281 and 289 amino acids in length. However, due to a short DNA insertion at the C-terminal region of the gene, the putative lysin of DT1 consists of only 200 amino acids (Tremblay and Moineau, 1999). Sheehan et al. (1999) have shown that the lysin of øO1205 is active specifically against streptococcal cell walls. Similar to other phage-encoded lysins, it was assumed that the carboxy-terminal domain is responsible for substrate specificity while the N-terminal domain mediates the enzymatic activity of the protein. Southern blotting experiments have indicated that a homologue of the lysin gene is present in most of the 30 *S. thermophilus* phages tested. The N-terminal region shows similarity to the amidase from the pneumococcal phage Dp-1 suggesting that the lysin of øO1205 may exhibit a similar cell wall-degrading activity (Sheehan et al., 1999).

Lactobacillus *Phage.* The first Lactobacillus phage lysin to be purified and characterized was that of the *Lb. casei* phage PL-1, which was identified as a muramidase (Watanabe et al., 1984; Hayashida et al., 1987). The lysin exibited a narrow spectrum of activity showing high activity against the host strain but very poor or no activity against a number of other Lb. casei strains. On the basis of similarity searches the lysin of the *Lb. bulgaricus* phage mv1 is likely to be a muramidase (Boizet et al., 1990).

The lytic genes of the *Lb. gasseri* phage øadh have also been identified and their protein products characterized (Henrich et al., 1995). The øadh lysin shows significant similarity to the lysin of mv4 as well as to the muramidases of the pneumococcal phages Cp-1, Cp-7, Cp-9, and the lactococcal phage øLC3 suggesting that it too is a muramidase (Henrich et al., 1995). When either the holin or the lysin of øadh was expressed in conjunction with the holin or lysin of lambda or the *B. subtilis* phage ø29, lysis of *E. coli* occurred indicating that the two enzyme activities required for phage-induced lysis from different phages are interchangeable (Henrich et al., 1995). The lysin of the *Lb. delbrueckii* subsp. *lactis* phage LL-H has a wide spectrum of activity and is active against other strains of *Lb. delbrueckii*, in addition to *Lb. acidophilus, Lb. helveticus*, and *Pediococcus damnosus* (Vasala et al., 1995). The enzyme has been characterized as a muramidase and the C-terminal domain was shown to be nonessential for catalytic activity. It shows high similarity to the putative or proven muramidases of the *Lb. delbrueckii* subsp. *bulgaricus* phages mv1 and mv4, the *S. pneumonia* phages Cp-1, Cp-7, and Cp-9 and the *L. lactis* phages Tuc2009 and øLC3. However, this similarity was restricted to approximately the first 200 N-terminally-located amino acids (except for mv4) and no similarity was observed in the C-terminal domain, which is assumed to determine substrate specificity (Vasala et al., 1995). The putative lysin of the *Lactobacillus* phage øg1e also displays significant similarity to the muramidases of the *Lactobacillus* phages mv1 and øadh, the lactococcal phage øLC3 and the *S. pneumonia* phages Cp-1, Cp-7, and Cp-9 (Oki et al., 1996). When either the lysin and/or the holin was expressed in *E. coli* a reduction in cell turbidity was noted, demonstrating their role in the lytic process (Oki et al., 1996). This reduction was most apparent when both the holin and lysin were expressed together, but a reduction was also noted when either of these two proteins were expressed individually.

Oe. oeni *Phage.* The putative lysins from the *Oe. oeni* phages fOg44 and ø10MC have recently been identified (Gindreau and Lonvaud-Funel, 1999; Parreira et al., 1999). They are almost identical to each other and also show high similarity to the lysin of Tuc2009. Both use an atypical start codon (TTG), which may be employed to control the timing of host lysis (Parreira et al., 1999).

Bacteriophage Evolution

Botstein (1980) and Campbell (1994) proposed that bacteriophage within the same interbreeding population evolve through the exchange of functional modules resulting in phage with mosaic or chimeric structures. Module exchanges are mediated by homologous recombination, site-specific recombination, or illegitimate recombination, the latter resulting in the joining of two non-homologous DNA segments (Casjen et al., 1992). Although rare, illegitimate recombination is considered to be an important process for acquiring new DNA material into the gene pool (Campbell, 1988, 1994). In addition, phage may evolve through point mutations and various deletions, inversions and duplications (Ackermann and Dubow, 1987; Campbell, 1988, 1994; Ackermann et al., 1995). The diversity of evolutionary approaches allows a bacteriophage population to constantly evolve and adapt to various environmental pressures.

Horizontal gene transfer may play an important role in the evolution of LAB phages. Several adjacent genes on the genome of the *S. thermophilus* phages øO1205 and Sfi11 show similarity to a gene cluster from the lactococcal P335 phages TP901-1 and Tuc2009 (Stanley et al., 1997; Lucchini et al., 1998). High similarities were also noted between a gene cluster from the *S. thermophilus* phage ø7201 and the *Oe. oeni* phage L10 (Stanley et al., 1999, unpublished results). Over a third of the ORFs identified on the øO1205 genome show significant similarity to ORFs from the lactococcal P335-type phages (Stanley et al., 1997).

The entire sequence of the genomes of the prolate lactococcal phages bIL67 and c2 (Schouler et al., 1994; Lubbers et al., 1995) have been determined and comparison at the nucleotide level has revealed 80% identity. One region that displayed the lowest level of sequence homology is a module, which encodes the phage-specific structural proteins of both phages (Lubbers et al., 1995).

Early reports by Jarvis (1984) concluded that lactococcal lytic and lysogenic phages were not related and therefore it had been believed that temperate phages do not contribute significantly to the emergence of new virulent lactococcal phages (Jarvis, 1989; Davidson et al., 1990). Nevertheless, subsequent analysis revealed that some relatedness between lactococcal phages with different life cycles does exist, leading to the definition of the P335 and BK5-T lactococcal phage types (Jarvis et al., 1991). All members of the lactococcal bacteriophage P335 species, containing both lytic and lysogenic phage, exhibit some degree of DNA homology, suggesting that some temperate and lytic phages may have some common ancestors (Lautier and Novel, 1987; Relano et al., 1987; Braun et al., 1989; Jarvis, 1989; Davidson et al., 1990). However, it may still be correct to conclude that lysogenic strains are an unlikely source of lytic lactococcal phages because of the paucity of strains on which lysogenic strains can propagate lytically (Josephsen and Neve, 1998).

There is some evidence to suggest that some of the lytic *Lactobacillus* and *S. thermophilus* phage may have evolved from lysogenic strains. A truncated integrase gene and two sites homologous to the temperate *Lactobacillus* phage mv4 *attP* site were identified on the lytic *Lactobacillus* phage LL-H, suggesting that the two phages may be derived from a common temperate ancestor (Mikkonen et al., 1996a). Sequencing of various lysogenic and lytic *S. thermophilus* phages has indicated that they are very closely related. Furthermore, Bruttin and Brüssow (1996) described how a single integrase-mediated deletion in a temperate phage, gave rise to a lytic phage. Also, *cro*-like genes have been observed in three completely sequenced lytic *S. thermophilus* phages, DT1 (Tremblay and Moineau, 1999), Sfi19 (Lucchini et al., 1999) and ø7201 (Proux et al., 2002). This suggests that these phages may have evolved from a temperate ancestor simply through loss of part of the lysogenic module. Fayard et al. (1993) reported that recombination of *S. thermophilus* phages can occur during infection. When a lysogenic host was infected with a lytic phage the DNA restriction pattern of the resulting progeny phage no longer matched the lytic phage or the prophage. These results provide a warning that care should therefore be taken when using a lysogenic strain as a starter culture. Hill et al. (1991) reported the genetic exchange of a functional domain from a type II A methylase between a lactococcal plasmid and a lytic, lactococcal phage, while Moineau et al. (1994) reported that a lytic, lactococcal phage acquired a large DNA fragment from the chromosome of its host leading to the generation of a new phage. Phages of LAB therefore appear to be able to acquire genetic information from unrelated sources with relative ease and as a result the similarities between phages may represent horizontal evolution rather than phylogenetic relationships.

Brüssow and coworkers have published several articles in which comparative genomics was employed to gain insights into the evolutionary history of bacteriophages (Desiere et al., 2000; Brüssow and Desiere, 2001; Deseire et al., 2001a,b; Brüssow and Hendrix, 2002; Desiere et al., 2002; Proux et al., 2002; Ventura et al., 2002).

These authors concluded that the relatedness of individual phages is not based on sequence similarity alone but also includes the topological organization of genomes. On the basis of these analyses a new taxonomic classification concept for bacteriophages infecting low-G+C content Gram-positive bacteria has been proposed. This system is based on the genetic organization of the structural gene module and members of the *Siphoviridae* are divided into one of two groups, Sfi21-like or Sfi11-like. Currently there are over 100 complete phage genomes available with a great many more in progress (Brüssow and Hendrix, 2002). With the increasing volume of phage sequence data available coupled with such technologies as microarray analysis, researchers are now, more than ever, in a position to gain detailed insights into the progress of bacteriophage evolution.

Bacteriophage Derived Tools

The availability of LAB phage sequence information and the understanding of some of the mechanisms underlying the molecular biology of these phages has provided the opportunity to exploit this knowledge for the development of a number of phage derived tools. This topic has recently been extensively reviewed (McGrath et al., 2002b), however a summary is included below.

Genetically Engineered Phage-Resistant Mechanisms

Sanford and Johnston (1985) hypothesized that the life cycle of a phage could be disrupted if phage gene products were present in the host in a dysfunctional form, in excess, or expressed at the wrong stage of development. This model was substantiated by Hill et al. (1990) who developed a phage resistance system, Phage-encoded resistance (Per), based on the origin of replication of the lactococcal phage ø50. These authors proposed that cloned origins could act as false targets for phage replication proteins, thereby competing with replicating phage genomes. This presumed competition, if effective, would ultimately cause reduced phage propagation and the phenotype was experimentally manifested as a reduction in efficiency of plaquing (EOP) and/or plaque diameter. A similar Per mechanism was generated by cloning the origin of ø31 (O'Sullivan et al., 1993). More recently, a Per phenotype was observed when the gene encoding the replisome organizer of Tuc2009 was cloned onto a high copy number vector (McGrath et al., 1999). More specifically, delineation studies proved that the Per phenotype was due to the titration of essential replication factors by a 160 bp DNA segment located within the gene, which was rich in direct repeats and which was proposed to be the origin of replication of Tuc2009. A similar system has been described in *S. thermophilus* phages, which are segregated into at least two distinct replication groups. A 302 bp fragment of the *S. thermophilus* phage Sfi21 genome, which is thought to act as the phage origin of replication, was shown to confer resistance against 17 of 25 phages which had been active on the host strain *S. thermophilus* Sfi1 (Foley et al., 1998). Additionally, a Per system derived from the *Lactobacillus casei* bacteriophage øA2 was developed (Moscoso and Suarez, 2000). Per systems are generally active only towards phage, which are closely related to the phage from which the origin is derived. Moreover, the efficiency of a Per system is very much dependent on the copy number of the plasmid carrying the *ori* (Hill et al., 1990; O'Sullivan et al., 1993).

An alternative method of engineered phage resistance is the use of antisense RNA technology (Kim and Batt, 1991c; Kim et al., 1992; Batt et al., 1995). When a lactococcal phage ORF of unknown function from the phage ø7–9 was cloned in the antisense orientation with respect to a strong lactococcal promoter the construct was shown to inhibit phage propagation. Weaker inhibitory effects were observed when antisense mRNA constructs were directed against two other ORFs from ø7–9 (Kim et al., 1992) or the major capsid protein from F4-1 (Chug et al., 1992). The antisense RNA-targeting of genes coding for essential DNA replication proteins, such as a putative replisome organizer protein or a putative helicase loader protein, was found to confer a highly effective phage resistance phenotype against a number of P335-type phages infecting *L. lactis* (McGrath et al., 2001). Recently, Sturino and Klaenhammer (2002) reported on the use of the antisense RNA methodology to target an essential replication gene, the putative helicase of the *S. thermophilus* phage Sfi21. This putative helicase gene is a component of the so-called Sfi21-type DNA replication module, which is found in the majority of *S. thermophilus* phages of industrial importance. The targeting of this conserved gene was shown to be effective at impeding the proliferation of a number of different *S. thermophilus* bacteriophages.

A third artificial, Abi-like resistance mechanism has been described which is based on a high-copy number, plasmid-located DNA cassette comprising of a phage-derived promoter, which drives the expression of a lethal restriction endonuclease. Transcription of the restriction cassette is only initiated when the host cell is infected by phage closely related to the phage from which the promoter is derived and results in the death of the bacterial host (Djordjevic and Klaenhammer, 1997; Djordjevic et al., 1997).

Alvarez et al. (1999) have demonstrated the potential use of phage repressors as a means of inhibiting temperate bacteriophages. In a subsequent study an elegant delivery and clearing system was developed and used in the construction of a stable food-grade *Lb. casei* strain completely immune to phage A2 infection during milk fermentation (Martín et al., 2000). A system providing a complete phage resistance phenotype on *L. lactis* against a number of 936-type phage has recently been reported (McGrath et al., 2002). Expression of a prophage-encoded gene, designated sie_{2009}, from a plasmid vector was shown to mediate this resistance phenotype. The Sie_{2009} protein was demonstrated to be associated with the cell membrane and evidence was presented to support the hypothesis that it interferes with the phage DNA injection process.

Phage-Derived Expression Systems

A phage-derived inducible expression system has been described based on the immunity region of the temperate lactococcal phage r1t (Nauta et al., 1996). The repressor/operator region was cloned upstream of *lacZ* such that the promoter for *tec* (Cro-like protein gene) was directed towards the reporter gene. Expression of the *lacZ* fusion could be induced upon the addition of mitomycin C and levels of β-galactosidase activity increased 70-fold. With a view to making this system suitable for applications in the food industry a number of thermolabile derivatives of the repressor of r1t were isolated. One of these mutants allowed a thermo-induction ratio of almost 500 relative to the wild type repressor (Nauta et al., 1997).

O'Sullivan et al. (1996) combined a phage specific promoter and an origin of replication from the lactococcal phage ø31, on a low copy number plasmid to construct a phage-specific, explosive expression system. The promoter was cloned upstream of the *lacZ* gene from *S. thermophilus* and showed low levels of constitutive β-gal activity. However >2000 β-gal units were detected after phage infection as compared to just 85 units obtained with a control plasmid which lacked the phage origin of replication. In a later study by Walker and Klaenhammer (1998), the DNA fragment containing the phage specific promoter was subcloned and a smaller, more tightly regulated promoter was identified which did not allow any detectable β-gal activity until after phage infection and expression levels of 11,000 β-gal units were obtained 120 min after induction.

Exploitation of Phage-Encoded Lysins

It is generally accepted that during cheese ripening, lysis of the starter culture results in the release of intracellular enzymes involved in flavor development (Crow et al., 1995). This prompted Shearman et al. (1992) to clone the lysin gene of øvML3 along with its upstream sequences, and introduce it into *L. lactis*. The strain grew normally during the log phase of growth, but once it entered into the stationary phase, it lysed spontaneously.

The lysin of øvML3 could therefore be used to construct recombinant starter cultures for accelerated cheese ripening.

More recently, De Ruyter et al. (1997) have cloned the holin and lysin genes of øUS3, under the tight control of the P_{nisA} promoter. In the absence of nisin expression of the lethal genes was completely repressed and so they were successfully maintained in *L. lactis*. Once nisin was added, the culture rapidly lysed, releasing its intracellular enzymes.

Site-Specific Integration Vectors

Development of strategies for the integration of DNA into the chromosome of LAB has relied on a cross-over event between the incoming cloned DNA on a non-replicating plasmid and a homologous segment of DNA on the host chromosome. However, integrative vectors have now been constructed based on the integration systems of the temperate lactococcal phages Tuc2009 (Van de Guchte et al., 1994b), TP901-1 (Christiansen et al., 1994), and øLC3 (Lillehaug et al., 1997). These systems are based on the integrase gene and phage attachment site sequence (*attP*) being cloned into suitable non-replicative vectors. Integration occurs between the cloned *attP* site and the chromosomal *attB* site. It has previously been described how the lactococcal phages r1t, øLC3, and Tuc2009 share identical *attB* sites indicating that integration vectors based on the integration systems of these phages may have widespread applications. Similar types of vectors have also been constructed based on the integration system of the *S. thermophilus* phage Sfi21 (Bruttin et al., 1997b) and the *Lactobacillus* phage mv4 (Dupont et al., 1995; Auvary et al., 1997), øadh (Raya et al., 1992; Fremaux et al., 1993) and A2 (Alvarez et al., 1998). Recently, the integrative apparatus of TP901-1 has been utilized to develop a system that facilitates integration into mammalian genomes (Stoll et al., 2002).

Concluding Remarks

Tremendous advances have been made in the last number of years into gaining a more thorough understanding of the biology of phages infecting LAB. This is due, in no small measure, to the accumulating sequence information currently available for these phages. The challenge now facing the food fermentation industry is how best to exploit this information to develop novel phage defence mechanisms which will target specific stages of the phage life-cycle, but which can also take into account the genetic plasticity of the phage genomes which allows it to rapidly counteract any resistance mechanisms that may be deployed against it.

References

Accolas, J. P., and Spillmann, H. (1979). The morphology of six bacteriophages of *Streptococcus thermophilus*. *Journal of Applied Bacteriology* 47: 135–144.

Ackermann, H.-W., and DuBow, M. S. (1987). *Viruses of prokaryotes* (Vol. I and II). Boca Raton, Florida: CRC Press, Inc.

Ackermann, H.-W., Elzanowski, A., Fobo, G., and Stewart, G. (1995). Relationships of tailed phages: A survey of protein sequence identity. *Archives of Virology* 140: 1871–1884.

Alatossava, T., and Klaenhammer, T. R. (1991). Molecular characterization of three small isometric-headed bacteriophages which vary in their sensitivity to the lactococcal phage resistance plasmid pTR2030. *Applied and Environmental Microbiology* 57: 1346–1353.

Alatossava, T., Forsman, P., and Ritzenthaler, P. (1995). Genome homology and superinfection immunity between temperate and virulent *Lactobacillus delbrueckii* bacteriophages. *Archives Virology* 140: 2261–2268.

Altermann, E., Klein, J. R., and Henrich, B. (1999). Primary structure and features of the genome of the *Lactobacillus gasseri* temperate bacteriophage øadh. *General* 236: 333–346.

Alvarez, M. A., Herrero, M., and Suárez, J. E. (1998). The site-specific recombination system of the *Lactobacillus* species bacteriophage A2 integrates in Gram-positive and Gram-negative bacteria. *Virology* 250: 185–193.

Alvarez, M. A., Rodriquez, A., and Suarez, J. E. (1999). Stable expression of the *Lactobacillus casei* bacteriophage A2 repressor blocks phage propagation during milk fermentation. *Journal of Applied Microbiology* 86: 812–816.

Arendt, E. K., and Hammes, W. P. (1992). Isolation and characterization of *Leuconostoc oenos* phages from German wines. *Applied Microbiology and Biotechnology* 37: 643–646.

Arendt, E. K., Daly, C., Fitzgerald, G. F., and Van de Guchte, M. (1994). Molecular characterisation of lactococcal bacteriophage Tuc2009 and identification and analysis of genes encoding lysin, a putative holin, and two structural proteins. *Applied and Environmental Microbiology* 60: 1875–1883.

Arendt, E. K., Lonvaud, A., and Hammes, W. P. (1991). Lysogeny in *Leuconostoc oenos*. *Journal of General Microbiology* 137: 2135–2139.

Auvray, F., Coddeville, M., Ritzenthaler, P., and Dupont, L. (1997). Plasmid integration in a wide range of bacteria mediated by the integrase of *Lactobacillus delbrueckii* bacteriophage mv4. *Journal of Bacteriology* 179: 1837–1845.

Axelsson, L. T. (1993). Lactic acid bacteria: Classification and physiology. In: S. Salminen and A. Wright (Eds.), *Lactic acid bacteria* (pp. 1–63). New York: Marcel Dekker, Inc.

Batt, C. A., Erlandson, K., and Bsat, N. (1995). Design and implementation of a strategy to reduce bacteriophage infection of dairy starter cultures. *International Dairy Journal* 5: 949–962.

Benbadis, L., Faelen, M., Slos, P., Fazel, A., and Mercenier, A. (1990). Characterisation and comparison of virulent bacteriophages of *Streptococcus thermophilus* isolated from yoghurt. *Biochimie* 72: 855–862.

Bidnenko, E., Ehrlich, S. D., and Chopin, M. C. (1995). Phage operon involved in sensitivity to *Lactococcus lactis* abortive infection mechanism AbiD1. *Journal of Bacteriology* 177: 3824–3829.

Birkeland, N.-K., and Holo, H. (1993). Transduction of a plasmid carrying the cohesive end region from *Lactococcus lactis* bacteriophage øLC3. *Applied and Environmental Microbiology* 59: 1966–1968.

Birkeland, N. K. (1994). Cloning, molecular characterization, and expression of the genes encoding the lytic functions of the lactococcal bacteriophage øLC3: A dual lysis system of modular design. *Canadian Journal of Microbiology* 40: 658–665.

Black, L. W. (1989). DNA packaging in dsDNA bacteriophages. *Annual Review of Microbiology* 43: 267–292.

Bläsi, U., and Young, R. (1996). Two beginnings for a single purpose: The dual start holins in the regulation of phage lysis. *Molecular Microbiology* 21: 675–682.

Blatny, J. M., Risoen, P. A., Lillehaug, D., Lunde, M., and Nes, I. F. (2001). Analysis of a regulator involved in the genetic switch between lysis and lysogeny of the temperate *Lactococcus lactis* phage phi LC3. *Molecular Genetic Genomics* 265: 189–197.

Boizet, B., Lahbibmansis, Y., Dupont, L., Ritzenthaler, P., and Mata, M. (1990). Cloning, expression and sequence analysis of an endolysin-encoding gene of *Lactobacillus bulgaricus* bacteriophage mv1. *General* 94: 61–67.

Boizet, B., Mata, M., Mignot, O., and Ritzenthaler, P. (1992). Taxonomic characterization of *Leuconostoc oenos* bacteriophage. *FEMS Microbiology Letters* 90: 211–216.

Botstein, D. (1980). A theory of modular evolution for bacteriophages. *Annuals of the New York Academy of Sciences* 354: 484–491.

Boyce, J. D., Davison, B. E., and Hillier, A. J. (1995a) Identification of prophage genes expressed in lysogens of the *Lactococcus lactis* bacteriophage BK5-T. *Applied and Environmental Microbiology* 61: 4099–4104.

Boyce, J. D., Davison, B. E., and Hillier, A. J. (1995b). Spontaneous deletion mutants of the *Lactococcus lactis* temperate bacteriophage BK5-T and localization of the BK5-T *attP* site. *Applied and Environmental Microbiology* 61: 4105–4109.

Boyce, J. D., Davison, B. E., and Hillier, A. J. (1995c). Sequence analysis of the *Lactococcus lactis* temperate bacteriophage BK5-T and demonstration that the phage DNA has cohesive ends. *Applied and Environmental Microbiology* 61: 4089–4098.

Bradley, D. E. (1967). A review: Ultrastructure of bacteriophage and bacteriocins. *Bacteriology Review* 31: 230–314.

Braun, V., Hertwig, S., Neve, H., Geis, A., and Teuber, M. (1989). Taxonomic differentiation of bacteriophages of *Lactococcus lactis* by electron microscopy, DNA–DNA-hybridisation, and protein profiles. *Journal of General Microbiology* 135: 2551–2560.

Brondsted, L., and Hammer, K. (1999). Use of the integration elements encoded by the temperate lactococcal bacteriophage TP901-1 to obtain chromosomal single-copy transcriptional fusions in *Lactococcus lactis*. *Applied and Environmental Microbiology* 65: 752–758.

Brüssow, H., and Bruttin, A. (1995). Characterisation of a temperate *Streptococcus thermophilus* bacteriophage and its genetic relationship with lytic phages. *Virology* 212: 532–640.

Brüssow, H., Bruttin, A., Desiere, F., Lucchini, S., and Foley, S. (1998). Molecular ecology and evolution of *Streptococcus thermophilus* bacteriophages-a review. *Virus Genes* 16: 95–109.

Brüssow, H., Frémont, M., Bruttin, A., Sidoti, J., Constable, A., and Fryder, V. (1994a). Detection and classification of *Streptococcus thermophilus* bacteriophages isolated from industrial milk fermentation. *Applied and Environmental Microbiology* 60: 4537–4543.

Brüssow, H., Probst, A., Frémont, M., and Sidoti, J. (1994b). Distinct *Streptococcus thermophilus* bacteriophages share an extremely conserved DNA fragment. *Virology* 200: 854–857.

Brüssow, H. (2001). Phages of dairy bacteria. *Annual Review of Microbiology* 55: 283–303.

Brüssow, H., and Hendrix, R. W. (2002). Phage genomics: Small is beautiful. *Cell* 108: 13–16.

Brüssow, H., and Desiere, F. (2001). Comparative phage genomics and the evolution of *Siphoviridae*: Insights from dairy phages. *Molecular Microbiology* 39: 213–222.

Breüner, A., Brøndsted, L., and Hammer, K. (1999) Novel organization of genes involved in prophage excision identified in the temperate lactococcal bacteriophage TP901-1. *Journal of Bacteriology* 181: 7291–7297.

Bruttin, A., and Brüssow, H. (1996). Site-specific spontaneous deletions in three genome regions of a temperate *Streptococcus thermophilus* phage. *Virology* 219: 96–104.

Bruttin, A., Desiere, F., Lucchini, S., Foley, S., and Brüssow, H. (1997a). Characterisation of the lysogeny DNA module from the temperate *Streptococcus thermophilus* bacteriophage øSfi21. *Virology* 223: 136–148.

Bruttin, A., Foley, S., and Brüssow, H. (1997b). The site-specific integration system of the temperate *Streptococcus thermophilus* bacteriophage øSfi21. *Virology* 237: 148–158.

Budde-Niekiel, A., and Teuber, M. (1987). Electron microscopy of the adsorption of bacteriophages to lactic acid streptococci. *Milchwissenschaft* 42: 551–554.

Callanan, M. J., O'Toole, P. W., Lubbers, M. W., and Polzin, K. M. (2001). Examination of lactococcal bacteriophage c2 DNA replication using two-dimensional agarose gel electrophoresis. *Gene* 278: 101–106.

Campbell, A. M. (1988). Phage evolution and speciation. In: R. Calendar (Ed.), *The bacteriophages* (pp. 1–14). New York: Plenum Press.

Campbell, A. M. (1992). Chromosomal insertion sites for phages and plasmids. *Journal of Bacteriology* 174: 7495–7499.

Campbell, A. M. (1994). Comparative molecular biology of lambdoid phages. *Annual Review of Microbiology* 48: 193–222.

Carminati, D., and Giraffa, G. (1992). Evidence and characterization of temperate bacteriophage in *Streptococcus salivarius* subsp. *thermophilus* St18. *Journal of Dairy Research* 59: 71–79.

Casjens, S., and Hendrix, R. (1974). Comments on the arrangement of the morphogenetic genes of bacteriophage lambda. *Journal of Molecular Biology* 90: 20–23.

Casjens, S., Hatful, G., and Hendrix, R. (1992). Evolution of dsDNA tailed-bacteriophage genomes. *Seminars in Virology* 3: 383–397.

Chai, S., Bravo, A., Lüder, G., Nedlin, A., Trauter, T. A., and Alonso, J. C. (1992). Molecular analysis of the *Bacillus subtilis* bacteriophage SPP1 region encompassing genes 1 to 6. *Journal of Molecular Biology* 224: 87–102.

Chandry, P. S., Moore, S. C., Boyce, J. D., Davidson, B. E., and Hillier, A. J. (1997). Analysis of the DNA sequence, gene expression, origin of replication and modular structure of the *Lactococcus lactis* bacteriophage sk1. *Molecular Microbiology* 26: 49–64.

Chandry, P. S., Moore, S. C., Davidson, B. E., and Hillier, A. J. (1994). Analysis of the *cos* region of the *Lactococcus lactis* bacteriophage sk1. *Gene* 138: 123–126.

Chopin, A., Bolotin, A., Sorokin, A., Ehrlich, S. D., and Chopin, M. C. (2001). Analysis of six prophages in *Lactococcus lactis* IL1403: Different genetic structure of temperate and virulent phage populations. *Nucleic Acids Research* 29: 644–651.

Christiansen, B., Brondsted, L., Vogensen, F. K., and Hammer, K. (1996). A resolvase-like protein is required for the site-specific integration of the temperate lactococcal bacteriophage TP901-1. *Journal of Bacteriology* 178: 5164–5173.

Christiansen, B., Johsen, M. G., Stenby, E., Vogensen, F. K., and Hammer, K. (1994). Characterization of the lactococcal temperate phage TP901-1 and its site specific integration. *Journal of Bacteriology* 176: 1069–1076.

Chung, D. K., Chung, S. K., and Batt, C. A. (1992). Antisense RNA directed against the major capsid protein of *Lactococcus lactis* subsp. *cremoris* bacteriophage 4–1 confers partial resistance to the host. *Applied Microbiological Biotechnology* 37: 79–83.

Chung, D. K., Kim, J. K., and Batt, C. A. (1991). Cloning and nucleotide sequences of the major capsid protein from *Lactococcus lactis* spp. *cremoris* bacteriophage F4-1. *Gene* 101: 121–125.

Crow, V. L., Coolbear, T., Gopal, P. K., Martley, F. G., McKay, L. L., and Riepe, H. (1995). The role of autolysis of lactic acid bacteria in the ripening of cheese. *International Dairy Journal* 5: 855–895.

Crutz-Le Coq, M., Cesselin, B., Commissaire, J., and Anba, J. (2002). Sequence analysis of the lactococcal bacteriophage bIL 170: Insights into structural proteins and HNH endonucleases in dairy phages. *Microbiology* 148: 985–1001.

d' Hérelle, F. (1917). Sur un microbe invisible antagonistic des bacilles dysenteriques. *Comptes Rendies de & ances de L'Academic des Sciences, Paris* 165: 373–375.

Daly, C., Fitzgerald, G. F., and Davis, R. (1996). Biotechnology of lactic acid bacteria with special reference to bacteriophage resistance. *Antonie van Leeuwenhoek* 70: 99–110.

Davidson, B. E., Kordias, N., Dobos, M., and Hillier, A. J. (1996). Genomic organization of lactic acid bacteria. *Antonie van Leeuwenhoek* 70: 161–183.

Davidson, B. E., Powell, I. B., and Hillier, A. J. (1990). Temperate bacteriophages and lysogeny in lactic acid bacteria. *FEMS Microbiology Review* 87: 79–90.

De Ruyter, P. G. G. A., Kuipers, O. P., Meijer, W. C., and de Vos, W. M. (1997). Food-grade controlled lysis of *Lactococcus lactis* for accelerated cheese ripening. *Nature Biotechnology* 15: 976–979.

Deane, D. D., Nelson, F. E., Ryser, F. C., and Carr, P. H. (1953). *Streptococcus thermophilus* bacteriophage from Swiss cheese whey. *Journal of Dairy Science* 36: 185–191.

Desiere, F., Lucchini, S., and Brüssow, H. (1998). Evolution of *Streptococcus thermophilus* bacteriophage genomes by modular exchanges followed by point mutations and small deletions and insertions. *Virology* 241: 345–356.

Desiere, F., Lucchini, S., and Brüssow, H. (1999). Comparative sequence analysis of the DNA packaging, head and tail morphogenesis modules in the temperate *cos*-site *Streptococcus thermophilus* bacteriophage Sfi21. *Virology* 260: 244–253.

Desiere, F., Lucchini, S., Bruttin, A., Zwahlen, M. C., and Brüssow, H. (1997). A highly conserved DNA replication module from *Streptococcus thermophilus* phages is similar in sequence and topology to a module from *Lactococcus lactis* phages. *Virology* 234: 372–382.

Desiere, F., Lucchini, S., Canchaya, C., Ventura, M., and Brüssow, H. (2000). Comparative genomics of phages and prophages in lactic acid bacteria. *Antoine van Leeuwenhoek* 82: 73–91.

Desiere, F., Mahanivong, C., Hillier, A. J., Chandry, P. S., Davidson, B. E., and Brüssow, H. (2001a). Comparative genomics of lactococcal phages: Insight from the complete genome sequence of *Lactococcus lactis phage* BK5-T. *Virology* 283: 240–252.

Desiere, F., McShan, W. M., van Sinderen, D., Ferretti, J. J., and Brüssow, H. (2001b). Comparative genomics reveals close genetic relationships between phages from dairy bacteria and pathogenic Streptococci: Evolutionary implications for prophage-host interactions. *Virology* 288: 325–341.

Desiere, F., Pridmore, R. D., and Brüssow, H. (2000). Comparative genomics of the late gene cluster from *Lactobacillus* phages. *Virology* 275: 294–305.

Días, E., Munthali, M., Lünsdorf, H., Höltje, J. V., and Timmis, K. N. (1996). The two step lysis system of pneumococcal bacteriophage Ej-1 is functional in Gram-negative bacteria: triggering of the major pneumococcal autolysin in *E. coli*. *Molecular Microbiology* 19: 667–681.

Díaz, E., López, R., and García, J. L. (1992). EJ-1, a temperate bacteriophage of *Streptococcus pneumoniae* with a *Myoviridae* morphotype. *Journal of Bacteriology* 174: 5516–5525.

Dicks, L. M. T., Dellaglio, F., and Collins, M. D. (1995). Proposal to reclassify *Leuconostoc oenos* as *Oenococcus oeni*. *International Journal of Systematic Bacteriology* 45: 375–397.

Djordjevic, G. M., and Klaenhammer, T. R. (1997). Bacteriophage-triggered defence systems: Phage adaptation and design improvements. *Applied and Environmental Microbiology* 63: 4370–4376.

Djordjevic, G. M., O'Sullivan, D. J., Walker, S. A., Conkling, M. A., and Klaenhammer, T. R. (1997). A triggered-suicide system designed as a defence against bacteriophage. *Journal of Bacteriology* 179: 6741–6748.

Dube, P., Tavares, P., Lurz, R., and van Heel, M. (1993). The portal protein of bacteriophage SPP1: A DNA pump with 13-fold symmetry. *EMBO Journal* 12: 1303–1309.

Dupont, L., Boizet-Bonhoure, B., Coddeville, M., Auvray, F., and Ritzenthaler, P. (1995). Characterisation of genetic elements required for site-specific integration of *Lactobacillus delbrueckii* subsp. *bulgaricus* bacteriophage mv4 and construction of an integration-proficient vector for *Lactobacillus plantarum*. *Journal of Bacteriology* 177: 586–595.

Duplessis, M., and Moineau, S. (2001). Identification of a genetic determinant responsible for host specificity in *Streptococcus thermophilus bacteriophages. Molecular Microbiology* 41: 325–336.

Engel, G., Altermann, E., Klein, J. R., and Henrich, B. (1998). Structure of a genome region of the *Lactobacillus gasseri* temperate phage øadh covering a repressor gene and cognate promoters. *Gene* 210: 61–70.

Fayard, B., Haeflinger, M., and Accolas, J. P. (1993). Interaction of temperate bacteriophages of *Streptococcus salivarius* subsp. *thermophilus* with lysogenic indicators affect phage DNA restriction patterns and host ranges. *Journal of Dairy Science* 60: 385–399.

Foley, S., Lucchini, S., Zwahlen, M.-C., Sidoti, J., and Brüssow, H. (1998). A short non-coding viral DNA element showing characteristics of a replication origin confers bacteriophage resistance to *Streptococcus thermophilus. Virology* 250: 377–387.

Foley, S., Bruttin, A., and Brüssow, H. (2000). Widespread distribution of a group I intron and its three deletion derivatives in the lysin gene of *Streptococcus thermophilus* bacteriophages. *Journal of Virology* 74: 611–618.

Forde, A., and Fitzgerald, G. F. (1999). Bacteriophage defence systems in lactic acid bacteria. In: W. N. Konings, O. P. Kuipers, and J. H. J. Huisin'tveld (Eds.), *Proceedings of the sixth symposium on Lactic acid bacteria*. Veldhoven, The Netherlands: Kluwer Academic Publishers.

Forsman, P. (1993). Characterization of a prolate-headed bacteriophage of *Lactobacillus delbrueckii* subsp. *lactis* and its DNA homology with isometric-headed phages. *Archives Virology* 132: 321–330.

Forsman, P., and Alatossava, T. (1991). Genetic variation of *Lactobacillus deldrueckii* subsp. *lactis* bacteriophage isolated from cheese processing plants in Finland. *Applied and Environmental Microbiology* 57: 1805–1812.

Fremaux, C., De Antoni, G. L., Raya, R. R., and Klaenhammer, T. (1993). Genetic organization and sequence of the region encoding integrative functions from *Lactobacillus gasseri* temperate bacteriophage øadh. *Gene* 126: 61–66.

Fuller, R. S., Funnell, B. E., and Kornberg, A. (1984). The DnaA protein complex with *E. coli* chromosomal replication origin (*ori*C) and other DNA sites. *Cell* 38: 889–900.

Furth, M. E., and Wickner, S. H. (1983). In: R. W. Hendrix, J. W. Roberts, F. W. Stahl, and R. A. Weisberg (Eds.), *LambdaII* (pp. 145–173). Cold Spring Harbor, NY: Cold Spring Harbor Laboratory Press.

García, P., Alonso, J. C., and Suárez, J. E. (1997). Molecular analysis of the *cos* region of the *Lactobacillus casei* bacteriophage A2. Gene product 3, gp3 specifically binds to its downstream *cos* region. *Molecular Microbiology* 23: 505–514.

García, P., García, J. L., García, E., Sánchez-Puelles, J. M., and López, R. (1990). Modular organisation of the lytic enzymes of *Streptococcus pneumoniae* and its bacteriophages. *Gene* 86: 81–88.

García, P., Ladero, V., Alonso, J. C., and Suárez, J. E. (1999). Cooperative interaction of CI protein regulates lysogeny of *Lactobacillus casei* by bacteriophage A2. *Journal of Virology* 73: 3920–3929.

Garvey, P., van Sinderen, D., Twomey, D. P., Hill, C., and Fitzgerald, G. F. (1995). Molecular genetics of bacteriophage and natural phage defence systems in the genus *Lactococcus*. *International Dairy Journal* 5: 905–947.

Gasson, M. J. (1996). Lytic systems in lactic acid bacteria and their bacteriophages. *Antonie van Leeuwenhoek* 10: 147–159.

Geis, A. (1992). Cloning and DNA sequence analysis of a lysin gene of lactococcal bacteriophage P001. In: *Annual report 1991* (p. B94). Kiel, Germany: Federal Dairy Research Centre.

Gindreau, E., and Lonvaud-Funel, A. (1999). Molecular analysis of the region encoding the lytic systems from *Oenococcus oeni* temperate bacteriophage ø10MC. *FEMS Microbiology Letters* 171: 231–238.

Gindreau, E., Torlois, S., and Lonvaud-Funel, A. (1997). Identification and sequence analysis of the region encoding the site-specific integration system from *Leuconostoc oenos (Œnococcus œni)* temperate bacteriophage ø10MC. *FEMS Microbiology Letters* 147: 279–285.

Gottesman, M. E., and Weisberg, R. A. (1971). Prophage insertion and excision. In: A. D. Hershey (Ed.), *The bacteriophage Lambda* (pp. 113–138). Cold Spring Harbor, NY: Cold Spring Harbour Laboratory.

Grainge, I., and Jayaram, M. (1999). The integrase family of recombinases: Organization and function of the active site. *Molecular Microbiology* 33: 449–456.

Graschopf, A., and Bläsi, U. (1999). Molecular function of the dual-start motif of the λ S holin. *Molecular Microbiology* 33: 569–582.

Guo, P., Grimes, S., and Anderson, D. (1986). A defined system for *in vitro* packaging of DNA-gp3 of the *Bacillus subtilis* bacteriophage ø29. *Proceding of the National Academy of Sciences, USA* 83: 3505–3509.

Hamada, K., Fujisawa, H., and Minagawa, T. (1986). A defined *in vitro* system for packaging of bacteriophage T3 DNA. *Virology* 151: 119–123.

Hatfull, G. F., and Sarkis, G. J. (1993). DNA sequence, structure and gene expression of mycobacteriophage L5: A phage system for mycobacterial genetics. *Molecular Microbiology* 7: 395–405.

Hauser, M. A., and Scocca, J. J. (1990). Location of the host attachment site for phage HP1 within a cluster of *Haemophilus influenza* tRNA genes. *Nucleic Acid Research* 18: 5305.
Hayashida, M., Watanabe, K., Muramatsu, T., and Goto, M. A. (1987). Further characterization of PL-1 phage-associated *N*-acetylmuramidase of *Lactobacillus casei*. *Journal of General Microbiology* 133: 1343–1349.
Henrich, B., Binishofer, B., and Bläsi, U. (1995). Primary structure and functional analysis of the lysis genes of *Lactobacillus gasseri* bacteriophage øadh. *Journal of Bacteriology* 177: 723–732.
Highton, P. J., Chang, Y., and Myers, R. (1990). Evidence for the exchange of segments between genomes during the evolution of lambdoid bacteriophages. *Molecular Microbiology* 4: 1329–1340.
Hill, C., Miller, L. A., and Klaenhammer, T. R. (1990). Cloning, expression, and sequence determination of a bacteriophage fragment encoding bacteriophage resistance in *Lactococcus lactis*. *Journal of Bacteriology* 172: 6419–6426.
Hill, C., Miller, L. A., and Klaenhammer, T. R. (1991). *In vitro* genetic exchange of a functional domain from a type II A methylase between lactococcal plasmid pTR2030 and a virulent bacteriophage. *Journal of Bacteriology* 173: 4363–4370.
Huggins, A. R., and Sandine, W. E. (1977). Incidence and properties of temperate bacteriophages induced from lactic streptococci. *Applied and Environmental Microbiology* 33: 184–191.
Jarvis, A. W. (1984). DNA–DNA homology between streptococci and their temperate and lytic phage. *Applied Environmental Microbiology* 47: 1031–1038.
Jarvis, A. W. (1989). Bacteriophages of lactic acid bacteria. *Journal of Dairy Science* 72: 3406–3428.
Jarvis, A. W., Fitzgerald, G. F., Mata, M., Mercenier, A., Neve, H., Powell, I. B., Ronda, C., Saxelin, M., and Teuber, M. (1991). Species and type phages of lactococcal bacteriophages. *Intervirology* 32: 2–9.
Jarvis, A. W., Lubbers, M. W., Beresford, T. P., Ward, L. J., Waterfield, N. R., Collins, L. J., and Jarvis, B. D. (1995a). Molecular biology of lactococcal bacteriophage c2. *Developments in Biological Standardization* 85: 561–567.
Jarvis, A. W., Lubbers, M. W., Waterfield, N. R., Collins, L. J., and Polzin, K. M. (1995b). Sequencing and analysis of the genome of Lactococcal phage c2. *International Dairy Journal* 5: 963–976.
Johnsen, M. G., Appel, K. F., Madsen, P. L., Vogensen, F. K., Hammer, K., and Arnau, J. (1996). A genomic region of the lactococcal temperate bacteriophage TP901-1 encoding major virion proteins. *Virology* 218: 306–315.
Johnsen, M. G., Neve, H., Vogensen, F. K., and Hammer, K. (1995). Virion positions and relationships of lactococcal temperate bacteriophage TP901-1 proteins. *Virology* 212: 595–606.
Josephsen, J., and Neve, H. (1998). Bacteriophages and lactic acid bacteria. In: Seppo Sabminen and Atte Von Wright (Eds.), *Lactic acid bacteria, microbiology and functional aspects* (pp. 385–436). New York: Marcel Dekker, Inc.
Kakikawa, M., Oki, M., Tadokoro, H., Nakamura, S., Taketo, A., and Kodaira, K.-I. (1996). Cloning and nucleotide sequence of the major capsid proteins of *Lactobacillus* bacteriophage øg1e. *Gene* 175: 157–165.
Kakikawa, M., Oki, M., Watanabe, N., Yasukawa, H., Masamune, Y., Taketo, A., and Kodaira, K.-I. (1997). Characterization of the genes encoding integrative and excisive functions of *Lactobacillus* phage øg1e: Cloning, sequence analysis, and expression in *Escherichia coli*. *Gene* 185: 119–125.
Kakikawa, M., Watanabe, N., Funawatashi, T., Oki, M., Yasukawa, H., Taketo, A., and Kodaira, K.-I. (1998). Promoter/repressor system of *Lactobacillus plantarum* phage øg1e: Characterization of the promoters *pR49–pR–pL* and overproduction of the Cro-like protein Cng in *Escherichia coli*. *Gene* 215: 371–379.
Kakikawa, M., Ohkubo, S., Sakate, T., Sayama, M., Taketo, A., and Kodaira, K. (2000a). Purification and DNA-binding properties of the cro-type regulatory repressor protein cng encoded by the *Lactobacillus plantarum* phage phi g1e. *Gene* 249: 161–169.
Kakikawa, M., Ohkubo, S., Syama, M., Taketo, A., and Kodaira, K. I. (2000b). The genetic switch for the regulatory pathway of *Lactobacillus plantarum* phage g1e: Characterization of the promoter P(L), the repressor gene *cpg*, and the *cpg*-encoded protein Cpg in *Escherichia coli*. *Gene* 242: 155–166.
Kiliç, A. O., Pavlova, S. I., Ma, W.-G., and Tao, L. (1996). Analysis of *Lactobacillus* phages and bacteriocins in American dairy products and characterisation of a phage isolated from yogurt. *Applied and Environmental Microbiology* 62: 2111–2116.
Kim, S. G., and Batt, C. A. (1991a). Identification of a nucleotide sequence conserved in *Lactococcus lactis* bacteriophages. *Gene* 98: 95–100.
Kim, S. G., and Batt, C. A. (1991b). Molecular characterisation of a *Lactococcus lactis* bacteriophage F4-1. *Food Microbiology* 8: 15–26.
Kim, S. G., and Batt, C. A. (1991c). Antisense mRNA-mediated bacteriophage resistance in *Lactococcus lactis*. *Applied and Environmental Microbiology* 57: 1109–1113.
Kim, S. G., Bor, Y.-C., and Batt, C. A. (1992). Bacteriophage resistance in *Lactococcus lactis* spp. *lactis* using antisense ribonucleic acid. *Journal of Dairy Science* 75: 1761–1767.

Kivi, S., Peltomaki, T., Luomala, K., and Sarimo, S. S. (1987). Some properties of *Streptococcus thermophilus* bacteriophages. *Folia Microbiology* 32: 106–106.

Klaenhammer, T. R., and Fitzgerald, G. F. (1994). Bacteriophages and bacteriophage resistance. In: M. J. Gasson and W. de Vos (Eds.), *Genetics and biotechnology of lactic acid bacteria* (pp. 106–168). Glasgow: Blackie Academic and Professional.

Kodaira, K.-I., Oki, M., Kakikawa, M., Watanabe, N., Hirakawa, M., Yamada, K., and Taketo, A. (1997). Genome structure of the *Lactobacillus* temperate phage øg1e: The whole genome sequence and the putative promoter repressor system. *Gene* 187: 45–53.

Kornberg, A., and Baker, T. A. (1992). In: *DNA replication*. New York: W. H. Freeman and Company.

Krusch, U., Neve, H., Luschei, B., and Teuber, M. (1987). Characterisation of a virulent bacteriophage of *Streptococcus salivarius* subsp. *thermophilus* by host specificity and electron microscopy. *Kiel Milchwirtsch Forschungsber* 39: 155–167.

Labrie, S., and Moineau, S. (2002). Complete genomic sequence of bacteriophage ul36: Demonstration of phage heterogeneity within the P335 quasi-species of lactococcal phages. *Virology* 296: 308–320.

Ladero, V., García, P., Bascarán, V., Herrero, M., Álvarez, M. A., and Suárez, J. E. (1998). Identification of the repressor-encoding gene of the *Lactobacillus* bacteriophage A2. *Journal of Bacteriology* 180: 3474–3476.

Ladero, V., Garcia, P., Alonso, J. C., and Suarez, J. E. (1999). A2 cro, the lysogenic cycle repressor, specifically binds to the genetic switch region of *Lactobacillus casei* bacteriophage A2. *Virology* 262: 220–229.

Lahbib-Mansais, Y., Mata, M., and Ritzenthaler, P. (1988). Molecular taxonomy of *Lactobacillus* phages. *Biochimie* 70: 429–435.

Landy, A., and Ross, W. (1977). Viral integration and excision. Structure of the λ *att* sites. *Science* 197: 1147–1160.

Larbi, D., Colurin, C., Rouselle, L., Decaris, B., and Simonet, J. M. (1990). Genetic and biological characterisation of nine *Streptococcus salivarius* subsp. *thermophilus* bacteriophages. *Lait* 70: 107–116.

Lautier, M., and Novel, G. (1987). DNA–DNA hybridization in lactic streptococcal temperate and virulent phages belonging to distinct groups. *Journal of Industrial Microbiology* 2: 151–158.

Le Marrec, C., van Sinderen, D., Walsh, L., Stanley, E., Vlegels, E., Moineau, S., Heinze, P., Fitzgerald, G., and Fayard, B. (1997). *Streptococcus thermophilus* bacteriophages can be divided into two distinct groups based on mode of packaging and structural protein composition. *Applied and Environmental Microbiology* 63: 3246–3253.

Lillehaug, D., and Birkeland, N.-K. (1993). Characterization of genetic elements required for site-specific integration of the temperate lactococcal bacteriophage øLC3 and construction of integration-negative øLC3 mutants. *Journal of Bacteriology* 175: 1745–1755.

Lillehaug, D., Lindqvist, B. H., and Birkeland, N. K. (1991). Characterization of øLC3, a *Lactococcus lactis* ssp. *cremoris* temperate bacteriophage with cohensive single-stranded ends. *Applied and Environmental Microbiology* 57: 3206–3211.

Lillehaug, D., Nes, I. F., and Birkeland, N. K. (1997). A highly efficient and stable system for site-specific integration of genes and plasmids into the phage øLC3 attachment site (*attB*) of the *Lactococcus lactis* chromosome. *Gene* 188: 129–136.

Little, J. W. (1993). LexA cleavage and other self-processing reactions. *Journal of Bacteriology* 175: 4943–4950.

Lubbers, M. W., Waterfield, N. R., Beresford, T. P. J., Le Page, R. W. J., and Jarvis, A. J. (1995). Sequencing and analysis of the prolate-headed lactococcal bacteriophage c2 genome and identification of the structural genes. *Applied and Environmental Microbiology* 61: 4348–4356.

Lucchini, S., Desiere, F., and Brüssow, H. (1998). The structural gene module in *Streptococcus thermophilus* bacteriophage øSfi11 shows a hierarchy of relatedness to Siphoviridae from a wide range of bacterial hosts. *Virology* 246: 63–73.

Lucchini, S., Desiere, F., and Brüssow, H. (1999a). The genetic relationship between virulent and temperate *Streptococcus thermophilus* bacteriophages: Whole genome comparison of *cos*-site phages øSfi19 and øSfi21. *Virology* 260: 232–243.

Lucchini, S., Desiere, F., and Brüssow, H. (1999b). Comparative genomics of *Streptococcus thermophilus* phage species supports a modular evolution theory. *Journal of Virology* 73: 8647–8656.

Lucchini, S., Desiere, F., and Brüssow, H. (1999c). Similarly organized lysogeny modules in temperate *Siphoviridae* from low GC content Gram-positive bacteria. *Virology* 263: 427–435.

Madsen, P. L., and Hammer, K. (1998). Temporal transcription of the lactococcal temperate phage TP901-1 and DNA sequence of the early promoter region. *Microbiology* 144: 2203–2215.

Madsen, P. L., Johansen, A. H., Hammer, K., and Brøndsted, L. (1999). The genetic switch regulating activity of early promoters of the temperate lactococcal bacteriophage TP901-1. *Journal of Bacteriology* 181: 7430–7438.

Madsen, S. M., Mills, D., Djordjevic, G., Israelsen, H., and Klaenhammer, T. R. (2001). Analysis of the genetic switch and replication region of a P335-type bacteriophage with an obligate lytic lifestyle on *Lactococcus lactis*. *Applied and Environmental Microbiology* 67: 1128–1139.
Marians, K. J. (1992). Prokaryotic DNA replication. *Annual Review of Biochemistry* 61: 673–719.
Mata, M., and Ritzenthaler, P. (1988). Present state of lactic acid bacteria phage taxonomy. *Biochimie* 70: 395–399.
Mata, M., Trautwetter, A., Luthaud, G., and Ritzenthaler, P. (1986). Thirteen virulent and temperate bacteriophages of *Lactobacillus bulgaricus* and *Lactobacillus lactis* belong to a single DNA homology group. *Applied and Environmental Microbiology* 52: 812–818.
Martín, A. C., López, R., and García P. (1996). Analysis of the complete nucleotide sequence and functional organisation of the genome of Streptococcus pneumonia bacteriophage cp-1. *Journal of Virology* 70: 3678–3687.
Martín, M. C., Alonso, J. C., Suárez, J. E., and Alvarez, M. A. (2000). Generation of food-grade recombinant lactic acid bacterium strains by site-specific recombination. *Applied and Environmental Microbiology* 66: 2599–2604.
Matthews, K. (1992). DNA looping. *Microbiology Review* 56: 123–136.
Matz, K., Schmandt, M., and Gussin, G. N. (1982). The rex gene of bacteriophage lambda is really two genes. *Genetics* 102: 319–327.
McGrath, S., Seegers, J. F. M., Fitzgerald, G. F., and van Sinderen, D. (1999). Molecular characterisation of a phage-encoded resistance system in *Lactococcus lactis*. *Applied and Environmental Microbiology* 65: 1891–1899.
McGrath, S., Fitzgerald, G. F., and van Sinderen, D. (2001). Improvement and optimization of two engineered phage resistance mechanisms in *Lactococcus lactis*. *Applied and Environmental Microbiology* 67: 608–616.
McGrath, S., Fitzgerald, G. F., and van Sinderen, D. (2002a). Identification and characterization of phage-resistance genes in temperate lactococcal bacteriophages. *Molecular Microbiology* 43: 509–520.
McGrath, S., van Sinderen, D., and Fitzgerald, G. F. (2002b). Bacteriophage-derived genetic tools for use in lactic acid bacteria. *International Dairy Journal* 12: 3–15.
McKay, L. L., and Baldwin, K. A. (1990). Applications for Biotechnology: Present and future improvements in lactic acid bacteria. *FEMS Microbiology Review* 87: 3–14.
McShan, W. M., Tang, Y. F., and Ferretti, J. J. (1997). Bacteriophage T12 of *Streptococcus pyogenes* integrates into the gene encoding a serine tRNA. *Molecular Microbiology* 23: 719–728.
Mercenier, A., Pouwels, P. H., and Chassy, B. M. (1994). Genetic engineering of lactobacilli, leuconostoc and *Streptococcus thermophilus*. In: M. J. Gasson and W. M. de Vos (Eds.), *Genetic and biotechnology of lactic acid bacteria* (pp. 252–293). Glasgow: Blackie Academic and Professional.
Mikkonen, M., and Alatossava, T. (1994). Characterization of the genome region encoding structural proteins of *Lactobacillus delbrueckii* subsp. *lactis* phage LL-H. *Gene* 151: 53–59.
Mikkonen, M., and Alatossava, T. (1995). A group I intron in the terminase gene of *Lactobacillus delbrueckii* subsp. *lactis* phage LL-H. *Microbiology* 141: 2183–2190.
Mikkonen, M., Dupont, L., Alatossava, T., and Ritzenthaler, P. (1996a). Defective site-specific integration elements are present in the genome of virulent bacteriophage LL-H of *lactobacillus delbrueckii*. *Applied and Environmental Microbiology* 62: 1847–1851.
Mikkonen, M., Räisänen, L., and Alatossava, T. (1996b). The early region completes the nucleotide sequence of *Lactobacillus delbrueckii* subsp. *lactis* phage LL-H. *Gene* 175: 49–57.
Missich, R., Weise, F., Chai, S., Lurz, R., Pedré, X., and Alonso, J. C. (1997). The replisome organizer (G38P) of *Bacillus subtilis* bacteriophage SPP1 forms specialized nucleoprotein complexes with two discrete distant regions of the SPP1 genome. *Journal of Molecular Biology* 270: 50–64.
Moineau, S., Fortier, J., Ackermann, H. W., and Pandian, S. (1992). Characterization of lactococcal bacteriophages from Quebec cheese plants. *Canadian Journal of Microbiology* 38: 875–882.
Moineau, S., Pandian, S., and Klaenhammer, T. R. (1994). Evolution of a lytic bacteriophage via DNA acquisition from the *Lactococcus lactis* chromosome. *Applied and Environmental Microbiology* 60: 1832–1841.
Moscoso, M., and Suarez, J. E. (2000). Characterization of the DNA replication module of bacteriophage A2 and use of its origin of replication as a defense against infection during milk fermentation by *Lactobacillus casei*. *Virology* 273: 101–111.
Nakashima, Y., Ikeda, H., Kakita, Y., Miake, F., and Watanabe, K. (1994). Restriction map of the genomic DNA of *Lactobacillus casei* bacteriophage PL-1 and nucleotide sequence of its cohesive single-stranded ends. *Journal of General Virology* 75: 2537–2541.
Nauta, A., van de Burg, B., Karsens, H., Venema, G., and Kok, J. (1997). Design of thermolabile bacteriophage repressor mutants by comparative molecular modeling. *Nature Biotechnology* 15: 980–983.

Nauta, A., van Sinderen, D., Karsens, H., Smit, E., Venema, G., and Kok, J. (1996). Inducible gene expression mediated by a repressor–operator system isolated from *Lactococcus lactis* bacteriophage r1t. *Molecular Microbiology* 19: 1331–1341.

Neve, H. (1996). Bacteriophage. In: T. M. Cogan and J. P. Accolas (Eds.), *Dairy starter cultures* (pp. 157–189). New York: VCH Publishers.

Neve, H., Krusch, U., and Teuber, M. (1989). Classification of virulent bacteriophages of *Streptococcus salivarius* subsp. *thermophilus* isolated from yoghurt and Swiss-type cheese. *Applied Microbiology and Biotechnology* 30: 624–629.

Neve, H., Zenz, K. I., Desiere, F., Koch, A., Heller, K. J., and Brüssow, H. (1998). Comparison of the lysogeny modules from the temperate *Streptococcus thermophilus* bacteriophages TP-J34 and øSfi21: Implications for the modular theory of phage evolution. *Virology* 241: 61–72.

O'Sullivan, D. J., Hill, C., and Klaenhammer, T. R. (1993). Effect of increasing the copy number of bacteriophage origins of replication, in *trans*, on incoming-phage proliferation. *Applied and Environmental Microbiology* 59: 2449–2456.

O'Sullivan, D. J., Walker, S. A., West, S. G., and Klaenhammer, T. R. (1996). Development of an expression strategy using a lytic phage to trigger explosive plasmid amplification and gene expression. *Biotechnology* 14: 82–87.

Oki, M., Kakikawa, M., Yamada, K., Taketo, A., and Kodaira, K. I. (1996). Cloning, sequence analysis, and expression of the genes encoding lytic functions of bacteriophage øg1e. *Gene* 176: 215–223.

Oram, J. D., and Reiter, B. (1965). Phage-associated lysins affecting group N and group D streptococci. *Journal of General Microbiology* 40: 57–70.

Parreira, R., São-José, C., Isidro, A., Domingues, S., Vieira, G., and Santos, M. A. (1999). Gene organization in a central DNA fragment of *Oenococcus oeni* bacteriophage fOg44 encoding lytic, integrative and non-essential functions. *Genetics* 226: 83–93.

Parreira, R., Valyasevi, R., Lerayer, A. L. S., Ehrlich, D. S., and Chopin, M. C. (1996). Gene organization and transcription of a late-expressed region of a *Lactococcus lactis* phage. *Journal of Bacteriology* 178: 6158–6165.

Pedré, X., Weise, F., Chai, S., Lüder, G., and Alonso, J. C. (1994). Analysis of *cis* and *trans* acting elements required for the initiation of DNA replication in the *Bacillus subtilis* bacteriophage SPP1. *Journal of Molecular Biology* 236: 1324–1340.

Perrin, R., Billard, P., and Branlant, C. (1997). Comparative analysis of the genomic DNA terminal regions of the lactococcal bacteriophages from species c2. *Research in Microbiology* 148: 573–583.

Platteeuw, C., and de Vos, W. M. (1992). Location, characterisation and expression of the lytic enzyme-encoding gene, *lytA*, of *Lactococcus lactis* bacteriophage øUS3. *Gene* 118: 115–120.

Poblet-Icart, M., Bordons, A., and Lonvaud-Funal, A. (1998). Lysogeny of *Oenococcus oeni* (syn. *Leuconostoc oenos*) and study of their induced bacteriophages. *Current Microbiology* 36: 365–369.

Prévots, F., Mata, M., and Ritzenthaler, P. (1990). Taxonomic differentiation of 101 lactococcal bacteriophages and characterization of bacteriophages with unusually large genomes. *Applied and Environmental Microbiology* 56: 2180–2185.

Prévots, F., Relano, P., Mata, M., and Ritzenthaler, P. (1989). Close relationship of virulent bacteriophages of *Streptococcus salivarius* subsp. *thermophilus* at both the protein and the DNA level. *Journal of General Microbiology* 135: 3337–3344.

Proux, C., van Sinderen, D., Suarez, J., Garcia, P., Ladero, V., Fitzgerald, G. F., Desiere, F., and Brussow, H. (2002). The dilemma of phage taxonomy illustrated by comparative genomics of sfi21-like *Siphoviridae* in lactic acid bacteria. *Journal of Bacteriology* 184: 6026–6036.

Ptashne, M. (1986). *A genetic switch: Gene control and phage lambda*. Palo Alto, USA: Blackwell Scientific Publications.

Raya, R. R., Fremaux, C., de Antoni, G. L., and Klaenhammer, T. R. (1992). Site-specific integration of the temperate bacteriophage ϕadh into the *Lactobacillus gasseri* chromosome and molecular characterization of the phage (*attP*) and bacterial (*attB*) attachment sites. *Journal of Bacteriology* 174: 5584–5592.

Reinbold, G. W., Reddy, M. S., and Hammond, E. G. (1982). Ultrastructures of bacteriophages active against *Streptococcus thermophilus, Lactobacillus bulgaricus, Lactobacillus lactis*, and *Lactobacillus helveticus*. *Journal of Food Protection* 45: 119–124.

Reiter, W. D., Palm, P., and Yeats, S. (1989). Transfer RNA genes frequently serve as integration sites for prokaryotic genetic elements. *Nucleic Acids Research* 17: 1907–1914.

Relano, P., Mata, M., Bonneau, M., and Ritzenthaler, P. (1987). Molecular characterisation and comparison of 38 virulent and temperate bacteriophages of *Streptococcus lactis*. *Journal of General Microbiology* 133: 3053–3063.

Roa, V. B., and Black, L. W. (1985). DNA packaging of bacteriophage T4 proheads in vitro: Evidence that prohead expansion is not coupled to DNA packaging. *Journal of Molecular Biology* 185: 565–578.

Rodgers, H. J., Perkins, H. R., and Ward, J. B. (1980). *Microbial cell walls and membranes*. London, UK: Chapman and Hall.

Sanford, J. C., and Johnston, S. A. (1985). The concept of parasite-derived resistance—Deriving resistance genes from the parasites own genome. *Journal of Bacteriology* 113: 395–405.

Schleif, R. F. (1992). DNA looping. *Annual Review of Biochemistry* 61: 199–223.

Schouler, C., Bouet, C., Ritzenthaler, P., Drouet, X., and Mata, M. (1992). Characterization of *Lactococcus lactis* phage antigens. *Applied and Environmental Microbiology* 59: 2470–2484.

Schouler, C., Ehrlich, D. S., and Chopin, M. C. (1994). Sequence and organisation of the lactococcal prolate headed bIL67 phage genome. *Microbiology* 140: 3061–3069.

Séchaud, L., Cluzel, P.-J., Rousseau, M., Baumgartner, A., and Accolas, J. P. (1988). Bacteriophages of lactobacilli. *Biochimie* 70: 401–410.

Séchaud, L., Rousseau, M., Fayard, B., Callegari, M. L., Quénée, P., and Accolas, J. P. (1992). Comparative study of 35 bacteriophages of *Lactobacillus helveticus*: Morphology and host range. *Applied Environmental Microbiology* 58: 1011–1018.

Sharples, Gary J., Bolt, Edward L., Lloyd, and Robert, G. (2002). RusA proteins from the extreme thermophile *Aquifex aeolicus* and lactococcal phage r1t resolve Holliday junctions. *Molecular Microbiology* 44: 549–559.

Shearman, C., Jury, K., and Gasson, M. J. (1994). Controlled expression and structural organisation of a *Lactococcus lactis* bacteriophage lysin encoded by two overlapping genes. *Applied and Environmental Microbiology* 60: 3063–3073.

Shearman, C., Underwood, H., Jury, K., and Gasson, M. (1989). Cloning and DNA sequence analysis of a *Lactococcus* bacteriophage lysin gene. *Molecular Genetics and Genomics* 218: 214–221.

Shearman, C. A., Jury, K., and Gasson, M. J. (1992). Autolytic *Lactococcus lactis* expressing a lactococcal bacteriophage lysin gene. *Biotechnology* 10: 196–199.

Sheehan, M., García, J. L., López, R., and García, P. (1996). Analysis of the catalytic domain of the lysin of the lactococcal bacteriophage Tuc2009 by chimeric gene assembling. *FEMS Microbiology Letters* 140: 23–28.

Sheehan, M. M., Stanley, E., Fitzgerald, G. F., and van Sinderen, D. (1999). Identification and characterisation of a lysis module present in a large proportion of bacteriophages infecting *Stretococcus thermophilus*. *Applied and Environmental Microbiology* 65: 569–577.

Smaczny, T., and Kramer, J. (1984). Acidification disturbance in manufacture of yoghurt. Bioghurt and Biogarde caused by bacteriocins and bacteriophages of *Streptococcus thermophilus*. 2. Distribution and characterization of bacteriophages. *Deutsche Molkerei-Zeitung* 105: 614–618.

Stanley, E., Fitzgerald, G. F., Le Marrec, C., Fayard, B., and van Sinderen, D. (1997). Sequence analysis and characterisation of øO1205, a temperate bacteriophage infecting *Streptococcus thermophilus* CNRZ1205. *Microbiology* 143: 3417–3429.

Stanley, E., Walsh, L., van der Zwet, A., Fitzgerald, G. F., and van Sinderen, D. (2000) Identification of four loci isolated from two *Streptococcus thermophilus* phage genomes responsible for mediating bacteriophage resistance. *FEMS Microbiology Letters* 182: 271–277.

Stanley, E., Walsh, L., Fitzgerald, G. F., and van Sinderen, D. Sequence analysis of ø7201, a lytic *cos*-site-containing bacteriophage infecting *Streptococcus thermophilus*. Unpublished results.

Stoll, S. M., Ginsburg, D. S., and Calos, M. P. (2002). Phage TP901-1 site-specific integrase functions in human cells. *Journal of Bacteriology* 184: 3657–3663.

Sturino, J. M., and Klaenhammer, T. R. (2002). Expression of antisense RNA targeted against *Streptococcus thermophilus* bacteriophages. *Applied and Environmental Microbiology* 68: 588–596.

Susskind, M. M., Botstein, D., and Wright, A. (1971). Superinfection exclusion by prophage P22 in lysogens of *Salmonella typhimurium* II. Genetic evidence for two exclusion systems. *Virology* 45: 638–652.

Sutherland, M., van Vuuren, H. J. J., and Howe, M. M. (1994). Cloning, sequence and in vitro transcription/translation analysis of a 3.2-kb *Eco*RI-*Hin*dIII fragment of *Leuconostoc oenos* bacteriophage L10. *Gene* 148: 125–129.

Tohyama, K., Sakurai, T., Arai, H., and Oda, A. (1972). Studies on temperate phages of *Lactobacillus salivarius*. I. Morphological, biological, and serological properties of newly isolated temperate phages of *Lactobacillus salivarius*. *Japaneses Journal of Microbiology* 16: 385–395.

Trautwetter, A., Ritzenthaler, P., Alatossava, T., and Mata-Gilsinger, M. (1986). Physical and genetic characterization of the genome of *Lactobacillus lactis* bacteriophage LL-H. *Journal of Virology* 59: 551–55.

Tremblay, D. M., and Moineau, S. (1999). Complete genomic sequence of the lytic bacteriophage DT1 of *Streptococcus thermophilus*. *Virology* 255: 63–76.

Twort, F. W. (1915). An investigation on the nature of ultra-microscopic viruses. *Lancet* 2: 1241–1243.

Van de Guchte, M., Daly, C., Fitzgerald, G. F., and Arendt, E. K. (1994a). Identification of the putative repressor-encoding gene cI of the temperate lactococcal bacteriophage Tuc2009. *Gene* 144: 93–95.

Van de Guchte, M., Daly, C., Fitzgerald, G. F., and Arendt, E. K. (1994b). Identification of *int* and *attP* on the genome of the Lactococcal bacteriophage Tuc2009 and their use for site-specific plasmid integration in the chromosome of Tuc2009-resistant *Lactococcus lactis* MG1363. *Applied and Environmental Microbiology* 60: 2324–2329.

van Sinderen, D., Creavan, M., Daly, C., Van de Guchte, M., Arendt, E. K., and Fitzgerald, G. F. (1999). Sequence analysis of the temperate lactococcal phage Tuc2009. Unpublished results.

van Sinderen, D., Karsens, H., Kok, J., Terpstra, P., Ruiters, M. H., Venema, G., and Nauta, A. (1996). Sequence analysis and molecular characterization of the temperate lactococcal bacteriophage r1t. *Molecular Microbiology* 19: 1343–1355.

Vasala, A., Dupont, L., Baumann, M., Ritzenthaler, P., and Alatossava, T. (1993). Molecular comparison of the structural proteins encoding gene clusters of two related *Lactobacillus delbrueckii* bacteriophages. *Journal of Virology* 67: 3061–3068.

Vasala, A., Välkkilä, M., Caldentey, J., and Alatossava, T. (1995). Genetic and biochemical characterisation of the *Lactobacillus delbrueckii* subsp. *lactis* bacteriophage LL-H lysin. *Applied and Environmental Microbiology* 61: 4004–4011.

Ventura, M., Foley, S., Bruttin, A., Chennoufi, S. C., Canchaya, C., and Brüssow, H. (2002). Transcription mapping as a tool in phage genomics: The case of the temperate *Streptococcus thermophilus* phage Sfi21. *Virology* 296: 62–76.

Walker, S. A., and Klaenhammer, T. R. (1998). Molecular characterization of a phage-inducible middle promoter and its transcriptional activator from the lactococcal bacteriophage ø31. *Journal of Bacteriology* 180: 921–931.

Walker, S. A., Drombroski, C. S., and Klaenhammer, T. R. (1998). Common elements regulating gene expression in temperate and lytic bacteriophages of *Lactococcus* species. *Applied and Environmental Microbiology* 64: 1147–1152.

Ward, L. J. H., Beresford, T. P. J., Lubbers, M. W., Jarvis, B. D. W., and Jarvis, A. W. (1993). Sequence analysis of the lysin gene region of the prolate lactococcal bacteriophage c2. *Canadian Journal of Microbiology* 39: 767–774.

Watanabe, K., Hayashia, M., Ishibashi, K., and Nakashima, Y. (1984). An *N*-acetylmuramidase induced by PL-1 phage infection of *Lactobacillus casei*. *Journal of General Microbiology* 130: 275–277.

Waterfield, N. R., Lubbers, M. W., Polzin, K. M., le Page, R. W. F., and Jarvis, A. W. (1996). An origin of DNA replication from *Lactococcus lactis* bacteriophage c2. *Applied and Environmental Microbiology* 62: 1452–1453.

Weerakoon, L. K., and Jayaswal, R. K. (1995). Sequence analysis of the region upstream of a peptidoglycan hydrolase-encoding gene from bacteriophage phi 11 of *Staphylococcus aureus*. *FEMS Microbiology Letters* 133: 9–15.

Weisberg, R. A., and Landy, A. (1983). Site-specific recombination in phage lambda. In: R. W. Hendrix, J. W. Roberts, F. W. Stahl, and R. A. Weisberg (Eds.), *LambdaII* (pp. 211–249). Cold Spring Harbor, NY: Cold Spring Harbor Laboratory Press.

Whitehead, H. R., and Cox, G. A. (1935). The occurrence of bacteriophages in starter cultures of lactic streptococci. *New Zealand Journal of Science and Technology* 16: 319–320.

Yasukawa, H., Kakikawa, M., Masamune, Y., Taketo, A., and Kodaira, K.-I. (1997). Purification and DNA-binding properties of the integrase protein Int encoded by *Lactobacillus plantarum* phage. *Gene* 204: 219–225.

Young, R. (1992). Bacteriophage lysis: Mechanism and regulation. *Microbiology Review* 56: 430–481.

Young, R., and Bläsi, U. (1995). Holins: Form and function in bacteriophage lysis. *FEMS Microbiology Review* 17: 191–205.

Zuniga, M., Franke-Fayard, B., Venema, G., Kok, J., and Nauta, A. (2000). Characterization of the Putative replisome organizer of the Lactococcal bacteriophage rlt. *Journal of Virology* 76: 10234–10244.

Zylicz, M., Arg, D., Liberek, K., and Georgopolous, C. (1987). Initiation of DNA replication with purified host- and bacteriophage-encoded proteins: The role of the *dnaK, dnaJ* and *dnaE* heat shock proteins. *EMBO Journal* 8: 1601–1608.

4

Genetics of the Metabolism of Lactose and Other Sugars

Elaine E. Vaughan, Michiel Kleerebezem,
and Willem M. de Vos

Introduction

The practice of fermentation is a fairly simple, cheap and safe way to preserve raw materials of plant and animal origin that is performed all over the world. The predominant microorganisms used in these fermentations are the lactic acid bacteria (LAB) that metabolize a variety of sugars present in the raw material as an energy source. These LAB are added as starter cultures or are selected during the fermentation process and added to the quality and functionality of the fermented raw materials. Moreover, many LAB have an important function in the animal gastro-intestinal tract where they metabolize a variety of sugars (Hudson and Marsh, 1995; Vaughan et al., 1999). They belong predominantly to the genera *Lactococcus, Lactobacillus, Leuconostoc*, and *Streptococcus*. All have a long history of safe use in the manufacture of foodstuffs and their primary function is the production of lactic acid that preserves the product and inhibits the growth of both spoilage and pathogenic bacteria. The metabolic routes by which sugars are converted into lactic acid have been well established and include the classical Embden–Meyerhof pathway for the homofermentative and the oxidative pentose phosphate pathway for the heterofermentative LAB (Kandler, 1983). Especially the conversion of lactose in milk into lactic acid is one of the most large-scale industrial applications of the LAB. In view of the economic importance of this dairy produce, lactose metabolism has been the subject of considerable research aimed at understanding, and, more recently, exploiting the process involved. The history of the genetics of lactose utilization stretches back to the 1930s when researchers observed the

Elaine E. Vaughan and Willem M. de Vos • Laboratory of Microbiology, Department of Agrotechnology and Food Sciences, Wageningen University, and Wageningen Centre for Food Sciences, Hesselink van Suchtelenweg 4, 6703 CT Wageningen, The Netherlands; e-mail: elaine.vaughan@algemeen.micr.wau.nl, willem.devos@algemeen.micr.wau.nl **Michiel Kleerebezem** • Wageningen Centre for Food Sciences, NIZO Food Research, P.O. Box 20, 6710 BA Ede, The Netherlands; e-mail: kleerebe@nizo.nl

loss of lactose metabolism in *Lactococcus lactis*, but it was the early 1970s before this was explained by the plasmid-located nature of the lactose genes (McKay, 1982). This paved the way for a detailed genetic analysis of these *lac* genes that has culminated in the first model for gene organization and regulation in *Lc. lactis* (van Rooijen and de Vos, 1993a). Subsequently, the genetics of the metabolism of lactose and the related sugar galactose has been the subject of several reviews (de Vos and Vaughan, 1994; Grossiord et al., 1998).

The aim of this chapter is to present the genetics and regulation of the metabolism of sugars in various relevant LAB using the well-studied *lac* and *gal* gene expression as a model. The reader is referred to previous reviews describing the establishment of the biochemical pathways for lactose transport and metabolism (Kandler, 1983; Thompson, 1987; de Vos, 1990). Special attention will be given to recent progress in the *lac* gene regulation that involves both specific and global control systems. Finally, the impact and potential of genomics on the study of sugar utilization will be demonstrated by surveying LAB genome sequences for the presence of genes encoding potential sugar transport systems.

Lactococcus lactis

Rapid Lactose Fermentation by the PEP-PTS

The lactococci typically found in dairy fermentations transport lactose into the cell via the highly efficient lactose phosphoenolpyruvate–phosphotransferase system (PEP-PTS) with concomitant phosphorylation of lactose. The structure and function of the enzymes involved in the lactose PEP-PTS have been reviewed extensively (Hengstenberg

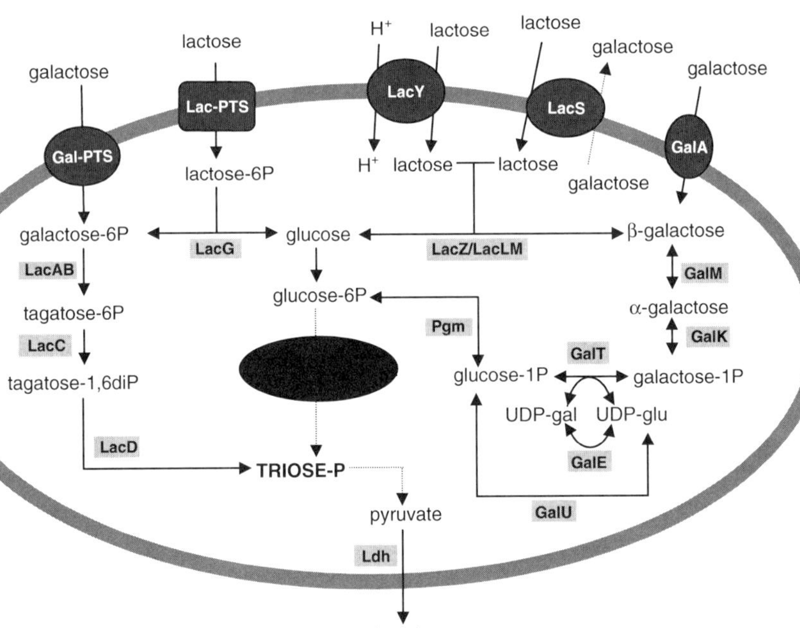

Figure 4.1. Lactose and galactose transport and metabolic systems described for LAB. The Leloir and tagatose phosphate pathways are illustrated on the right and left sides, respectively.

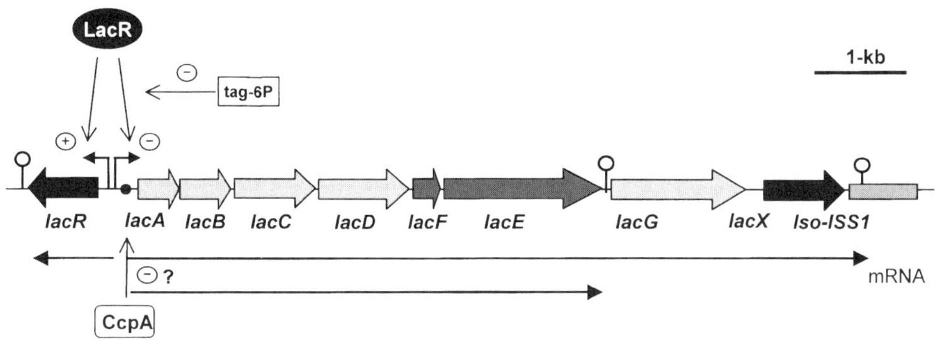

Figure 4.2. Model for regulation of the lactose PTS and tagatose 6-phosphate genes in *Lactococcus lactis* MG1820. Arrows indicate position and direction of mapped promoters; hairpin structures indicate potential transcription terminators. The *cre* site is illustrated with a black circle. Positive and negative regulation by LacR or CcpA is indicated with a plus and minus symbol, respectively. Binding of tagatose-6-phosphate (tag-6P) to LacR causes dissociation of the LacR–*lacO1O2* complex and transcription of the *lacA* promoter proceeds. The sizes of mRNAs are indicated below the genes with arrows.

et al., 1989; Postma et al., 1993). Briefly, the PEP-PTS is a multicomponent system comprising the general nonsugar specific proteins, enzyme I (EI) and heat stable protein (HPr), in combination with sugar-specific enzyme II proteins. Enzyme IIs may consist of a single membrane-bound protein composed of three domains (EIIA, EIIB, and EIIC), or two or more proteins at least one of which is membrane bound (e.g., EIIBC and EIIC), and one of which is soluble (EIIA) (Saier and Reizer, 1992). EI, which is autophosphorylated at the expense of PEP, catalyzes the phosphorylation of HPr on a conserved histidyl residue 15 to generate HPr(His-P). HPr(His-P) in turn transfers the phosphate to the sugar-specific EII that transports and phosphorylates the sugar. The internalized disaccharide is hydrolyzed by the phospho-β-galactosidase into galactose-6-phosphate and glucose, and the latter is converted by the enzymes of the tagatose-6-phosphate pathway into triose-phosphate (Figure 4.1) (Bisette and Andersen, 1973, 1974).

Genetics of the Lactose-PTS in Lactococci

In the model strain *Lc. lactis* NCDO712 and its derivatives, the genes encoding the PEP-PTS and the tagatose-6-phosphate pathway have been located to plasmids, the smallest of which is the 23.7-kb mini-plasmid pMG820 in *Lc. lactis* strain MG1820 (Gasson, 1983; Maeda and Gasson, 1986). The genes comprise the PTS translocation system, EIIBC (*lacE*) and EIIA (*lacF*), the phospho-β-galactosidase (*lacG*) and the tagatose-6-phosphate enzymes, galactose 6-phosphate isomerase (*lacAB*), tagatose 6-phosphate kinase (*lacC*), and the tagatose 1,6-diphosphate aldolase (*lacD*) (de Vos and Gasson, 1989; de Vos et al., 1990; van Rooijen and de Vos, 1990; van Rooijen et al., 1991). The genes are organized in a 7.8-kb operon with the gene order *lacABCDFEGX* that is followed by an *iso*-ISS*1* element (Figure 4.2) (van Rooijen and de Vos, 1993b). The *lacX* gene appears to be dispensable for growth on lactose and has been implicated in signal transduction of the SOS response, which includes resistance to DNA-damaging agents, in another *Lc. lactis* strain (Huang et al., 1995). The transcriptional regulator (LacR) of the *lac* operon, product of the 0.8-kb *galR* gene, is positioned upstream and in a divergent orientation to the operon such that the two promoters are in a back-to-back configuration (van Rooijen and de Vos, 1990). The *lac* metabolic genes are transcribed as two transcripts, comprising the 6-kb *lacABCDFE* and the 8-kb *lacABCDFEGX* genes. An inverted repeat located between the *lacE* and *lacG* genes appears to cause intercistronic termination. The *lac* operon is induced up to 10-fold by growth on lactose while *lacR* is similarly induced during growth on glucose. LacR belongs to the DeoR family of repressors and is both responsible for repression of the *lac* operon and activating its own transcription (van Rooijen and de Vos, 1990; van Rooijen et al., 1992). There are two operons present in the *lac* region with different affinities for LacR, a high affinity operator *lacO1* located in the *lac* operon promoter, and the second lower affinity operator *lacO2* that is positioned near the start codon of the *lacR* gene (van Rooijen and de Vos, 1990). The model for *lac* gene regulation, based on substantial genetic and biochemical analysis, is as follows. During growth on glucose (or uninduced state) the binding of LacR to the *lacO1* operator represses transcription of the *lac* promoter but activates transcription of *lacR*. As LacR increases in concentration, both the *lac* operon and *lacR* gene expression will be repressed because *lacO2* has a lower affinity for LacR than *lacO1*, and therefore, will become susceptible at rising LacR concentrations. Binding of the inducer, that is, tagotose-6-phosphate generated during growth on lactose, to LacR, results in dissociation of the LacR-operator complex and expression of the *lac* operon may proceed (van Rooijen and de Vos, 1993a; van Rooijen et al., 1993b).

Chromosomally Encoded *gal* Operon

The plasmid-free *Lc. lactis* MG1363 strain, hence lacking the lactose PEP-PTS system, could no longer grow effectively on lactose but fermented galactose via the Leloir pathway (Figure 4.1). This complete *gal* operon has been characterized and comprises the galactose permease (*galP*), mutarotase (*galM*), galactokinase (*galK*), galactose 1-phosphate uridylyltransferase (*galT*), and UDPgalactose 4-epimerase (*galE*) genes in a novel order that reflects the biochemical degradation of galactose (Figure 4.3; Grossiord et al., 1998). The genes were transcribed together on a 7-kb transcript that appeared to terminate occasionally after the *galP* gene resulting in an extra 1.4-kb mRNA, and undergo processing between the *galK* and *galT* genes to generate 4- and 2.5-kb mRNAs (Grossiord,

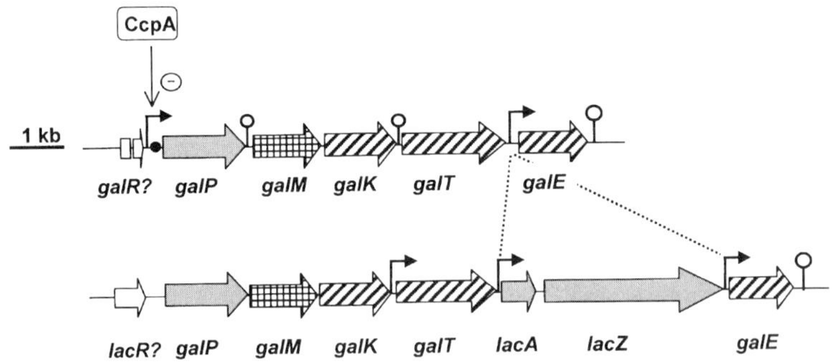

Figure 4.3. Comparison of the genetic organization of (A) the *gal* operon in *Lactococcus lactis* MG1363 (GenBank Accession No. AJ011653), and (B) the *lac–gal* operon of *Lactococcus lactis* NCDO 2054 (GenBank Accession No. U60828; Vaughan et al., 1998). Direction of genes and mapped promoters are indicated with arrows; hairpins indicate potential transcription terminators. The *cre* site is illustrated with a black circle. Negative regulation by CcpA at *cre* due to catabolite repression is indicated with a minus symbol. The point in the MG1363 operon at which the intervening *lacA–lacZ* genes are present in NCDO 2054 is illustrated with dashed lines.

1998). The *galP* (also referred to as *galA*) promoter was induced by galactose and a strong catabolite repression was observed with growth on glucose (Luesink et al., 1998; see below). The *galE* gene was also transcribed from its own promoter but appears to be constitutively expressed which may be related to the other function of the UDPgalactose 4-epimerase (Grossiord, 1998). The latter enzyme interconverts UDP-sugars that are building blocks for the biosynthesis of cell wall carbohydrate polymers. A *galE* disruption mutant of *L. lactis* MG1363 became galactose-negative and also demonstrated an unusual long-chain phenotype instead of the normal coccoid growth when cells were grown on glucose as the sole carbon source (Grossiord et al., 2003). Electron microscopy revealed the cells no longer attached to each other but were connected by bridges of possibly peptidoglycan. It was speculated that GalE was necessary for the appropriate configuration of cell envelope polymers, especially lipoteichoic acid, and the *Lc. lactis* autolysin may not be able to act on the incorrect form. Recovery of the wild-type phenotype for the *galE* mutant was obtained by either genetic complementation or by adding trace amounts of galactose to the medium.

GalE mediated interconversion of UDP-glucose and UDP-galactoses was also shown to be essential for the production of the galactose containing exopolysaccharide EPS-B40 (Boels et al., 2001) when glucose was the sole carbon source. The levels of these sugar nucleotides could be increased by engineered overproduction of the phosphoglucomutase (Pgm) (Boels et al., 2003) or the UDP-glucose pyrophosphorylase (GalU) (Boels et al., 2001) without affecting the ratio between UDP-glucose and UDP-galactose, indicating that the endogenous GalE enzyme activity levels are more than sufficient to maintain a constant UDP-sugar balance under normal conditions.

The galactose permease of *Lc. lactis* MG1363 belongs to a family of transporter proteins (GPH family) that transport galactosides, pentoses, or hexuronides that are discussed in more detail below (Grossiord et al., 2003). While the predicted protein sequence of GalP was more homologous (44%) with the lactose permease (LacS) of *Strep. thermophilus* in the GPH family, it lacks the carboxy terminal regulatory domain. A plasmid harboring the *galA* gene could complement a melibiose permease (*melB* gene) deficient *Escherichia coli* mutant DW2 but not a lactose permease deficient mutant. Disruption of *galP* in *Lc. lactis* MG1363 confirmed its role in galactose transport. Interestingly, disruption of *galA* in *Lc. lactis* NZ3900, a lactose positive derivative of MG1363 that contains the *lac* PTS genes integrated in the chromosome, indicated the presence of a second galactose permease system that may be enzyme II of the lactose PTS.

Lc. lactis can metabolize the galactose moiety of lactose via the tagatose-6-phosphate pathway but galactose may also be transported via a PTS system that has a 10-fold lower affinity for galactose than the permease (Thompson, 1980). The latter system is unrelated to the lactose-PTS at least in some strains since mutations in *lacE* or *lacF*, or inactivation of the *lac* operon in the case of *Lc. lactis* MG1820, indicated the presence of a distinct galactose-PTS (Park and McKay, 1982; Crow et al., 1983; de Vos and van Alen-Boerrigter, unpublished data).

Carbon Catabolite Repression in Global Metabolic Control in LAB

Carbon catabolite repression in bacteria is a regulatory mechanism whereby a rapidly metabolisable carbon source, usually glucose, in the growth medium inhibits utilization of other substrates (reviewed by Stülke and Hillen, 1999 and Gunnewijk et al., 2001). In low G + C Gram-positive bacteria, the catabolite control protein A (CcpA) that was first described for *Bacillus subtilis* is one of the central regulators of catabolite repression (Stulke and Hillen, 2000). CcpA is a member of the LacI-GalR family of transcriptional regulator proteins and it typically exerts its action via a catabolite responsive element (*cre*) that is usually positioned near the promoter region and either represses or activates transcription (Weickert and Chambliss, 1990). CcpA functions as a transcriptional regulator involved in the global metabolic control. Another critical factor in catabolite repression is HPr, which has additional functions besides acting as an intermediate in the phosphate-transfer chain of the sugar PEP-PTS. It has been shown for Gram-positive bacteria that HPr may be phosphorylated by the bifunctional enzyme HPr kinase/phosphatase on serine residue 46, generating HPr(Ser-P) (Galinier et al., 1998; Kravanja et al., 1999). This ATP-dependent phosphorylation that is stimulated by fructose-1,6-biphosphate triggers a regulatory cascade that culminates in catabolite repression. CcpA in combination with HPr(Ser-P) or NADP and possibly with other glycolytic intermediates forms a complex that stimulates binding to the *cre* site and regulates the transcription of the associated genes (Deutscher et al., 1995; Fujita et al., 1995; Kim et al., 1998). Since ATP-dependent phosphorylation at Ser-46 is a prerequisite for the HPr interaction with CcpA, whereas PEP-dependent phosphorylation at His-15 prevents the interaction, PTS-mediated sugar transport is linked to catabolite repression.

HPr(Ser-P) has also been implicated in inducer exclusion, a phenomenon whereby the cell immediately reduces the uptake of a sugar upon introduction of a rapidly metabolizable carbon source to the environment, such as the inhibition of the glucose and lactose-specific non-PTS permeases (Ye and Saier, 1995a,b), and the galactose : H^+ symporter of *Lactobacillus brevis* (see below; Djordjevic et al., 2001). Inducer expulsion, a mechanism by which the cell can reduce the intracellular concentration of sugar phosphates may also involve HPr(Ser-P); this is suggested by its stimulation of sugar-phosphate phosphatases in LAB (Ye et al., 1994).

Catabolite Repression in *Lc. lactis*

The first support for the functionality of such a *cre* site in catabolite repression in LAB came from studies in the *Lc. lactis* MG1820 *lac* operon that contains a near consensus *cre* in the promoter region (Figure 4.2) (van Rooijen et al., 1993a). Introduction of a multicopy plasmid containing the potential *cre* sequence in the *lacA* promoter into a LacR deficient mutant resulted in constitutive LacG activity, suggesting that a transacting factor that binds *cre* was titrated (van Rooijen et al., 1993a). The *ccpA* gene of *Lc. lactis* strain NZ9800, that is a derivative of strain MG1363, has been characterized and is constitutively expressed on a single transcript (Luesink et al., 1998). Disruption of *ccpA* reduced the catabolite repression of the *gal* operon that contains a *cre* at the transcriptional start site. In contrast, CcpA activates transcription of the *las* operon encoding the glycolytic enzymes phosphofructokinase, pyruvate kinase, and lactate dehydrogenase. These enzymes convert pyruvate to compounds that can easily be expelled from the cell and possibly prevent toxic accumulation of end products (Luesink et al., 1998).

The genes encoding enzyme I (*ptsI*) and HPr (*ptsH*) have been characterized in *Lc. lactis* and are located in an operon with the order *ptsHI* (Luesink et al., 1999a). The *ptsH* gene was transcribed as a single 0.3-kb mRNA but also as part of a longer 2.0-kb mRNA with the *ptsI* gene. Expression of the operon was regulated at the transcriptional level and glucose-inducible but the regulatory elements have not yet been identified. Disruption of the genes abolished growth on sucrose and fructose, indicating the dominant role of the PTS system in transport of these sugars, and caused reduced growth rates on glucose, galactose, and maltose. Construction of a HPr mutant that contains an aspartic acid at residue 46, which mimics a phosphorylated serine, was used to show the role of HPr(Ser-P) as a co-activator in the CcpA-mediated catabolite repression of the *gal* operon, and a co-activator of the *las* operon (Luesink et al., 1999a).

An Alternative Lactose Metabolic System in Lactococci

Some lactococci, notably of non-dairy origin, ferment lactose more slowly than the industrial starter strains (Farrow, 1980). Furthermore, while fermenting galactose alone lactococci may produce end products such as acetate, formate, and ethanol in addition to lactate (Thomas et al., 1980). *Lc. lactis* ATCC 7962 (also known as NCDO 2054), the best studied slow lactose fermenter, transports lactose into the cell via a permease and hydrolyzes the disaccharide to glucose and galactose with the β-galactosidase enzyme (Figure 4.1). The galactose moiety is metabolized via the enzymes of the Leloir pathway to triose-phosphate. Several of the *lac* and *gal* genes of *Lc. lactis* ATCC 7962, including the β-galactosidase (*lacZ*), *galK, galT, galE*, and putative galactoside acetyltransferase (*lacA*) are located in an operon that has been partly characterized with the gene order *galK–galT–lacA–lacZ–galE* (Figure 4.2; Vaughan et al., 1998). A surprisingly large number of transcripts ranging from 11 to 1.1 kb for presumably the complete operon to the *galE* gene alone have been demonstrated. The transcripts were induced to a greater extent by galactose than lactose, except the *galE* gene that was constitutively expressed on glucose and galactose and induced by lactose. Three lactose inducible intergenic promoters identified within the operon, as well as mRNA processing, are believed to be responsible for this unusual transcriptional organisation (Vaughan et al., 1998).

Further DNA sequence analysis of the *lac–gal* region of *Lc. lactis* ATCC 7962 (GenBank Accession no. U60828) and the genome sequence of *Lc. lactis* IL403 (Bolotin et al., 1999) revealed an identical organization for these genes within both strains. Both analyses revealed *galA, galM, galK, galT, lacA, lacZ*, and *galE* genes in that order (Figure 4.3). The predicted protein sequence of the *galA* gene homologue was 96% identical to *galA* of *Lc. lactis* MG1363. It is more than likely that this GalA permease is identical to the proton coupled galactoside transporter that is highly specific for galactose and shows minimal affinity for lactose, as was previously described for *Lc. lactis* strain ATCC 7962, representing the first characterization of a lactose transporter (Kashket and Wilson, 1973).

The organization of the *gal* genes in both *Lc. lactis* ATCC 7962 and IL1403 is essentially the same as that of MG1363 described above except for the intervening *lacA* and *lacZ* genes (Figure 4.3) (Vaughan et al., 1998; Bolotin et al., 1999, 2001; GenBank Accession no. U60828). The greater similarity of the predicted LacA and LacZ proteins to homologues in Gram-negative bacteria, especially in comparison to the surrounding *gal* genes, suggest they may have been recently acquired. Thus, it has been proposed that the *lac* genes may have engaged the *gal* operon promoters in order to direct and regulate their expression (Vaughan et al., 1998). One important point to note is that *Lc. lactis* ATCC 7962 can grow on lactose, although slowly, while strain IL1403 like MG1363 cannot. Thus, other differences related to lactose utilization exist between these strains and one is the presence of an active β-galactosidase, since the expression of the *E. coli lacZ* gene in *Lc. lactis* MG1363 shows slow but significant growth in lactose (de Vos and Simons, 1988).

Finally, the question of the regulator of these *lac* and *gal* genes must be addressed. Upstream of the *galP* gene in *Lc. lactis* ATCC 7962 (GenBank Accession no. U60828) and IL1403, and in the same orientation, an open reading frame that can encode a protein of 244 animoacids, which has approximately 45% similarity with transcriptional regulators of the SIS family, was found. The ORF contains DNA binding and phosphosugar-binding motifs (Bateman, 1999), and in combination to its close association with the *lac–gal* genes makes it a strong candidate for their regulation. The 5′end of an ORF encoding a similar protein was found upstream of the *galP* gene in *Lc. lactis* MG1363 that is likely to be the GalR regulator (Grossiord, B., personal communication).

It is notable that indirect evidence for another lactose permease has been obtained for *Lc. lactis* strain MG1363 whereby a chromosomal fragment could weakly complement the *lacY1* (lactose permease) mutation of *E. coli* HB101 (Ross et al., 1987). The genetics and mode of action have not been characterised yet but it seems different from the *galA* encoded permease since this gene only complements a *melB* deficient *E. coli* strain (see above).

Streptococcus thermophilus

Lactose–Galactose Exchange during Transport

The lactose transporter (LacS) of *Streptococcus thermophilus* is remarkable in that it operates as a lactose–galactose antiporter, although it may also function as a galactoside/proton symport system (Poolman et al., 1989; Foucaud and Poolman, 1992). *Strep. thermophilus* and also *Lactobacillus bulgaricus* do not metabolize the galactose moiety of lactose nor the free sugar like the other LAB but excrete it into the medium in amounts stoichiometric with the uptake of lactose (Figure 4.1; Hutkins and Morris, 1987; Hickey et al., 1996). The galactoside/H^+ reaction is a slower reaction than the lactose/galactose exchange that is driven by the concentration gradients of both sugars across the membrane (Foucaud and Poolman, 1992). LacS is the sole galactoside transporter in *Strep. thermophilus*, and therefore, is also responsible for galactose transport (Poolman et al., 1995). The secretion of galactose in the medium is due to the lactose/galactose exchange mode of transport and the inability of *Strep. thermophilus* to utilize galactose. Other LAB such as *Leuconostoc* possess a LacS homologue but have the capacity to metabolize the galactose (see below; Vaughan et al., 1996).

The LacS proteins are classified as a subgroup of members of the galactoside–pentose–hexuronide family based on the primary sequence identity of their amino-terminal hydrophobic carrier domains (Poolman et al., 1996). Other members of this family include the MelB and GusB subfamilies, represented by the melibiose and glucuronide transporters, respectively, of *E. coli*. The LacS proteins are chimeric as they also possess a carboxy-terminal hydrophilic region of 180 amino acids that is homologous to the enzyme IIA domains of various PTS enzymes (Poolman et al., 1989). This IIA domain can be phosphorylated on His-552 by HPr(His-P) which affects the activity of LacS (Poolman et al., 1995; Gunnewijk et al., 1999; Gunnewijk and Poolman, 2000a). Using purified LacS reconstituted into proteoliposomes, it was demonstrated that the HPr (His-P)-mediated phosphorylation of LacS increased the lactose/galactose transport reaction while lactose/H^+ symport was unaffected (Gunnewijk and Poolman, 2000a).

The *lacS* gene of *Strep. thermophilus* forms an operon with the downstream β-galactosidase (*lacZ*) gene and the genes are regulated on the transcriptional level with induction of a 5.5-kb mRNA during growth on lactose (Figure 4.4; Poolman et al., 1990; Schroeder et al., 1991). In fact, galactose and galactose analogues rather than lactose are the inducers of this *lac* operon (Poolman, 1993), while glucose represses their expression. A *cre* site is present in the *lac* operon promoter, suggesting regulation by CcpA and HPr(Ser-P) (Poolman, 1993). Immediately upstream of the *lac* operon, the mutarotase gene (*galM*) was located (Poolman et al., 1990). Although expression was very weak as

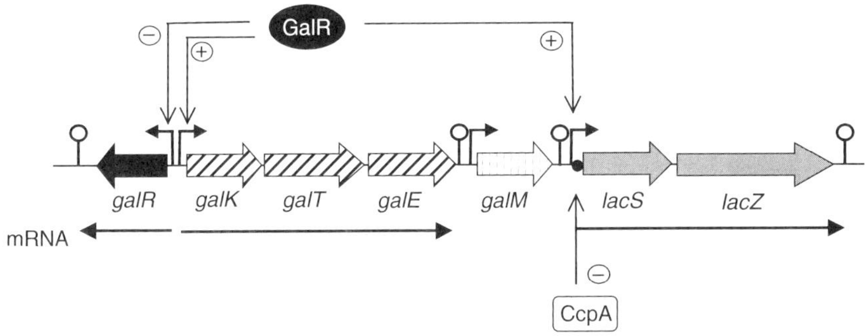

Figure 4.4. Model of *gal* and *lac* gene regulation in *Streptococcus thermophilus*. Direction of genes and mapped promoters are indicated with arrows; hairpins indicate potential transcription terminators. The *cre* site is illustrated with a black circle. Positive and negative regulation by GalR or CcpA is indicated with a plus and minus symbol. The sizes of mRNAs are indicated below the genes with arrows.

measured by mRNA detection, significant activity was obtained from cell lysates of *E. coli* cells containing plasmids encoding *galM*.

Fine Tuning of Lactose Metabolism by CcpA/HPr(Ser-P) and HPr(His-P)

Unlike many other Gram-positive bacteria, *Strep. thermophilus* prefers lactose over glucose as the primary carbon and energy source (Poolman, 1993). The *ccpA* gene of *Strep. thermophilus* has been characterized and is located in a back-to-back configuration with the *pepQ* gene coding for a putative proline peptidase (van den Bogaard et al., 2000). Disruption of the *ccpA* gene resulted in at least 4-fold increased lactose transport during fermentation and the *lac* operon showed a 7-fold increase in expression compared to the wild type. Surprisingly, the *ccpA* disruption strain secreted substantial amounts of glucose into the medium during growth on lactose that was not utilized after lactose depletion, and a lower quantity of lactate was produced. CcpA is a positive regulator of the lactate dehydrogenase (*ldh*) gene that is induced 2-fold during growth on lactose compared to glucose or galactose. The *ccpA* disruption mutant also showed a reduced rate of glycolysis that in combination with the increased lactose transport would overburden the glycolytic pathway and could explain the expulsion of glucose. Apparently, *Strep. thermophilus* possesses an overcapacity for lactose uptake that is controlled by CcpA to match its capacity for glycolysis (van den Bogaard et al., 2000). This is rather exceptional among the LAB and in low G + C Gram-positive bacteria whereby non-PTS carbon sources induce catabolite repression at the transcriptional level. In general, CcpA mediates catabolite repression when cells are cultured on PTS carbon sources.

Thus, in addition to HPr(His-P) affecting the activity of LacS, CcpA/HPr(Ser-P) mediates control of *lacS* gene expression presumably at the *cre* site (Gunnewijk and Poolman, 2000b; van den Bogaard et al., 2000). The phosphorylation state of HPr at different stages of growth of *Strep. thermophilus* was correlated with the expression level and phosphorylation state of LacS (Gunnewijk and Poolman, 2000b). The results indicated that *Strep. thermophilus* maintains a high lactose transport capacity at relatively adverse lactose/galactose ratios (in the late log and stationary phase) by synthesizing more LacS and stimulating its transport capacity. This dual regulation revolving around the phosphorylation state of HPr adjusts lactose uptake to its metabolic needs.

The genes encoding HPr (*ptsH*) and enzyme I (*ptsI*) are under the control of one strong promoter that generates two transcripts, one encompassing the *ptsHI* genes and one specific for *ptsH* (van den Bogaard, 2002). Effects of mutations in the *Strep. thermophilus* HPr were investigated by complementation of the *Lc. lactis* HPr negative background as deletion mutants in the *Strep. thermophilus ptsH* gene could not be obtained. Amino acid residues His-15 and Arg-17 were found to be essential for PTS sugars transport. Interestingly, galactose metabolism, whereby transport is via the GalA permease, was also inhibited suggesting a phosphotransfer independent modulation of GalA by HPr (van den Bogaard, 2002).

Activation of Silent Gal Genes

Although *Strep. thermophilus* has a galactose-negative phenotype, strain CNRZ 302 was demonstrated to contain structurally intact genes for the Leloir pathway enzymes (Vaughan et al., 2001). These were organized into an operon with the order the *galKTE*, which was preceded by a divergently transcribed regulator gene *galR*, and followed by the *galM* gene and the *lac* operon (Figure 4.4). These *gal* genes were transcribed, but very weakly, with transcripts detected only in medium containing lactose but this was insufficient for utilization of galactose. However, galactose-fermenting mutants of CNRZ 302 could be isolated either spontaneously or by mutagenesis (Benetaya et al., 1991; Vaughan et al., 2001). One spontaneous mutant, designated NZ302G, was studied in more detail, that showed the *galKTE* genes were efficiently transcribed as a 3.5-kb transcript in cells grown on lactose or galactose (Vaughan et al., 2001). In both CNRZ 302 and the Gal^{+} mutant NZ302G, the transcription of the *galR* gene on a 1.1-kb mRNA was induced by growth on lactose. Disruption of *galR* indicated that it functioned as a transcriptional activator of both the *gal* and *lac* operons while negatively regulating its own expression. Sequence analysis of the *gal* promoter regions of NZ302G and nine other spontaneous Gal^{+} mutants of CNRZ 302 revealed mutations at three positions in the *galK* promoter region. One class of mutations resulted in a -10 box with greater homology to the consensus, the second generated a TG doublet 1 bp upstream of the -10 sequence that is a feature present in the promoters of Gram-positive bacteria. The third class consisted of an adenine insertion in a homopolymeric run of adenine residues upstream of the -35 box in a potential operator sequence that may enhance intrinsic DNA curvature and consequently increase promoter strength. Galactokinase activity measurements and analysis of *gusA* reporter gene fusions in strains containing the mutated promoters supported the hypothesis that they were *gal* promoter-up mutations. The inducible phenotype of the *gal* genes suggests that *Strep. thermophilus* had been Gal^{+} but became Gal^{-} in the recent past. Therefore, it seems likely that poor expression of the *gal* genes in the galactose-negative *Strep. thermophilus* CNRZ 302 was caused by naturally occurring mutations in the *galK* promoter.

The *gal–lac* gene cluster of a *Strep. thermophilus* strain SMQ-301 shared the same organization as that of CNRZ 302 above and as that of *Streptococcus salivarius* (Vaillancourt et al., 2002). The *galK* promoters were highly similar but both the *Strep. thermophilus* sequences showed mismatches in the potential operator upstream of the -35 box, in the -10 box, and the Shine–Delgarno sequences compared to the *Strep. salivarius* sequence. Poor translation of the *galK* gene was suggested to also play a role in the Gal^{-} phenotype of *Strep. thermophilus*.

The *galK* gene of a galactose-fermenting *Strep. thermophilus* strain F410 isolated from a yogurt starter culture was also characterized (Mustapha et al., 1995), and showed 58% identity with the *galK* gene of strain CNRZ 302. The F410 *galK* gene did not appear to be linked to other *gal* genes. Further studies on location and expression of *gal* genes in *Strep. thermophilus* will undoubtedly reveal interesting insights into their galactose phenotype.

Leuconostoc lactis

Plasmid Encoded lac Genes of *Leuconostoc lactis*

Like *Streptococcus thermophilus, Leuconostoc* species transport lactose into the cell using a permease, and following hydrolysis by β-galactosidase, glucose is metabolized via the phosphoketolase pathway while the galactose moiety is converted to glycolytic intermediates via the Leloir pathway (Figure 4.1). In *Leuconostoc lactis* NZ6009, lactose transport and hydrolysis were linked to the native plasmid pNZ63 (David et al., 1989; David, 1992). The β-galactosidase of *Leuc. lactis* was unusual in that it was encoded by two genes, *lacL* and *lacM*, that are probably translationally coupled (David et al., 1992). This type of two subunit β-galactosidase, which was first discovered in *Leuc. lactis* has since been found in several *Lactobacillus* species, and is believed to have been generated by an internal deletion in an ancestral β-galactosidase gene. The lactose permease gene (*lacS*) was separated from the downstream *lacLM* genes by 2 kb of DNA that contained an IS*3*-like insertion sequence (Vaughan et al., 1996). Preceding *lacS* was an ORF that could encode a peptide of 95 amino acids with an amino-terminal sequence similar to that of β-galactosidase I from *Bacillus stearothermophilus*. The *lacS* gene was designated as such because of the strong similarity to the LacS permease of *Strep. thermophilus*. Both the *lacLM* and *lacS* genes were constitutively expressed.

In addition to lactose uptake, the LacS protein could also transport galactose like the *Strep. thermophilus* LacS. However, galactose uptake and metabolism still occurred in a pNZ63-cured derivative of *Leuc. lactis* indicating that another transport system for this sugar was present (Vaughan et al., 1996). The *galK* gene has been identified on the chromosome and appears to be flanked by the *galT* gene downstream and an α-galactosidase gene (*agaA*) immediately upstream (Vaughan, E. E., Catzeddu, P., and de Vos, W. M., unpublished data).

Lactobacillus

Among the LAB, usually the lactobacilli have a greater capacity to ferment a broader range of carbohydrates. Again the genetics of lactose metabolism and transport has dominated the research so far in the lactobacilli. Since the *Lactobacillus* genus is very large and heterogenous, there is interesting variety in the regulation of these systems. Especially the recent progress within the genetics of the system for *Lactobacillus casei* is described below, as well as the more recently characterized systems for other sugars.

Lactose PEP-PTS in *Lactobacillus casei*

The operon for the lactose-specific PEP-PTS of *Lactobacillus casei* may be plasmid or chromosomally located but does not contain the tagatose 6-phosphate genes as in *Lactococcus lactis* (Chassy and Alpert, 1989; Gosalbes et al., 1997; Shimuzu-Kadota, 1987). It is interesting that lactose specific PEP-PTS systems have only been described for the Gram-positive *Lactococcus, Lactobacillus, Streptococcus*, and *Staphylococcus* genera. The lactose-PTS system and phospho-β-galactosidase gene (*lacG*) of *Lb. casei* was characterized from the lactose plasmid pLZ64 of *Lb. casei* 64H (reviewed by Chassy and Alpert, 1989). Lactose-PTS genes were also found to be chromosomally located in some *Lb. casei* strains, and some of the latter contained a plasmid encoded β-galactosidase gene. *Lb. casei*

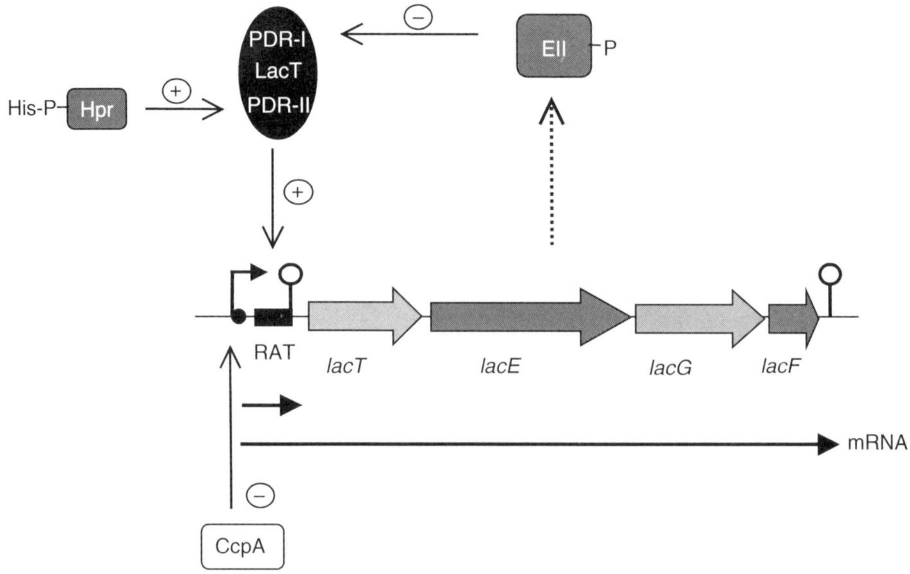

Figure 4.5. Model of *lac* gene regulation in *Lactobacillus casei*. The promoter is indicated with an arrow and the hairpin a potential transcription terminator. Positive and negative regulation is indicated with plus and minus symbols. The sizes of mRNAs are indicated below the genes with arrows.

may also transport galactose by a distinct galactose-PTS that can be induced by growth on either galactose or lactose (Chassy and Thompson, 1983; Bettenbrock et al., 1999).

An almost identical *lac* operon to that of strain 64H was present in single copy on the chromosome of *Lb. casei* strain ATCC 393, and therefore was chosen as a model for expression studies of the *lac* genes (Gosalbes et al., 1997). The *lac* operon consists of *lacTEGF* that encode LacT, EIICB, phospho-β-galactosidase, and EIIA proteins (Figure 4.5). The promoter region contains a *cre* element overlapping the −35 region that is followed by a ribonucleic antiterminator (RAT) sequence, and a terminator structure (Alpert and Siebers, 1997; Gosalbes et al., 1997).

LacT belongs to a family of transcriptional terminator proteins designated the BglR family on the basis of sequence homology, cross-complementation, and the fact that their DNA targets share a consensus ribonucleic antiterminator (RAT) sequence (Alpert and Siebers, 1997). Such antiterminator proteins may be regulated through phosphorylation by sugar-specific PTS components or Hpr at PTS-regulation domains (PRD), one of which is specialized in induction and the other in catabolite repression, that result in different consequences (Rutberg, 1997; Stülke et al., 1998). In the first case, in the absence of inducer, the phoshorylated EII donates its phosphate to PRD-I, thereby inactivating the regulator, whereas when the inducer is present the phosphate is transferred to the sugar and the active regulator induces the operon. The second mechanism, that is essentially a novel form of carbon catabolite repression, has so far been demonstrated only in Gram-positive bacteria. Briefly, HPr is phosphorylated by EI at His-15 in the absence of PTS sugars, and HPr(His-P) can phosphorylate the regulator at PRD-II and stimulate its activity. In the presence of rapidly metabolizable carbon sources, phosphorylation of HPr at Ser-46 inhibits phosphorylation by EI, and the regulator remains inactive.

The expression of the *lac* operon of *Lb. casei* is induced by lactose that is mediated by LacT (Gosalbes et al., 1999). It is proposed that in the presence of the inducer the binding of the antiterminator protein to the RAT sequence prevents the formation of the following more stable terminator structure and allows the transcription to proceed beyond the stop signal. In accordance with this model, a transcript corresponding to the *lacTEFG* genes was induced in lactose-grown *L. casei* cells, whereas in the absence of inducer, a mRNA of about 100 nucleotides was produced that would commence at the transcriptional start site, span the RAT sequence and end at the terminator (Gosalbes et al., 1999). When *lacE* and *lacF* were inactivated, the antiterminator LacT remained active and antiterminator activity occurred independent of inducer, indicating that EII negatively regulates LacT, possibly by phosphorylation at PDR-I as described above.

The *lac* operon is also subject to catabolite repression by CcpA. The *ccpA* gene of *Lb. casei* has been characterized and is transcribed as a single transcript that was constitutively expressed from a chromosomal location (Monedero et al., 1997). Inactivation of *ccpA* resulted in derepression of transcription initiation of the *lac* operon but no elongation through the terminator was found in the presence of glucose and lactose, and so glucose repression was not overcome. Full derepression of the operon was observed only in glucose and lactose-grown double CcpA-EII^{man} (glucose-specific PTS) deficient mutant cells in which event LacT was active (Gosalbes et al., 1999). A model for the regulation of LacT activity has been proposed, based on the model of PTS-mediated control of PRD-containing regulators (Stülke et al., 1998) whereby LacT would exist in three forms: (a) LacT is active when dephosphorylated at PDR-I and phosphorylated at PDR-II in the presence of inducer; (b) inactive when PRD-II is dephosphorylated by HPr, that is, under catabolite repression conditions; and (c) inactive when phosphorylated at both domains (Gosalbes et al., 1999). In conclusion, in addition to the catabolite repression mediated by CcpA, the *lac* operon is regulated by a second CcpA-independent catabolite repression mechanism that involves LacT (Gosalbes et al., 1999). Site-directed mutagenesis of LacT identified specific PRD-I and PRD-II histidyl residues to be responsible for induction of the *lac* operon and playing a role in CcpA-independent carbon catabolite repression, respectively (Gosalbes et al., 2002). Differences in the affinity of different phosphotransfer elements for PRD-I and PRD-II histidines were further suggested.

The *ptsH* and *ptsI* genes encoding Hpr and EI of *Lb. casei* ATCC 393 have been characterized and are transcribed together in that order in an operon (Viana et al., 2000). EI-deficient *Lb. casei* mutants lost the ability to ferment a large number of sugars such as lactose, fructose, mannose, cellobiose, and others. Several HPr mutants were constructed in which phosphorylation of HPr at serine residue 46 was either inhibited or reduced using replacement by alanine or threonine, or replacing isoleucine residue 47 with threonine, resulting in significant loss of catabolite repression. Furthermore, when the three *ptsH* mutants were grown on an non-PTS sugar maltose, the addition of glucose lost its usual inhibitory effect on maltose uptake. The *hprK* gene encoding the bifunctional Hpr kinase/P-Ser-HPR phosphatase has also been characterized in *Lb. casei* (Dossonnet et al., 2000). Inactivation of *hprK* also resulted in loss of catabolite repression and inducer exclusion exerted by glucose over maltose transport. However, inducer expulsion of methyl β-D-thiogalactoside caused by rapidly metabolizable carbon sources still operated in the mutants, suggesting another mechanism for this regulatory process.

Genetics of Lactose and Galactose Utilization in Other Lactobacilli and Bifidobacteria

Phospho-β-galactosidase genes (*lacG*) have also been characterized or reported for other lactobacilli besides *Lb. casei*. In *Lactobacillus acidophilus* LTF42 a gene encoding phospho-β-galactosidase with high similarity to LacG of *Lactococcus lactis* is present, indicating metabolism of lactose by the PTS system, but the genes for transport have not been identified yet (Kanatani and Oshimura, 1994). Two *lacG* genes have been characterized for a human intestinal *Lactobacillus gasseri* isolate that encode phospho-β-galactosidase I and II (Saito et al., 1998). However, it is mainly genes encoding β-galactosidases that are been isolated and characterized for lactobacilli.

Lactobacillus delbrueckii subsp. *bulgaricus* contains a *lacSZ* operon highly homologous to that of *Streptococcus thermophilus* described above, in which the β-galactosidase (*lacZ*) gene is located downstream from the *lacS* gene encoding a lactose permease (LacS) but the genes appear to be constitutively expressed (Schmidt et al., 1989; Leong-Morgenthaler et al., 1991). The *lacA* gene, whose product is similar to the *E. coli* thiogalactosyl-transacetylase, appears to be transcribed alone, and was found upstream of *lacSZ* in *Lb. bulgaricus* but separated by a series of insertion sequence (IS) elements (Lapierre et al., 2002). The *lac* gene cluster of *Lactobacillus delbrueckii* subsp. *lactis* has a similar arrangement consisting of *lacA*, IS element(s) (different to those found in *Lb. bulgaricus*) followed by *lacS–lacZ–lacR*, the latter encoding the lactose repressor. Characterization of the clusters in the two species indicated that the lactose repressor was inactivated by a series of mutations in *Lb. bulgaricus* resulting in constitutive expression of the *lac* genes, while the insertion of IS elements appeared to increase the activity of the *lac* promoter (Lapierre et al., 2002). Like *Strep. thermophilus, Lb. bulgaricus* does not grow on galactose and ferments only the glucose portion of lactose, while the galactose is excreted into the medium (Hickey et al., 1986) and *gal* genes have not been reported for *Lb. bulgaricus*.

Gene(s) encoding β-galactosidases have been reported for several other *Lactobacillus* species. Two subunit β-galactosidase enzymes encoded by *lacL* and *lacM* genes, which was first described for *Leuconostoc lactis*, have since been characterized or reported for *Lactobacillus helveticus* (Zwahlen and Mollet, 1993), a human intestinal *Lb. acidophilus* isolate (Genbank accession No. AB004867 and AB004868), and *Lactobacillus sakei* (Obst et al., 1995). In a dairy *Lactobacillus plantarum* a plasmid-encoded *lacLM* cluster has been described, and a structurally related chromosomal copy was also detected that appears to be ubiquitous among *Lb. plantarum* strains from a variety of environments (Mayo et al., 1994; Fernández et al., 1999).

Unlike *Lb. bulgaricus, Lb. helveticus* metabolizes the galactose moiety of lactose that is fermented via the Leloir pathway (Figure 4.1), and *gal* genes have been described that are clustered at two locations on the chromosome. One cluster contains the *galK, galT*, and *galM* genes that are probably transcribed as an operon with a promoter upstream of *galK* (Mollet and Pilloud, 1991; Vaughan, 1991). At another locus the *galE* was found positioned downstream of the *lacLM* genes (Zwahlen and Mollet, 1993). Two adjacent divergently transcribed *lac–gal* operons have been characterized for the probiotic *Lactobacillus johnsonii* La1 (Pridmore et al., 1999). One contains a split β-galactosidase (*lacLM*) and a *galE* gene, while the second comprises genes coding for putative proteins with similarities to a regulator, a lactose permease (*lacS*), a second β-galactosidase gene (*bgaB*), and the Leloir pathway genes *galK, galT*, and *galM*. Also a second *galE* was found at an alternative location on the genome.

The *gal* genes have been characterized for the *Lb. casei* strain 64H and they are arranged in an operon with order *galKETRM* (Bettenbrock and Alpert, 1998). The genes are transcribed from two promoters, one upstream of *galK* that is galactose inducible, and the other semiconstitutive promoter is located within the *galK* gene. The predicted proteins of the *gal* genes are very similar to the corresponding proteins of other LAB such as *Lb. helveticus* and *Strep. thermophilus*. It is interesting that the *galR* gene, which encodes a regulator related to *galR* of *Strep. thermophilus*, is transcribed in this operon rather than being separately located as in *Strep. thermophilus*. The presence of a permease-type galactose uptake system has been demonstrated using PTS-deficient *Lb. casei* mutants that grow on galactose but the gene(s) has not yet been characterized (Bettenbrock et al., 1999).

The galactose : H^+ symporter of *Lactobacillus brevis* encoded by the *galP* gene was followed by the *galK* gene on a chromosomal location (Djordjevic et al., 2001). GalP is a member of the GPH family like LacS of *Strep. thermophilus*, but shared most similarity with the galactose permease (GalA) of *Lc. lactis*, the only two members of this family to lack the IIA^{glc}-like carboxy-terminal regulatory domain. Integration of *galP* into the chromosome of *Bacillus subtilis* was used to demonstrate allosteric regulation of GalP by phosphorylated HPr on Ser-46 via HPr(Ser) kinase resulting in uncoupling of sugar transport from proton symport that is, inducer exclusion (Djordjevic et al., 2001).

More recently, genetic determinants for β-galactosidase enzymes are being characterized for the bifidobacteria that are gaining importance because of their probiotic potential. Although *Bifidobacterium* are not strictly members of the LAB, they produce lactic acid in high amounts like the LAB. The *lacZ* gene of *Bifidobacterium longum* was cloned by functional complementation of an *E. coli* mutant and demonstrated very high similarity with its counterparts in LAB such as *Lb. bulgaricus* and *Strep. thermophilus* (Rossi et al., 2000). The high activity of this LacZ enzyme could complement bifidobacteria strains that do not grow on lactose to use this sugar as a sole carbon source. Three β-galactosidase genes of *Bifidobacterium bifidum* and one from *Bifidobacterium infantis* were cloned, characterized, and expressed in the *E. coli* background (Moller et al., 2001). All exhibited little resemblance to each other and one appeared to be an extracellular enzyme. It is with interest we await the characterization of the genes involved in prebiotic degradation such as the novel β-galactosidase described for *Bifidobacterium adolescentis* involved in the metabolism of transgalactooligosaccharides (van Laere et al., 2000).

Power of Genomics

Comparative genomics is a powerful tool for the analysis of gene function and regulation in bacterial genomes. The number of bacterial genome sequences projects is rapidly increasing and genomes of certain LAB are among these (Klaenhammer et al., 2002). The availability of complete genomes allows one to make a prediction of the metabolic potential of a certain microbe. These predictions include a complete inventory of the metabolic conversions that can be performed by the microbe, allowing the prediction of all metabolites it can potentially produce. Thereby, whole genome sequence information generates an important database for metabolic engineering purposes that aim at increasing the production level of a desired metabolite. Another feature that can directly be extracted from complete genome sequence information is a prediction of the sugars that can be utilized by a specific microbe, which can be done by analysis of all genes that are predicted to encode sugar transport systems. By comparing such a prediction with relevant experimental data, one can confirm the predicted function of the genes found. Comparison of complete genome information from different microbes could generate insight into their respective functionalities that are related to their natural habitats. An example of such an approach is given here by the analysis of PTS genes present in the genomes of *Lb. plantarum* (Kleerebezem et al., 2003) and *Lc. lactis* (Bolotin et al., 2001). The total number of PTS sugar transport systems found in *Lb. plantarum* is much larger than that found in *Lc. lactis* (27 vs. 6; Figure 4.6). This finding primarily confirms the larger flexibility in sugar usage displayed by *Lb. plantarum* compared to *Lc. lactis*. Interestingly, in many cases these PTS

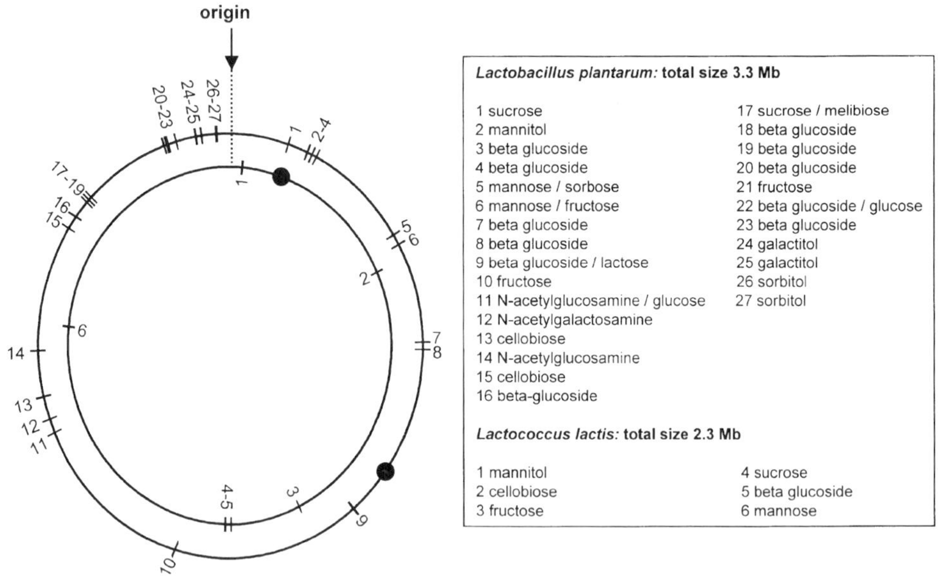

Figure 4.6. Illustration of the predicted PTS systems in the *Lactobacillus plantarum* and *Lactococcus lactis* genomes. The outer and inner circles represent the genomes of the *Lb. plantarum* and *Lc. lactis*, respectively, and the origin of replication is indicated with an arrow. The position of a particular PTS system, which is numbered in the box with its predicted substrate, is marked on the circle. The position of the *ptsHI* gene, encoding EI, is marked with a black circle.

genes are genetically linked to genes that are predicted to encode enzymes involved in degradation of the sugar that is transported by the PTS system encoded by the neighboring genes. This genetic linkage can be used to provide a more accurate prediction of the sugar specificity of the PTS system involved. Moreover, analysis of the location of these PTS systems in the chromosome reveals that the PTS genes of *Lb. plantarum* are relatively clustered around the chromosomal origin of replication, which is a feature that is not shared by *Lc. lactis* (Figure 4.6). Such a preferential localization might reflect the relative importance of these genes for the survival of *Lb. plantarum* in its natural habitat. Detailed analysis of promoter elements driving the expression of sugar transport system-encoding genes and the correlated genes involved in utilization of these sugars, might reveal regulatory motifs involved in preferential sugar utilization, including global catabolite repression and specific sugar regulation. The potential of high throughput technologies was recently implied by a study of the physiological response of *Lc. lactis* IL1403 grown on glucose or galactose containing medium (Even et al., 2001). The specific metabolic rates of a variety of enzymes and measurement of intracellular intermediates, as well as transcript profiling of all genes encoding glycolytic enzymes and lactate and mixed-acid fermentative pathways by a DNA macroarray technique were determined. Furthermore, results indicated that translational regulation occurred with 3-fold higher translational efficiency in cells grown on glucose compared to galactose (Even et al., 2001). Thus, the use of genomics, proteomics, and metabolomics may contribute enormously to this field of research.

Overall, the impact of whole genome sequence analysis on our understanding of the behavior of a certain microbe has many aspects, including global insight in metabolic potential and sugar utilization, but might very well be extended to the prediction of regulatory pathways involved into regulation of its metabolism.

Perspectives

The last decade has seen significant progress in understanding the control of sugar transport and degradation by LAB. In most cases the initial steps in the metabolic pathway, which involve the reactions from sugar transport to phosphorylation, are controlled by sugar-specific systems that react to the availability of the sugar. In the foregoing, ample attention has been given to the specific control of lactose transport, hydrolysis, and phosphorylation. These include modulation of the initiation and termination of transcription that is mediated by dedicated DNA binding proteins. The well-characterized lactose systems may serve as paradigms for the unity and diversity in organization, expression and control of other sugar-specific genes. This is supported by the genetic analyses of the utilization of other sugars that show the presence of similar dedicated DNA binding proteins (see Table 4.1). Hence it is expected that this also holds for other sugar-specific systems that will be studied. Moreover, these paradigms will be of significant help in the annotation of complete or even partial genome sequences of LAB that are now emerging (Klaenhammer et al., 2002). In other systems such approaches have showed their potential and resulted in the identification of two presumably functional PTS permease genes in the complete genome of *Mycoplasma genitalium* (Reizer et al., 1996) while that of *Bacillus subtilis* was found to contain 15 different PTS permeases (Reizer et al., 1999). The first analysis of the genomes of LAB presented here suggest the presence of a panoply of PTS-permease genes that show an unusual organization in the large genome of *Lactobacillus plantarum* (Figure 4.6). However, the functional analysis of these and other systems is needed to determine the significance of these observations.

While the specific control of sugar-related genes is mediated by sugar-specific dedicated proteins, the CcpA-mediated catabolite control is a global system that is relevant for all genetic systems involved in sugar transport and also affects the general metabolism. Also in this case the utilization of lactose or its component sugars have served to discover the functionality of this global control system in LAB. An unexpected finding has been the transcriptional activation of genes and operons involved in glycolysis and lactic acid production (Luesink et al., 1998; van den Bogaard et al., 2000). By screening the genomes of LAB for *cis*-acting CcpA operator sequences, various genes involved in major sugar degradation pathways have been found to be preceded by consensus *cre* elements. Similar approaches also have been applied to the *Bacillus subtilis* genome that revealed the presence of 126 known and putative *cre*-like elements (Miwa et al., 2000). However, also here the functionality of many of these sequences need to be demonstrated. The availability of the complete genome and the high throughput methodologies allows for the analysis of global effects. Notably, it would be of great interest to determine, understand, and subsequently model the effect of the inactivation or conditional expression of the *ccpA* gene on the transcriptome, proteome, and metabolome of LAB.

The fundamental analysis of the sugar-specific genes and their control have already shown several avenues for new applications. The exploitation of sugar-specific gene expression systems is an obvious one and has been developed based on the lactose genes in *Lc. lactis* (van Rooijen et al., 1992), *Strep. thermophilus* (Mollet et al., 1993) and more recently *Lb. casei* (Gosalbes et al., 2000). The latter two capitalize on integrative gene expression obviating the need for a selection marker. However, as a consequence the copy number of the new genetic combination is low and this can be obviated by the use of multicopy plasmid-based systems. To realize this, another use can be made of the sugar-specific genes, that is, their application as selection marker. This concept has been shown

Table 4.1. Sugar Gene Clusters and Operons besides Lactose and Galactose Characterized for Lactic Acid Bacteria

Species	Substrate and Function	Gene Clusters	Remarks	Reference
Lc. lactis[a]	Sucrose uptake & use	*sacBK sacAR*	SacR, DeoR family member; PTS[b]	Luesink et al. (1999b)
	Maltose & trehalose uptake & use	*malRP trePP-pgmB malEFG*	Part of larger operon/cluster	Nilsson and Radstrom (2001), Andersson et al. (2001), Andersson (2002)
Lb. casei	Sorbose uptake & use	*sorRE sorFABCDG*	SorR, novel in Gram-positives; PTS	Yebra et al. (2000)
Lb. brevis	Xylose uptake & use	*xylAB xylT*	XylT, Na^+-symporter	Bor et al. (1992;), Chaillou et al. (1998)
Lb. curvatus	Glucose/mannose uptake	*manABCD*	PTS system	Veyrat et al. (1996)
Lb. delbrueckii ssp. *lactis*	Arbutin metabolism	*arbZ*	Probable phospho-β-glycosidase	Weber et al. (2000)
Lb. pentosus	Isoprimeverose uptake & use	*xylPQ xylAB xylR*	Xylose intermediate; symporter	Lokman et al. (1991, 1994, 1997)
	Pentoses & gluconate uptake & use	*xpkA*	Central enzyme of phosphoketolase pathway	Posthuma et al. (2002)
Lb. plantarum	β-glucosides uptake & use	*bglGPT bglH*	BglT, BglG family antiterminators; PTS	Marasco et al. (1998, 2000)
Lb. sakei	Ribose uptake & use	*rbsUDKR*	RbsR similar to *S. aureus* GltA transporter	Stentz and Zagorec (1999)

[a]*Lc.* and *Lb.* indicate *Lactococcus* and *Lactobacillus*, respectively.
[b]Genes encode part of PTS system for uptake of sugar.

to be applicable on a large scale in the food-grade selection system based on the lactose complementation in *Lc. lactis* (Platteeuw et al., 1996). Furthermore, the use of genes involved in sugar degradation has shown potential in various applications, such as the production of oligosaccharides by specific β-galactosidases (de Vos et al., 1998) or improved EPS production (Kleerebezem et al., 1999). Finally, metabolic effects can be realized by affecting the global CcpA-mediated control and the change from homolactic to mixed acid fermentation in *ccpA* deficient mutants of *Lc. lactis* represents a new approach in metabolic engineering (Luesink et al., 1998). In addition, the global regulator CcpA and also the general PTS component HPr seem to be involved in response to cold-shock, illustrating new possibilities for exploiting sugar-related genes (Wouters et al., 2000).

In conclusion, many of the main concepts on the genetics of sugar utilization have been worked out. However, LAB are entering a new phase where the sequence of their genomes and that of their plasmids and other mobile elements is becoming available. Application of this knowledge in combination with the analysis of their transcriptome, proteome, and metabolome will allow for the further understanding and exploitation of sugar metabolism in LAB. Moreover, it will allow for the analysis of the functionality of LAB in their man-made and natural ecosystems, that include fermented food as well as the animal gastro-intestinal tract.

Acknowledgments

We are grateful to the European Community for financial support: EU grants NUTRACELLS QLRT-1999-00053, and PROGID (QKL1-2000-00536) and EU MICROFUNCTION (QKL1-2001-00135).

References

Alpert, C. A., and Siebers, U. (1997). The *lac* operon of *Lactobacillus casei* contains *lacT*, a gene coding for a protein of the BglG family of transcriptional antiterminators. *Journal of Bacteriology* 179: 1555–1562.

Andersson, U. (2002). β-Glucose 1-phosphate interconverting enzymes in *Lactococcus lactis*: Physiological role and regulation in maltose, trehalose and glucose metabolism. PhD Thesis. Lund University, Sweden

Andersson, U., Levander, F., and Radstrom, P. (2001). Trehalose-6-phosphate phosphorylase is part of a novel metabolic pathway for trehalose utilization in *Lactococcus lactis*. *Journal of Biological Chemistry* 276: 42707–42713.

Bateman, A. (1999). The SIS domain: a phosphosugar-binding domain. *Trends in Biochemical Sciences* 24: 94–95.

Benataya, A., Bracquart, P., and Linden, G. (1991). Galactose-fermenting mutants of *Streptococcus thermophilus*. *Canadian Journal of Microbiology* 35: 136–140.

Bettenbrock, K., and Alpert, C. A. (1998). The *gal* genes for the Leloir pathway of *Lactobacillus casei* 64H. *Applied and Environmental Microbiology* 64: 2013–2019.

Bettenbrock, K., Siebers, U., Ehrenreich, P., and Alpert, C. A. (1999). *Lactobacillus casei* 64H contains a phosphoenolpyruvate-dependent phosphotransferase system for uptake of galactose, as confirmed by analysis of *ptsH* and different *gal* mutants. *Journal of Bacteriology* 181: 225–230.

Bisset, D. L., and Anderson, R. L. (1973). Lactose and D-galactose metabolism in *Staphylococcus aureus*: Pathway of D-galactose 6-phosphate degradation. *Biochemical and Biophysical Research Communications* 52: 641–647.

Bisset, D. L., and Anderson, R. L. (1974). Lactose and D-galactose metabolism in group N streptococci: Presence of enzymes for both the D-galactose-1-phosphate and D-tagatose 6-phosphate pathways. *Journal of Bacteriology* 117: 318–320.

Boels, I. C., Kleerebezem, M., and de Vos, W. M. (2003). Engineering of carbon distribution between glycolysis and sugar nucleotide biosynthesis in *Lactococcus lactis*. *Applied Environmental Microbiology* 69: 1129–1135.

Boels, I. C., Ramos, A., Kleerebezem, M., de Vos, W. M. (2001). Functional analysis of the *Lactococcus lactis galU* and *galE* genes and their impact on sugar nucleotide and exopolysaccharide biosynthesis. *Applied Environmental Microbiology* 67: 3033–3040.

Bolotin, A., Mauger, S., Malarme, K., Ehrlich, S. D., and Sorokin, A. (1999). Low-redundancy sequencing of the entire *Lactococcus lactis* IL1403 genome. *Antonie Van Leeuwenhoek* 76: 27–76.

Bolotin, A., Wincker, P., Mauger, S., Jaillon, O., Malarme, K., Weissenbach, J., Ehrlich, S. D., and Sorokin, A. (2001). The complete genome sequence of the lactic acid bacterium *Lactococcus lactis* ssp. *lactis* IL1403. *Genome Research* 11: 731–753.

Bor, Y. C., Moraes, C., Lee, S. P., Crosby, W. L., Sinskey, A. J., and Batt, C. A. (1992). Cloning and sequencing the *Lactobacillus brevis* gene encoding xylose isomerase. *Gene* 114: 127–132.

Chaillou, S., Bor, Y. C., Batt, C. A., Postma, P. W., and Pouwels, P. H. (1998). Molecular cloning and functional expression in *Lactobacillus plantarum* 80 of *xylT*, encoding the D-xylose-H+ symporter of *Lactobacillus brevis*. *Applied and Environmental Microbiology* 64: 4720–4728.

Chassy, B. M., and Alpert, C. A. (1989). Molecular characterization of the plasmid-encoded lactose- PTS of *Lactobacillus casei*. *FEMS Microbiology Reviews* 5: 157–165.

Chassy, B. M., Gibson, E. V., and Giuffrida, A. (1978). Evidence for plasmid associated lactose metabolism in *Lactobacillus casei* subsp. *casei*. *Current Microbiology* 1: 141–144.

Chassy, B. M., and Thompson, J. (1983). Regulation of lactose-phosphoenolpyruvate-dependent phosphotransferase system and ß-D-phosphogalactoside galactohydrolase activities in *Lactobacillus casei*. *Journal of Bacteriology* 154: 1195–1203.

Crow, V. L., Davey, G. P., Pearce, L. E., and Thomas, T. D. (1983). Plasmid linkage of the D-tagatose 6-phosphate pathway in *Streptococcus lactis*: Effect on lactose and galactose metabolism. *Journal of Bacteriology* 153: 76–83.

David, S. (1992). Genetics of mesophilic citrate fermenting lactic acid bacteria. PhD Thesis, Wageningen Agriculture University, Wageningen, The Netherlands.

David, S., Simons, G., and de Vos, W. M. (1989). Plasmid transformation by electroporation in *Leuconostoc paramesenteroides*. *Applied and Environmental Microbiology* 55: 1483–1489.

David, S., Stevens, H., Van Riel, M., Simons, S., and de Vos, W. (1992). *Leuconostoc lactis* ß-galactosidase is encoded by two overlapping genes. *Journal of Bacteriology* 174: 4475–4481.

Deutscher, J., Kuster, E., Bergstedt, U., Charrier, V., and Hillen, W. (1995). Protein kinase-dependent HPr/CcpA interaction links glycolytic activity to carbon catabolite repression in Gram-positive bacteria. *Molecular Microbiology* 15: 1049–1053.

de Vos, W. M. (1990). Disaccharide utilization in lactic acid bacteria. In: J. Heslot, J. Davies, J. Florent, L. Bobichon, G. Durant, and L. Penasse (Eds.), *Proceedings of the 6th Symposium on the genetics of industrial microorganisms, GIM90* (pp. 447–457). Paris: Societe Francaise de Microbiologie.

de Vos, W. M., Boerrigter, I., van Rooijen, R. J., Reiche, B., and Hengstenberg, W. (1990). Characterization of the lactose-specific enzymes of the phosphotransferase system in *Lactococcus lactis*. *Journal of Biological Chemistry* 265: 22554–22560.

de Vos, W. M., and Gasson, M. J. (1989). Structure and expression of the *Lactococcus lactis* gene for phospho-ß-galactosidase (*lacG*) in *Escherichia coli* and *L. lactis*. *Journal of General Microbiology* 135: 1833–1846.

de Vos, W. M., Hols, P., van Kranenurg, R., Luesink, E. J., Kuipers, O. P., van der Oost, J., Kleerebezem, M., and Hugenholtz, J. (1998). Making more of milk sugar by engineering lactic acid bacteria. *International Dairy Journal* 8: 227–233.

de Vos, W. M., and Simons, G. (1988). Molecular cloning of lactose genes in dairy lactic streptococci: The phospho-ß-galactosidase and ß-galactosidase genes and their expression products. *Biochimie* 70: 461–475.

de Vos, W. M., and Vaughan, E. E. (1994). Genetics of lactose utilization in lactic acid bacteria. *FEMS Microbiological Reviews* 15: 217–237.

Djordjevic, G. M., Tchieu, J. H., and Saier M. H., Jr. (2001). Genes involved in control of galactose uptake in *Lactobacillus brevis* and reconstitution of the regulatory system in *Bacillus subtilis*. *Journal of Bacteriology* 183: 3224–3236.

Dossonnet, V., Monedero, V., Zagorec, M., Galinier, A., Perez-Martinez, G., and Deutscher, J. (2000). Phosphorylation of HPr by the bifunctional HPr Kinase/P-ser-HPr phosphatase from *Lactobacillus casei* controls catabolite repression and inducer exclusion but not inducer expulsion. *Journal of Bacteriology* 182: 2582–2590.

Even, S., Lindley, N. D., and Cocaign-Bousquet, M. (2001). Molecular physiology of sugar catabolism in *Lactococcus lactis* IL1403. *Journal of Bacteriology* 183: 3817–3824.

Farrow, J. A. (1980). Lactose hydrolysing enzymes in *Streptococcus lactis* and *Streptococcus cremoris* and also in some other species of streptococci. *Journal of Applied Bacteriology* 49: 493–503.

Fernández, M., Margolles, A., Suarez, J. E., and Mayo, B. (1999). Duplication of the beta-galactosidase gene in some *Lactobacillus plantarum* strains. *International Journal of Food Microbiology* 48: 113–123.

Foucaud, C., and Poolman, B. (1992). Lactose transport system of *Streptococcus thermophilus*. Functional reconstitution of the protein and characterization of the kinetic mechanism of transport. *Journal of Biological Chemistry* 267: 22087–22094.

Fujita, Y., Miwa, Y., Galinier, A., and Deutscher, J. (1995). Specific recognition of the *Bacillus subtilis gnt cis*-acting catabolite-responsive element by a protein complex formed between CcpA and seryl-phosphorylated HPr. *Molecular Microbiology* 17: 953–960.

Galinier, A., Kravanja, M., Engelmann, R., Hengstenberg, W., Kilhoffer, M. C., Deutscher, J., and Haiech, J. (1998). New protein kinase and protein phosphatase families mediate signal transduction in bacterial catabolite repression. *Proceedings of the National Academy of Science USA* 95: 1823–1828.

Gasson, M. J. (1983). Plasmid complements of *Streptococcus lactis* NCDO 712 and other lactic streptococci after protoplast-induced curing. *Journal of Bacteriology* 154: 1–9.

Gosalbes, M. J., Esteban, C. D., Galan, J. L., and Perez-Martinez, G. (2000). Integrative food-grade expression system based on the lactose regulon of *Lactobacillus casei*. *Applied and Environmental Microbiology* 66: 4822–4828.

Gosalbes, M. J., Esteban, C. D., and Perez-Martinez, G. (2002). *In vivo* effect of mutations in the antiterminator LacT in *Lactobacillus casei*. *Microbiology* 148: 695–702.

Gosalbes, M. J., Monedero, V., Alpert, C. A., and Perez-Martinez, G. (1997). Establishing a model to study the regulation of the lactose operon in *Lactobacillus casei*. *FEMS Microbiological Letters* 148: 83–89.

Gosalbes, M. J., Monedero, V., and Perez-Martinez, G. (1999). Elements involved in catabolite repression and substrate induction of the lactose operon in *Lactobacillus casei*. *Journal of Bacteriology* 181: 3928–3934.

Grossiord, B. (1998). Métabolisme du galactose par la voie de Leloir: l'óperon *gal* de *Lactococcus lactis*. PhD thesis. École Nationale Supérieure Agronomique de Montpellier, France.

Grossiord, B. P., Luesink, E. J., Vaughan, E. E., Arnaud A., and de Vos W. M. (2003). Characterization, expression, and mutation of the *Lactococcus lactis galPMKTE* genes, involved in galactose utilization via the Leloir pathway. *Journal of Bacteriology* 185: 870–878.

Grossiord, B., Vaughan, E. E., Luesink, E., and de Vos, W. M. (1998). Genetics of galactose utilisation via the Leloir pathway in lactic acid bacteria. *Lait* 78: 77–84.

Gunnewijk, M. G., and Poolman, B. (2000a). HPr(His approximately P)-mediated phosphorylation differently affects counterflow and proton motive force-driven uptake via the lactose transport protein of *Streptococcus thermophilus*. *Journal of Biological Chemistry* 275: 34080–34085.

Gunnewijk, M. G., and Poolman, B. (2000b). Phosphorylation state of HPr determines the level of expression and the extent of phosphorylation of the lactose transport protein of *Streptococcus thermophilus*. *Journal of Biological Chemistry* 275: 34073–34079.

Gunnewijk, M. G., Postma, P. W., and Poolman, B. (1999). Phosphorylation and functional properties of the IIA domain of the lactose transport protein of *Streptococcus thermophilus*. *Journal of Bacteriology* 181: 632–641.

Gunnewijk, M. G., van den Bogaard, P. T., Veenhof, L. M., Heuberger, E. H., de Vos, W. M., Kleerebezem, M., Kuipers, O. P., and Poolman, B. (2001). Hierarchical control versus autoregulation of carbohydrate utilisation in bacteria. *Journal of Molecular Microbiology and Biotechnology* 3: 401–413.

Hengstenberg, W., Reiche, B., Eiserman, R., Fischer, R., Kessler, U., Tarrach, A., de Vos, W. M., Kalbitzer, H. R., and Glaser, S. (1989). Structure and function of proteins involved in sugar transport by the PTS of Gram-positive bacteria. *FEMS Microbiological Reviews* 63: 35–42.

Hickey, M. W., Hillier, A. J., and Jago, G. R. (1986). Transport and metabolism of lactose, glucose, and galactose in homofermentative lactobacilli. *Applied Environmental Microbiology* 51: 825–831.

Huang, X. F., Huang, D. C., Novel, G., and Novel, M. (1995). Two *Lactococcus lactis* genes, including *lacX*, cooperate to trigger an SOS response in a *recA*-negative background. *Journal of Bacteriology* 177: 283–289.

Hudson, M. J., and Marsh, P. D. (1995). Carbohydrate metabolism in the colon. In: G. R. Gibson and G. T. Macfarlane (Eds.), *Human colonic bacteria: Role in nutrition, physiology, and pathology* (pp. 61–73). CRC Press.

Hutkins, R. W., and Morris, H. A. (1987). Carbohydrate metabolism by *Streptococcus thermophilus*: A review. *Journal of Food Protection* 50: 876–884.

Kanatani, K., and Oshimura, M. (1994). Isolation and structural analysis of the phospho-beta-galactosidase gene from *Lactobacillus acidophilus*. *Journal of Fermentation and Bioengineering* 78: 123–129.

Kandler, O. (1983). Carbohydrate metabolism in the lactic acid bacteria. *Antonie van Leeuwenhoek* 49: 209–224.

Kashket, E. R., and Wilson, T. H. (1973). Proton-coupled accumulation of galactoside transport in *Streptococcus lactis* 7962. *Proceedings of the National Academy of Science USA* 70: 2866–2869.

Kim, J. H., Voskuil, M. I., and Chambliss, G. H. (1998). NADP, corepressor for the *Bacillus* catabolite control protein CcpA. *Proceedings of the National Academy of Science USA* 95: 9590–9595.

Klaenhammer, T. R. (1998). Functional activities of *Lactobacillus* probiotics: Genetic mandate. *International Dairy Journal* 8: 497–505.
Klaenhammer, T. R. K., Altermann, E., Arigoni, F., Bolotin, A., Breidt, F., Broadbent, J., Cano, R., Chaillou, S., Deutscher, J., Gasson, M., van de Guchte, M., Guzzo, J., Hartke, A., Hawkins, T., Hols, P., Hutkins, R., Kleerebezem, M., Kok, J., Kuipers, O., Lubbers, M., Maguin, E., McKay, L., Mills, D., Nauta, A., Overbeek, R., Pel, H., Pridmore, D., Saier, M., van Sinderen, D., Sorokin, A., Steele, J., O'Sullivan, D., de Vos, W., Weimer, B., Zagorec, M., and Siezen, R. (2002). Discovering lactic acid bacteria by genomics. *Antonie Van Leeuwenhoek* 82: 29–58.
Kleerebezem, M., Boekhorst, J., van Kranenburg, R., Molenaar, D., Kuipers, O. P., Leer, R., Tarchini, R., Peters, S. A., Sandbrink, H. M., Fiers, M. W., Stiekema, W., Lankhorst, R. M., Bron, P. A., Hoffer, S. M., Groot, M. N., Kerkhoven, R., de Vries, M., Ursing, B., de Vos, W. M., and Siezen R. J. (2003). Complete genome sequence of *Lactobacillus plantarum* WCFS1. *Proceedings of the National Academy of Science USA* 18: 1990–1995.
Kleerebezem, M., van Kranenburg, R., Tuinier, R., Boels, I. C., Zoon, P., Looijesteijn, E., Hugenholtz, J., and de Vos, W. M. (1999). Exopolysaccharides produced by *Lactococcus lactis*: From genetic engineering to improved rheological properties? *Antonie Van Leeuwenhoek* 76: 357–365.
Kravanja, M., Engelmann, R., Dossonnet, V., Bluggel, M., Meyer, H. E., Frank, R., Galinier, A., Deutscher, J., Schnell, N., and Hengstenberg, W. (1999). The *hprK* gene of *Enterococcus faecalis* encodes a novel bifunctional enzyme: The HPr kinase/phosphatase. *Molecular Microbiology* 31: 59–66.
Lapierre, L., Mollet, B., and Germond, J. E. (2002). Regulation and adaptive evolution of lactose operon expression in *Lactobacillus delbrueckii*. *Journal of Bacteriology* 184: 928–935.
Leong-Morgenthaler, P., Zwahlen, M. C., and Hottinger, H. (1991). Lactose metabolism in *Lactobacillus bulgaricus*: Analysis of the primary structure and expression of the genes involved. *Journal of Bacteriology* 173: 1951–1957.
Lokman, B. C., Heerikhuisen, M., Leer, R. J., van den Broek, A., Borsboom, Y., Chaillou, S., Postma, P. W., and Pouwels, P. H. (1997). Regulation of expression of the *Lactobacillus pentosus* xylAB operon. *Journal of Bacteriology* 179: 5391–5397.
Lokman, B. C., Leer, R. J., van Sorge, R., and Pouwels, P. H. (1994). Promoter analysis and transcriptional regulation of *Lactobacillus pentosus* genes involved in xylose catabolism. *Molecular and General Genetics* 245: 117–125.
Lokman, B. C., van Santen, P., Verdoes, J. C., Kruse, J., Leer, R. J., Posno, M., and Pouwels, P. H. (1991). Organization and characterization of three genes involved in D-xylose catabolism in *Lactobacillus pentosus*. *Molecular and General Genetics* 230: 161–169.
Luesink, E. J., Beumer, C. M., Kuipers, O. P., and de Vos, W. M. (1999a). Molecular characterization of the *Lactococcus lactis ptsHI* operon and analysis of the regulatory role of HPr. *Journal of Bacteriology* 181: 764–771.
Luesink, E. J., Maragg, J. D., Kuipers O. P., and de Vos, W. M. (1999b). Characterization of the divergent *sacBK* and *sacAR* operons, involved in sucrose utilization by *Lactococcus lactis*. *Journal of Bacteriology* 181: 1924–1926.
Luesink, E. J., van Herpen, R. E., Grossiord, B. P., Kuipers, O. P., and de Vos, W. M. (1998). Transcriptional activation of the glycolytic *las* operon and catabolite repression of the *gal* operon in *Lactococcus lactis* are mediated by the catabolite control protein CcpA. *Molecular Microbiology* 30: 789–798.
Maeda, S., and Gasson, M. J. (1986). Cloning, expression and location of the *Streptococcus lactis* gene for phospho-beta-D-galactosidase. *Journal of General Microbiology* 132: 331–340.
Marasco, R., Muscariello, L., Varcamonti, M., De Felice, M., and Sacco, M. (1998). Expression of the *bglH* gene of *Lactobacillus plantarum* is controlled by carbon catabolite repression. *Journal of Bacteriology* 180: 3400–3404.
Marasco, R., Salatiello, I., De Felice, M., and Sacco, M. (2000). A physical and functional analysis of the newly-identified *bglGPT* operon of *Lactobacillus plantarum*. *FEMS Microbiology Letters* 186: 269–273.
Mayo, B., Gonzalez, B., Arca, P., and Suarez, J. E. (1994). Cloning and expression of the plasmid encoded beta-D-galactosidase gene from a *Lactobacillus plantarum* strain of dairy origin. *FEMS Microbiology Letters* 122: 145–151.
McKay, L. L. (1982). Regulation of lactose metabolism in dairy streptococci. In: R. Davies (Ed.), *Developments in food microbiology* (Vol. 1, pp. 153–182). London: Elsevier Applied Science Publishers.
McKay, L. L., Walter, L. A., Sandine, W. E., and Elliker, P. R. (1969). Involvement of phosphoenolpyruvate in lactose utilization by Group N streptococci. *Journal of Bacteriology* 99: 603–610.
Miwa, Y., Nakata, A., Ogiwara, A., Yamamoto, M., and Fujita, Y. (2000). Evaluation and characterization of catabolite-responsive elements of *Bacillus subtilis*. *Nucleic Acids Research* 28: 1206–1210.

Moller, P. L., Jorgensen, F., Hansen, O. C., Madsen, S. M., and Stougaard, P. (2001). Intra- and extracellular β-galactosidases from *Bifidobacterium bifidum* and *B. infantis*: Molecular cloning, heterologous expression, and comparative characterization. *Applied and Environmental Microbiology* 67: 2276–2283.

Mollet, B., and Pilloud, N. (1991). Galactose utilization in *Lactobacillus helveticus*: Isolation and characterization of the galactokinase (*galK*) and galactose-1-phosphate uridyl transferase (*galT*) genes. *Journal of Bacteriology* 173: 4464–4473.

Mollet, B., Knol, J., Poolman, B., Marciset, O., and Delley, M. (1993). Directed genomic integration, gene replacement, and integrative gene expression in *Streptococcus thermophilus*. *Journal of Bacteriology* 175: 4315–4324.

Monedero, V., Gosalbes, M. J., and Perez-Martinez, G. (1997). Catabolite repression in *Lactobacillus casei* ATCC 393 is mediated by CcpA. *Journal of Bacteriology* 179: 6657–6664.

Mustapha, A., Hutkins, R. W., and Zirnstein, W. (1995). Cloning and characterization of the galactokinase gene from *Streptococcus thermophilus*. *Journal of Dairy Science* 78: 989–997.

Nilsson, U., and Radstrom, P. (2001). Genetic localization and regulation of the maltose phosphorylase gene, *malP*, in *Lactococcus lactis*. *Microbiology* 147: 1565–1573.

Obst, M., Meding, E. R., Vogel, R. F., and Hammes, W. P. (1995). Two genes encoding the β-galactosidase of *Lactobacillus sake*. *Microbiology* 141: 3059–3066.

Park, Y. H., and McKay, L. L. (1982). Distinct galactose phosphoenolpyruvate-dependent phosphotransferase system in *Streptococcus lactis*. *Journal of Bacteriology* 149: 420–425.

Platteeuw, C., van Alen-Boerrigter, I., van Schalkwijk, S., and de Vos, W. M. (1996). Food-grade cloning and expression system for *Lactococcus lactis*. *Applied and Environmental Microbiology* 62: 1008–1013.

Poolman, B. (1993). Energy transduction in lactic acid bacteria. *FEMS Microbiological Reviews* 4: 1629–1636.

Poolman, B., Knol, J., Mollet, B., Nieuwenhuis, B., and Sulter, G. (1995). Regulation of bacterial sugar-H^+ symport by phosphoenolpyruvate-dependent enzyme I/HPr-mediated phosphorylation. *Proceedings of the National Academy of Science USA* 92: 778–782.

Poolman, B., Knol, J., van der Does, C., Henderson, P. J., Liang, W. J., Leblanc, G., Pourcher, T., and Mus-Veteau, I. (1996). Cation and sugar selectivity determinants in a novel family of transport proteins. *Molecular Microbiology* 19: 911–922.

Poolman, B., Royer, T. J., Mainzer, S. E., and Schmidt, B. F. (1989). Lactose transport system of *Streptococcus thermophilus*: A hybrid protein with homology to the melibiose carrier and enzyme III of phosphoenolpyruvate-dependent phosphotransferase systems. *Journal of Bacteriology* 171: 244–253.

Poolman, B., Royer, T. J., Mainzer, S. E., and Schmidt, B. F. (1990). Carbohydrate utilization in *Streptococcus thermophilus*: Characterization of the genes for aldose 1-epimerase (mutarotase) and UDPglucose 4-epimerase. *Journal of Bacteriology* 172: 4037–4047.

Posthuma, C. C., Bader, R., Engelmann, R., Postma, P. W., Hengstenberg, W., and Pouwels, P. H. (2002). Expression of the xylulose 5-phosphate phosphoketolase gene, *xpkA*, from *Lactobacillus pentosus* MD363 is induced by sugars that are fermented via the phosphoketolase pathway and is repressed by glucose mediated by CcpA and the mannose phosphoenolpyruvate phosphotransferase system. *Applied and Environmental Microbiology* 68: 831–837.

Postma, P. W., Lengeler, J. W., and Jacobson, G. R. (1993). Phosphoenolpyruvate: Carbohydrate phosphotransferase systems of bacteria. *Microbiological Reviews* 57: 543–594.

Pridmore, R. D., Pittet, A.-C., Zwahlen, M.-C., Walker, C., and Mollet, B. (1999). The lactose/galactose operons of *Lactobacillus johnsonii* La1. *Sixth Symposium on Lactic Acid Bacteria—Genetics, Metabolism and Applications, Veldhoeven, The Netherlands*. Abstract H20.

Reizer, J., Bachem, S., Reizer, A., Arnaud, M., Saier, M. H., Jr., and Stülke, J. (1999). Novel phosphotransferase system genes revealed by genome analysis—the complete complement of PTS proteins encoded within the genome of *Bacillus subtilis*. *Microbiology* 145: 3419–3429.

Reizer, J., Paulsen, I. T., Reizer, A., Titgemeyer, F., and Saier, M. H., Jr. (1996). Novel phosphotransferase system genes revealed by bacteria genome analysis: The complete complement of PTS genes in *Mycoplasma genitalium*. *Microbial Comparative Genomics* 1: 151–163.

Ross, P., O'Gara, F., and Condon, S. (1987). Cloning of chromosomal genes by heterologous complementation: Partial characterization of a putative lactose transport gene of *Lactococcus lactis* subsp. *lactis*. *FEMS Microbiological Letters* 61: 183–188.

Rossi, M., Altomare, L., Gonzalez Vara y Rodriguez, A., Brigidi, P., and Matteuzzi, D. (2000). Nucleotide sequence, expression and transcriptional analysis of the *Bifidobacterium longum* MB 219 *lacZ* gene. *Archives in Microbiology* 174: 74–80.

Rutberg, B. (1997). Antitermination of transcription of catabolic operons. *Molecular Microbiology* 23: 413–421.

Saier, M. H., Jr., and Reizer, J. (1992). Proposed uniform nomenclature for the proteins and protein domains of the bacterial phosphoenolpyruvate: Sugar phosphotransferase system. *Journal of Bacteriology* 174: 1433–1438.

Saito, T., Suzuki, M., Konno, K., Kitazawa, H., Kawai, Y., Itoh, T., and Kamio, Y. (1998). Molecular cloning and sequencing of two phospho-beta-galactosidase I and II genes of *Lactobacillus gasseri* JCM1031 isolated from human intestine. *Bioscience Biotechnology Biochemistry* 62: 2318–2327.

Schmidt, B. F., Adams, R. M., Requadt, C., Power, S., and Mainzer, S. E. (1989). Expression and nucleotide sequence of the *Lactobacillus bulgaricus* ß-galactosidase gene cloned in *Escherichia coli. Journal of Bacteriology* 171: 625–635.

Schmidt, B. F., Royer, T. J., Yoast, S., and Poolman, B. (1990). The lactose transport gene from *Lactobacillus delbrueckii* subsp. *bulgaricus*: Part of the lactose operon as in *Streptococcus thermophilus*. In: G. Venema, B. Poolman, and J. T. M. Wouters (Eds.), *FEMS microbiological reviews* (Vol. 87), P18 A26. Amsterdam: Elsevier Science Publishers.

Schroeder, C. J., Robert, C., Lenzen, G., McKay, L. L., and Mercienier, A. (1991). Analysis of the *lacZ* sequences from two *Streptococcus thermophilus* strains: Comparison with the *Escherichia coli* and *Lactobacillus bulgaricus* ß-galactosidase sequences. *Journal of General Microbiology* 137: 369–380.

Shimuzu-Kadota, M. (1987). Properties of lactose plasmid pLY101 in *Lactobacillus casei. Applied and Environmental Microbiology* 53: 2987–2991.

Stentz, R., and Zagorec, M. (1999). Ribose utilization in *Lactobacillus sakei*: Analysis of the regulation of the *rbs* operon and putative involvement of a new transporter. *Journal of Molecular Microbiology and Biotechnology* 1: 165–173.

Stülke, J., and Hillen, W. (1999). Carbon catabolite repression in bacteria. *Current Opinion in Microbiology* 2: 195–201.

Stülke, J., and Hillen, W. (2000). Regulation of carbon catabolism in *Bacillus* species. *Annual Review of Microbiology* 54: 849–880.

Stülke, J., Arnaud, M., Rapoport, G., and Martin-Verstraete, I. (1998). PRD—a protein domain involved in PTS-dependent induction and carbon catabolite repression of catabolic operons in bacteria. *Molecular Microbiology* 28: 865–874.

Thomas, T. D., Turner, K. W., and Crow, V. L. (1980). Galactose fermentation by *Streptococcus lactis* and *Streptococcus cremoris*: Pathways, products, and regulation. *Journal of Bacteriology* 144: 672–682.

Thompson, J. (1980). Galactose transport systems in *Streptococcus lactis. Journal of Bacteriology* 144: 683–691.

Thompson, J. (1987). Regulation of sugar transport and metabolism in lactic acid bacteria. *FEMS Microbiological Reviews* 46: 221–231.

Vaillancourt, K., Moineau, S., Frenette, M., Lessard, C., and Vadeboncoeur, C. (2002). Galactose and lactose genes from the galactose-positive bacterium *Streptococcus salivarius* and the phylogenetically related galactose-negative bacterium *Streptococcus thermophilus*: Organization, sequence, transcription, and activity of the *gal* gene products. *Journal of Bacteriology* 184: 785–793.

van den Bogaard, P. T. C. (2002). Catabolite control of sugar metabolism in *Streptococcus thermophilus*. PhD Thesis. Wageningen University, The Netherlands.

van den Bogaard, P. T. C., Kleerebezem, M., Kuipers, O. P., and de Vos, W. M. (2000). Control of lactose transport, β-galactosidase activity, and glycolysis by CcpA in *Streptococcus thermophilus*: Evidence for carbon catabolite repression by a non-phosphoenolpyruvate-dependent phosphotransferase system sugar. *Journal of Bacteriology* 182: 5982–5989.

van Laere, K. M., Abee, T., Schols, H. A., Beldman, G., and Voragen, A. G. (2000). Characterization of a novel β-galactosidase from *Bifidobacterium adolescentis* DSM 20083 active towards transgalactooligosaccharides. *Applied and Environmental Microbiology* 66: 1379–1384.

van Rooijen, R. J., Dam, W., and de Vos, W. M. (1993a). Deletion of the *Lactococcus lactis lacR* repressor gene and its effect on the regulation of lactose operon expression. In: R. J. van Rooijen (Ed.), *Characterization of the* Lactococcus lactis *lactose genes and regulation of their expression* (pp. 119–134). PhD thesis Wageningen Agricultural University.

van Rooijen, R. J., Dechering, K. J., Wilmink, C. N. J., and de Vos, W. M. (1993b). Lysines 72, 80, 213, and aspartic acid 210 of the *Lactococcus lactis* LacR repressor are involved in the response to the inducer tagatose-6-phosphate leading to induction of *lac* operon expression. *Protein Engineering* 6: 208–215.

van Rooijen, R. J., and de Vos, W. M. (1990). Molecular cloning, transcriptional analysis and nucleotide sequence of *lacR*, a gene encoding the repressor of the lactose phosphotransferase system of *Lactococcus lactis. Journal of Biological Chemistry* 265: 18499–18503.

van Rooijen, R. J., and de Vos, W. M. (1993a). Purification of the *Lactococcus lactis* LacR repressor gene and characterization of its DNA binding. In: R. J. van Rooijen (Ed.), *Characterization of the Lactococcus lactis lactose genes and regulation of their expression* (pp. 101–118). PhD thesis Wageningen Agricultural University, The Netherlands.

van Rooijen, R. J., and de Vos, W. M. (1993b). Nucleotide sequence of an *iso*-IS*S1* element flanking the 3′ end of the *Lactococcus lactis lac operon*. In: R. J. van Rooijen (Ed.), *Characterization of the Lactococcus lactis lactose genes and regulation of their expression* (pp. 59–61). PhD thesis Wageningen Agricultural University, The Netherlands.
van Rooijen, R. J., Gasson, M. J., and de Vos, W. M. (1992). Characterization of the promoter of the *Lactococcus lactis* lactose operon: Contribution of flanking sequences and LacR repressor to its activity. *Journal of Bacteriology* 174: 2273–2280.
van Rooijen, R. J., van Schalkwijk, S., and de Vos, W. M. (1991). Molecular cloning, characterization, and nucleotide sequence of the tagatose 6-phosphate pathway gene cluster of the lactose operon of *Lactococcus lactis*. *Journal of Biological Chemistry* 266: 7176–7181.
Vaughan, E. E. (1991). Characterization of a bacteriocin produced by *Lactobacillus helveticus* and cloning of chromosomal genes by heterologous complementation. PhD Thesis, National University of Ireland.
Vaughan, E. E., and Mollet, B. (1999). Probiotics in the new millenium. *Nahrung* 43: 148–153.
Vaughan, E. E., David, S., and de Vos, W. M. (1996). The lactose transporter in *Leuconostoc lactis* is a new member of the LacS subfamily of galactoside–pentose–hexuronide translocators. *Applied and Environmental Microbiology* 62: 1574–1582.
Vaughan, E. E., de Vries, M. C., Zoetendal, E. G., Ben-Amor, K., Akkermans, A. D. L., and de Vos, W. M. (2002). The Intestinal LABs. *Antonie Van Leeuwenhoek* 82: 341–352.
Vaughan, E. E., Mollet, B., and de Vos, W. M. (1999). Functionality of probiotics and intestinal lactobacilli: Light in the intestinal tract tunnel. *Current Opinion in Biotechnology* 10: 505–510.
Vaughan, E. E., Pridmore, R. D., and Mollet, B. (1998). Transcriptional regulation and evolution of lactose genes in the *galactose–lactose* operon of *Lactococcus lactis* NCDO2054. *Journal of Bacteriology* 180: 4893–4902.
Vaughan, E. E., van den Bogaard, P. T. C., Catzeddu, P., Kuipers, O. P., and de Vos, W. M. (2001). Activation of silent *gal* genes in the *lac-gal* regulon of *Streptococcus thermophilus*. *Journal of Bacteriology* 183: 1184–1194.
Veyrat, A., Gosalbes, M. J., and Perez-Martinez, G. (1996). *Lactobacillus curvatus* has a glucose transport system homologous to the mannose family of phosphoenolpyruvate-dependent phosphotransferase systems. *Microbiology* 142: 3469–3477.
Viana, R., Monedero, V., Dossonnet, V., Vadeboncoeur, C., Perez-Martinez, G., and Deutscher, J. (2000). Enzyme I and HPr from *Lactobacillus casei*: Their role in sugar transport, carbon catabolite repression and inducer exclusion. *Molecular Microbiology* 36: 570–584.
Weber, B. A., Klein, J. R., and Henrich, B. (2000). Expression of the phospho-beta-glycosidase ArbZ from *Lactobacillus delbrueckii* subsp. *lactis* in *Lactobacillus helveticus*: Substrate induction and catabolite repression. *Microbiology* 146: 1941–1948.
Weickert, M. J., and Chambliss, G. H. (1990). Site-directed mutagenesis of a catabolite repression operator sequence in *Bacillus subtilis*. *Proceedings of the National Academy of Science USA* 87: 6238–6242.
Wouters, J. A., Kamphuis, H. H., Hugenholtz, J., Kuipers, O. P., de Vos, W. M., and Abee, T. (2000). Changes in glycolytic activity of *Lactococcus lactis* induced by low temperature. *Applied and Environmental Microbiology* 66: 3686–3691.
Ye, J. J., and Saier, M. H., Jr. (1995a). Allosteric regulation of the glucose:H+ symporter of *Lactobacillus brevis*: Cooperative binding of glucose and HPr(ser-P). *Journal of Bacteriology* 177: 1900–1902.
Ye, J. J., and Saier, M. H., Jr. (1995b). Cooperative binding of lactose and the phosphorylated phosphocarrier protein HPr(Ser-P) to the lactose/H^+ symport permease of *Lactobacillus brevis*. *Proceedings of the National Academy Science USA* 92: 417–421.
Ye, J. J., Reizer, J., Cui, X., and Saier, M. H., Jr. (1994). Inhibition of the phosphoenolpyruvate : Lactose phosphotransferase system and activation of a cytoplasmic sugar-phosphate phosphatase in *Lactococcus lactis* by ATP-dependent metabolite-activated phosphorylation of serine 46 in the phosphocarrier protein HPr. *Journal of Biological Chemistry* 269: 11837–11844.
Yebra, M. J., Veyrat, A., Santos, M. A., and Perez-Martinez, G. (2000). Genetics of L-sorbose transport and metabolism in *Lactobacillus casei*. *Journal of Bacteriology* 182: 155–163.
Zwahlen, M.-C., and Mollet, B. (1993). Characterization of the *lacZ* gene and discovery of a novel IS element (ISL2) in *Lactobacillus helveticus*. In: W. M. de Vos, J. H. R. Huis in't Veld, and B. Poolman (Eds.), *FEMS microbiological reviews* (Vol. 12), P27 B9. Amsterdam: Elsevier Science Publishers.

5

Regulation of Gene Expression in *Lactococcus lactis*

Oscar P. Kuipers and Kees J. Leenhouts

Introduction

Undoubtedly, the second-best genetically characterized Gram-positive bacterium is *Lactococcus lactis*, following behind the unchallenged model system *Bacillus subtilis*. Although there are quite a number of similarities between these two organisms with respect to gene regulation and gene expression in general, it is important to realize there are also important differences. *Lactococcus* can be regarded as a simpler organism lacking the potential to sporulate or, so far as we know, to be naturally competent, possessing only a very limited number of sigma factors (in known cases one to four), and being fully fermentative organisms, without electron transport chains. Studying such an organism also has some advantages for the researcher: the genome is relatively small, without great numbers of paralog genes, metabolic engineering can be straightforward since there are relatively few regulatory and metabolic pathways present, and the bacterium lacks the great number of proteases that can affect the success of homologous and heterologous gene expression. Another specific property of *Lc. lactis* is that it is a bacterium ingested in high numbers by humans in the form of fermented foods and subsequently resides for some time in the gastro-intestinal (GI) tract. Studying the behavior of *Lc. lactis* in the GI-tract poses an interesting challenge for molecular biologists, immunologists, and other researchers. There are several reasons why molecular studies of *Lc. lactis* are important.

Application of *Lactococcus* as an oral vaccine can be foreseen. Attack by phages is a common problem, recognized, and worked on for a long time by several groups (see Chapter 3). In the past years, some excellent reviews have been published on gene expression in *Lc. lactis* (Kok, 1996; Rallu et al., 1996; de Vos et al., 1997; Sanders et al., 1999; de Vos, 1999), while more specific ones have appeared, for example, on phage

Oscar P. Kuipers • Department of Genetics, Groningen Biomolecular Sciences and Biotechnology Institute (GBB), University of Groningen, P.O. Box 14, 9750 AA Haren, The Netherlands; e-mail: o.p.kuipers@biol.rug.nl
Kees J. Leenhouts • BioMaDe Technology, Nijenborgh 4, 9747 AG Groningen, The Netherlands; e-mail: leenhouts@biomedical.nl

(resistance) (Dinsmore and Klaenhammer, 1995; Forde and Fitzgerald, 1999; Chapter 3), regulation of proteolysis (see Chapter 7), on introns and intron homing (Dunny and McKay, 1999), on behavior in the GI-tract (Blum et al., 1999; Dunne et al., 1999; Tannock, 1999), and on inducible gene expression systems (Kuipers et al., 1997; Djordjevic and Klaenhammer, 1998). For this reason we will in this chapter focus further on those subjects that have gained increased attention in the literature quite recently, that is, stress responses, regulation of sugar utilization (see also Chapter 4), metabolic pathways (see also Chapter 6), bacteriocin biosynthesis (see also Chapter 8), synthetic promoters, and RNA stability. Finally, we will discuss the novel possibilities that functional genomics studies, making use of DNA-microarrays for transcriptional profiling and 2D-gel electrophoresis combined with MALDI-TOF MS for proteomics studies are offering.

Stress Responses in *Lc. lactis*

Like virtually all-biological systems lactococci exhibit an inducible biochemical response when subjected to a physiologically abnormal environment. One of the first steps in this biochemical response is usually the induced expression of one or more genes. Although post-transcriptional or post-translational regulation or a combination of these may also play an important role, the identification and isolation of possible regulatory genes and DNA elements involved in stress responses is an important driving force in the study of the response of lactococci to (semi-) detrimental environmental conditions. Various stress response genes in *Lc. lactis* have been identified through homologies with known genes of other organisms. Nevertheless, the analysis of the stress response in *Lc. lactis* thus far, provided also indications of the presence of unique regulatory circuits.

Among the stress conditions cells encounter during a life cycle we can distinguish those imposed by the environment, for example, temperature, oxygen, salt, and mutagens, and those resulting from cell growth, for example, low pH and starvation. The response to environmental changes is often complex, it may consist of specific responses and of general or overlapping responses induced both when cells undergo a particular stress and suffer from nutrient depletion. Other factors complicating the data generated in this field are the different experimental conditions applied in each study and the different stress resistance properties exhibited by the two lactococcal subspecies *Lc. lactis* ssp. *lactis* and ssp. *cremoris*. It has been determined that *Lc. lactis* ssp. *lactis* is more heat, acid, bile salt, and freezing resistant than *Lc. lactis* ssp. *cremoris* and that these traits can be used to phenotypically distinguish the two (Kim et al., 1999). A detailed recent overview of the responses of *Lc. lactis* to environmental stress was given by Sanders et al. (1999).

High Temperature Stress

Lc. lactis has been found to elicit a heat-shock response similar to that of other bacteria (Batt, 1995; Hartke et al., 1996; Rallu et al., 1996). Exposure of *Lc. lactis* to lethal temperatures such as 42°C increases expression of 12–17 proteins (Whitaker and Batt, 1991; Auffrey et al., 1992; Kilstrup et al., 1997). Among these are the well conserved heat-shock proteins (HSPs) GroEL, GroES (Kim and Batt, 1993), DnaK, GrpE (Eaton et al., 1993), and DnaJ (van Asseldonk et al., 1993), which act as protein chaperones and function in proper (re)folding and maturation of new or denatured proteins (Georgopolous and Welch, 1993). Regulation of the heat-shock response has focused so far mainly on the expression of HSP encoding operons. The levels of these HSPs are usually elevated not more than 2- to 10-fold (Sanders et al., 1999), while mRNA levels may increase up to 100-fold (Arnau et al., 1996). The organization of the HSPs encoding genes is partially different from other bacteria. The lactococcal *dnaJ* is transcribed independently from *dnaK*, whereas these genes form one operon in most other cases. In *Lc. lactis dnaK* is part of the *hcrA–grpE–dnaK* operon.

HcrA negatively regulates the dnaK operon in *B. subtilis* that contains the same genes as in the *Lc. lactis* operon and includes *dnaJ* and some other genes. The activity of the HcrA repressor in this bacterium is dependent on the chaperone function of the GroELS complex that acts as the central sensor for denatured proteins. It has been shown that inactivation of *dnaK* of *B. subtilis* does not result in an increase in expression of other genes in both the *dnaK* and the *groESL* operon. Therefore, DnaK plays no role in the regulation of the expression of general HSPs in *B. subtilis* (Mogk et al., 1997). This is in contrast to the role of DnaK in *Escherichia coli*. In this bacterium it acts as a negative factor in the regulation of the heat-shock response by modulating the activity of the heat-shock protease HflB that degrades in consort with the DnaK chaperone complex, the heat-shock sigma factor σ^{32} at normal temperatures. At elevated growth temperatures DnaK interacts with misfolded proteins rather than with HflB, resulting in inhibition of the degradation of the heat-shock sigma factor (Straus et al., 1990).

Mutational analysis of the lactococcal *dnaK* revealed a temperature sensitive phenotype and elevated levels of other heat-shock proteins, but not HflB, at normal growth temperatures. This is similar to *dnaK* inactivation in *E. coli*, suggesting a regulatory role for DnaK in *Lc. lactis* (Koch et al., 1998). However, unlike *E. coli, Lc. lactis dnaK* mutants were able to develop thermotolerance. These data suggest a role for DnaK as a sensor of misfolded proteins. Since *Lc. lactis* seems to lack a specific heat-shock sigma factor, but does contain an HcrA homolog, it is presently thought that if DnaK acts as a molecular thermometer in *Lc. lactis*, then the HcrA heat-shock repressor would be expected to be dependent upon the DnaK complex for activity (Koch et al., 1998).

From studies in *B. subtilis* it is known that the HrcA repressor can bind to operator regions upstream of the *dnaK* and *groELS* operons. These operators consist of two highly conserved 9 bp inverted repeats separated by a 9 bp loop and are termed CIRCE (controlling inverted repeat of chaperone expression) elements (Zuber and Schuman, 1994). CIRCE elements are present upstream of heat-shock genes in many different bacteria (Hecker et al., 1996) and have a role as negatively acting *cis*-elements. Deletion of the CIRCE upstream of the *Lc. lactis dnaJ* promoter resulted in constitutive expression of *dnaJ* (van Asseldonk et al., 1993).

A heat-shock gene in *Lc. lactis* that does not contain a CIRCE regulatory element is *clpP*. ClpP is most likely involved in the degradation of misfolded proteins. Cells lacking ClpP constitutively synthesized heat shock proteins in the absence of stress (Frees and Ingmer, 1999). This observation would fit in the assumption that DnaK acts as a sensor for unfolded proteins and is involved in HcrA stabilization. Inactivation of *clpP* results in accumulation of misfolded protein, which complexes with DnaK. This in turn prevents the interaction of DnaK with HcrA resulting in inactive HcrA repressor, which causes constitutive expression of CIRCE regulated operons (Figure 5.1). The observation that the inactivation of *clpE*, which was shown also to be involved in the degradation of misfolded proteins and is part of the recently cloned *clpC–clpE–clpB* heat-shock operon, does not result in an altered expression pattern of the CIRCE regulated HSP operons (Ingmer et al., 1999), suggests that ClpE interacts with misfolded proteins in a way different from ClpP or that ClpE degrades other types of misfolded proteins than those recognized by DnaK.

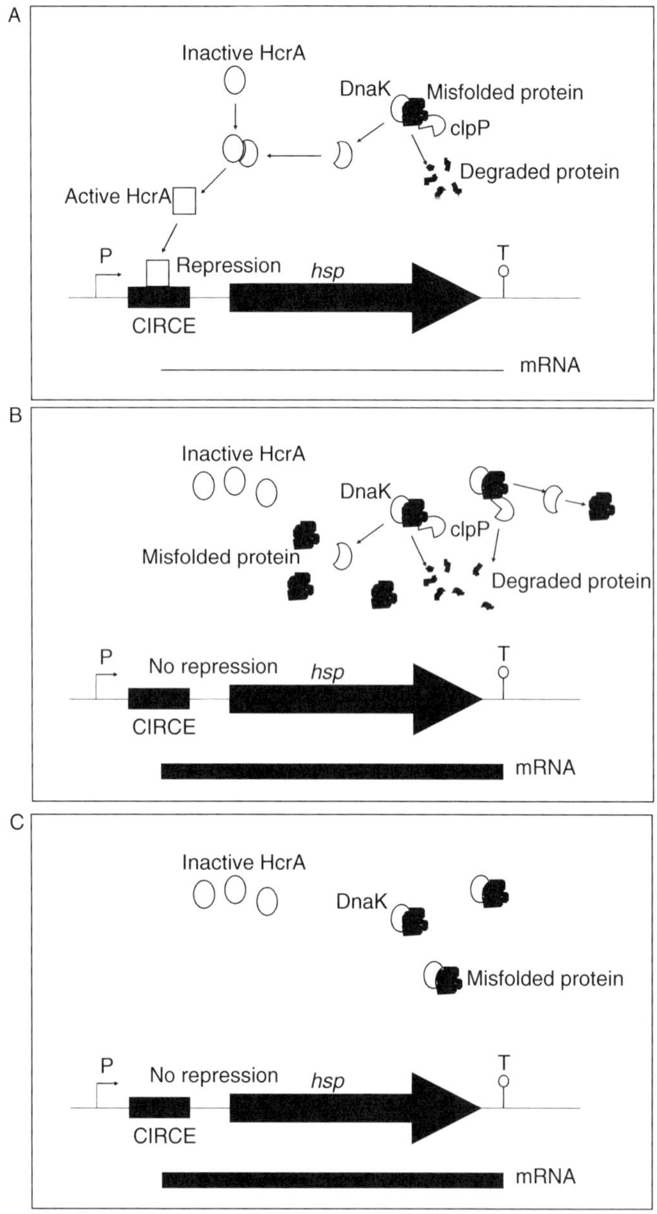

Figure 5.1. Model for the regulation of heat shock protein genes (*hsp*). Panel A: normal growth conditions. Panel B: heat shock. Panel C: *clpP* mutant. P: promoter; T: transcriptional terminator. The level of transcription is indicated by the thickness of the line representing the mRNA.

The regulation of *clpP* in *Lc. lactis* might be similar to that in *B. subtilis* where CtsR acts as a repressor *clpP*. The −35 region of the lactococcal *clpP* promoter contains sequences resembling a motif that was recently found to be bound by the stress regulator CtsR in *B. subtilis* (Derré et al., 1999). The identification of the *Lc. lactis ctsR* homolog has not been reported yet.

A regulatory role for heat-shock genes in *Lc. lactis* has also been proposed for RecA. A *recA* mutant showed reduced levels of DnaK, GroEL, and GrpE and induction of these proteins by heat shock was delayed, whereas HflB levels were 3-fold higher in the mutant strain (Duwat et al., 1995a,b). Therefore, the reduced levels of the HSPs in the *recA* strain may be caused by the increased HflB level. However, the exact roles of RecA and HflB are not clear and other control circuits may be involved in the HSP expression in *Lc. lactis*. Indeed, several other proteins and genes have been shown to be induced under heat-shock conditions, among which are a number of as yet unidentified proteins (Kilstrup et al., 1997) and putative *Lc. lactis* homologs of the cell division gene *ftsZ*, the heat-shock gene *hsp86*, the alkaline-shock protein *asp23*, and a transcriptional repressor of the *deoR*-like family (Arnau and Sørrensen, 1997). Their role in the regulation of the heat-shock response awaits further analysis. Some other genes that may also be involved in the heat-shock regulatory circuit were identified by mutagenesis of a *recA* strain and screening for heat-resistant mutants (Duwat et al., 1999). Improved heat-stress resistance was reported for mutations in seven genes, *pnpA, pstB, trmA, deoB, guaA, htp*, and *tktA*, for the last four mentioned genes not only in the *recA* but also in the wild-type context. These four genes play a role in guanine and phosphate metabolism and point at an intimate link between cellular metabolic pathways and stress responses. The expression of the HSPs is also induced at low pH and high salt conditions, as well as by UV irradiation (Hartke et al., 1995, 1996, 1997; Kilstrup et al., 1997). The latter indicates towards an interactive relation between the response to DNA damage and the HSP response mediated through RecA.

Low Temperature Stress

In *Lc. lactis* five genes, *cspABCDE*, directly involved in cold adaptation have been cloned, sequenced, and partially characterized (Wouters et al., 1999b). Interestingly, two tandem repeats comprising *cspAB* and *cspCD* were identified at different loci, which encode proteins of 7 kDa with unusual high isoelectric point (pI) values between 9 and 10 (CspA and CspC) and between 4 and 5 (CspB and D), respectively. The *cspE* gene seems to be constitutively expressed, whereas at a temperature shift from 30°C to 10°C, CspA and CspC were induced 10-fold after 2 hr, followed by a 30–40-fold induction of CspB and CspD after 4 hr, as shown by Northern blotting and 2D-gel-electrophoresis. Highest expression levels were obtained 6–8 hr following cold-shock. Individual promoters controlled all genes and transcription start sites could unambiguously be identified (Wouters et al., 1998). Induction of *csp* gene expression by incubation at 10°C in mid-exponential growth phase for a period of 2 or 4 hr gave rise to an approximately 100-fold increased survival after freezing (Figure 5.2), providing an attractive method for improved performance of frozen starter cultures (Wouters et al., 1999a). In the pretreated cells increased expression levels of at least three other proteins was observed, suggesting a role for these proteins in cryoprotection. Also overexpression of *cspD* by the nisin inducible system at 30°C did result in a 2–10-fold increase in survival after freezing compared to control cells (Wouters et al., 1999a). The mechanisms by which the *csp* and other promoters are induced upon cold-shock and the factors influencing mRNA stability and translation efficiency at different temperatures are largely unknown. Use of alternative sigma factors is unlikely since in strain *Lc. lactis* MG1363 only one sigma factor encoding gene, that is, *rpoD*, has been identified. Single stranded DNA-binding motifs are present in CspB, CspD, and CspE. The RNA-binding motifs RNP1 and RNP-2 are found in all lactococcal Csp proteins, although some sequence differences are observed. The high pI's of CspA and CspC

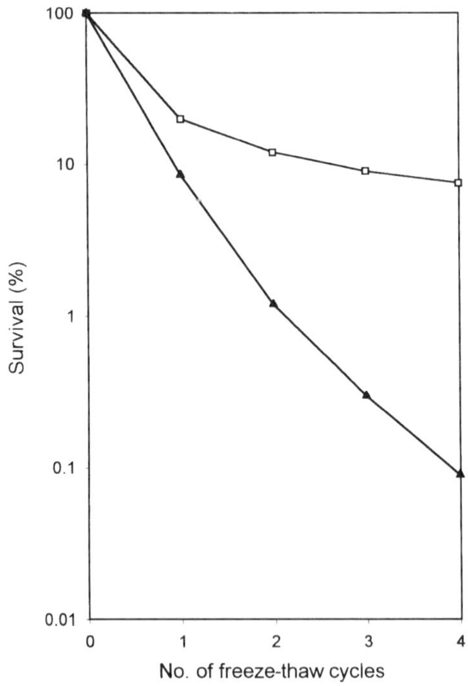

Figure 5.2. Effect of cold adaptation on survival after freezing. Adapted and modified from Wouters et al. (1999a). Survival after freezing of *Lc. lactis* cultured without (closed triangle) or with (open square) a cold-shock treatment from 30°C to 10°C for 4 hr.

might allow improved binding of DNA, thereby enhancing transcription rates. Since CspB and CspD are expressed at a later stage it is tempting to speculate that CspA and CspC are involved in the regulation of their respective counterparts in the tandem. Also the 5′ untranslated regions of the lactococcal *csp*'s might play a role in determining the stability of the mRNA at various temperatures, thereby influencing Csp levels at different temperatures. Multiple knock-out strains have been constructed showing only limited effects of the removal of one tandem (*cspAB* or *cspCD*), while the removal of one tandem and cspE shows significantly reduced survival after freezing and altered overall expression profiles (Wouters, personal communication). It cannot be excluded that more than five *csp* genes are present in *Lc. lactis* MG1363, since 2D-gel-electrophoresis experiments showed another two likely 7 kDa candidates, which await further analysis (Wouters, thesis 2000).

Osmotic Stress

Lc. lactis encounters osmotic challenges in both industrial and natural environments. To cope with hyperosmotic conditions this bacterium reacts by the cytoplasmic accumulation of compatible solutes, mostly betaine and proline (Molenaar et al., 1993). Recent work revealed the presence of a high-affinity betaine uptake system, with low affinity for proline, which is regulated at the levels of both expression and transport activity (Obis et al., 1999; van der Heide and Poolman, 2000). The cloned *busA* operon contains two genes, *busAA* and *busAB*, encoding an ATP-binding protein fused to a transmembrane domain or a substrate-binding domain, respectively. RNA studies revealed a strong induction of this system in growth medium containing 0.3 M NaCl and betaine transport activity was shown to be 5-fold higher under these conditions. Surprisingly, the BusAB protein appeared to be present in equal amounts in the membrane of both induced and uninduced cells. This observation suggests that additional mechanisms are involved in the regulation of BusAB besides the transcriptional control exerted by external osmolality on *busA* expression (Obis et al., 1999). Further analysis of the biochemical regulation and the genetic elements involved in the regulation of this system is expected in the near future.

2D-PAA-gel-electrophoresis revealed that hyperosmotic growth conditions also induce the HSPs DnaK, GroEL, GroES, and ClpP, although to a somewhat lower level than under heat-shock conditions. An additional eight other unknown proteins were identified as being salt induced. One of them, designated Ssp21, demonstrated a 35-fold increase of expression upon salt stress (Kilstrup et al., 1997). In addition, *hflB* of Lc lactis was shown to be involved in salt tolerance. Since *hflB* expression was not induced at high osmolarity, it was suggested that HflB supports proper assembly of membrane proteins that may be essential for salt tolerance (Nilsson et al., 1994). In this respect it is tempting to speculate on a possible role of HflB in the regulation of BusAB activity. However, further analysis of these systems is required to corroborate this assumption.

Oxidative Stress and DNA Damage

Growth of *Lc. lactis* is not affected by aeration. However, under aerobic growth conditions highly toxic oxygen compounds may be generated, such as superoxide (O_2^-), hydrogen peroxide (H_2O_2) and hydroxyl radicals (•OH) (Hansson and Häggström, 1984; Duwat et al., 1995a,b). Although a number of enzymes are known to be involved in the neutralization of toxic oxygen intermediates, their regulation is largely unknown. It has been shown that in aerated cultures 5-fold higher levels of the NADH oxidase/NADH peroxidase and 2-fold higher levels of superoxide dismutase (*sodA*) occur (Hansson and Häggström, 1984; Sanders et al., 1995). The inactivation of *sodA* results in a markedly reduced growth rate during aerobic growth, suggesting that this enzyme is important in oxygen stress survival. Also *recA* is induced in aerated cultures and a *recA* mutant is highly sensitive to aeration. This observation clearly suggests an important role for *recA* in the oxidative stress response (Duwat et al., 1995a,b).

As in other bacteria *Lc. lactis* RecA plays a key role in the SOS response to DNA damage induced by UV light or drugs like mitomycin C (Duwat et al., 1995a,b). The latter compound induced the transcription of recA, but the protein level remained unchanged (Rallu et al., 1996). Again this points into the direction of multiple levels of regulation, which awaits further analysis. In *Lc. lactis recA* is located in an operon with *fpg* that encodes an enzyme involved in releasing 8-oxoguanine from oxidatively damaged DNA (Duwat et al., 1995b). The observation that the *fpg–recA* operon is also induced by aeration supports its role in oxygen stress (Duwat et al., 1995b).

A number of genes involved in the response to DNA-damaging agents have been identified by transposon mutagenesis. One of these mutants lacked exonuclease activity, was affected in *rexAB*, was more UV sensitive than wild-type cells and was recombination deficient. A *recBCD*-like role was postulated for *rexAB* (El Karoui et al., 1998). Other mutants sensitive to UV light and mitomycin C appeared to carry inactivated genes that are involved in DNA metabolism (*polA*, *hexB*, *deoB*), cell envelope formation (*gerC* and *dltD*) and various metabolic pathways (*arcD*, *bglA*, *gidA*, *hgrP*, *metB*, and *proA*). These results suggest that factors other than DNA repair enzymes may be important in mediating resistance to DNA damage (Duwat et al., 1997). The regulation of these genes or the regulatory role of their products in the response to DNA damage, if any, remains to be established.

Low pH Stress

During growth *Lc. lactis* produces lactic acid, which at low pH is not charged and can easily pass the cell membrane in the protonated form. In the cell it dissociates and this lowers the internal pH in a linear fashion relative to the external pH, which strongly stresses the cells. Acidification of the external pH by HCl, for example, in gastric juices, has a less dramatic effect on the internal pH (Poolman et al., 1987; Cook and Russell, 1994). It was found that the intracellular pH is a major factor in the induction of a stress response to acidification of the environment of *Lc. lactis* (O'Sullivan and Condon, 1997).

One of the best characterized pH-inducible promoters in *Lc. lactis* was isolated using an integrative reporter system based on Tn*917*, but the downstream gene (*orfX*) encodes a protein with an unknown function in acid stress response (Israelsen et al., 1995a,b). It was shown that the promoter, designated P170, was induced approximately 20-fold between pH6.5 and pH6.0, but only at the onset of the stationary phase. P170 contains an extended consensus −10 promoter region (TGNTATAAT) but lacks a consensus −35 region. The region required for pH inducibility could be minimized to a *cis*-acting 27-bp sequence located 15 bp upstream of the extended −10 region (Madsen et al., 1999). This sequence may represent the recognition target for a transcriptional activator or a specific sigma factor that alters the specificity of the core RNA polymerase. The latter possibility is not very likely since sigma factors other than the vegetative sigma factor σ^{39} (RpoD) seem to be absent in *Lc. lactis*. Interestingly, the mRNA of *orfX* contains a long leader sequence that contains a 72-bp fragment that acts as a negative regulator. However, this element is not regulated by stress conditions (Madsen et al., 1999).

Another promoter that was isolated using an integrative plasmid reporter system and that responded to acidification of the medium is one that drives the expression of the lactococcal *gadCB* operon. The induction of the promoter is also dependent on glutamate and chloride (Sanders et al., 1998a,b). The promoter region of the *gadCB* operon (P_{gad}) contains a well-defined −10 region without an extended motif and also lacks the −35 consensus sequence. Instead, a 21-bp inverted repeat is located in this region. Furthermore, it was shown that directly upstream of *gadCB* a third gene encodes the regulator GadR. Expression of *gadR* appeared to be constitutive, but its gene product positively regulates P_{gad}. It was speculated that GadR acts directly or indirectly upon the inverted repeat in P_{gad}, however, no experimental evidence has been provided to corroborate this supposition (Sanders et al., 1998a). The *gadC* gene encodes an antiporter that internalizes glutamate. The glutamate is then converted by GadB, a glutamate decarboxylase, into γ-aminobutyrate that is expelled by GadC. The conversion of glutamate into γ-aminobutyrate removes a proton from the cytoplasm and, thus, may contribute in this way to pH homeostasis (Figure 5.3).

Other systems that have been implicated in pH homeostasis in *Lc. lactis* are an H^+-ATPase and enzymes involved in the arginine deiminase (ADI) pathway. The ATPase system is induced at low pH both at the activity and expression level (Kobayashi et al., 1986; Nannen and Hutkins, 1991). Its activity expels protons from the cytoplasm at the expense of ATP and has, therefore, a negative effect on growth (Susuki et al., 1988; Nannen and Hutkins, 1991). The activity of the ADI pathway, a unique property of *Lc. lactis* ssp. *lactis* (but also present in strain MG1363, which is a ssp. *cremoris*), generates metabolic energy. This pathway consists of three cytoplasmic enzymes active at low pH: arginine deiminase,

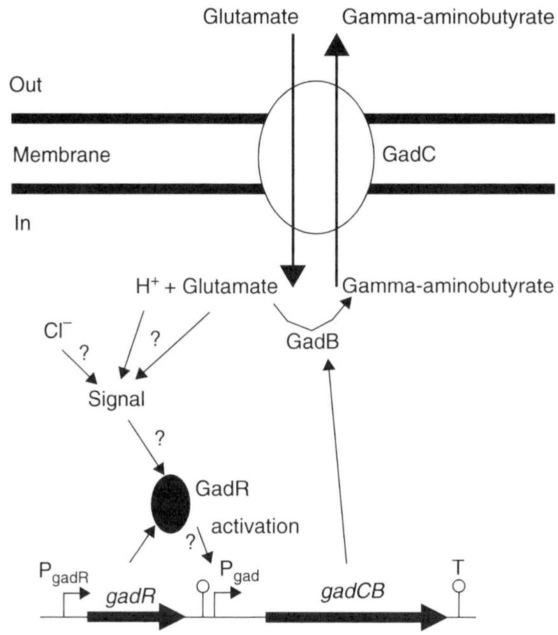

Figure 5.3. Model for the pH-regulating GadCB system. T: transcriptional terminator.

ornithine carbamoyltransferase, and carbamate kinase, that convert arginine to ammonia, ornithine, and carbon dioxide. The activity of the ADI pathway is induced up to 5-fold in the presence of arginine. The ammonia produced by this system neutralizes the pH and this is likely to contribute to survival at acid stress conditions (Poolman et al., 1987; Casiano-Colón and Marquis, 1988). A mutant in the putative regulator gene of the ADI pathway, *ahrC*, shows increased arginine metabolism which increases the pH (Rallu et al., 1996). Recently the genes of this pathway have been completely sequenced (Gasson, M., personal communication). The genes encoding the lactococcal H^+-ATPase system have been identified (Koebmann et al., 2000), but both systems need further characterization.

Several other genes have been reported to respond to low acid conditions, including: *citP* of *Lc. lactis* ssp. *lactis* biovar. *diacetylactis* (Garcia-Quintans et al., 1998), some of the *hsp* and UV-inducible genes (Hartke et al., 1996, 1997). Rallu et al. (2000) reported the partial characterization of 18 genes after selection of acid-resistant mutants, which are involved in glutamate/glutamine transport (*glnH*, *glnP*), high-affinity phosphate transport (*pstS*, *pstB*), purine nucleotide metabolism (*hpt*, *relA*, *guaA*, *deoB*, and possibly *arl7*), DNA repair (*recN*), or have a yet unknown function (*arl1–7*). The important aspect of this work is that many of these mutants demonstrate resistance to various types of stress, such as oxidative stress (*arl1*, *arl2*, *arl4*, *relA*, *hpt*, *guaA*, and *pstS*) and heat shock (*recN*, *relA*, *deoB*, *hpt*, *guaA*, *arl7*, and *arl5*) and points to the importance of intracellular phosphate and guanine nucleotide pools as signals in the response to acid and other stress.

Cross Protection and Global Regulation

The response of *Lc. lactis* to different types of environmental stress seems to be very complex. Some genes induced by stress are truly specific, while others are induced by multiple types of stress. The regulatory circuits that are beginning to be unraveled show interesting differences when compared to other bacteria. In *E. coli* and *B. subtilis*, specific sigma factors (σ^S and σ^B, respectively) are involved in the general stress response (Loewen and Hengge-Aronis, 1994; Hecker et al., 1996). Thus far, no other sigma factor than the vegetative sigma factor σ^{39} (RpoD) has been identified in *Lc. lactis* (Gansel et al., 1993). Nevertheless, there is ample evidence that multiple stress resistance can be induced after exposure of cells to a given stress. For example, salt stress induces HSPs (Kilstrup et al., 1997); UV irradiation results in improved protection against acid, oxidative, and heat stress (Hartke et al., 1996); acid adaptation results in increased survival from heat, oxidative, and salt stress (O'Sullivan and Condon, 1997). A possible new regulatory role in the heat-shock response has been suggested for RecA, also involved in the response to oxidative stress, in which HflB, implicated both in heat shock and acid response, may also play an important role (Duwat et al., 1995a,b).

Furthermore, carbon starvation renders cells more resistant to other forms of stress (Hartke et al., 1994), indicating that a general stress response is induced both during starvation and a particular stress. Recent work on the FNR-like proteins FlpA and FlpB in *Lc. lactis*, their homologs in *E. coli* are involved in regulation of carbon metabolism, revealed that inactivation of *flpA* and *flpB* resulted in sensitivity to oxidative stress. Therefore, FlpA and FlpB may provide a link carbon regulatory circuits and stress response (Gostick et al., 1999). A link between the physiological state of the cell and the level of stress response is becoming increasingly apparent from the works of Duwat et al. (1999) and Rallu et al. (2000). In these studies, mutants were selected under different stress conditions. Mutations in *pstS* and *pstB* (high affinity phosphate transport system), and *guaA* and *deoB* (purine metabolism) were isolated in both studies and demonstrate the importance of intracellular phosphate and purine nucleotide pools as signals in stress response. Genes like *deoB*, *hpt*, *guaA*, *relA* encode enzymes involved in the synthesis of (p)ppGpp. This compound is a known regulatory signal of the stringent response in *E. coli*. The stringent response is involved in starvation and stationary phase survival and, therefore, provides an intimate link between cellular metabolic pathways and stress response. The challenge remains to unravel the regulation of these complex overlapping networks by using existing and new technologies.

Biosynthetic Pathways

Amino Acid Biosynthesis

In most bacteria amino acid biosynthesis is a tightly controlled process. Extracellular levels of amino acids usually determine the transcriptional activity of the biosynthesis pathways. Three large clusters of biosynthesis operons for histidine, tryptophan, and branched-chain amino acids (BCAA: isoleucine, leucine, and valine) have been characterized in *Lc. lactis* (Chopin, 1993; Renault et al., 1995). The *his* operon is controlled at the level of transcriptional attenuation and at the level of initiation of transcription (Delorme et al., 1999). The *trp* operon is regulated through transcription antitermination in which the $tRNA^{trp}$ plays a key role (Frenkiel et al., 1998; Raya et al., 1998; van de Guchte et al., 1998). The BCAA biosynthesis operon is regulated at the level of transcription initiation at multiple promoters in which alpha-acetolactate decarboxylase AldB, an enzyme not involved in BCAA biosynthesis but encoded by a gene in the BCAA operon, has a key regulatory role in BCAA biosynthesis, in addition to its catalitic function in the

2,3-butanediol pathway (Goupil-Feuillerat et al., 1997). The regulation of these three amino acid biosynthesis pathways is described in more detail in Chapter 3.

The cloning of genes involved in threonine biosynthesis in *Lc. lactis* has been described as well. Two genes, encoding homoserine dehydrogenase (*hom*) and homoserine kinase (*thrB*), are located in a bicistronic operon (Madsen et al., 1996). The promoter region of the *hom–thrB* operon contains a consensus −10 region but no consensus −35 region. Interestingly, the *hom–thrB* promoter showed no threonine dependent regulation. In *Corynebacterium glutamicum* expression of the *hom–thrB* operon is repressed by methionine and the activity of Hom is feedback inhibited by threonine. It is presently unknown whether the regulation in *Lc. lactis* is similar.

Nucleotide Biosynthesis

Also the biosynthesis of nucleotides is an energy requiring process and, therefore, a highly regulated process in bacteria. The regulation of the *de novo* purine biosynthesis pathway in *Lc. lactis* differs from that described for *E. coli* and *B. subtilis*. The purine biosynthetic genes are scattered around the chromosome of *E. coli*, but the transcription of all these genes is repressed by a single regulatory protein, PurR (Meng et al., 1990). The *E. coli* PurR repressor binds to a specific target DNA sequences, indicated as PurBox, and requires the co-repressors guanine and hypoxanthine (Meng and Nygaard, 1990). In *B. subtilis* all purine biosynthesis genes are organized in a single purine operon that is regulated by two independent mechanisms (Zalkin, 1993). Initiation of transcription is controlled by the repressor PurR (not homologous to the *E. coli* PurR), which requires low concentrations of 5-phosphoribosyl-1-pyrophosphate (PRPP; an intermediate in the purine biosynthesis pathway) to bind specifically to the promoter region. In addition, transcription is regulated by a mechanism of premature termination of transcription that involves an unidentified RNA binding protein in the presence of guanine and hypoxanthine (Christiansen et al., 1997).

Two operons involved in *de novo* purine biosynthesis have been identified thus far, *purDEK* and *purC(orf)QLF* (Kilstrup et al., 1998; Nilsson and Kilstrup, 1998; Peltonen and Mantsala, 1999). The expression of these operons is decreased approximately 35-fold at the transcriptional level when purine is available in the growth medium. The promoter regions of both operons contain consensus −10 sequences but lack the conventional −35 consensus element. Instead both promoters contain consensus PurBox sequences (AWWWCCGAACWWT) 79 bp upstream of the transcriptional start points, while the *purC* promoter region contains one additional PurBox. Deletion analysis of these regions resulted in low levels of transcription and loss of purine-mediated regulation suggesting that transcription of the *purDEK* and *purC(orf)QLF* operons are regulated by a transcriptional activator binding to the PurBox. The gene encoding this activator, *purR*, is located elsewhere in the *Lc. lactis* chromosome and the protein it encodes shows a high degree of homology to the *B. subtilis* PurR repressor. The promoter of the *Lc. lactis purR* gene also contains a PurBox consensus sequence and the gene is autoregulated. Presently it is thought that PurR forms a complex with RNA polymerase in the presence of PRPP in order to activate the *pur* promoters (Kilstrup and Martinussen, 1998).

Much less is known about the regulation of pyrimidine biosynthesis in *Lc. lactis*. Two transcriptional units that play a role in pyrimidine biosynthesis have been identified, the *pyrKDbF* operon and the monocistronic *carB* gene (Andersen et al., 1996; Martinussen and Hammer, 1998). Only in the case of *carB* was it shown that transcription of the gene is regulated by pyrimidines, most probably by an attenuation mechanism.

Clearly, much more can be learned from the regulation of these biosynthesis pathways and their relation to catalytic and salvage pathways.

Carbon Metabolism

Sugar utilization in *Lc. lactis* has been studied for many years (see Chapter 4). The *lac*-operon for lactose utilization and the mode of gene regulation by a *lac*-repressor has been thoroughly studied and extensively reviewed (van Rooijen and de Vos, 1990; de Vos, 1996; de Vos et al., 1998; de Vos, Chapter 4). In more recent years also other sugar utilization operons were characterized, among which those for galactose and sucrose (Grossiord et al., 1998; Vaughan et al., 1998; de Vos, Chapter 4). An important aspect of sugar utilization is the regulatory mechanism by which the operon expression is controlled. Diauxic growth can be observed in various cases when cells are grown on a combination of preferred (e.g., glucose) and less favorable sugar sources (e.g., sucrose, galactose). It has been shown in *B. subtilis*, *Bacillus megaterium* and other Gram-positive bacteria that a common mechanism for control of sugar utilization pathways is exerted by carbon catabolite control protein A (CcpA), together with allosteric factors such as HPr-Ser46-P and internal levels of fructose-1,6-biphosphate and/or glucose-6-phosphate (Deutscher et al., 1995; Hueck et al., 1995). Also in *Lc. lactis* this carbon catabolite repression (CCR) mechanism was shown to occur via CcpA and HPr-Ser46-P in case of galactose fermentation (Luesink et al., 1998a,b, 1999a). Various gene clusters encoding genes for sugar utilization are controlled at two levels: first by specific repressor or activator proteins embedded in the same gene cluster (e.g., LacR; SacR, Luesink et al., 1999b) and second by the general mechanisms of CCR involving CcpA and HPr-Ser46-P. Apart from the known repression functions of CcpA it was also found that CcpA could exert an activating function in the expression of several glycolytic genes present in the *las*-operon, that is, *pfk, pyk*, and *ldh*. By the combination of catabolite repression and glycolytic activation cells are able to rapidly adjust to any alterations in relative sugar concentrations in their growth medium, for example, to avoid the occurrence of bottlenecks impeding growth. For a more extensive and complete overview of regulation of sugar utilization the reader is referred to Chapter 4 by Willem M. de Vos.

Bacteriocin Production

Undoubtedly the best characterized bacteriocin-encoding gene cluster of *Lc. lactis* is the nisin gene cluster, comprising the genes *nisABTCIPRKFEG* on approximately 11 kb located on conjugative transposon *Tn*5276. Biosynthesis, mode of action and protein engineering for various purposes have been described in detail by a number of groups (for a review see van Kraaij et al., 1999). The report of autoregulation by nisin itself, being sensed and transduced to stimulate transcription of two promoters within the gene cluster by a two-component regulatory unit comprising NisK and NisR (Kuipers et al., 1995) has stimulated a lot of follow-up work, not least in the applied field of developing strictly regulated and food-grade gene expression systems for a wide range of Gram-positive hosts (de Ruyter et al., 1996a,b; Kleerebezem et al., 1997a,b, 1998; Kuipers et al., 1997, 1998; Eichenbaum et al., 1998). Since nisin is a food grade molecule and the nisin genes are derived from *Lc. lactis* itself, expression systems fully based on self-cloning can be developed, bringing real applications of GMOs closer to reality. At the molecular level it is now clear that direct interaction between nisin and the sensor histidine kinase take place, as was indicated by elegant NisK/SpaK domain swapping studies of Kleerebezem et al. (1998). Figure 5.4 presents an outline of the gene clusters of nisin and subtilin. Interestingly, a SpaK/NisK hybrid could be constructed that responded to subtilin concentrations in the medium, but in the reciprocal way: induction was constitutive without subtilin in the medium, whereas controlled decrease of expression resulted from increased subtilin. The current working model for this is that the conformational state of the hybrid dimer is frozen in the activated state without inducer, enabling continuous phosphorylation of NisR, giving rise to activation of *nisA*-promoter controlled gene expression. Upon addition of the recognized inducer, in this case subtilin, the sensor might resume the state resembling wildtype SpaK (NisK), thereby stimulating the dephosphorylation of NisR and reducing transcription. Also the interaction of the response regulator NisR with its *cis*-acting element has been studied, first by gel retardation using partially purified NisR and a nisA promoter fragment. A specific shift was observed in the presence of NisR albeit that the concentrations required were unexpectedly high, perhaps caused by the lack of phosphorylation of NisR (Kleerebezem, personal communication). Mutation analysis of the *nisA* and the *nisF* promoters revealed a common pentanucleotide repeat located at the presumed −35 region and 6 bp downstream (Figure 5.5). Several of the residues within any of the two repeats were indispensible for inducibility of the promoter, while also the spacing between putative −35 and −10 boxes was critical (de Ruyter, Kleerebezem, and Kuipers, unpublished results). This indicates that these boxes are involved in the binding of NisR, a notion also strengthened by the fact that a minimal promoter fragment that was still controllable was just starting 1 bp upstream of the putative −35 region.

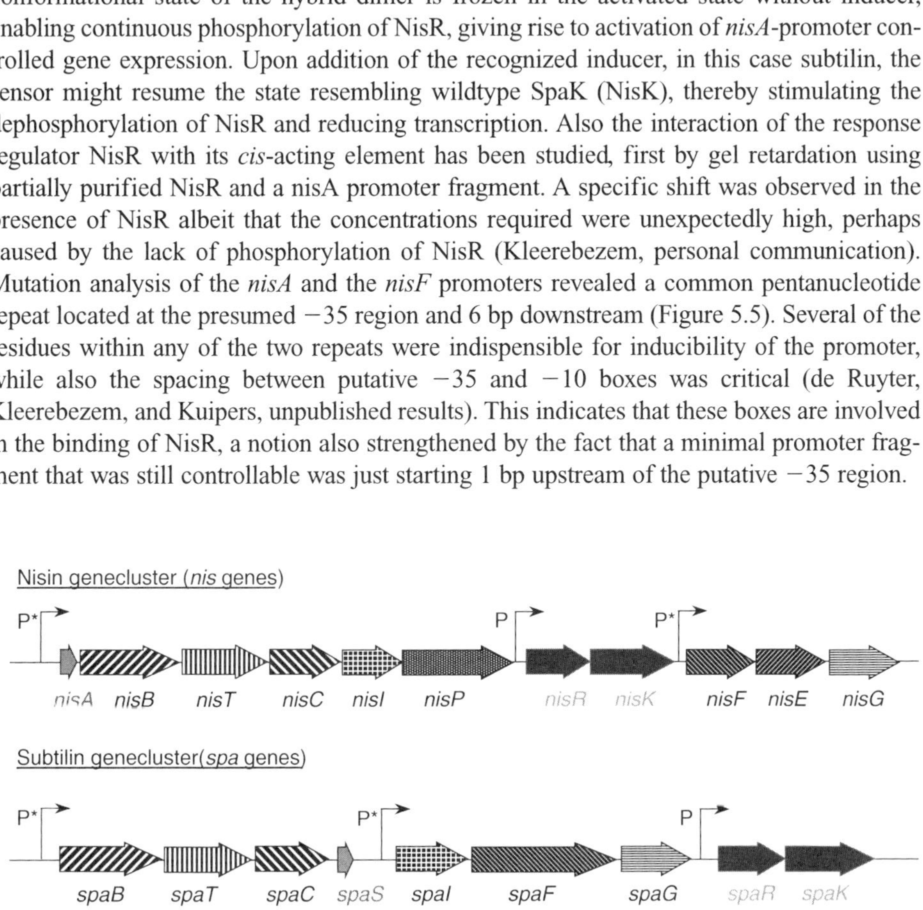

Figure 5.4. Comparison of the biosynthetic gene clusters for nisin A and subtilin. Homologous genes are shaded similar. P: promoter.

−10 ↓

AAACGGC**TCTGA**TTAAAT**TCTGA**AGTTTGTTAGATACAATGATTTCGTTCGAAGGA *nisA*

↓↓

TTTTGTT**TCTGA**ATAGAT**TCTGA**AAATTGTTTATATACTTTTTTAACATAAAAT *nisF*

Figure 5.5. Alignment of the *nisA* and *nisF* promoter sequences. Dashed lines denote the conserved pentanucleotide repeats, which are also depicted in bold. The arrows indicated the transcriptional start points.

More recently, several other gene clusters of lactococcal bacteriocins have been analyzed, for example, those encoding the lantibiotic lacticin 481, the linear bacteriocins lactococcin A, B, G, and M/N and the two component lantibiotic lacticin 3147. The last shows some very interesting features with regard to its biosynthesis: the peptides LtnA1 and LtnA2 act synergistically, contain dehydrated residues, lanthionine residues and D-alanine residues, a type of modification also found in lactocin S which probably arises from dehydroalanine being hydrogenated (Ryan et al., 1999). The encoding gene cluster contains 10 genes in two divergently arranged gene clusters. The genes *ltnRIFE* confer immunity, of which *ltnI* seems to be the most important (McAuliffe et al., 2000). The functional role of the *ltnR* gene might be that of a repressor for both sets of divergently transcribed genes, since knockout of this gene induced a hyperimmune phenotype and since it shares sequence similarity with Xre repressor of the defective prophage PBSX of *B. subtilis* (McAuliffe et al., 2000). Elucidation of the full regulatory mechanism still awaits completion, but it is evident that the mechanism is different from the two-component regulatory system operational in nisin biosynthesis and several other bacteriocin biosyntheses.

Artificial Promoters

Although several useful constitutive and regulated promoters have been described for *Lc. lactis* (van de Guchte et al., 1992; Kuipers et al., 1997), a constitutive-promoter library would be most useful for experimental control analysis in a wide range of biological systems. The great advantage of such a library is that it facilitates the choice of the best promoter to optimize gene expression after measuring the flux or yield with each of the constructs from the library and calculating the control efficient. This goal has been achieved by Jensen and Hammer (1998a,b), who succeeded in the construction of a library of synthetic promoters in which the consensus sequences were maintained, while the sequences of the separating spacers were randomized. The differences in promoter strengths varied between 0.3 and 2,000 arbitrary units in a gradual way, which makes these promoters perfectly suited for quantitative physiological studies and for optimizing gene expression under various conditions.

In another study an interesting finding was that the higher expressed genes in the recently cloned and characterized H^+-ATPase operon had TTG as the start codon (Koebmann et al., 2000). It would be interesting to see by a proteomic approach whether this is a general phenomenon in *Lc. lactis* or not.

A number of hybrid promoters were made by Madsen et al. (1999). They replaced the consensus −35 region of promoter CP25 (Jensen and Hammer, 1998b) by the 27-bp cis-acting element located 15 bp upstream of the extended −10 region of the pH-inducible promoter P170 (see also the section low *p*H Stress of this chapter). This converted the constitutive promoter into a pH-inducible one with a 30-fold inducibility. Replacing the −35 hexamer of this hybrid pH-inducible promoter by the consensus −35 sequence TTGACA, converted this promoter again to a constitutive one with an expression level even 3-fold higher than that of the induced state of the hybrid pH-inducible promoter. These studies provide the proof of concept that artificial promoters can be tailor made for specific applications.

RNA Stability

It is known from work in *E. coli* that regulation of gene expression can be modulated at the level of mRNA stability (Arraiano, 1993). In this bacterium the RNase E degradosome complex and RNase III play important roles in the degradation of mRNA (Nierlich and Murakawa, 1996; Vanzo et al., 1998). The investigation of the influence of mRNA stability on gene expression in *Lc.lactis* has only just started. Santos et al. (1997) and Drider et al. (1998) used the *citQRP* operon of *Lc. lactis* ssp. *lactis* biovar *diacetylactis*, involved in citrate metabolism, as a model to study its mRNA stability in *E. coli* RNase E and RNase III mutant strains and in *Lc. lactis*. They established that RNase III is crucial for the decay process of the *citQRP* messenger in *E. coli* and that the chemical half-life for the *citQRP* mRNA in *Lc. lactis* was unusually long for bacteria and even longer than in the *E. coli* mutants. The endonucleotide cleavage sites in the mRNA of *citQRP* were determined in *E. coli* and *Lc. lactis*. A number of these cleavage sites appeared to be the same for both organisms and could be attributed to the action of RNAse III in *E. coli* (Drider et al., 1999). However, at present it is unknown whether *Lc. lactis* contains an RNase III-type enzyme.

A gene that was recently identified in a screening of thermoresistant insertional mutants in a *recA* lactococcal background, *pnpA*, could play a role in mRNA stability (Duwat et al., 1999). PnpA of *B. subtilis* (Luttinger et al., 1996) and other organisms is involved in mRNA degradation by hydrolyzing single stranded polynucleotides progressively in the 3′ to 5′direction. Further analysis is required to determine its role in *Lc. lactis*.

Functional Genomics and the Future

Exciting developments are taking place in the field of global functional analysis of living cells, especially in transcriptome-, proteome-, and metabolome analysis, in bioinformatics and in high throughput structure determination. Relevant to the study of complex regulatory pathways in bacteria and their interrelatedness are the use of tools for transcript profiling, for example, DNA-microarrays, and for the determination of the whole protein complement of a cell, for example, 2D-electrophoresis combined with MALDI-TOF MS. A prerequisite for genomic transcript profiling is to have access to the full genomic sequence of the species of interest. Recently, the low-redundancy sequencing of *Lc. lactis* IL1403 was published and the full DNA sequence is expected to appear in the public domain in 2000 (Bolotin et al., 1999). This offers great possibilities for production of full-genome DNA-microarrays, sub-arrays, or arrays containing intergenic regions for studying regulatory protein binding. An outline of transcript profiling by DNA-microarrays is presented in Figure 5.6. There are many ways in which this tool can be applied to elucidate complex regulatory mechanisms and pathways (see also Kuipers, 1999; Kuipers et al., 1999). Also novel computational methods for the identification of differential gene expression are being developed to aid the interpretation of the data (Claverie, 1999). As an example of the application of DNA-microarrays, the resistance mechanisms occurring in bacteriocin resistant strains could be clarified by using genomic arrays and hybridizing them with cDNA of sensitive and resistant strains. This will immediately point to those genes involved in biosynthetic pathways underlying the resistance. Subsequently, detailed analyses of the genes involved have to take place. Another attractive application of arrays could be their use for safety assessment of GMOs, which is of particular relevance to facilitate real applications of genetically modified LAB in food. Wild-type industrial strains could be profiled for "acceptable" levels of expression of all genes, followed by the same procedure for classically or genetically modified strains. The profiles of the industrial strains provide a window, which can be used as a discriminator for genes in a GMO the expression of which are falling outside this window. Subsequently, the risk of the unusual high or low expression of such genes should be determined on an individual basis. The study of stress responses in

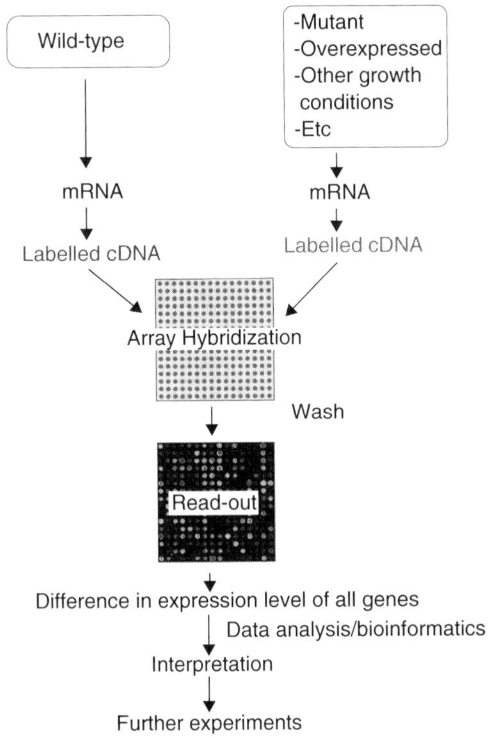

Figure 5.6. Principle of transcript profiling by DNA-microarrays. Whole genomic arrays can be obtained by high density spotting of all amplicons in the annotated genome sequence. mRNA can conveniently be labeled by making cDNA with incorporated Cy3 and Cy5 dyes for detection using specific primer mixes.

Lc. lactis could also greatly benefit from a genomic approach, since several stress-effects seem to be interrelated and many regulatory factors are pleiotropic. Especially when a large number of genes are expected to have altered transcription during stress, a global analysis approach will be very powerful. In all cases proteomic analyses will complement the transcriptome analyses, since protein levels might very well vary from levels of expressed genes. Finally, DNA-arrays can also be used for rapid identification of spoilage or pathogenic bacteria provided that the right probes are spotted on the glass slides. This will provide a method for establishing the identity of microorganisms in a sample (even when it contains a mix of species) within a few hours after DNA isolation. In conclusion, functional genomics will enable the molecular biologist to have a total view of the cell, opening the (long) way to *in silico* experimenting using simulation models of all cellular processes. It should be stressed that further development of a large variety of bioinformatics tools to be able to handle the overwhelming amount of experimental data is indispensable to reach this goal.

Acknowledgments

The authors want to thank Drs P. Renault, E. Johansen, P. R. Jensen, and J. Kok for making available data prior to publication and to all our colleagues who have contributed to the field in the past years.

References

Andersen, P. S., Martinussen, J., and Hammer, K. (1996). Sequence analysis and identification of the pyrKDbF operon from *Lactococcus lactis* including a novel gene, pyrK, involved in pyrimidine biosynthesis. *Journal of Bacteriology* 178(16): 5005–5012.

Arnau, J., Sörrensen, K. I., Appel, K. F., Vogensen, F. K., and Hammer, K. (1996). Analysis of heat shock gene expression in *Lactococcus lactis* MG1363. *Microbiology* 142: 1685–1691.

Arnau, J., and Sörrensen, K. I. (1997). The isolation of novel heat shock genes in *Lactococcus lactis* using RNA subtractive hybridisation. *Gene* 188: 229–234.

Arraiano, C. M. (1993). Post-transcriptional control of gene expression: Bacterial mRNA degradation. *World Journal of Microbiology and Biotechnology* 9: 421–432.

Auffrey, Y., Gansel, X., Thammavongs, B., and Boutibonnes, P. (1992). Heat shock-induced protein synthesis in *Lactococcus lactis* subsp. *lactis*. *Current Microbiology* 24: 281–284.

Batt, C. A. (1995). Stress response in *Lactococcus lactis*. *Developments in Biological Standardization* 85: 449–454.

Blum, S., Alvarez, S., Haller, D., Perez, P., and Schiffrin, E. J. (1999). Intestinal microflora and the interaction with immunocompetent cells. *Antonie van Leeuwenhoek* 76: 199–205.

Bolotin, A., Mauger, S., Malarme, K., Ehrlich, S. D., and Sorokin, A. (1999). Low-reduncancy sequencing of the entire *Lactococcus lactis* IL1403 genome. *Antonie van Leeuwenhoek* 76: 27–76.

Casiano-Colón, A., and Marquis, R. E. (1988). Role of the arginine deiminase system and bacterial adaptation to acid environments. *Applied and Environmental Microbiology* 54: 1318–1324.

Chopin, A. (1993). Organization and regulation of genes for amino acid biosynthesis in lactic acid bacteria. *FEMS Microbiology Reviews* 12: 21–38.

Christiansen, L. C., Schou, S., Nygaard, P., and Saxild, H. H. (1997). Xanthine metabolism in *Bacillus subtilis*: characterization of the *xpt-pbuX* operon and evidence for purine- and nitrogen-controlled expression of genes involved in xanthine salvage and catabolism. *Journal of Bacteriology* 179: 2540–2550.

Claverie, J. M. (1999). Computational methods for the identification of differential and coordinated gene expression. *Human Molecular Genetics* 8: 1821–1832.

Cook, G. M., and Russell, J. B. (1994). The effect of extracellular pH and lactic acid on pH homeostasis in *Lactococcis lactis* and *Streptococcus bovis*. *Current Microbiology* 28: 165–168.

Delorme, C., Ehrlich, S. D., and Renault, P. (1999). Regulation of expression of the *Lactococcus lactis* histidine operon. *Journal of Bacteriology* 181(7): 2026–2037.

Derré, I., Rapoport, G., and Msadek, T. (1999). CtsR, a novel regulator of stress and heat shock response, controls *clp* and molecular chaperone gene expression in Gram-positive bacteria. *Molecular Microbiology* 31(1): 117–131.

De Ruyter, P. G. G. A., Kuipers, O. P., Beerthuyzen, M. M., van Alen-Boerrigter, I. J., and de Vos, W. M. (1996a). Functional analysis of promoters in the nisin gene cluster of *Lactococcus lactis*. *Journal of Bacteriology* 178: 3434–3439.

De Ruyter, P. G. G. A., Kuipers, O. P., and de Vos, W. M. (1996b). Controlled gene expression systems for *Lactococcus lactis* with the food-grade inducer nisin. *Applied and Environmental Microbiology* 62: 3662–3667.

Deutscher, J., Kuester, E., Bergstedt, U., Charrier, V., and Hillen, W. (1995). Protein kinase-dependent HPr/CcpA interaction links glycolytic activity to carbon catabolite repression in Gram-positive bacteria. *Molecular Microbiology* 15: 1049–1053.

de Vos, W. M. (1999). Gene expression systems for lactic acid bacteria. *Current Opinion in Microbiology* 2: 289–329.

de Vos, W. M. (1996). Metabolic engineering of sugar catabolism in lactic acid bacteria. *Antonie van Leeuwenhoek* 70: 223–242.

de Vos, W. M., Hols, P., van Kranenburg, R., Luesink, E., Kuipers, O. P., van der Oost, J., Kleerebezem, M., and Hugenholz, J. (1998). Making more of milk sugar by engineering lactic acid bacteria. *International Dairy Journal* 8: 227–233.

de Vos, W. M., Kleerebezem, M., and Kuipers, O. P. (1997). Expression systems for industrial Gram-positive bacteria with low guanine and cytosine content. *Current Opinion in Biotechnology* 8: 547–553.

Dinsmore, P. K., and Klaenhammer, T. R. (1995). Bacteriophafe resistance in *Lactococcus*. *Molecular Biotechnology* 4(3): 297–314.

Djordjevic, G. M., and Klaenhammer, T. R. (1998). Inducible gene expression systems in *Lactococcus lactis*. *Molecular Biotechnology* 9(2): 127–139.

Drider, D., Garcia-Quintans, N., Santos, J. M., Arraiano, C. M., and Lopez, P. (1999). A comparative analysis of the citrate permease P mRNA stability in *Lactococcus lactis* biovar diacetylactis and *Escherichia coli*. *FEMS Microbiology Letters* 172(2): 115–122.

Drider, D., Santos, J. M., Arraiano, C. M., and Lopez, P. (1998). RNA processing is involved in the post-transcriptional control of the citQRP operon from *Lactococcus lactis* biovar diacetylactis. *Molecular and General Genetics* 258(1–2): 9–15.

Dunne, C., Murphy, L., Flynn, S., O'Mahony, L., O'Halloran, S., Feeney, M., Morrissey, D., Thornton, G., Fitzgerald, G., Daly, C., Kiely, B., Quigley, E. M. M., O'Sullivan, G. C., Shanahan, F., and Collins, J. K. (1999). Probiotics: From myth to reality. Demonstration of functionality in animal models of disease and in human clinical trials. *Antonie van Leeuwenhoek* 76: 279–292.

Dunny, G. M., and McKay, L. L. (1999). Group II introns and expression of conjugative transfer functions in lactic acid bacteria. *Antonie van Leeuwenhoek* 76: 77–88.

Duwat, P., Cochu, A., Ehrlich, S. D., and Gruss, A. (1997). Characterization of *Lactococcus lactis* UV-sensitive mutants obtained by ISS1 transposition. *Journal of Bacteriology* 179(14): 4473–4479.

Duwat, P., Ehrlich, S. D., and Gruss, A. (1999). Effects of metabolic flux on stress response pathways in *Lactococcus lactis*. *Molecular Microbiology* 31(3): 845–858.

Duwat, P., Ehrlich, S. D., and Gruss, A. (1995). The recA gene of *Lactococcus lactis*: Characterization and involvement in oxidative and thermal stress. *Molecular Microbiology* 17(6): 1121–1131.

Duwat, P., Sourice, S., Ehrlich, S. D., and Gruss, A. (1995). RecA Gene involvement in oxidative and thermal stress in *Lactococcus lactis*. *Developments in Biological Standardization* 85: 455–467.

Eaton, T., Shearman, C., and Gasson, M. (1993). Cloning and sequence analysis of the *dnaK* gene region of *Lactococcus lactis* subsp. *lactis*. *Journal of General Microbiology* 139: 3253–3264.

Eichenbaum, Z., Federle, M. J., Marra, D., De Vos, W. M., Kuipers, O. P., Kleerebezem, M., and Scott, J. R. (1998). Use of the lactococcal *nisA* promoter to regulate gene expression in Gram-positive bacteria: Comparison of induction level and promoter strength. *Applied and Environmental Microbiology* 64: 2763–2769.

El Karoui, M., Ehrlich, D., and Gruss, A. (1998). Identification of the lactococcal exonucluease/recombinase and its modulation by the putative Chi sequence. *Proceedings of the National Academy of Science USA* 95: 626–631.

Forde, A., and Fitzgerald, G. F. (1999). Bacteriophage defence systems in lactic acid bacteria. *Antonie van Leeuwenhoek* 76: 89–113.

Frees, D., and Ingmer, H. (1999). ClpP participates in the degradation of misfolded protein in *Lactococcus lactis*. *Molecular Microbiology* 31(1): 79–87.

Frenkiel, H., Bardowski, J., Ehrlich, S. D., and Chopin, A. (1998). Transcription of the trp operon in *Lactococcus lactis* is controlled by antitermination in the leader region. *Microbiology* 144(Pt 8): 2103–2111.

Gansel, X., Hartke, A., Boutibonnes, P., and Auffray, Y. (1993). Nucleotide sequence of *Lactococcus lactis* NCDOO763 (ML3) *rpoD* gene. *Biochimica Biophysica Acta* 1216: 115–118.

Garcia-Quintans, N., Magni, C., de Mendoza, D., and Lopez, P. (1998). The citrate transport system of *Lactococcus lactis* subsp. lactis *biovar diacetylactis* is induced by acid stress. *Applied and Environmental Microbiology* 64(3): 850–857.

Georgopoulos, C., and Welch, W. J. (1993). Role of the major heat shock proteins as molecular chaperones. *Annual Review of Cellular Biology* 9: 601–634.

Gostick, D. O., Griffin, H. G., Shearman, C. A., Scott, C., Green, J., Gasson, M. J., and Guest, J. R. (1999). Two operons that encode FNR-like proteins in *Lactococcus lactis*. *Molecular Microbiology* 31(5): 1523–1535.

Goupil-Feuillerat, N., Cocaign-Bousquet, M., Godon, J. J., Ehrlich, S. D., and Renault, P. (1997). Dual role of alpha-acetolactate decarboxylase in *Lactococcus lactis* subsp. *lactis*. *Journal of Bacteriology* 179(20): 6285–6293.

Grossiord, B., Vaughan, E. E., Luesink, E., and de Vos, W. M. (1998). Genetics of galactose utilisation via the Leloir pathway in lactic acid bacteria. *Lait* 78: 77–84.

Hansson, L., and Häggström, M. H. (1984). Effects of growth conditions on the activities of superoxide dismutase and NADH-oxidase/NADH-peroxidase in *Streptococcus lactis*. *Current Microbiology* 10: 345–352.

Hartke, A., Bouche, S., Gansel, X., Boutibonnes, P., and Auffrey, Y. (1994). Starvation-induced stress resistance in *Lactococcus lactis* subsp. *lactis* IL1403. *Applied and Environmental Microbiology* 60: 3474–3478.

Hartke, A., Bouche, S., Giard, J. C., Benachour, A., Boutibonnes, P., and Auffray, Y. (1996). The lactic acid stress response of *Lactococcus lactis* subsp. *lactis*. *Current Microbiology* 33(3): 194–199.

Hartke, A., Bouche, S., Laplace, J. M., Benachour, A., Boutibonnes, P., and Auffray, Y. (1995). UV-inducible proteins and UV-induced cross-protection against acid, ethanol, H_2O_2 or heat treatments in *Lactococcus lactis* subsp. *lactis*. *Archives of Microbiology* 163: 329–336.

Hartke, A., Frere, J., Boutibonnes, P., and Auffrey, Y. (1997). Differential induction of the chaperonin GroEL and the Co-chaperonin GroES by heat, acid, and UV-irradiation in *Lactococcus lactis* subsp. *lactis*. *Current Microbiology* 34(1): 23–26.

Hecker, M., Schumann, W., and Völker, W. (1996). Heat-shock and general stress response in *Bacillus subtilis*. *Molecular Microbiology* 19: 417–428.

Hueck, C. J., Kraus, A., Schmiedel, D., and Hillen, W. (1995). Cloning, expression and functional analysis of the catabolite control protein CcpA from *Bacillus megaterium*. *Molecular Microbiology* 16: 855–864.

Ingmer, H., Vogensen, F. K., Hammer, K., and Kilstrup, M. (1999). Disruption and analysis of the clpB, clpC, and clpE genes in *Lactococcus lactis*: ClpE, a new Clp family in gram-positive bacteria. *Journal of Bacteriology* 181(7): 2075–2083.

Isrealsen, H., Madsen, S. M., Johansen, E., Vrang, A., and Hansen, E. B. (1995a). Environmentally regulated promoters in lactococci. *Developments in Biological Standardization* 85: 443–448.

Isrealsen, H., Madsen, S. M., Vrang, A., Hansen, E. B., and Johansen, E. (1995b). Cloning and partial characterization of regulated promoters from *Lactococcus lactis* Tn*917-lacZ* integrants with the new promoter probe vector pAK80. *Applied and Environmental Microbiology* 61: 2540–2547.

Jensen, P. R., and Hammer, K. (1998a). Artificial promoters for metabolic optimization. *Biotechnology and Bioengineering* 58: 191–195.

Jensen, P. R., and Hammer, K. (1998b). The sequence of spacers between the consensus sequences modulates the strength of prokaryotic promoters. *Applied and Environmental Microbiology* 64(1): 82–87.

Kilstrup, M., Jacobsen, S., Hammer, K., and Vogensen, F. K. (1997). Induction of heat shock proteins DnaK, GroEL, and GroES by salt stress in *Lactococcus lactis*. *Applied and Environmental Microbiology* 63(5): 1826–1837.

Kilstrup, M., Jessing, S. G., Wichmand-Jprgensen, S. B., Madsen, M., and Nilsson, D. (1998). Activation control of *pur* gene expression in *Lactococcus lactis*: Proposal for a consensus activator binding sequence based on deletion analysis and site-directed mutagenesis of *purC* and *PurD* promoter regions. *Journal of Bacteriology* 180(15): 3900–3906.

Kilstrup, M., and Martinussen, J. (1998). A transcriptional activator, homologous to the *Bacillus subtilis* PurR repressor, is required for expression of purine biosynthetic genes in *Lactococcus lactis*. *Journal of Bacteriology* 180(15): 3907–3916.

Kim, S. G., and Batt, C. A. (1993). Cloning and sequencing of the *Lactococcus lactis* subsp. *lactis* groESL operon. *Gene* 127(1): 121–126.

Kim, W. S., Ren, J., and Dunn, N. W. (1999). Differentiation of *Lactococcus lactis* subspecies *lactis* and subspecies *cremoris* strains by their adaptive response to stresses. *FEMS Microbiology Letters* 171(1); 57–65.

Kleerebezem, M., Beerthuyzen, M. M., Vaughan, E. E., De Vos, W. M., and Kuipers, O. P. (1997a). Controlled gene expression systems for lactic acid bacteria: Transferable nisin inducible expression cassettes for *Lactococcus*, *Leuconostoc* and *Lactobacillus* spp. *Applied and Environmental Microbiology* 63: 4581–4584.

Kleerebezem, M., de Vos, W. M., and Kuipers, O. P. (1998). The lantibiotics nisin and subtilin act as extracellular regulators of their own biosynthesis. In: G. M. Dunny and S. C. Winans (Eds.), *Cell–cell signaling in bacteria* (pp. 159–174). Washington: American Society for Microbiology.

Kleerebezem, M., Quadri, L. E. N., Kuipers, O. P., and de Vos, W. M. (1997b). Quorum sensing by peptide pheromones and two-component signal-transduction systems in Gram-positive bacteria. *Molecular Microbiology* 24: 895–904.

Kobayashi, H., Suzuki, T., and Unemoto, T. (1986). Streptococcal cytoplasmic pH is regulated by changes in amount and activity of a proton-translocating ATPase. *Journal of Biological Chemistry* 261: 627–630.

Koch, B., Kilstrup, M., Vogensen, F. K., and Hammer, K. (1998). Induced levels of heat shock proteins in a dnaK mutant of *Lactococcus lactis*. *Journal of Bacteriology* 180(15): 3873–3881.

Koebmann, B., Nilsson, D., Kuipers, O. P., and Jensen, P. R. (2000). The membrane-bound H(+)-ATPase complex is essential for growth of *Lactococcus lactis*. *Journal of Bacteriology* 182(17): 4738–4743.

Kok, J. (1996). Inducible gene expression and environmentally regulated genes in lactic acid bacteria. *Antonie van Leeuwenhoek* 70: 129–145.

Kuipers, O. P. (1999). Genomics for food biotechnology: prospects of the use of high-throughput technologies for the improvement of food microorganisms. *Current Opinion in Biotechnology* 10: 511–516.

Kuipers, O. P., Beerthuyzen, M. M., de Ruyter, P. G. G. A., Leusink, E. J., and de Vos, W. M. (1995). Autoregulation of nisin biosynthesis in *Lactococcus lactis* by signal transduction. *Journal of Biological Chemistry* 270: 27299–27304.

Kuipers, O. P., de Jong, A., Holsappel, S., Bron, S., Kok, J., and Hamoen, L. W. (1999). DNA-microarrays and food-biotechnology. *Antonie van Leeuwenhoek* 76: 353–355.

Kuipers, O. P., de Ruyter, P. G. G. A., Kleerebezem, M., and de Vos, W. M. (1997). Controlled overproduction of proteins by lactic acid bacteria. *Tibtech* 15: 135–140.

Kuipers, O. P., de Ruyter, P. G. G. A., Kleerebezem, M., and de Vos, W. M. (1998). Quorum sensing-controlled gene expression in lactic acid bacteria [review]. *Journal of Biotechnology* 64: 15–21.

Loewen, P. C., and Hengge-Aronis, R. (1994). The role of sigma factor σ^S (KatF) in bacterial global regulation. *Annual Review of Microbiology* 48: 53–80.

Luesink, E. J., Beumer, C. M. A., Kuipers, O. P., and de Vos, W. M. (1999a). Molecular characterization of the *Lactococcus lactis ptsHI* operon and analysis of the regulatory role of HPr. *Journal of Bacteriology* 181(3): 764–771.

Luesink, E. J., Kuipers, O. P., and de Vos, W. M. (1998a). Regulation of the carbohydrate metabolism in *Lactococcus lactis* and other lactic acid bacteria. *Lait* 78: 69–76.

Luesink, E. J., Marugg, J. D., Kuipers, O. P., and de Vos, W. M. (1999b). Characterization of the divergent *sacBK* and *sacAR* operons, involved in sucrose utilization by *Lactococcus lactis*. *Journal of Bacteriology* 181(6): 1924–1926.

Luesink, E. J., van Herpen, R. E. M. A., Grossiord, B. P., Kuipers, O. P., and de Vos, W. M. (1998b). Transcriptional activation of the glycolytic *las* operon and catabolite repression of the *gal* operon in *Lactococcus* lactis are mediated by the catabolite control protein CcpA. *Molecular Microbiology* 30(4): 789–798.

Luttinger, A., Hahn, J., and Dubnau, D. (1996). Polynucleotide phosphorylase is necessary for competence development in *Bacillus subtilis*. *Molecular Microbiology* 19(2): 343–356.

Madsen, S. M., Albrechtsen, B., Hansen, E. B., and Israelsen, H. (1996). Cloning and transcriptional analysis of two threonine biosynthetic genes from *Lactococcus lactis* MG1614. *Journal of Bacteriology* 178(13): 3689–3694.

Madsen, S. M., Arnau, J., Vrang, A., Givskov, M., and Israelsen, H. (1999). Molecular characterization of the pH-inducible and growth phase-dependent promoter P170 of *Lactococcus lactis*. *Molecular Microbiology* 32(1): 75–87.

Martinussen, J., and Hammer, K. (1998). The carB gene encoding the large subunit of carbamoylphosphate synthetase from *Lactococcus lactis* is transcribed monocistronically. *Journal of Bacteriology* 180(17): 4380–4386.

McAuliffe, O., Hill, C., and Ross, R. P. (2000). Identification and overexpression of *ltnl*, a novel gene which confers immunity to the two-component lantibiotic lacticin 3147. *Microbiology* 146: 129–138.

Meng, L. M., Kilstrup, M., and Nygaard, P. (1990). Autoregulation of PurR repressor synthesis and involvement of *purR* in the regulation of *purB*, *purC*, *purL*, *purMN* and *guaAB* expression in *Escherichia coli*. *European Journal of Biochemistry* 187: 373–379.

Meng, L. M., and Nygaard, P. (1990). Identification of hypoxanthine and guanine as the corepressors for the purine regulon genes of *Escherichia coli*. *Molecular Microbiology* 4: 2187–2192.

Mogk, A., Homuth, G., Scholz, C., Kim, L., Schmid, F. X., and Schumann, W. (1997). The GroE chaperonin machine is a major modulator of the CIRCE heat shock regulon of *Bacillus subtilis*. *EMBO Journal* 16: 4579–4590.

Molenaar, Hagting, A., Alkema, H., Driessen, A. J. M., and Konings, W. N. (1993). Characteristics and osmoregulatory roles of uptake systems for proline and glycine betaine in *Lactococcus lactis*. *Journal of Bacteriology* 175: 5438–5444.

Nannen, N. L., and Hutkins, R. W. (1991). Proton-translocating adenosine triphosphate activity in lactic acid bacteria. *Journal of Dairy Science* 74: 747–751.

Nierlich, D. P., and Murakawa, G. J. (1996). The decay of bacterial messenger RNA. *Annual Review of Biochemistry* 52: 153–216.

Nilsson, D., and Kilstrup, M. (1998). Cloning and expression of the *Lactococcus lactis purDEK* genes, required for growth in milk. *Applied and Environmental Microbiology* 64(11): 4321–4327.

Nilsson, D., Lauridsen, A. A., Tomoyasu, T., and Ogura, T. (1994). A *Lactococcus lactis* gene encodes a membrane protein with putative ATPase activity that is homologous to the essential *Escherichia coli* ftsH gene product. *Microbiology* 140(10): 2601–2610.

Obis, D., Guillot, A., Gripon, J.-C., Renault, P., Bolotin, A., and Mistou, M.-Y. (1999). Genetic and biochemical characterization of a high-affinity betaine uptake system (BusA) in *Lactococcus lactis* reveals a new functional organization within bacterial ABC transporters. *Journal of Bacteriology* 181(20): 6238–6246.

O'Sullivan, E., and Condon, S. (1997). Intracellular pH is a major factor in the induction of tolerance to acid and other stresses in *Lactococcus lactis*. *Applied and Environmental Microbiology* 63(11): 4210–4215.

Peltonen, T., and Mantsala, P. (1999). Isolation and characterization of a purC(orf)QLF operon from *Lactococcus lactis* MG1614. *Molecular and General Genetics* 261(1): 31–41.

Poolman, B., Driessen, A. J. M., and Konings, W. N. (1987). Regulation of arginine-ornithine exchange and the arginine deiminase pathway in *Streptococcus lactis*. *Journal of Bacteriology* 169: 5597–5604.
Rallu, F., Gruss, A., Ehrlich, S. D., and Maguin, E. (2000). Acid- and multistress-resistant mutants of *Lactococcus lactis*: Identification of intracellular stress signals. *Molecular Microbiology* 35(3): 517–528.
Rallu, F., Gruss, A., and Maguin, E. (1996). *Lactococcus lactis* and stress. *Antonie Van Leeuwenhoek* 70(2–4): 243–251.
Raya, R., Bardowski, J., Andersen, P. S., Ehrlich, S. D., and Chopin, A. (1998). Multiple transcriptional control of the *Lactococcus lactis trp* operon. *Journal of Bacteriology* 180(12): 3174–3180.
Renault, P., Godon, J. J., Goupil, N., Delorme, C., Corthier, G., and Ehrlich, S. D. (1995). Metabolic operons in lactococci. *Developments in Biological Standerdization* 85: 431–441.
Ryan, M. P., Jack, R. W., Josten, M., Sahl, H. G., Jung, G., Ross, R. P., and Hill, C. (1999). Extensive post-translational modification, including serine to D-alanine conversion, in the two-component lantibiotic, lacticin 3147. *Journal of Biological Chemistry* 274: 37544–37550.
Sanders, J. W., Leenhouts, K., Burghoorn, J., Brands, J. R., Venema, G., and Kok, J. (1998a). A chloride-inducible acid resistance mechanism in *Lactococcus lactis* and its regulation. *Molecular Microbiology* 27(2): 299–310.
Sanders, J. W., Leenhouts, K. J., Haandrikman, A. J., Venema, G., and Kok, J. (1995). Stress response in *Lactococcus lactis*: Cloning, expression analysis, and mutation of the lactococcal superoxide dismutase gene. *Journal of Bacteriology* 177(18): 5254–5260.
Sanders, J. W., Venema, G., and Kok, J. (1999). Environmental stress responses in *Lactococcus lactis*. *FEMS Microbiology Reviews* 23: 483–501.
Sanders, J. W., Venema, G., Kok, J., and Leenhouts, K. (1998b). Identification of a sodium chloride-regulated promoter in *Lactococcus lactis* by single-copy chromosomal fusion with a reporter gene. *Molecular and General Genetics* 257(6): 681–685.
Santos, J. M., Drider, D., Marujo, P. E., Lopez, P., and Arraiano, C. M. (1997). Determinant role of *E. coli* RNase III in the decay of both specific and heterologous mRNAs. *FEMS Microbiology Letters* 157: 31–38.
Straus, D., Walter, W., and Gross, C. A. (1990). DnaK, DnaJ and GrpE heat shock proteins negatively regulate heat shock gene expression by controlling the synthesis and stability of sigma 32. *Genes and Development* 4(12A): 2202–2209.
Suzuki, T., Unemoto, T., and Kobayashi, H. (1988). Novel streptococcal mutants defective in the regulation of H^+-ATPase biosynthesis and in F_0 complex. *Journal of Biological Chemistry* 263: 11840–11843.
Tannock, G. W. (1999). Analysis of the intestinal microflora: A renaissance. *Antonie van Leeuwenhoek* 76: 265–278.
Van Asseldonk, M., Simons, A., Visser, H., de Vos, W. M., and Simons, G. (1993). Cloning, nucleotide sequence, and regulatory analysis of the *Lactococcus lactis dnaJ* gene. *Journal of Bacteriology* 175: 1637–1644.
Van de Guchte, M., Ehrlich, S. D., and Chopin, A. (1998). $tRNA^{Trp}$ as a key element of antitermination in the *Lactococcus lactis trp* operon. *Molecular Microbiology* 29(1): 61–74.
Van de Guchte, M., Kok, J., and Venema, G. (1992). Gene expression in *Lactococcus lactis*. *FEMS Microbiology Reviews* 88: 73–92.
Van der Heide, T., and Poolman, B. (2000). Glycine betaine transport in *Lactococcus lactis* is osmotically regulated at the level of expression and translocation activity. *Journal of Bacteriology* 182(1): 203–206.
Van Kraaij, C., de Vos, W. M., Siezen, R. J., and Kuipers, O. P. (1999). Lantibiotics: Biosynthesis, mode of action and applications. *Natural Product Reports* 16(5): 575–587.
Van Rooijen, R. J., and De Vos, W. M. (1990). Molecular cloning, transcriptional analysis, and nucleotide sequence of *lacR*, a gene encoding the repressor of the lactose phosphotransferase system of *Lactococcus lactis*. *Journal of Biological Chemistry* 265: 18499–18503.
Vanzo, N. F., Li, Y. S., Py, B., Blum, E., Higgins, C. F., Raynal, L. C., Krisch, H. M., and Carpouis, A. J. (1998). Ribonuclease E organizes the protein interactions in the *Escherichia coli* RNA degradosome. *Genes and Development* 12(17): 2770–2781.
Vaughan, E. E., David, R., and Mollet, B. (1998). Transcriptional regulation and evolution of lactose genes in the galactose-lactose operon of *Lactococcus lactis* NCDO2054. *Journal of Bacteriology* 180(18): 4893–4902.
Whitaker, R. D., and Batt, C. A. (1991). Characterization of the heat shock response in *Lactococcus lactis* subsp. *lactis*. *Applied and Environmental Microbiology* 57: 1408–1412.
Wouters, J. A., Jeynov, B., Rombouts, F. M., de Vos, W. M., Kuipers, O. P., and Abee, T. (1999a). Analysis of the role of 7 kDa cold-shock proteins of *Lactococcus lactis* MG1363 in cryoprotection. *Microbiology* 145: 3185–3194.
Wouters, J. A., Rombouts, F. M., de Vos, W. M., Kuipers, O. P., and Abee, T. (1999b). Cold shock proteins and low-temperature response of *Streptococcus thermophilus* CNRZ302. *Applied and Environmental Microbiology* 65(10): 4436–4442.

Wouters, J. A., Sanders, J.-W., Kok, J., de Vos, W. M., Kuipers, O. P., and Abee, T. (1998). Clustered organization and transcriptional analysis of a family of five *csp* genes of *Lactococcus lactis* MG1363. *Microbiology* 144: 2885–2893.

Zalkin, H. (1993). De novo purine nucleotide biosynthesis. In: A. L. Sonenshein, J. A. Hoch, and R. Losick (Eds.), *Bacillus subtilis and other Gram-positive Bacteria: Biochemistry, physiology, and molecular genetics* (1st ed., pp. 335–339). Washington: American Society for Microbiology.

Zuber, U., and Schuman, W. (1994). CIRCE, a novel heat shock element involved in regulation of heat shock operon *dnaK* of *Bacillus subtilis*. *Journal of Bacteriology* 176: 1359–1363.

6

Gene Expression in Lactobacilli

Peter H. Pouwels and Stéphane Chaillou

Introduction

Lactobacilli have always occupied an important place in food production. Their properties are widely exploited all over the world, in particular, in the preparation of food products and beverages (Table 6.1). Lactic acid fermentation is one of the oldest techniques used for the preservation of highly perishable raw materials like milk, meat, and vegetables. This method of food conservation dates back to ancient times, before recorded history. Food products fermented by lactic acid bacteria have an increased nutritive value, they are rich in flavor and are considered as hygienically safe. The unique properties of lactic acid bacteria in fermented food mainly result from their carbohydrate metabolism. Lactic acid, the main product formed during sugar metabolism, is responsible for the characteristic fresh acid taste of the fermented product. It also contributes to a "clean" fermentation process by preventing the outgrowth of pathogenic or putrefactive organisms. The preservation of food products by lactic acid bacteria is also exerted by the production of bacteriocins, antibacterial polypeptides acting on undesired pathogenic bacteria such as *Listeria* and *Clostridium* (Klaenhammer, 1988). But the most interesting aspect of lactic acid bacteria regarding food fermentation is certainly the establishment of a characteristic flavor, texture, and wholesomeness as a result of their metabolic activities, which give unique sensory properties to the fermented product.

Nowadays, the economic importance of lactic acid bacteria is beyond doubt since fermented food is industrially manufactured on a large scale. For many of the food-fermented products, made by modern industrial technology, so-called starter cultures (defined cultures containing strains with known properties) are now added to the fermenting material. The use of starter cultures has progressively replaced the traditional, often uncontrolled, fermentation processes. As a direct consequence, there is a growing interest in the development of new starter cultures, whose specific properties would make them better adapted

Peter H. Pouwels • TNO Prevention and Health, Special Programme Infectious Diseases, Postbox 2215, Leiden, The Netherlands; e-mail: p.pouwels@pg.tno.nl **Stéphane Chaillou** • Flore Lactique et Environnement Carné (FLEC), INRA-CRJ, Domaine de Vilvert, 78350 Jouy-en-Josas, France

Table 6.1. Lactic Acid Bacteria Associated with Fermented Foods, Beverages, and Feed

Products	Lactic Acid Bacteria Species
Dairy products	
Gouda-type cheeses	*Lactococcus lactis* subsp. *cremoris* and subsp. *lactis*, *Leuconostoc lactis* subsp. *cremoris*
Swiss-type cheeses	*Lactobacillus delbrueckii* subsp. *lactis*, *Lactobacillus helveticus*
Fermented milks and yogurts	*Streptococcus thermophilus*, *Lactobacillus delbrueckii* subsp. *bulgaricus*, *Lactobacillus acidophilus*, *Lactobacillus casei*, *Lactobacillus kefir*, *Lactococcus lactis* subsp. *diacetylactis*
Fermented meat	
Sausages	*Lactobacillus sake*, *Lactobacillus curvatus*, *Pediococcus acidilactici*, *Leuconostoc carnosum*
Fermented vegetables	
Sauerkraut (white cabbage)	*Leuconostoc mesenteroides*, *Lactobacillus plantarum*, *Lactobacillus pentosus*, *Lactobacillus bavaricus*
Soy sauce	*Tetragenococcus halophilus* (formerly called: *Pediococcus halophilus*)
Pickles, cucumbers	*Lactobacillus plantarum*, *Lactobacillus pentosus*, *Pediococcus pentosaceus*, *Leuconostoc mesenteroides*
Olives	*Leuconostoc mesenteroides*, *Lactobacillus pentosus*
Other products of plant origin	
Sourdough bread	*Lactobacillus sanfransisco*, *Lactobacillus brevis*
Silage	*Lactobacillus plantarum*
Wines and ciders	*Oenococcus oeni* (formerly called: *Leuconostoc oenos*), *Lactobacillus plantarum*

to a given food environment, or would allow them to produce, for example, new flavors that are attractive to the consumer.

Research carried out in recent years has led to the conviction that certain strains of lactic acid bacteria, in particular, strains from the genera *Lactobacillus* and *Bifidobacterium*, may promote health in man and animals. It was suggested that lactobacilli or products made by these organisms have antagonistic effects against undesirable intestinal infections and certain forms of cancer (Adachi, 1992). Lactobacilli or their products may also have an anticholesteremic effect by lowering the blood serum cholesterol level (de Roos and Katan, 2000). Some strains of *Lactobacillus* are found as natural commensals of the gastrointestinal tract (GIT), the oral cavity, and the female uro-genital tract of animals and humans. The ability to adhere to specific regions of the GIT has prompted research aimed at the use of lactobacilli as vehicles for the delivery of biologically active compounds, such as immunomodulators, antibodies, enzymes, and vaccines (Wells et al., 1996; Pouwels et al., 1998; Mercenier, 1999; Mercenier et al., 2000; Havenith et al., 2002).

The genus *Lactobacillus* comprises more than 50 species widely differing in biochemical, ecological, molecular–biological, and immunological properties. This large variation is reflected, amongst other things, by the large differences in the G + C content of their DNA. Whereas species like *Lactobacillus acidophilus* and *Lactobacillus helveticus* contain DNA with a G+C content of approximately 36 mol%, that of *Lactobacillus delbrueckii* and *Lactobacillus fermentum* is 52 mol%. Control of transcription and translation may differ greatly from one species to the other, implying that knowledge generated for one organism may not simply be extrapolated to another. This means, for example, that genes that are efficiently expressed in one *Lactobacillus* species are not necessarily expressed in (all) other species, or are expressed with a different efficiency (Pouwels and Leer, 1993; Savijoki et al., 1997; McCracken and Timms, 1999). This review will summarize more recent advancements of our knowledge regarding control of gene expression in lactobacilli. For previous reviews on this topic, the reader is referred to Pouwels and Leer (1993) and Kok (1996).

Genetic Tools for Studying Gene Expression in Lactobacilli

During the past few years, the assortment of genetic instruments for studies of gene expression and metabolic pathway engineering in lactobacilli have considerably increased. Protocols were developed to genetically modify strains from species so far inaccessible or poorly accessible to electro-transformation, for example, species of the *L. acidophilus* group and the *L. delbrueckii* group (Walker et al., 1996; Russell and Klaenhammer, 2001; Serror et al., 2002). New small-size plasmids from different *Lactobacillus* species were isolated and sequenced (Pridmore et al., 1994; Kanatani et al., 1995). Some of these plasmids carry antibiotic resistance genes rendering such plasmids in principle suitable for the development of vectors for transformation experiments (Tannock et al., 1994; Fons et al., 1997).

For different species like *L. acidophilus, Lactobacillus casei, L. helveticus, Lactobacillus pentosus, Lactobacillus plantarum*, and *Lactobacillus sakei*, gene replacement and gene disruption by site-specific integration into the chromosome has been demonstrated (Bhowmik et al., 1993; Dupont et al., 1995; Lin et al., 1996; Auvray et al., 1997; Leloup et al., 1997; Lokman et al., 1997; Alvarez et al., 1998; Chaillou et al., 1998b; Malleret et al., 1998; Gosalbes et al., 2000; Martin et al., 2000). Site-specific integration either relies on general (RecA dependent) recombination or on site-specific recombination systems identified in several bacteriophages. Integration mediated by RecA requires the presence on the (non-replicative) plasmid of a DNA fragment of at least 400 nt homologous to that of the gene where integration should occur. Single-crossover integration in *L. sakei* was found to take place with a frequency which was logarithmically proportional to the extent of homology between 0.3 and 1.2 kb, reaching a maximum efficiency value of 1.4×10^3 integrants/μg of DNA (Leloup et al., 1997).

Gene disruption by site-specific recombination was, for example, used to construct *L. plantarum* strains deficient either in L-LDH, D-LDH, or both enzymes (Ferain et al., 1994, 1996b). These mutant organisms have been instrumental in analyzing the role of these enzymes in the formation of secondary end products. Unlike the wild-type strain that produced lactate as the major end product under all conditions tested, an *ldh* null mutant strain mainly produced acetoin. A variety of secondary end products was found, including succinate, acetate, pyruvate and lactate, and ethanol-2,3-butanediol and mannitol (Ferain et al., 1996b). In many lactic acid bacteria D-lactate is a constituent of the cell wall. Consequently, elimination of the two *ldh* genes in *L. plantarum* also had a major impact on peptidoglycan precursor synthesis (Ferain et al., 1996a). A similar approach involving a two-step homologous recombination process in which the wild-type gene was replaced by an *in vitro* inactivated mutant allele, was used to construct two isogenic strains of *L. helveticus* deficient in the formation of either D- or L-lactate (Ferain, personal communication). Such strains might be useful to determine whether lactate isomers have a significant impact on propionic fermentation in Emmental cheese. In another study, vector-free cloning of a bacterial endo-1,4-β-glucanase into the chromosome of *L. plantarum* was demonstrated to exploit its use as a silage inoculant (Rossi et al., 2001).

A second class of integration vectors was constructed that rely on elements of lysogenic phage for integration at a specific locus of the bacterial chromosome (*attB*). Nonreplicative vectors comprising the integrative elements (*attP* site and integrase encoding gene, *int*) of the *L. delbrueckii* bacteriophage mv4 are capable of integrating at a specific locus of the chromosome of a wide range of bacterial hosts, including *L. plantarum, L. casei, Lactococcus lactis* subsp. *cremoris, Enterococcus faecalis*, and *Streptococcus pneumoniae* (Auvray et al., 1997). Similarly, plasmids harboring the *int* gene and *attP* site of the *L. casei* bacteriophage A2 were found to integrate into the chromosome of *L. plantarum, L. casei, Lc. lactis*, and *Escherichia coli* (Alvarez et al., 1998). Integrative recombination of such vectors into the chromosomes of these species is dependent on the *int* gene product and occurs specifically at the $tRNA^{Ser}$ gene (CGA; mv4) or $tRNA^{Leu}$ gene (CAA; A2) of lactobacilli. In other bacterial species where this tRNA gene is less or not conserved, secondary integration sites either in protein encoding regions or in intergenic DNA were used. Comparison of the integration sites in the different hosts indicates that some flexibility is permitted in the *attB* sequence, since *Lc. lactis* and *E. coli* only share 13 and 11 nt, respectively, with the 19-nt core sequence of *attB* of lactobacilli (Auvray et al., 1997; Alvarez et al., 1998). The integrative *att* sites specific for *Lactobacillus gasseri* phage ΦADH have been analyzed (Raya et al., 1992) and site-specific integration via high-frequency plasmid transduction was reported (Fremaux et al., 1993). The integration system based on phage A2 was validated by the construction of a stable food-grade *L. casei* ATCC 393-derived strain completely immune to phage A2 infection during milk fermentation (Martin et al., 2000).

By applying prophage integration and subsequent excision, a method to stably maintain introduced DNA sequences in the chromosome of *L. case*i strain Shirota was developed. For this purpose, the prophage integration system of phage phi FSW was modified and a chloramphenicol (Cm)-resistance gene was used as passenger DNA. On the integration plasmid harboring an erythromycin (Em)-resistance gene as a selection marker, N- and C-terminally-truncated Cm-resistance genes were inserted on both sides of the *attP* of phi FSW, within which site-specific recombination took place with *attB* of phi FSW on the recipient chromosome through the phi FSW integrase. Primary integrants of the modified plasmid (integration-excision vector) exhibiting Em-resistant and Cm-sensitive phenotype generated Em-sensitive and Cm-resistant derivatives under nonselective conditions. Homologous recombination resulted in the presence of one copy of the complete Cm-resistance gene residing at the attachment site on the host chromosome while the other vector-derived sequences were excised. The Cm-resistant phenotype of the final integrants was stable for more than 50 generations under nonselective conditions. Since prophage integration and homologous recombination are prevalent among bacteria, the procedure is expected to be applicable also to other *Lactobacillus* strains (Shimizu-Kadota, 2001).

To investigate transcriptional regulation of expression in *L. sakei*, a plasmid integration system was developed which allowed replacement of the *lacLM* locus by the *E. coli lacZ* gene. The *lacZ* gene could then be used as a reporter gene to investigate regulation of expression of promoters that are cloned upstream of *lacZ* (Stentz et al., 2000).

It should be emphasized, however, that many *Lactobacillus* strains are not or poorly transformable. In particular, species found in the gastrointestinal tract of humans and animals like *L. crispatus*, as well as strains used in dairy industry like some *L. delbrueckii* strains and *L. helveticus* strains were found to be refractory to genetic manipulation. To circumvent these problems, methods were developed to introduce foreign genes by conjugation (Langella et al., 1993). This method was used successfully to deliver the genetic determinants for β-glucanase, β-glucuronidase, and green fluorescent protein to

L. helveticus. Although expression of two of the three genes could be demonstrated, all recombinant plasmids were segregationally unstable in *L. helveticus* and there was some evidence for structural instability. The instability in the vector could be reduced by replacing the duplicated pBluescript polylinker with that from pUC19 (Thompson et al., 2001).

Expression Vectors

Although expression of foreign proteins in *Lactobacillus* had been demonstrated a decade ago, the yields were in most cases low (less than 0.2% of total soluble protein) (Roy et al., 1993; Brurberg et al., 1994; Wanker et al., 1995; Gold et al., 1996; Rush et al., 1997). A breakthrough in the expression of foreign proteins in lactobacilli was obtained by isolating and characterizing a number of highly efficient promoters, translation initiation sequences, and secretion sequences. By combining such elements in expression vectors, the yield of protein produced could be increased 10- to 100-fold, reaching levels equivalent to those obtained in other bacterial hosts, or even better. The expression vectors constructed at TNO were designed in such a way that antigens can be expressed either intracellularly, extracellularly, or secreted and anchored to the surface (Pouwels et al., 1996; Pouwels et al., 2000). All vectors are comprised of cassettes, enabling easy exchange of different expression signals between different plasmids. The cassette structure also enables workers to easily adapt the vectors for the expression of non-fused proteins, for example, enzymes, as demonstrated by the efficient expression in *L. plantarum* of a xylose proton motive force-driven transport protein from *Lactobacillus brevis* (Chaillou et al., 1998a). The expression signals and replication elements of the vectors are all derived from *Lactobacillus* DNA sequences (Figure 6.1). Replacement of current antibiotic resistance markers by *Lactobacillus* sequences will result in completely food-grade vectors. Such a replacement can be achieved by homologous or site-specific recombination (Gosalbes et al., 2000; Martin et al., 2000). An example of the first approach is provided by Gosalbes et al. (2000) who constructed an integrative vector allowing stable gene insertion in the chromosomal lactose operon of *L. casei*. The vector was based on a nonreplicative plasmid and contained two DNA fragments corresponding to the 3′ end of *lacG* and the complete *lacF* gene. By integration of cloned sequences through homologous recombination, highly stable food-grade integrants were obtained. The procedure was successfully used for the expression of the *E. coli gusA* gene and the *L. lactis ilvBN* genes in *L. casei* (Gosalbes et al., 2000). The use of food-grade vectors is expected to facilitate the application, as a food additive, of the products made by lactobacilli by minimizing safety and environmental concerns to regulatory authorities.

The TNO expression vectors have been successfully used to construct different antigen expressing *Lactobacillus* strains. Full-size proteins such as the tetanus toxin fragment C (TTFC), several rota virus surface proteins with sizes ranging from 37 to 87 kD, urease A and B subunits from *Helicobacter pylori*, and some small peptide epitopes (e.g., from influenza virus and encephalitogenic myelin peptides fused to a carrier protein (β-glucuronidase) have been successfully expressed (Maassen et al., 1999; Shaw et al., 2000). Synthesis in *L. casei* of intracellular antigens yielded levels of production ranging from 1% to 5%, those in *L. plantarum* being, in general, slightly lower. Efficient production levels were also obtained in this and other *Lactobacillus* species when the products were directed to the bacterial surface. Using fluorescence-activated cell sorter (FACS) analysis, it was shown that the heterologous antigens are exposed to the environment at the surface of the bacteria, by staining recombinant bacteria with specific antisera. FACS staining indicated

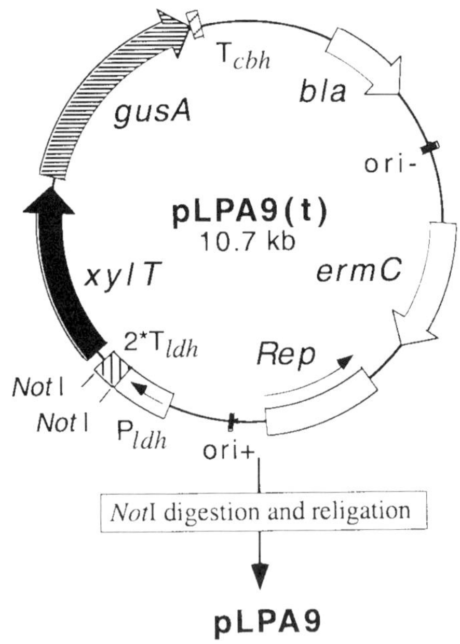

Figure 6.1. Structure of the *xylT Lactobacillus–E. coli* shuttle expression vector pLPA9(t). The expression cassette of this vector comprises the strong *ldh* promoter (P_{ldh} from *L. casei* ATCC 393), the *xylT* gene, the *E. coli* β-glucuronidase gene (*gusA*) used as a marker for gene expression, and the terminator region of the *L. plantarum* 80 *cbh* gene (T_{cbh}). The two terminator sequences (T_{ldh} from *L. casei* ATCC 393) downstream from the strong P_{ldh} promoter are used to circumvent instability of the vector in *E. coli*. These two T_{ldh} sequences can be removed by digestion of the plasmid with *Not*I and religation, yielding pLPA9. After transformation of *Lactobacillus* with plasmid pLPA9, transformants expressing the *gusA* reporter gene can be selected based on their capacity to form blue colonies on agar medium containing the chromogenic substrate X-gluc.

that mean levels of fluorescence corresponded to approximately 0.5×10^4 molecules of TTFC per cell for *ldh*-promoter-driven vectors and approximately 1×10^3 TTFC molecules per cell for the α-*amy*-promoter-driven vectors. Staining of TTFC-β-glucuronidase fusion proteins on the surface of the cells suggested that lower levels of these larger proteins were synthesized and that a proportion of the cells did not express detectable levels of TTFC. Removal of *gusA* resulted in higher antigen expression levels as well as a higher proportion of expressor cells within the population. Staining of late log phase or stationary phase cells indicated either reduced levels of expression or degradation of proteins (Pouwels et al., 1996; Shaw et al., 2000).

Following a conventional FACS staining, the highest 20–25% of expressing cells were sorted and re-inoculated into fresh medium to attempt selection and enrichment for high-level expressors. The results have indicated that this strategy does indeed result in a population of cells with a higher mean channel fluorescence value than cells obtained directly from a stock culture. However, this difference was not stable and following two further rounds of growth mean, channel fluorescence values for all sorted groups returned to equivalent levels. A further analysis has identified which sub-population of cells within the total population were most appropriate for sorting cells based upon "real" differences in levels of antigen expression. Further sorting experiments may, therefore, identify mutants which have higher promoter activities or higher plasmid copy numbers, enabling the immediate selection of efficient expression vectors from a heterogeneous population obtained directly following transformation (Tielen, Shaw, Leer and Pouwels, unpublished results).

Expression vectors comprising the expression signals of the L-*ldh* gene of *L. plantarum* yielded similar results (Hols et al., 1997). Expression of TTFC was studied in *L. plantarum* NCIMB 8826 carrying the expression cassette on a replicative plasmid or in strains with a single copy of the expression cassette integrated either into the L-*ldh* locus or the $tRNA^{Ser}$ locus. The amounts of TTFC estimated by western blotting appeared to be 4–5 times lower, when the vector was inserted into the chromosome compared to a strain with a multi-copy plasmid, and ranged from 2% to 6% of the total protein (Mercenier, 1999; Grangette et al., 2001).

A secretion cassette, based on the expression and secretion signals of an S-protein encoding gene from *L. brevis*, was used to efficiently express and secrete *E. coli* β-lactamase in *L. plantarum, L. brevis*, and in *Lc. lactis* (Savijoki et al., 1997). In *L. gasseri*, the *slp* promoter appeared to be recognized less efficiently (lower levels of both β-lactamase activity and mRNA), while in *L. casei*, very low levels of β-lactamase activity were found and no β-lactamase-specific messenger RNA could be detected. In all bacterial species tested, all β-lactamase activity was secreted into the medium. Elevated levels of β-lactamase activity (up to 80 mg/L in *Lc. lactis*) were obtained when the pH was kept constant at 5.5 and a rich medium was used for growth. Apparently, proteolytic degradation of β-lactamase was reduced at the stationary phase under these conditions. The kinetics of β-lactamase accumulation in *L. plantarum* and *Lc. lactis* showed that its production is restricted to the exponential phase of growth. The rate of synthesis and secretion was found to be 5×10^5 molecules/cell/hr, a value comparable to that found for the synthesis, secretion, and assembly of the S-protein in S-layer containing bacteria (Sleytr and Messner, 1983). The rate of production and secretion of β-lactamase in *L. brevis* was lower, probably because of competition with the formation of S-protein (Savijoki et al., 1997).

In experiments aimed at determining the relative strength of different promoters in *L. casei* by measuring chloramphenicol acetyl transferase (product of *cat* gene) activity directed by these promoters, it was found that the promoter of the S-protein gene of *L. acidophilus* resulted in an approximately 3-fold higher activity compared to a vector with the L-*ldh* promoter of *L. casei* (Boot et al., 1996). The apparent efficiency with which the S-protein promoter drives the expression of the *cat* gene could be due to a higher rate of transcription or to a more efficient translation of mRNA, or both. It has been shown that the presence of a long untranslated region of the *slpA* gene results in an exceptionally long half-life of the *slp* mRNA, enabling a more efficient translation. The efficient synthesis of β-lactamase directed by the *slp* promoter of *L. brevis* (Savijoki et al., 1997) may be explained in a similar fashion. Regulatory signals of S-layer protein encoding genes may thus be very useful for the development of highly efficient expression vectors.

The efficient expression in *L. casei* of the *cat* gene under control of the *slpA* promoter of *L. acidophilus* contrasts with the finding that expression in *L. casei* of the *slp* promoter of *L. brevis* was found to be extremely inefficient, although the promoter was found to be "strong" in other bacteria (Savijoki et al., 1997). It will be interesting to determine whether initiation of transcription of the *slp* promoter of *L. brevis* is less efficient in *L. casei* than in other bacteria or that the mRNA is very unstable.

A novel type of regulatable expression vector (NICE) originally designed for use in lactococci may also be useful for other Gram-positive bacteria, including lactobacilli. Expression in these vectors is based on the auto-inducible nisin promoter of *Lc. lactis* (de Ruyter et al., 1996). The nisin auto-induction system is an example of quorum sensing (cell-density-dependent gene expression) employed by *Lc. lactis* for the production of the antimicrobial peptide nisin. The induction of expression of a gene of interest cloned behind the nisin promoter, which can either take place in a nisin-producing or a nisin non-producing strain, requires the presence of two genes, *nisR* and *nisK* for signal transduction. These genes should be present on a compatible plasmid or need first to be integrated into the chromosome. Preliminary experiments with *L. plantarum* NCIM 8826 using the *gusA* gene of *E. coli* to monitor levels of gene expression showed low levels of gene expression and some clonal variation. However, integration of the *nisR* and *nisK* genes into the chromosome by site-specific recombination at the $tRNA^{Ser}$ locus solved the variability problems observed with the two-plasmid system. By optimizing the induction conditions, levels of *gusA* expression were obtained that are similar to those in *Lc. lactis* (Pavan et al., 2000). In *L. sakei*, a *pldh*L :: *gfp*UV fusion was constructed enabling efficient production of the GFP protein, either when present on a single copy in the chromosome (integration in *lac*LM locus) or when carried on a multicopy plasmid. Although the expression efficiency is difficult to assess for such proteins, it is a reliable marker to monitor *L. sakei* in fermented meat products (Gory et al., 2001).

Analysis of Expression Signals

Promoter

Since the previous review on this topic (Pouwels and Leer, 1993), the rapid advancement of DNA sequencing techniques has yielded sequence information about numerous genes and an increasing number of promoter sequences have been experimentally determined. To date, transcription start sequences have been identified for approximately 80 *Lactobacillus* genes originating from 9 different species (Table 6.2). The data confirm and extend our previous conclusions. Nearly all promoters show typical −35 and −10 sequences which, when aligned, enable us to define a consensus sequence (Figure 6.2). This result is in line with the observation that the main sigma factor, σ^A in *Bacillus* or σ^{70} in *E. coli*, which specifies transcription initiation, is conserved in both Gram-negative bacteria like *E. coli* and in low GC-content Gram-positive bacteria.

A TG motif has been found in *B. subtilis* and *E. coli* promoters, which is located one base upstream of the −10 region. This −16 region is moderately conserved in *B. subtilis* (45% of 142 promoters examined) but was observed only in a limited number of *E. coli* promoters. In *E. coli* the presence of a −16 TG motif was found in what are referred to as extended −10 promoters that lack an identifiable −35 region but are transcribed by $E\sigma^{70}$, indicating that the need for a −35 region can be bypassed in the presence of a TG motif. In *B. subtilis*, however, promoters with a TG motif contain the highly conserved −35 region (Voskuil and Chambliss, 1998). In approximately 30% of all *Lactobacillus* promoters examined, a TG motif was found. (Table 6.3). T and G residues at these two positions are conserved in more than 50% of the promoters in such a way that the motif can be seen in the graph when all promoters are included in the analysis (Figure 6.2). It has been suggested that the TG motif together with the −10 region was an early promoter configuration from which contemporary promoters have evolved, as it is the minimum sequence necessary for promoter function in *E. coli* (Brown et al., 1997). If so, most *Lactobacillus* species, and in particular species other than *L. delbrueckii*, have lost the TG motif (Table 6.2). Except for

Table 6.2. Sequence of Promoters of Chromosomal *Lactobacillus* Genes Lacking TG Motif

Species	Gene	Upstream Region	−35		−10		GenBank
acidophilus	*acdT*	gattcaaattataaacaacgttttaa	TTGAAA	ttatgaaaactagac	TATACT	gtaatag	D43626
	groESL	ttataaagagtgctaatttttc	TTGCTT	tttttagtaaacgggt	TATTAT	catatttgt	AF300645
	slpA	aatagtatttttcggtcattttaac	TTGCTA	tttcttgaagaggttag	TACAAT	atgaatc	X89375
brevis	*slpA*	tccaacgacaatcagagcgtaatcc	TTGTAT	ctccttaaggaaatcgc	TATACT	tatct	Z14250
	slpA	cgctaatgttatgaaaataaaattc	TTAACA	aaagcgctaacttcggt	TATACT	attct	Z14250
casei	*groES*	aagtataacattccacggtttgggg	TTGCAT	tcaaccgcaaaactcgt	TATAGT	tacttct	AF010281
	*hic*DH	gcggccaatttttaaagatgcttt	TTCACA	gaggcatcttgta	TACGGT	gagtgg	M26929
delbrueckii	*arbZ*	cttgcacctgcatgagaacgatgac	TTGTTA	aacgaatacctcaagttaaaaga	TCAACT	atagtta	Z86115
	aroP	caaccataaa	TTCTTA	ttttattttaatttac	TTTTAT	ttttcta	[a]
	brnQ	gcacaatagttttcaaatttatatt	TTCTAG	tttttaatttctatgtat	TGTTAT	tttaact	Z48676
	gap	gtcccgcatattctggcaattgccc	TTGGCA	cgagaaaggccaaggc	CATCAA	ggccta	AJ000339
	lacP	actaaaaatattttagtaaaacatc	TTGGTT	tatttagtaaacaagtc	TATACT	gtaattat	M55068
	oppD	aaaagcactagaagataattaagaaactg	TTGCAA	aatatttgaaaaaggt	TAAAAT	ctactagtgtggt	AY040221
	oppA2	cctttttctgttctcccggcttaggcccggtc	TTGCCG	cttttgttatggtaaac	TACATT	atgtagcaattta	AY040221
	pepC	aaaccaacaaattaagctacttga	TAGACG	gccttgcttttatgggc	TAAAAT	gggctta	X80643
	ORF	ttgccctttcttaaaggattttat	TTTACA	aaaaagactgaatcc	TATATT	atacaac	Z31377
	pepX	aaggaagcggtttgcttgcattaac	TTGAGA	acttgcttaaaaaacagc	TAAAAA	aactgg	Z14230
	pepW	gagaagcccgctacggcttctttt	TTGCCC	tctttagcgtaagattattc	TATAAT	catctattg	Z71782
helveticus	*helJ*	aataagtattttactaaaatgta	TTGACA	atattagtctttggacg	TAATAT	aagaact	M39360
	htrA	aaatttagcgtttttgtatagatta	TTCATA	tatttttcaaatttgccgtg	TATAGT	taataca	AJ005672
	D-*ldh*	ttttgtgttttg	TTGAGC	aaagtgaagcg	TATAAT	gaggaatg	[b]
	mvk	tgggtcagtttgtcgtcctgttaaatt	TTGATC	atttgttcgcacttccttgtt	TATTAT	tttatcata	AJ279018
	ndt2	gttaacaagacgttt	TTTTCA	atcgaaaatatgttaaag	TTAATT	cgtca	AB039914
	pepC	ttatcgtgatatattcatctagaga	TAGACT	acttccttttatcagc	TAAAAT	atagaat	Z30340
	pepD	atttcgtagaaattaattatattct	TTGCTT	aactcaggcttctttgca	TACAAT	atatagt	Z38063
	pepE	aagcgagttcatta	TTGAAC	ccgcttttattttggtt	TAAAAT	aaggag	[b]
	pepI	actgaaatgacccttttacggcag	TAGACA	ggcaaaaaatcattttg	TACAAT	cagaatt	Z56283
	pepN	cggcactcttacaatcagaaagaaa	TTGCCT	tttttaagcacttttaccga	TATTTT	ggtaaaa	Z30323
	pepN	aaagaaattgcctttttaagcact	TTTACC	gatattttggtaaaatt	TAGAAT	gaattat	Z30323

(continued)

Table 6.2. (*continued*)

Species	Gene	Upstream Region	−35		−10		GenBank
	pepT	ccgcccatttatt	TTGCAA	gaaaaaaaatcctgtttttt	ATCAAA	aaatg	AJ243321
	pepX	tttcatttttat	TGGTTC	tctctctttaaacggg	TAAAAT	ataagg	[b]
	pro	ttattaaaacattatacccgctatc	TTGCCT	ttttctcaatctgatac	AATAAT	taaagta	Z30709
pentosus	*ccpA*	aaaaataacaatctccgtgtggtaaatc	TTGCAT	tttgaaaacagataggg	TATTAT	tttcatg	AF176799
	xylA	ttttattttt ttgttctagaaagcg	TTTACA	aaaataagccaatgccgc	TGTAAT	cttacttg	M57384
	xylP	gataattttttaaacgaaaaaggc	TTGCAA	tcaaaaatgaaacgg	TATACT	cttctttg	U89276
	xylR	gcggaagtaacgctttagtaagaat	TTGACA	ggtaattgagcggtcat	CACATT	cttgtgacgg	M57384
plantarum	*argC*	aaagtgaatattttttcaataaagc	TTGCAA	tttaaaagcgatgagaa	TATAGT	gtgaatc	X99978
	bglGTP	gagatgatagaaattggactttaacgc	TTGCAA	tgcttttccgaaaccgc	TATACT	agctaattgtaa	AJ250202
	bglT	gaagatttgggatagttattaataa	TTGATA	ttcagaccaatgattgat	TATACT	tgttgta	Y15954
	carA	tgcaagcttta	TTGAAA	aaatattcacttttat	TCTATT	aattgca	X99978
	L-*ldh*	gcttattgacgcccgccaaagggtt	TTGCGG	acattgttaataattg	TATTAA	aagcatg	X70926
	L-*ldh*	cgcccgccaaagggttttgcggaca	TTGTTA	ataattgtattaaaag	CATGCT	caatcta	X70926
	pdc	ttttgcgccattggaaattcctcct	TGACGA	ttccttgataacagta	TACACT	aaccttg	U63827
	plsA	tgtagtagtaaagaaggtagacaat	TCGTCA	atactttttggaaatgtaagagt	TATACT	aatttca	Y15127
	kat	attatttgcatgattatttgcatga	TAAACA	agcattttcagagttcaatg	TATAAT	gcacatt	D87070
	pyr	agttgattagtccgttgattagtcc	TTGACA	gttgtggtggagttcgt	TACACT	taatcca	Z54240
Reuteri	*mub*	ctgcaattaa ctttaaagaa g	TTGCAA	cagcaaatgccaa	TAATTG	ttggttg	AF120104
	mub	gttgcaacagcaaatgccaataattgttgg	TTGCTG	aatgaatgttgatttttca	TAATGC	aaaaattt	AF120104
Sakei	*katA*	taacttgttgagcaagctctttcat	TTGACG	gttgcctgttgaaggtcc	TATAGT	gactagg	M84015
	lacML	tgacactaattgtgtagggttcttt	TTGACA	tcccagcggcaaacttc	TATACT	caaaaat	X82287
	las	ccctaaaatttaatatattatccct	TTGCAC	tcaatattaacatataaatt	TACCCT	taagtca	Z54312
	sppA	ataaagttgaacgttaatatttttt	TTGCGC	agaaatggtaaattgaag	CATAAT	agtcttg	X75081
	sppK	gatccgcttgtgaattatgtataat	TTGATT	agactaaagaataggagaaag	TATGAT	gatattt	Z48542
	sppT	tttaaatgcagcattaacgttaatt	TTGATA	aacgtaacgttaatg	GATAAT	catcctg	Z48542
Other	L-*hicDH*	aaaataatgatgagatgttgttcag	TGGTGA	acaacgtctctttttttg	TATAAT	gaacat	M28050
	hdcA	atatagataaagttcaataaaacgc	TTTACT	tttttattttttgaggt	TATAAT	gaaaatcg	J02613
Consensus[c]			TTG – a		TATAAT		

[a]Matern, H. T. et al. (1994). *FEMS Microbiology Letters* 122: 121–128.
[b]Chen and Steele, personal communication.
[c]Consensus sequence; upper case letters > 70%; lower case letters > 50%.

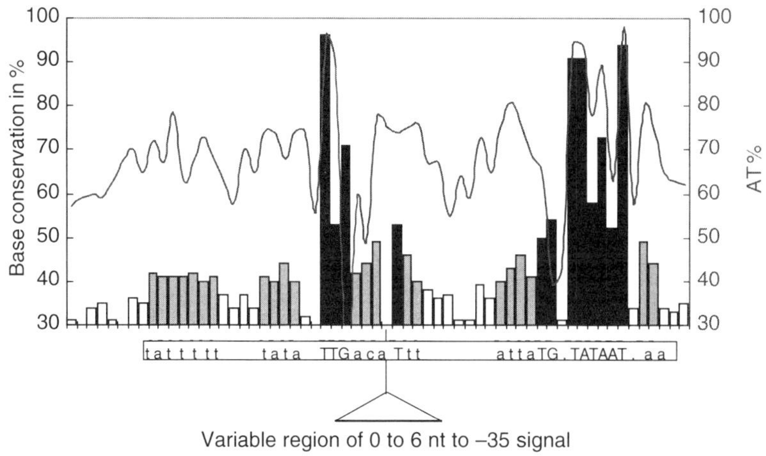

Figure 6.2. Statistical analysis of *Lactobacillus* promoter sequences. Curved line indicates AT% at each position of the promoter region. Nucleotides conserved in more than 50% of the promoters are in black, nucleotides conserved in more than 40% of the promoters are shaded in gray.

two cold-shock promoters (*cspC* and *cspL*) that show no typical −35 region, conservation of nucleotides was observed in promoters with a TG motif (Table 6.3). The first T residue of the hexamer (TTGACA) is present in more than 70% and the second T residue in more than 50% of the promoters. In position 4, no conservation of nucleotides was observed while in positions 3, 5, and 6, C and T residues were found in 50% or more of the promoters. In promoters lacking a TG motif, the first three nucleotides (TTG) are present in more than 75% of all promoters, whereas conservation of the last three residues (ACA) is weak. These results suggest that a TG motif is not essential for promoter activity but might enhance a rate limiting reaction, for example, docking of RNA polymerase near the −35 region.

Interestingly, substitution of −35 and −10 hexamers of the S-protein encoding gene of *L. acidophilus* by consensus sequences and introduction of a TG motif resulted in considerable improvement of the promoter in *L. fermentum* BR11 but in decreased transcription in *L. rhamnosus* GG. The TG motif was found to be important in *L. fermentum* BR11 when the −35 deviated from the consensus sequence, and in *L. rhamnosus* GG with a weaker −10 region. From these results the authors concluded that the efficiency of transcription initiation is both strain- and context-dependent (McCracken and Timms, 1999). In an independent study it was observed that the promoter-like sequence P15 from *L. acidophilus* ATCC 4356 is active in *L. reuteri, L. plantarum, L. acidophilus*, and *E. coli*, but not in *Lc. lactis*. By deletion of a 90 bp sequence deletion and a T→A transversion, a mutant promoter was obtained (P16) with putative −35 and −10 hexamers identical to the consensus promoter sequence. Based on chloramphenicol resistance determinations, P16 was found to be more active than P15 in *L. reuteri* and *L. plantarum* (3-fold and 9-fold, respectively) but 7-fold less active in *L. acidophilus* (Arsenijevic and Topisirovic, 2000).

Promoters in *Bacillus* are characterized by the presence of A- and T-rich regions upstream of the −35 region. Many of the *Lactobacillus* promoters also show the presence of A_n and T_n tracts upstream of the −35 region (Table 6.2). In contrast to *B. subtilis*, where the T_n tracts are found largely from positions −50 to −47 and the A_n tracts from −54 to −51, the positions in *Lactobacillus* promoters vary highly between −63 and −38. In *B. subtilis* promoters lacking the TG motif less conserved sequences were found

Table 6.3. Sequence of Promoters of Chromosomal *Lactobacillus* Genes with TG Motif

Species	Gene	Upstream Region	−35		−10		GenBank
acidophilus	*acdA*	ccatgtggcttacgattatatc	TTGTAT	ttatttatactata TG c	TATAAT	aaaaccttc	D37881
casei	*fgs*	tgaaaacgtaaattggctggctaag	CTCATA	agttagacccatttttc TG g	TATGAT	gaagcta	J05221
	L-*ldh*	acaatcacatgagaagcatgttcaat	TCCACA	cttgcctggcgcaaata TG t	TACAAT	acaaccgtaaa	M37466
delbrueckii	*oppA1*	ctaaaataattagcattaaattaaatttctca	TTGACT	ttaaaaaatgaaaa TG t	TAAAGT	aaaaggcat	AY040221
	pepG	agccgatcgaacttgatccttggga	TTCCTT	aatttaagcaggta TG t	TAACAT	tgactta	Z71782
	pepI	ttgcttaatcattgctgtccccacc	TTAATT	ttactcattattca TG a	TACCAT	ttttttg	Z26948
	pepN	ctgcaaacagatattttgcgttaaa	TGGGCT	ttatttagcctttt TG c	TAGAAT	agagaag	Z21701
	pepQ	ttttgtgcaatcgcttacagctatt	TTTTCA	acttttttcagttttttttag TG c	TATACT	gaggtta	Z34896
	pepR	aaaaagttgaaaaaatagctgtaagcga	TTGCAC	caaaaatgttctca TG g	TATCAT	taaatcagta	Y13385
	pepV	gcggcttttttgcttggcgtcttgt	TTGCCA	gggctggcgaagat TG a	TAGAAT	tttattta	Z31377
helveticus	*pepO*	aagaacgt	TTGGCT	aatcctcagacgttctttt TG c	TATAAT	gaattta	[a]
pentosus	*ackA*	tggttatgaaagaaataatatgctgacgaatcgg	TTTACA	atgttatgaaaatcatgagtttg TG a	ATAAAT	ccttgaaag	AJ309012
	ccpA	aaagcgatttcaatagcattcttaag	TTGCAT	tgagaccgtaattt TG c	TATATT	ggttgatgt	AF176799
	D-*ldh*	aatttagcaaagttttcacaattta	TGATTT	tatttctggcatttac TG t	TATAAT	gtttaat	D90339
	L-*ldh*	caatcacatgagaagcatgttcaat	TCCACA	cttgcctggcgcaaata TG t	TACAAT	acaaccg	D90340
	xpkA	tttaaaaattggaccgttccaattaacaaaaagg	TTGATT	tttaaaaataact TG g	TAGAAT	agaactt	AJ309011
plantarum	*cspC*	atttcatggaaatcatggtgtttgg	CTACCC	tttttagaaacaata TG c	TACAAT	tgttcttg	Y19217
	cspL	gtcatacgttatgcacaccgttttca	GCGATT	aaaaactagggatg TG a	TATACT	taagcca	Y19218
	cspP	tttttttgaattaatttgtgttctga	TTGGAA	attactgggtgagtg TG t	TAATCT	atataatg	Y19219
sakei	*hcrA*	atccgtgaaaattacagttcaattc	TTGACT	ttatttgacgttct TG c	TATATT	aatactt	AJ006274
	L-*ldh*	tagttttctgaaaatttaaacaaaa	TTAGCG	aactttcatgcaaatta TG c	TATACT	ggttttc	AF054624
	ptsH	atcattaattttgttagcgaagctg	TTGTAG	tacttgtctccaca TG g	TAATCT	taatatt	U82366
	sakB	ggtttcagacactgttagaattaaa	TATGCT	agctcctaaatt TG g	TATACT	gaattac	Z21855
Consensus[b]			TT g − c t		TA t AaT		

[a]Chen and Steele (personal communication).

[b]Upper case letters: >70%; lower case letter: >50%.

upstream of the −35 region compared with the TG motif-containing promoters. Typically, A_n and T_n tracts were only found in promoters with a TG motif (Voskuil and Chambliss, 1998). In *Lactobacillus* promoters no obvious difference was found between promoters containing the TG motif and those that lacked this sequence (Table 6.2).

Codon Usage

In previous studies codon usage was analyzed in *L. acidophilus, L. casei, L. delbrueckii, L. helveticus*, and the *L. plantarum/L. pentosus* group (Pouwels and Leer, 1993; Pouwels and Leunissen, 1994). A more than 3-fold increase in the number of sequenced genes from these species have now been analyzed. The results confirm and extend our previous conclusions. The greatly increased number of sequenced genes has also enabled us to perform a statistically reliable analysis for *Lactobacillus* species for which in the past no or insufficient information was available. Novel codon usage information has now become available for *L. brevis, L. reuteri*, and *L. sakei* (Table 6.4).

Codon usage of *Lactobacillus* genes shows a clear bias for specific codons. All possible codons are used by lactobacilli although some of them very rarely. The Arg codon AGG and the Ile codon ATA are very infrequently used in all species examined. Interestingly, rare codons in one species are used at moderate or even frequent rates in other species. For example, the Arg codon AGA is rarely used in *L. brevis, L. casei, L. plantarum*, and *L. reuteri*, but is used at normal frequencies in *L. acidophilus, L. delbrueckii, L. helveticus*, and *L. sakei*.

Codon usage in *L. acidophilus* is similar to that in *L. helveticus* and *L. reuteri*, but dissimilar to that in *L. brevis, L. casei, L. delbrueckii*, the *L. plantarum/L. pentosus* group, and *L. sakei*. Codon usage in *L. brevis* and *L. delbrueckii* is similar, but different from that in all other species. *L. brevis, L. delbrueckii*, and *L. fermentum* (data not shown) show GC drift reflected by a higher GC content at the third position of codons (GC3), whereas all other species show AT drift. In the latter organisms T residues are preferentially used over C residues at the third position of codons in two-codon sets. *L. acidophilus, L. helveticus*, and *L. reuteri* rarely use the codon NNG in family-box (four synonymous) codons, in contrast to all other species. In *L. reuteri* the codon CGG (Arg) forms an exception to this rule, where it is used with a very high frequency (Table 6.4).

Amino Acid Biosynthesis

Lactobacilli are known for their multiple nutritional requirements. Many lactic acid bacteria, including lactobacilli cannot synthesize all amino acids that are required for protein biosynthesis or for the formation of other metabolites (Morishita et al., 1974, 1981). Amino acid auxotrophy varies from strain to strain. Strains from *L. helveticus, L. casei*, or *L. plantarum*, for example, require between 7 and 14 exogenously supplied amino acids. Most lactobacilli used in dairy fermentation depend for growth in milk on a proteolytic system that allows degradation of milk proteins (caseins). The proteolytic systems of lactic acid bacteria can functionally be grouped into (a) proteinases that degrade casein into peptides, (b) peptidases that degrade peptides, and (c) transport systems that translocate the peptides and amino acids across the cell membrane. The proteolytic system of lactococci has been studied in great detail and many genes involved in each of these processes have been cloned and characterized (Kunji et al., 1996). During the last decade,

Table 6.4. Codon Frequencies in *Lactobacillus* Species

Amino		*L. acidophilus*		*L. brevis*		*L. casei*		*L. delbrueckii*		*L. helveticus*		*L. plantarum*		*L. reuteri*		*L. sakei*	
Acid	Codon	Number	(%)	Number	(%)	Number	(%)	Number	(%)	Number	(%)	Number	(%)	Number	(%)	Number	(%)
Gly	GGA	20	10	43	23	131	15	246	21	25	03	153	17	26	11	446	20
Gly	GGA	47	24	19	10	91	10	68	06	73	10	148	17	58	25	242	11
Gly	GGT	86	44	82	44	316	35	224	19	418	57	330	38	112	47	907	40
Gly	GGC	42	22	43	23	357	40	622	54	216	30	244	28	40	17	653	29
Glu	GAG	26	17	12	14	177	26	154	14	62	09	129	21	26	16	242	12
Glu	GAA	130	83	74	86	515	74	911	86	597	91	475	79	135	84	1716	88
Asp	GAT	136	75	76	60	507	66	254	24	479	64	514	69	125	74	1445	75
Asp	GAC	45	25	51	40	267	34	783	76	266	36	226	31	43	26	470	25
Val	GTG	31	19	29	19	248	26	155	14	58	09	188	21	12	6	460	19
Val	GTA	31	19	17	11	60	06	130	12	147	22	109	12	44	23	314	13
Val	GTT	76	47	74	49	410	43	444	41	372	57	367	42	108	57	1019	42
Val	GTC	24	15	32	21	226	24	362	33	80	12	216	25	24	13	614	26
Ala	GCG	19	11	36	15	275	22	139	11	55	07	312	28	25	10	542	20
Ala	GCA	47	28	43	18	262	21	192	15	256	32	247	22	79	33	776	28
Ala	GCT	64	38	107	45	340	28	431	33	365	46	322	29	90	37	817	30
Ala	GCC	39	23	53	22	346	28	554	42	119	15	240	21	47	20	607	22
Arg	AGG	4	05	0	0	14	03	29	05	10	03	4	01	2	2	40	03
Arg	AGA	17	19	1	02	9	02	85	15	98	28	29	07	3	3	153	12
Ser	AGT	36	27	28	20	113	20	80	09	98	17	197	29	43	25	542	27
Ser	AGC	18	14	21	15	111	20	308	34	110	19	100	15	16	9	234	12
Lys	AAG	53	30	92	74	329	47	911	82	480	58	273	48	129	60	701	34
Lys	AAA	124	70	33	26	376	53	201	18	346	42	298	52	87	40	1364	66
Asn	AAT	112	71	29	36	261	54	167	25	303	53	363	66	92	59	996	64
Asn	AAC	46	29	52	64	222	46	504	75	274	47	186	34	65	41	553	36
Met	ATG	70	100	53	100	326	100	365	100	257	100	297	100	77	100	984	100
Ile	ATA	23	13	0	0	23	03	12	01	32	04	48	06	7	3	242	9
Ile	ATT	117	68	74	64	472	61	223	27	471	62	473	63	154	72	1648	62
Ile	ATC	33	19	41	36	279	36	577	71	255	34	235	31	54	25	762	29
Thr	ACG	9	07	54	28	205	27	142	16	49	08	294	34	17	9	291	22
Thr	ACA	31	24	26	13	149	20	60	07	84	14	188	22	70	36	476	35

Thr	ACT	69	53	79	41	131	17	354	40	340	58	227	26	76	40	752	24
Thr	ACC	22	17	34	18	276	36	322	37	109	19	153	18	29	15	394	18
Trp	TGG	48	100	30	100	124	100	190	100	141	100	142	100	25	100	366	100
End	TGA	1	08	0	0	11	34	1	03	2	08	6	19	1	10	7	7
Cys	TGT	14	74	6	67	25	50	18	19	27	49	51	67	8	89	135	71
Cys	TGC	5	26	3	33	25	50	76	81	28	51	25	33	1	11	55	29
End	TAG	6	50	1	20	3	09	9	26	4	16	8	25	1	10	14	14
End	TAA	5	42	4	80	18	56	25	71	19	76	18	56	8	80	78	79
Tyr	TAT	97	70	29	32	283	66	120	21	195	46	307	67	52	56	773	65
Tyr	TAC	42	30	61	68	149	34	453	79	227	54	152	33	41	44	414	35
Leu	TTG	43	19	62	34	381	35	463	32	236	25	303	28	40	15	694	20
Leu	TTA	94	41	50	28	201	18	125	09	317	34	392	37	97	37	1599	46
Phe	TTT	102	69	47	50	299	59	276	39	265	61	317	66	77	75	930	64
Phe	TTC	45	31	47	50	209	41	426	61	172	39	160	34	26	25	530	36
Ser	TCG	7	05	5	04	73	13	20	02	16	03	75	11	15	9	207	10
Ser	TCA	28	21	39	28	115	20	218	24	181	32	173	25	44	26	604	30
Ser	TCT	37	28	29	21	75	13	91	10	130	23	97	14	34	20	294	15
Ser	TCC	7	05	18	13	76	13	195	21	35	06	40	06	18	11	121	06
Arg	CGG	5	06	22	34	137	27	206	36	11	03	114	28	47	39	258	20
Arg	CGA	13	15	11	17	57	11	11	02	16	05	72	18	14	12	156	12
Arg	CGT	37	42	23	35	124	25	65	11	161	46	117	29	43	36	365	29
Arg	CGC	12	14	8	12	158	32	178	31	54	15	71	17	11	9	294	23
Gln	CAG	7	09	28	35	253	44	268	49	59	14	200	35	24	21	317	18
Gln	CAA	73	91	53	65	318	56	274	51	360	86	369	65	88	79	1459	82
His	CAT	64	79	13	37	215	64	66	20	120	50	202	66	41	60	462	65
His	CAC	17	21	22	63	122	36	262	80	120	50	105	34	27	40	249	35
Leu	CTG	10	04	22	12	214	20	483	34	56	06	110	10	15	6	178	05
Leu	CTA	26	11	17	09	64	06	40	03	42	04	116	11	32	12	350	10
Leu	CTT	40	17	18	10	161	15	158	11	248	26	82	08	62	24	358	10
Leu	CTC	16	07	11	06	76	07	165	12	41	04	64	06	15	6	278	08
Pro	CCG	9	09	10	15	221	40	166	29	26	07	113	25	19	15	192	15
Pro	CCA	46	45	27	40	193	35	261	46	210	58	197	43	70	56	601	48
Pro	CCT	37	36	19	28	92	17	85	15	113	31	82	18	30	24	293	24
Pro	CCC	10	10	11	16	43	08	58	10	11	03	66	14	7	6	158	13
Total number of codons		2650		2154		12339		15461		10547		11931		12948		34399	

considerable progress has also been made in the identification and characterization of the proteolytic system of some *Lactobacillus* species. For a number of species like *L. helveticus, L. casei, L. rhamnosus*, and *L. delbrueckii*, genes involved in casein degradation, in peptide degradation, and in amino acid transport have been isolated and in some cases characterized. Our knowledge about the control of expression of the genes involved in the proteolytic system is, however, rudimentary (Kok, 1996; see Chapter 7 by Kok).

Amino Acid Biosynthesis in Lactobacilli: Tryptophan

Although, as mentioned, many strains of lactobacilli are multiple amino acid auxotrophs, in a number of cases such strains were found to carry rudimentary parts or a complete set of, inactive, amino acid biosynthetic genes (Morishita et al., 1981). This implies that isolated lactobacilli originate from parent strains with entirely functional genes. Such strains, most likely as a result of environmental conditions, have stopped the expression of anabolic pathways for amino acids that are not strictly essential under the given growth conditions. Morishita showed that strains of *L. acidophilus, L. casei*, and *L. helveticus* incapable of growing in the absence of certain amino acids, including tryptophan, could be rendered prototrophic by mutagenic treatment. The reversion of a mutation after successive transfers and the inverse relationship of growth rate and mutational steps support the hypothesis that lactobacilli restrict their expression capacity, thereby increasing their chances to compete with other microorganisms in circumstances where energy is not limited for which the growth rate and not the growth yield is of strategic importance (Vandevoorde et al., 1992). Tryptophan biosynthetic genes of *L. casei* were indeed found and their sequences were determined (Natori et al., 1990). Interestingly, a structure highly reminiscent of the terminator–antiterminator structure and T-box sequence was found to be contained within the 5′ untranslated region of the *L. casei trp* operon (Grundy et al., 1994). This finding suggests that the *trp* genes might be controlled by a mechanism of transcription termination–antitermination. No studies on the mode of expression of the tryptophan genes have been reported for this organism.

Arginine

In bacteria, arginine is synthesized from glutamate via ornithine. Ornithine is converted into citrulline by the enzyme ornithine transcarbamylase (OTCase) that couples carbamoyl phosphate (CP) to ornithine (Cunin et al., 1986). The arginine biosynthetic pathway in bacteria is particularly interesting because it is intimately linked with pyrimidine biosynthesis. Both pathways share CP as an intermediate. *L. plantarum* contains two CP synthetases (CPSase). One is CPSase P that is encoded by the *pyrAA* and *pyrAB* genes located in the *pyr* operon and is repressed by exogenous pyrimidines (Elagoz et al., 1996). The other enzyme, CPSase A also consists of two subunits and is encoded by the *carA* and *carB* genes that are part of an operon repressed by arginine (Bringel et al., 1997). A deletion of the CPSase P encoding genes rendered *L. plantarum* unable to grow in the absence of uracil and arginine, suggesting that CPSase A is unable to provide CP for the two biosynthetic pathways. The mutant strain did not grow in the presence of arginine that repressed CPSase A showing that apart from CPSase P and CPSase A, *L. plantarum* does not contain a system capable of synthesizing CP. When cultured in the presence of uracil, either wild-type or mutant bacteria only grew when the air was enriched with 4% CO_2.

Thus, *L. plantarum* CPSase A is capable of providing CP for arginine biosynthesis, although CPSase A may have a low affinity for one of its substrates, bicarbonate (Bringel et al., 1997; Nicoloff et al., 2000; Bringel, personal communication).

The arginine biosynthetic apparatus which is present in *L. plantarum* is as yet the only amino acid biosynthetic pathway studied at the molecular level. A cluster of genes involved in citrulline biosynthesis (*argCJBDF*) in *L. plantarum* was isolated by complementation of a *B. subtilis argF* mutation and chromosome walking. The genes were found to be closely linked, with opposite polarity, to *carA*, encoding CP synthase A, that catalyzes the conversion of glutamate plus ATP into CP (Bringel et al., 1997). Bacterial OTCases can be divided into two groups based on their primary structure. The *L. plantarum* ArgF group contains both anabolic and catabolic OTCases from both Gram-positive and Gram-negative bacteria, while the other group which includes *B. subtilis* ArgF also harbors catabolic and anabolic enzymes. Interestingly, the cloned *L. plantarum argF* gene complemented the OTCase deficiency of a *B. subtilis argF* strain. Conversely, the *B. subtilis argF* gene could complement the deficiency of an *L. plantarum argF* strain. In other words, the two OTCases are functionally similar. It appears, therefore, that the OTCases of *L. plantarum* and *B. subtilis* are paralogous enzymes (Bringel et al., 1997).

Sequence analysis of the *arg* gene cluster has revealed the presence of a promoter before the *carA* gene.The distance of the −35 region of the putative *carA* promoter to the −35 region of the putative promoter of the *argC* gene is only 6 nt. The translational stop and initiation codons of *argD/argF* are 2 nt apart while those of *argB/argD* are overlapping. These data strongly suggest translational coupling and are taken as evidence for stoichiometric translation of *argBDF* (Oppenheim and Yanofsky, 1980). OTCase synthesis was repressed in the presence of arginine. Multiple putative operator sites structurally similar to the consensus *E. coli arg* operator sites (ARG boxes) were identified in the promoter region for *carA* and *argC*, in line with the hypothesis that regulation of arginine biosynthesis is transcriptionally controlled. Transcription analysis of the *argCJBDF* operon has confirmed this hypothesis (Bringel, personal communication). The promoter region of *argC* contained seven putative ARG boxes, while there were four such sites for *carA*. In many cases the distance between the putative operator sites was found to be 11 nt or a multiple of 11 nt, one turn of the DNA helix. No functional analysis of the ARG boxes has as yet been reported.

Amino Acid Degradation

In some bacterial species, arginine is catabolized via the arginine deaminase (ADI) pathway. The ADI pathway catalyzes the conversion of arginine into ornithine, ammonia, and carbon dioxide, generating 1 mol of ATP per mol of arginine. In arginine catabolism, OTCase catalyzes the reverse but thermodynamically less favorable reaction of that in arginine biosynthesis whereby citrulline is split into CP and ornithine. In some bacteria, like *Pseudomonas aeruginosa*, the ADI pathway co-exists with the arginine biosynthetic pathway. In other bacteria, only one pathway is found. For example, *L. sakei* contains the ADI pathway but not the arginine biosynthetic pathway, while for *L. plantarum* it is the reverse (Montel and Champomier, 1987; Zuniga et al., 1998). The ADI pathway, which has been detected in several lactic acid bacteria, includes ADI, OTCase, and carbamate kinase (CK). A transport protein catalyzing the electroneutral exchange between arginine and ornithine has been found in some heterofermentative lactobacilli and other lactic acid bacterial strains (Poolman et al., 1987). A DNA fragment was isolated from *L. sakei* comprising all four genes involved in arginine catabolism, as well as a gene (*arcT*) encoding a putative transaminase. The gene order is *arcA* (ADI), *arcB* (OTCase), *arcC* (CK), *arcT*, and *arcD* (transporter). Transcription studies indicated that *arcA* is co-transcribed with *arcB* or together with all other *arc* genes. Transcription of the *arc* genes was found to be subject to glucose repression. Arginine induced the transcription of *arcA*. In the presence of arginine, glucose repressed transcription, while galactose had no effect (Zuniga et al., 1998). Transcriptional activation of the *arc* cluster under anaerobiosis has been shown, suggesting the involvement of more than one regulatory protein (Champomier-Verges et al., 1999). A repressive effect of glucose on ADI has also been observed in other lactic acid bacteria such as *L. leichmanii* (Manca de Nadra et al., 1986) and *Lc. lactis* (Poolman et al., 1987). The repressive effect of glucose may be mediated by the phosphoenolpyruvate: sugar phosphotransferase (PTS)-catabolite control protein A (CcpA) signal pathway, since two putative *cre* sites were found upstream of *arcA* (Zuniga et al., 1998).

Oenococcus oeni, the main species that induces malolactic fermentation in wine, uses arginine via the arginine deaminase pathway. A putative binding site for the regulation for fumarate and nitrate reduction (FNR) and cAMP receptor protein (CRP) transcriptional regulators was found in the promoter region of the *arcA* gene. Moreover, expression of a CRP-like gene that is present immediately upstream of *arcA* was stimulated by arginine, like that of the *arc* genes. These data suggest that a CRP-like regulator is involved in arginine metabolism in *O. oeni* (Tonon et al., 2001).

Genetics of Sugar Metabolism

Lactobacilli mostly utilize carbohydrates for the production of energy, which can be used to facilitate the synthesis of cell material from other components obtained from the growth medium. Energy is obtained in the form of ATP, generated by substrate-level phosphorylation, the dominating route of production being the anaerobic glycolysis. Some lactobacilli are also capable of fermenting sugars by obligate or facultative heterofermentation. All carbohydrates metabolized by the heterolactic pathway, also called the phosphoketolase pathway (PKP), are first converted by appropriate enzymes into xylulose 5-phosphate that is then fermented into equimolar amounts of lactic acid and acetic acid. This process requires the presence of two enzymes specific for the heterolactic pathway: xylulose 5-phosphate phosphoketolase (Xpk) and acetate kinase (Kandler, 1983). The production of lactic acid and flavor compounds from the metabolism of sugars plays an important role in the food industry, and considerable efforts have been devoted worldwide to study gene expression of catabolic pathways that might be useful for the improvement of starter strains. Until recently, however, we had little understanding of the regulation of carbon metabolism in lactobacilli. One of the major problems was the lack of model systems to study, as well as a lack of genetic tools to investigate global regulatory pathways. This section will present the main studies on regulation of carbon metabolism at the level of gene expression.

Carbon Catabolite Repression Mechanisms in Lactobacilli

The knowledge about carbon catabolite repression (CR) mechanisms in lactobacilli, or in lactic acid bacteria in general, is still limited compared to what is known for the model Gram-positive organism, *B. subtilis*. However, recent years have seen a significant increase in the number of studies dealing with this topic. To date, CR pathways have been

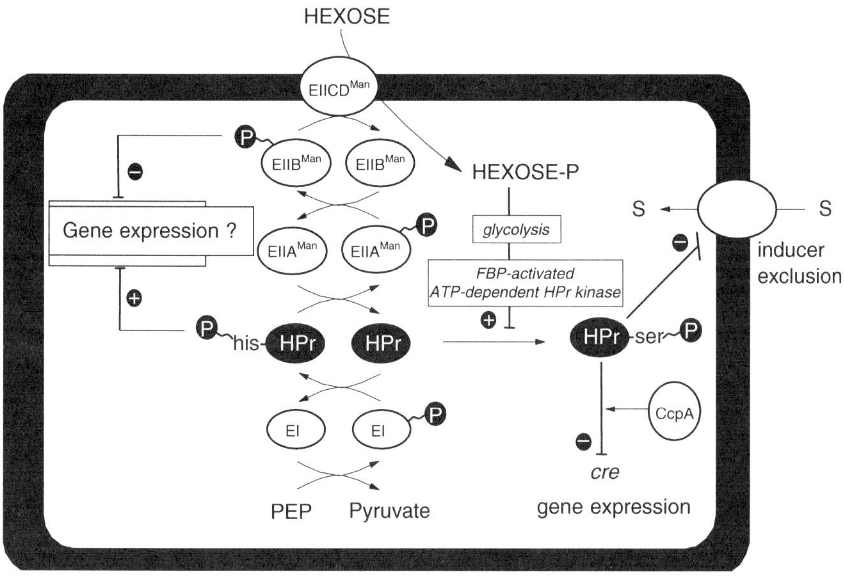

Figure 6.3. Schematic representation of CR mechanisms in lactobacilli by protein phosphorylation. The catabolism of hexose phosphate via the glycolytic pathway activates (+) the phosphorylation of the HPr protein on a serine 46 residue. The HPr(Ser-P) can interact with the transcriptional regulator CcpA, and this complex inhibits (−) the transcription of numerous genes after binding to *cre* sequences. Furthermore, HPr(Ser-P) can also regulate the activity of sugar transporters by a mechanism called inducer exclusion or favor the expulsion of preaccumulated solute. The transport of hexoses via the mannose-PTS (comprising the EII^{Man} complex and the general enzymes of the PTS, HPr, and EI) can also regulate, directly or indirectly, the expression of metabolic genes. One of the roles of the mannose-PTS in CR may involve the phosphorylation state of HPr(His-P) and of the substrate-specific $EIIB^{Man}$ subunit, but the mechanism, as well as the targets, remain to be characterized (see text for more details). EII^{Man} indicates the substrate-specific cytosolic ($EIIA^{Man}$ and $EIIB^{Man}$) or membrane-bound ($EIICD^{Man}$) enzymes of the mannose-PTS.

investigated in four species, *L. brevis, L. casei, L. pentosus*, and *L. sakei*. Some components involved in CR mechanisms have now been characterized. Given the wealth of information available on CR pathways in *B. subtilis* and the studies carried out with *Lactobacillus* species, it is now possible to outline a hypothetical sketch for the global control of carbon utilization in lactobacilli (Figure 6.3). CR mechanisms occurring in lactobacilli show extensive similarities with those of *Bacillus* species, but as will be shown in the following paragraphs, slight differences might be found for these two genera. Studying these differences is probably the key to the understanding of the mechanisms regulating carbon metabolism in lactobacilli.

CcpA-Mediated CR

The dominant CR pathway in *B. subtilis* involves one of the components of the PTS, the HPr protein. HPr can be phosphorylated at a Ser-46 residue by an ATP-dependent HPr kinase, activated by fructose-1,6-bisphosphate (FBP) and other glycolytic intermediates (Galinier et al., 1998; Reizer et al., 1998). The seryl-phosphorylated form of HPr, HPr(Ser-P), regulates the expression of ~10% of all genes in *B. subtilis* (Moreno et al., 2001). These genes are implicated in as different functions as carbon CR, nitrogen metabolism, stress response, and glycolysis (Deutscher et al., 1994, 2001). HPr(Ser-P) carries out this control by interacting with the trans-acting factor catabolite control protein A (CcpA) (Deutscher et al., 1995), which is a member of the GalR-LacI family of transcriptional regulators (Weickert and Adhya, 1992). Further investigations demonstrated that the HPr(Ser-P)/CcpA complex can bind to *cis*-acting catabolite responsive elements (*cre*), located in the promoter region of many catabolic operons (Deutscher et al., 1995; Fujita et al., 1995; Jones et al., 1997), thereby preventing their transcription. HPr(Ser-P) does not interact with CcpA when phosphorylation of HPr occurs on the His-15 residue, the site of phosphorylation involved in the phosphoryl transfer from PEP to the sugar (Deutscher et al., 1995). During growth on a PTS-dependent carbon source, the phosphoryl group bound to His-15 of HPr will constantly be used to phosphorylate the carbohydrate, and therefore, the transport of a PTS sugar will facilitate the complex formation between HPr(Ser-P) and CcpA. Thus, transport and phosphorylation of PTS sugars is an important mechanism to mediate CcpA-dependent CR in *Bacillus* species. It has also been shown that NADP can interact with CcpA and slightly stimulate the binding of the regulator to the *cre* site of the *amyO* operator in *B. subtilis* without the need for interaction with the co-repressor HPR(Ser-P) (Kim et al., 1998). The affinity of the CcpA/NADP complex for the *amyO cre* site was 7-fold lower than that found for the CcpA/HPR(Ser-P) complex. However, the inhibition of the *in vitro* transcription from the *amyE* promoter was only 2-fold lower in the presence of CcpA/NADP complex compared to the CcpA/HPR(Ser-P). The authors have concluded that the efficiency of CcpA binding to the *cre* site of the *amyO* may not correlate with the level at which transcription is inhibited and suggested that interaction of CcpA with the transcription machinery is also influenced by other factors such as NADP. The intracellular concentration of NADP may increase during the exponential growth and when there is a high glycolytic flux in *B. subtilis*. Therefore, NADP could serve, in addition to FDP, as an intracellular effector of CR.

The *ccpA* gene has been cloned and characterized in *L. casei* ATCC 393 and *L. plantarum* (Monedero et al., 1997; Muscariello et al., 2001) and was also detected by PCR, and inactivated in *L. pentosus* (Lokman et al., 1997). In both cases, a set of primers derived from the *Bacillus megaterium ccpA* gene was used to isolate the corresponding *Lactobacillus* homologue, indicating a strong conservation of the *ccpA* gene amongst low-GC content Gram-positive microorganisms. Analysis of *ccpA* mutants in *L. casei* ATCC 393, *L. plantarum*, and *L. pentosus* gave consistent results to support the role of CcpA as a common regulatory protein in lactobacilli. Indeed, inactivation of the *ccpA* gene resulted in relief of the negative effect mediated by glucose on the activity of several catabolic enzymes such as phospho-β-galactosidase and N-acetyl-glucosaminidase in *L. casei* (Monedero et al., 1997), β-glucosidase and β-galactosidase for *L. plantarum* and xylose isomerase, α-xylosidase, β-galactosidase, β-glucosidase, phosphoketolase, and acetate kinase in *L. pentosus* (Lokman et al., 1997; Chaillou et al., 1998b, 2001; Posthuma et al., 2002). A *cre* sequence was detected overlapping the transcription start site of the *bglH* gene encoding phospho-β-glucosidase of *L. plantarum*. Gel retardation experiments and direct mutagenesis of the *cre* site were used to demonstrate the role of this element in the glucose-mediated repression of the *bglH* gene (Marasco et al., 1998). Finally, the increasing number of putative *cre* sites detected in the promoter region of many *Lactobacillus* genes suggest the presence of CcpA-mediated CR in these species (Table 6.5).

There is still few data at the molecular or biochemical level on the role of HPr(Ser-P) as the co-repressor of CcpA in lactobacilli. However, it was recently observed that the extent of repression mediated by glucose, mannose, and fructose on the activities of

Table 6.5. Putative *cre* Sequences Identified in Lactobacilli

Species	Gene	Function	*cre* Sequence	Reference
amylovorus	*amyA*	α-amylase	TGAAATTGTTCACT TGAAAACGGTTGCA	Giraud (1997)
brevis	*xylAB*	Xylose catabolism	CGAAAACGCTTGCA	Chaillou et al. (1998a)
	xylT	Xylose transport	AGAAAACGGTTTCA	Chaillou et al. (1998b)
casei	*lacTEGF*	Lactose PTS	ATAAAACGTTTACA	Gosalbes et al. (1997)
	ccpA	Regulator of CR	GTAAAACGCTTGCA	Monedero et al. (1997)
delbrueckii	*pepR*1	Unknown	TGTAAGCGATTGCA	Stucky et al. (1996)
pentosus	*xylAB*	Xylose catabolism	AGAAAGCGTTTACA	Lokman et al. (1997)
	xylPQ	Isoprimeverose catabolism	TGAAACGGTATACT	Chaillou et al. (1998b)
	ccpA	Regulator of CR	TGAAAGCGATTTC	Mahr et al. (2000)
plantarum	*bglH*	Phospho-β-glucosidase	TGTAAGGGCTATCA	Marasco et al. (1998)
	amyA	α-amylase	TGAAAGTGTTTCAC TGAAAACGGTCGCA	Giraud and Cuny, (1997)
sakei	*arcABCTD*	ADI pathway	AGTAAGTGTTATTA TGAAAGCGATTTAC	Zuniga et al. (1998)

β-galactosidase and β-glucosidase in *L. pentosus* increased proportionally with the rates at which these hexoses were taken up and phosphorylated (Chaillou et al., 2001). Thus, the degree of CcpA-dependent repression on the activities of these two enzymes may correlate with the rate of hexose metabolism via the glycolytic pathway in *L. pentosus*. This result would agree with the finding that HPr(Ser-P)/CcpA-mediated CR is activated by phosphorylated glycolytic intermediates in *B. subtilis*. Thus, at first glance, the mechanisms underlying CcpA-mediated CR are likely to be similar in *Bacillus* and *Lactobacillus*. Is NADP also an effector of CR in *Lactobacillus* ? Unfortunately, this point has not yet been addressed in the few studies carried out to investigate the role of CcpA in CR in *Lactobacillus*. It should be noted that the NADH/NAD+ ratio was found to control the shift from homolactic to heterolactic fermentation in *Lc. lactis* (Garrigues et al., 1997). In lactic acid bacteria, the concentration of NADH may increase during high glycolytic fluxes. It thus seems plausible to assume that this co-factor could also stimulate the inhibition of transcription of non-glycolytic genes after interaction with CcpA.

A major difference was found between the two genera as to the location of the *ccpA* gene, however. In *B. subtilis* and *B. megaterium*, the *ccpA* gene is linked to *motA* and *motB*, the deduced products of which are presumably involved in cell motility (Hueck et al., 1994). Recently, the locus containing the *ccpA* gene of several lactobacilli was cloned and sequenced. In contrast to what was found in *Bacillus* species, the *ccpA* gene of *L. pentosus* is oriented in a back-to-back configuration with the *pepQ* gene, whose product shows high similarity to PepQ *of L. delbrueckii* subsp. *lactis*, which has been characterized as an aminoacyl-L-proline dipeptidase (Stucky et al., 1995; Mahr et al., 2000). Interestingly, the *pepR*1 gene of *L. delbrueckii* subsp. *lactis* encoding a potential transcriptional regulator similar to CcpA was found upstream of the *pepQ* gene (Stucky et al., 1996), in a configuration identical to that of the *pepQ-ccpA* locus of *L. pentosus* (Figure 6.4). It was found that expression of the *pepR*1 gene from an *E. coli/B. subtilis* shuttle vector in a *ccpA*

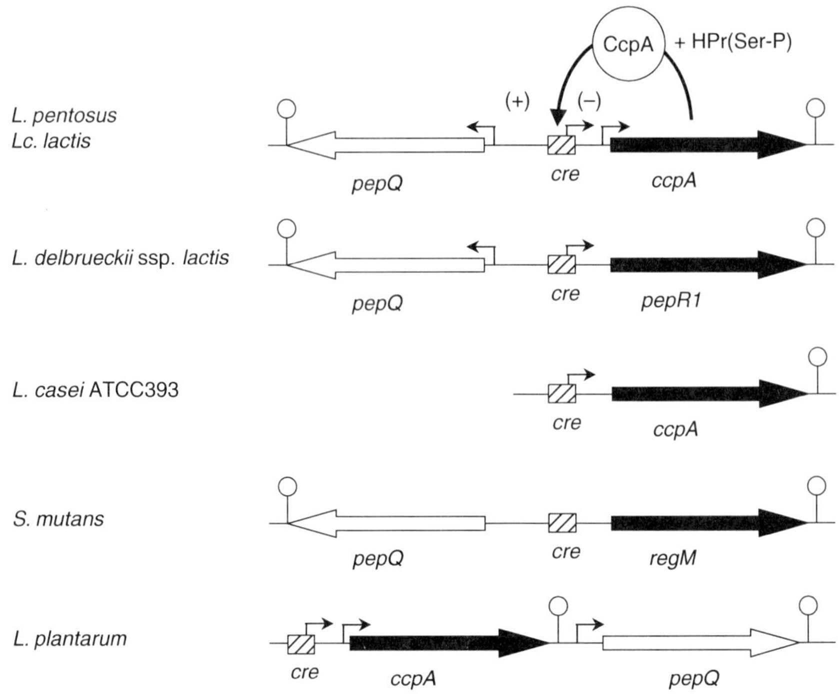

Figure 6.4. Schematic representation of the *ccpA* gene cluster of *L. pentosus*, *L. plantarum*, and *L. casei*, and comparison with other similar gene clusters from *L. delbrueckii* and *S. mutans*. The regulation of expression of the *L. pentosus ccpA* gene by its own product is indicated. Arrows with a straight angle indicate promoters; stem-loop structure indicates potential terminators of transcription. The *cre* sequence overlapping with one of the promoter elements is shown as a shaded box.

deletion mutant of *Staphylococcus xylosus* partially complemented the defect (Schick et al., 1999). Therefore, *pepR1* presumably encodes the *ccpA*-homologue of *L. delbrueckii* subsp. *lactis*. Moreover, in both *L. delbrueckii* subsp. *lactis* and *L. pentosus*, a putative *cre* site is present in the promoter region between *ccpA* and *pepQ*. In *L. pentosus*, this *cre* site partially overlaps the −35 element of the distal *ccpA* promoter, the activity of which is strongly repressed in the presence of glucose in the medium and is enhanced in a *ccpA* mutant. This finding suggests that CcpA may bind to this *cre* site to autoregulate its own expression. However, the use of antibodies directed against the *L. pentosus* CcpA revealed that the amount of CcpA protein detected in *L. pentosus* cells grown under various conditions is constant. The role of the two promoters in the expression of *ccpA* has to be further analyzed in order to explain the discrepancy found between *ccpA* expression and the amount of CcpA protein measured in cell-free extracts. Whether expression of the *pepQ* gene in *L. pentosus* is controlled by CcpA is not yet known, but PepR1 was postulated to be an activator of *pepQ* expression in *L. delbrueckii* subsp. *lactis*, since it was shown to increase slightly the expression of a *pepQ-lacZ* fusion when over-expressed. However, this study was carried out in a heterologous bacterium (*E. coli*) in which the activity of PepR1 may be different from that in lactobacilli, especially if PepR1 requires transduction of signals from carbon metabolism and/or interactions with other components such as HPr(Ser-P) for its binding to *cre*. Nevertheless, Schick et al. showed that transcription initiation of the *pepQ-lacZ* fusion required the integrity of the intergenic *cre* site located 73 bp upstream of *pepQ*. Moreover, in gel mobility assays, the purified PepR1 protein specifically interacted with the *pepQ* promoter region (Schick et al., 1999). Thus, the results suggest that under certain conditions of growth, PepR1 may activate transcription of *pepQ* in *L. delbrueckii* subsp. *lactis*. It may still be too early to conclude that the *pepQ-ccpA* locus is a general feature in lactobacilli. Indeed, the upstream region of the *L. casei* ATCC 393 *ccpA* gene is not yet cloned and characterized. However, a putative *cre* site could be detected in the promoter region of the *L. casei ccpA* gene at a position similar to that found in the *L. pentosus pepQ-ccpA* intergenic region. Transcriptional analysis of the *ccpA* gene by Northern blot revealed that the regulator from *L. casei* is expressed constitutively under various growth conditions and from a single promoter (Monedero et al., 1997).

In *L. plantarum, ccpA* is linked to the *pepQ* gene in the order *ccpA-pepQ*, with the two genes transcribed in tandem from the same strand as distinct transcriptional units. Two *ccpA* transcription start sites corresponding to two functional promoters were found, expression from the upstream promoter being autogenously regulated through a *cre* sequence overlapping the upstream +1 site. During growth on ribose, the upstream promoter showed maximal expression, while growth on glucose led to transcription from the downstream promoter. In a *ccpA* mutant strain, the gene was transcribed mainly from the upstream promoter in both repressing and non-repressing conditions.

A *ccpA-pepQ* gene cluster has also been found in *Lc. lactis*. Like in *L. pentosus*, the promoters of both genes are situated back-to-back and a *cre* site overlaps the promoter of *ccpA* (Hellendoorn et al., 1999). Using a PepQ assay and a gene expression analysis vector, it was shown that the expression of *pepQ* was reduced in a *ccpA* mutant. Furthermore, CcpA was shown to repress its own transcription as was found for *L. pentosus*.

Therefore, the *ccpA-pepQ* structure might be a general situation amongst lactic acid bacteria and not only amongst lactobacilli. Indeed, it should be noted that a locus containing *pepQ* and a gene homologous to *ccpA (regM)* was also found in *Streptococcus mutans* (Simpson and Russell, 1998). However, functional analysis of a *regM* mutant showed that the product of this gene did not influence the expression of the *pepQ* gene. On the other hand, inactivation of the *regM* gene decreased the growth rate of *S. mutans* on glucose (an effect observed with most *ccpA* mutants in Gram-positive bacteria). A *regM* inactivation in *S. mutans* also affected CR, though by increasing the glucose effect on several catabolic enzyme activities in this case.

In the light of this discussion, it appears clear that additional experiments are required to fully establish the similarities and differences between the *pepQ-ccpA* (*pepR1* or *regM*) locus described above. Interestingly, proline is an abundant residue in casein, the main protein in milk. Efficient growth of lactobacilli in milk must result in high proteolytic activity, thereby providing large amounts of exogenous proline-derived polypeptides. This observation raises an interesting question on the possible influence of carbon metabolism on proteolysis via CcpA in lactobacilli.

The HPr Protein and the ptsHI Operon

HPr(Ser-P) not only functions as the co-repressor in controlling carbon fluxes by activating or repressing metabolic enzymes, it also regulates the uptake of sugars that are transported via the PTS, since HPr(Ser-P) is a poor substrate for phosphorylation at His-15 by the PEP-dependent protein kinase enzyme I (E1) (Deutscher et al., 1994). In addition, HPr(Ser-P) has been reported to inhibit the activity of several non-PTS permeases (Ye, 1996; Dossonet et al., 2000; Viana et al., 2000). To demonstrate the regulatory role of HPr(Ser-P), membrane vesicles containing the lactose H^+-symporter of *L. brevis* were electrophorated with *B. subtilis* HPr, with or without glucose (or various glycolytic phosphorylated metabolites). These studies revealed that HPr(Ser-P) stimulates the efflux of preaccumulated thiomethyl β-galactoside (inducer expulsion), and uncouples the active TMG transport from H^+-symport, into a process of facilitated diffusion (inducer exclusion; Ye et al., 1994c). The authors have further shown that HPr(Ser-P) binds directly to inside-out membrane vesicles that contain the *L. brevis* lactose H^+-symporter suggesting an allosteric control of lactose transporter activity (Ye and Saier, 1995b). This phenomenon is, therefore, believed to control sugar accumulation in lactobacilli when readily metabolizable energy sources such as glucose are present in the growth medium. However, regulation of the *L. brevis* glucose H^+-symporter and galactose H^+-symporter by HPr (Ser-P) was also observed (Ye et al., 1994a; Ye and Saier, 1995a; Djordjevic et al., 2001).

To elucidate the molecular mechanism of inducer control in *L. brevis*, the genes encoding the HPr(Ser) kinase, HPr, enzyme I, and the galactose : H(+) symporter were cloned and characterized. Mutant HPr derivatives in which the regulatory serine was changed to either alanine or aspartate were constructed. The cloned galP gene was integrated into the chromosome of *B. subtilis*, and synthesis of the mutant HPr proteins in this organism was shown to promote regulation of GalP, as expected for a direct allosteric mechanism. By expression of mutant HPr genes inducer control was reconstituted in an organism that does not otherwise exhibit this phenomenon. These results are consistent with the conclusion that inducer exclusion and expulsion in *L. brevis* operates via a multicomponent signal transduction mechanism wherein the presence of glycolytic intermediates such as FBP (the intracellular effector), derived from exogenous glucose (the extracellular effector), activates HPr(Ser) kinase (the sensor) to phosphorylate HPr on Ser-46 (the messenger), which binds to the galactose : H(+) symporter (the target), resulting in uncoupling of sugar transport from proton symport (the response). This cascade allows bacteria to quickly respond to changes in external sugar concentrations (Djordjevic et al., 2001).

The *ptsHI* operon (encoding the proteins HPr and Enzyme I of the PTS, respectively) of *L. brevis, L. casei, L. pentosus*, and *L. sakei* has been cloned and sequenced. In the latter two species, transcription of the *ptsHI* operon is independent of the carbon source, while in *L. casei* a moderate induction in the presence of glucose was observed (Lokman and Pouwels, unpublished observations; Stentz et al., 1997; Viana et al., 2000). PtsI deficient mutants were unable to ferment a number of PTS sugars. In *L. casei* mutants were constructed in which phosphorylation of HPr at Ser-46 was either prevented or diminished (replacement of Ser-46 of HPr with Ala or Thr, respectively). In a third mutant, Ile-47 of HPr was replaced with a threonine, which was assumed to reduce the affinity of HPr(Ser-P) for its target protein, CcpA. The ptsH mutants exhibited a less pronounced lag phase during diauxic growth in a mixture of glucose and lactose. Diauxic growth was absent in a mixture of glucose and the non-PTS sugars ribose or maltose. The *ptsH* mutants synthesizing Ser-46-Ala or Ile-47-Thr mutant HPr were completely or partly relieved from CR suggesting that the HPr(Ser-P)/CcpA-mediated mechanism of CR is also present in lactobacilli. In addition, in the three *ptsH* mutants, glucose had lost its inhibitory effect on maltose transport, suggesting that HPr(Ser-P) also plays a role in inducer exclusion (Viana et al., 2000).

The evidence presented so far suggests that phosphorylation and dephosphorylation of HPr at Ser-46 plays a major role in inducer exclusion and CR. To prove or disprove this hypothesis, the gene encoding the bifunctional enzyme HPr kinase/P-Ser-HPr phosphatase (HprK/P) from *L. casei* and *L. brevis* was cloned and analyzed (Dossonet et al., 2000; Djordjevic et al., 2001). The two opposing activities of HprK/P (ATP-dependent phosphorylation of HPr and dephosphorylation of P-Ser-HPr) were regulated by FBP, which stimulated HPr phosphorylation, and by inorganic phosphate, which stimulated the P-Ser-HPr phosphatase activity. A mutant producing truncated HprK/P was found to be devoid of both HPr kinase and P-Ser-HPr phosphatase activities. When *hprK* was inactivated, carbon CR of N-acetyl-glucosaminidase disappeared, and the lag phase observed during diauxic growth of the wild-type strain on media containing glucose plus either lactose or maltose was strongly diminished. In addition, inducer exclusion exerted by the presence of glucose on maltose transport in the wild-type strain was abolished in the hprK mutant. However, inducer expulsion of methyl β-D-thiogalactoside triggered by rapidly metabolizable carbon sources was still operative in *ptsH* mutants altered at Ser-46 of HPr and the *hprK* mutant, suggesting that, in contrast to the model proposed for inducer expulsion in Gram-positive bacteria, P-Ser-HPr might not be involved in this regulatory process (Dossonet et al., 2000).

The three-dimensional structure of the bi-functional enzyme encoded by *hprK* of *L. casei*, was recently determined. HprK/P is unrelated to eukaryotic protein kinases, but contains the Walker motif A characteristic of nucleotide-binding proteins. The protein is a hexamer, with each subunit containing an ATP-binding domain similar to nucleoside/nucleotide kinases, and a putative HPr-binding domain unrelated to the substrate-binding domains of other kinases (Fieulaine et al., 2001).

To further characterize the bi-functional enzyme encoded by *hprK* of *L. casei*, alleles encoding mutant HprK/Ps exhibiting strongly reduced phosphatase, but almost normal kinase activity were analyzed. Two mutations affected the Walker motif A of HprK/P and four a conserved C-terminal region in contact with the ATP-binding site of an adjacent subunit in the hexamer. Kinase and phosphatase activity appeared to be closely associated and linked to the Walker motif A, but dephosphorylation HPr(Ser-P) is not simply a reversal of the kinase reaction. Expression of the *hprK* allele in *B. subtilis* led to increased amounts of HPr(Ser-P). The *hprK* mutants were unable to grow on most PTS and non-PTS carbohydrates. This inability could be related to the increased amounts of HPr(Ser-P) since *ptsHI* mutations or replacing Ser46 in HPr with alanine restored growth on PTS substrates. Introduction of a *ccpA* mutation restored growth on non-PTS but not, or poorly, on PTS carbohydrates, although the mutation was reported not to diminish the increased level of HPr(Ser-P). It appears that the *ccpA* mutation alleviates the repressing effects on permeases that transport non-PTS sugars while PTS transporters are also regulated by HPr(Ser-P) at the activity level in a CcpA independent manner (Monedero et al., 2001).

The Glucose/Mannose PTS of Lactobacilli

In several lactic acid bacteria and oral streptococci, the glucose/mannose PTS is the main transport system for glucose. This PTS was characterized in *Lc. lactis, Tetragenococcus halophila, L. casei, L. curvatus, L. pentosus, L. sakei*, and *Streptococcus salivarius*, and in most cases it was described as an active transport system for glucose, mannose, 2-deoxyglucose, and sometimes N-acetyl-glucosamine and fructose (Thompson, 1987; Abe and Uchiba, 1989; Bourassa et al., 1990; Veyrat et al., 1994, 1996; Lauret et al., 1996; Chaillou et al., 1999, 2000). Amongst the species mentioned above, the gene cluster encoding the EII^{Man} complex of the mannose PTS has been cloned and characterized for *L. curvatus* only (Veyrat et al., 1996). The gene cluster of *L. curvatus* comprises the *manABCD* genes encoding the sugar-specific EIIA, EIIB, and EIICD domains of the EII^{Man} complex. These proteins showed a high degree of homology with the EIIAB and EIICD domains of the *E. coli* EII^{Man}

(Erni et al., 1989) and to domains of other PTS elements of the mannose class (Postma et al., 1993). Several 2DG-resistant mutants with an inactive EII^{Man} complex were isolated from *Lc. lactis, T. halophila, L. casei, L. pentosus*, and *L.sakei*, and the role of EII^{Man} in the regulation of carbon utilization was investigated for some of these mutants. Interestingly, strains defective in the activity of EII^{Man} lacked the negative regulation mediated by glucose on the activity of several catabolic enzymes, such as xylose isomerase in *T. halophila* (Abe and Uchiba, 1989), P-β-galactosidase in *L. casei* (Gosalbes et al., 1997), β-galactosidase, and β-glucosidase in *L. pentosus* (Chaillou et al., 2001) or several catabolic enzymes in *S. salivarius* (Gauthier et al., 1990; Lapointe et al., 1993). These results indicated a possible regulatory role for EII^{Man}. As shown in Figure 6.3, the EII^{Man} complex is providing strong signals for CcpA-mediated CR, by first increasing the glycolytic flux, and second by promoting dephosphorylation of HPr on the His-15 residue (the forms HPr(His-P) or HPr (His-P, Ser-P) of HPr do not interact with CcpA). Thus, the phenotype of the 2DG-resistant mutants from the various species can be explained by the main role of the EII^{Man} complex in the transport of glucose. The finding that β-galactosidase and β-glucosidase activities in *L. pentosus* and phospho-β-galactosidase activity in *L. casei* are also negatively regulated by CcpA corroborates this view. One or more regulatory role(s) of EII^{Man} that are independent of the global CcpA pathway may also exist. Indeed, the activity of a fructose-specific PTS in *L. pentosus* and *S. salivarius* is negatively regulated by glucose. In *L. pentosus*, glucose repression of the fructose-specific PTS is relieved in a mutant with an inactive EII^{Man} but not in a *ccpA* mutant. Moreover, overexpression of the *manB* gene from *L. curvatus* in *L. pentosus* resulted in a strong repression of the fructose PTS suggesting a critical role of the $EIIB^{Man}$ subunit in this regulation (Chaillou et al., 2000). Similarly, several $EIIB^{Man}$ defective mutants of *S. salivarius* showed a derepression of the fructose PTS. The $EIIB^{Man}$ subunit of both species could possibly play a role in the regulation of the fructose PTS. Moreover, as it will be shown below, a mutation rendering the EII^{Man} complex inactive is required in addition to the inactivation of the *ccpA* gene in order to fully derepress the expression of the lactose PTS in *L. casei* ATCC 393. Therefore, in lactic acid bacteria, the EII^{Man} complex may regulate the expression of secondary PTS. In *E. coli* and *B. subtilis* for instance, several PTS encoding genes are regulated by HPr(His-P) and one of the EII components belonging to these PTS, via phosphorylation of antiterminators (Stülke et al., 1998). Whether HPr(His-P) and $EIIB^{Man}$ play such a role in lactobacilli remains to be demonstrated, however. It should be noted that EII^{Man} is found in both *E. coli* and *B. subtilis* but so far no regulatory functions for this PTS have been described in these bacteria. In contrast, the glucose-specific PTS, EII^{Glc}, which is present in *E. coli* and *B. subtilis* and which was shown to undertake regulatory roles in *E. coli*, has not been found in lactic acid bacteria. To conclude, these studies strongly indicate that the EII^{Man} complex of lactobacilli is involved in CcpA-independent CR pathways. However, additional studies are necessary to understand in more detail the mechanisms of this PTS-mediated regulation of carbon utilization.

Genetics of Lactose Utilization

At least three different systems for lactose utilization have been found in lactobacilli (Figure 6.5). Transport and phosphorylation of lactose via the PTS appears to be limited to *L. casei* species. The functions of the lactose PTS in *L. casei* is generally plasmid-encoded, with the exception of strain ATCC 393 which possesses a chromosome-encoded lactose PTS (Chassy et al., 1978; Gosalbes et al., 1997). Although strain ATCC 393 has long been considered as the species type-strain, it was recently reclassified as *Lactobacillus zeae* (Dicks et al., 1996). The *lac* operon of *L. casei* 64H was characterized in more details. It is

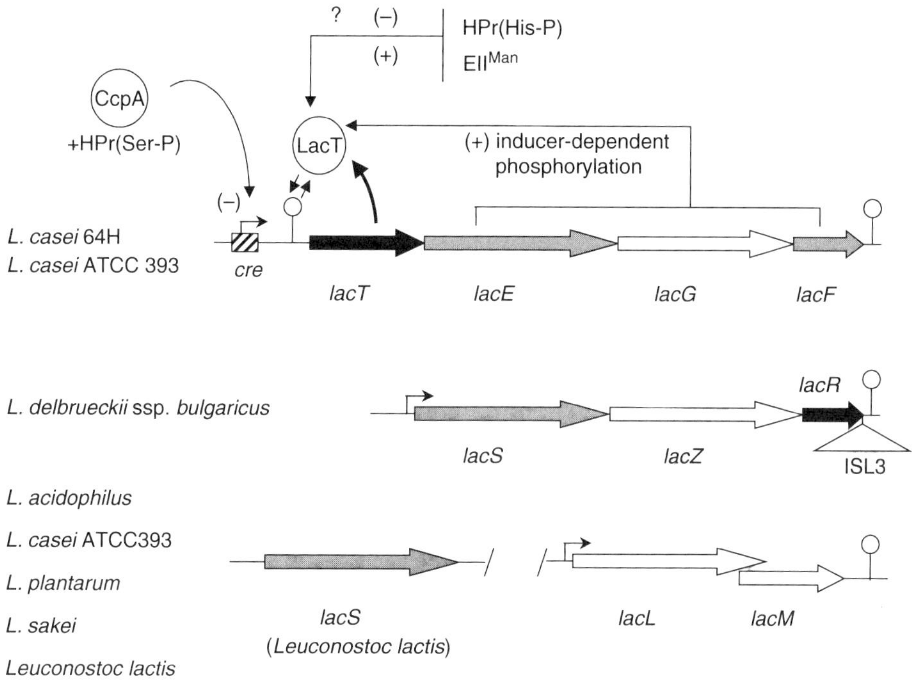

Figure 6.5. Schematic representation of the three types of *lac* operon in lactobacilli. The role of CcpA in the regulation of the *L. casei* lactose PTS as well as in the putative regulation of the antiterminator LacT are depicted. The non-contiguous lactose permease LacS of the LacL–LacM system, so far only characterized in *Lc. lactis*, is shown separated by a break in the line.

composed of the *lacTEGF* genes, encoding, respectively, the antiterminator of the operon (LacT; Alpert and Siebers, 1997), the integral membrane EIILac (LacE) of the PTS (Alpert and Chassy, 1990a,b), the phospho-β-galactosidase (LacG; Porter et al., 1988), and the cytoplasmic factor EIIILac (LacF) of the PTS (Alpert and Chassy, 1990a,b). The product of the *lacT* gene is similar to a family of proteins that have been identified as transcriptional antiterminators, the activities of which are regulated after phosphorylation by one or more components of the PTS. HPr(His-P), for instance, can transfer its phosphoryl group to a PRD-II domain of the transcriptional antiterminator proteins, such as LevR, LicT, or SacT, which are then activated, allowing transcription of the linked PTSs encoding genes (for reviews, see Deutscher et al., 1997; Stülke et al., 1998). Moreover, these antiterminator proteins are also subject to a negative regulation. This regulation involves a mechanism by which the antiterminator protein is phosphorylated at a second site, PRD-I domain, by one of the EII components belonging to its corresponding PTS: LevE, BglP, and SacP in the case of LevR, LicT, or SacT, respectively. When the antiterminator protein is phosphorylated at this second site, its binding to the terminator loop is inhibited and transcription of the PTSs encoding genes does not take place. As a result, the production of the PTS proteins is stimulated when no PTS-dependent sugar is transported (HPr phosphorylated on its his residue), and inhibited if the substrate of the corresponding PTS is not present in the growth environment (EIIB is then phosphorylated).

It is known that the lactose PTS of *L. casei* is induced by lactose in the growth medium and is subject to glucose-mediated CR (Gosalbes et al., 1997). A *L. casei* ATCC 393 *lacT* deletion strain has been constructed. This strain displayed a constitutive expression of the *lac* genes (Gosalbes et al., 1997). In the same study, *lacE* and *lacF* mutants were analyzed and showed an inducer-independent antiterminator activity. These results indicated that in the absence of functional EIILAC components, the antiterminator LacT was active, possibly because it cannot be phosphorylated at one of the conserved PTS regulation domains (PRD-I). Finally, the expression of the lactose PTS in *L. casei* 64H was shown to become constitutive in a *ptsH* mutant (Bettenbrock et al., 1999). Moreover, mutations in the EII^{Man} complex and deletion of the *ccpA* gene were found to partially relieve the glucose-mediated repression of the *lac* genes in *L. casei* ATCC 393 (Gosalbes et al., 1997). A putative *cre* site could be found overlapping the −35 element of the P_{lac} in strains 64H and ATCC 393 suggesting that CR of the *lac* genes in *L. casei* is mediated by the CcpA/HPr(Ser-P) pathway. It appears, however, that a total relief of the glucose-mediated CR is obtained only with a double inactivation of both CcpA and the EII^{Man} complex, indicating that these two components of CR are acting via independent pathways. It is thus possible that HPr(His-P) or that one or more domains of the EII^{Man} complex, such as $EIIB^{Man}$, could regulate the activity of LacT by phosphorylation on the PRD-II domain. Altogether these observations strongly support that fact that the phosphorylation state of the LacT protein is important to mediate the regulation of expression of the *lac* genes in *L. casei*.

By site-directed mutagenesis of LacT, four histidines (His-101, His-159 in PRD-I, and His-210, His-273 in PRD-II) were replaced by alanine and aspartate, mimicking non-phosphorylated and phosphorylated forms, respectively. *L. casei* strains with a deletion of *lacT* carrying the replacement of His-101 or His-159 by Ala showed phospho-β-galactosidase activity in the absence of the inducer (lactose), indicating that these amino acids, located in PRD-I, are essential for EII-dependent induction of the *lac* operon, possibly by dephosphorylation. Moreover, expression of a *L. casei lacT* strain carrying mutations in PRD-II (H210A and H273A) showed that these two histidyl residues could have a role in LacT-dependent carbon CR of this system. Overexpression of LacT in a *ccpA* background rendered the *lac* operon insensitive to CR, but it was still sensitive to lactose induction. This suggests that the transfer of phosphate groups from PTS elements, which controls these two regulatory processes (CR and substrate induction), could have different affinity for PRD-I and PRD-II histidines (Gosalbes et al., 2002).

L. casei ATCC 393 also possesses a plasmid-encoded (pLZ15) β-galactosidase (Mercenier et al., 1994). Surprisingly, the protein is encoded by two genes, *lacL* encoding a protein showing similarity to the N-terminal two third of the *lacZ* gene product of other microorganisms, and *lacM*, encoding a small protein corresponding to the C-terminal end of LacZ. The two genes overlap by 15 nt and are out of frame, suggesting a coordinate regulation at the level of translation in order to produce equal amounts of both polypeptides (Oppenheim and Yanofsky, 1980). A plasmid-encoded *lacLM* gene cluster has also been found in *Leuconostoc lactis* and *L. plantarum* (David et al., 1992; Mayo et al., 1994), whereas it is chromosome-encoded in *L. sakei* (Obst et al., 1995) and *L. acidophilus* (GenBank AB004867 and AB004868). Studies carried out with *Lc. lactis* and *L. sakei* showed that the expression of both polypeptides is required to obtain β-galactosidase activity. The *lacLM* genes are expressed from a promoter that is located upstream of the *lacL* gene. This promoter region is also highly conserved amongst the three species described above (Mayo et al., 1994). Unfortunately, limited information is available on the regulation of expression of the *lacLM* genes. Experiments carried out with the *L. plantarum* promoter region showed that the *lacLM* genes are expressed in glucose and lactose, with a 6-fold increase of activity in the presence of lactose compared to that found for glucose. The mechanism of induction by lactose (or repression by glucose) remains unknown, however (Mayo et al., 1994). In *Lc. lactis*, the *lacS* gene encoding a protein highly similar to the lactose transporter LacS of *S. thermophilus* has been identified on the lactose plasmid, approximately 2 kb upstream of the *lacLM* genes. An uncharacterized lactose transporter has also been reported to be present on pLZ15 in *L. casei* ATC 393 (Mercenier et al., 1994). In these organisms, the lactose transport determinant seems, therefore, associated with the *lacLM* genes although it is not contiguous to them.

The third example of *lac* genes identified in lactobacilli concerns the *lacS* and *lacZ* genes of *L. bulgaricus* strains 131 and ATCC 11842, encoding, respectively, the lactose permease (which is extended with a regulatory hydrophilic carboxy-terminal end similar to EIIA of several PTS) and β-galactosidase (Schmidt et al., 1989; Leong-Morgenthaler et al., 1991). Thus, the *lacSZ* gene cluster of *L. bulgaricus* shows structural similarity with that of *S. thermophilus* with the exception that it is not linked to the *gal* genes of the Leloir pathway. Another difference between *S. thermophilus* and *L. bulgaricus* is the constitutive expression and the absence of glucose-mediated repression of the *lacSZ* operon in the last organism (Schmidt et al., 1989). Downstream of *lacZ*, a remnant *lacR* gene is located encoding a product similar to the *E. coli* lactose repressor LacI. An IS element, designated ISL3 has been identified within the coding sequence of the *L. bulgaricus lacR* gene, approximately 1 kb downstream from the *lacZ* gene (Germond et al., 1993). Therefore, *lacR* is believed not to function as a repressor of the *lacSZ* operon, as shown by the constitutive expression of the *lacSZ* operon. Finally, no biochemical data is available about the function of the *L. bulgaricus* LacS. Nevertheless, this protein is expected to encode a lactose H^+-symporter, the activity of which might be regulated by phosphorylation of the EIIA-like domain by HPR(His-P), which was shown to mediate the partial inhibition of LacS activity in *S. thermophilus* (Poolman et al., 1995).

Genetics of Xylose Metabolism

The catabolism of xylose is a rare property amongst lactobacilli, but several species that are found consistently on a variety of plant materials can utilize this compound as a sole source of energy. The most common xylose fermenting species are *L. brevis* and *L. pentosus*. The chromosome-encoded *xyl* gene cluster of these two species has been cloned and characterized (Figure 6.6). The *xyl* genes of *L. pentosus* are organized in a regulon that comprises five genes (Lokman et al., 1991, 1994). The *xylP* and *xylQ* genes are the first genes of the regulon and are involved in isoprimeverose metabolism (Chaillou et al., 1998b,c). The disaccharide isoprimeverose (α-D-xylopyranosyl-[1,6]-D-glucopyranose) is the major building block of xyloglucan, a widely distributed hemicellulose which occurs in the primary cell wall in plants. *L. pentosus*, a species mostly isolated from fermented vegetables is capable of fermenting this disaccharide, once it is liberated from the cell wall by other scavenging microorganisms. The *xylP* gene encodes an isoprimeverose cation-symporter, whereas the *xylQ* gene encodes a membrane-associated α-xylosidase that is responsible for the hydrolysis of isoprimeverose into glucose and xylose.

Functional characterization of the isoprimeverose transporter, XylP was also studied with the aid of a spectroscopy-based assay system. Purified XylP was incorporated into liposomes, in which the glucose dehydrogenase from *Acinetobacter calcoaceticus* (sGDH) was entrapped. sGDH can oxidize aldose sugars in the presence of dichlorophenol-indophenol as electron acceptor. The coupled assay thus involves XylP-mediated isoprimeverose uptake followed by internal oxidation of the sugar by sGDH, which can be

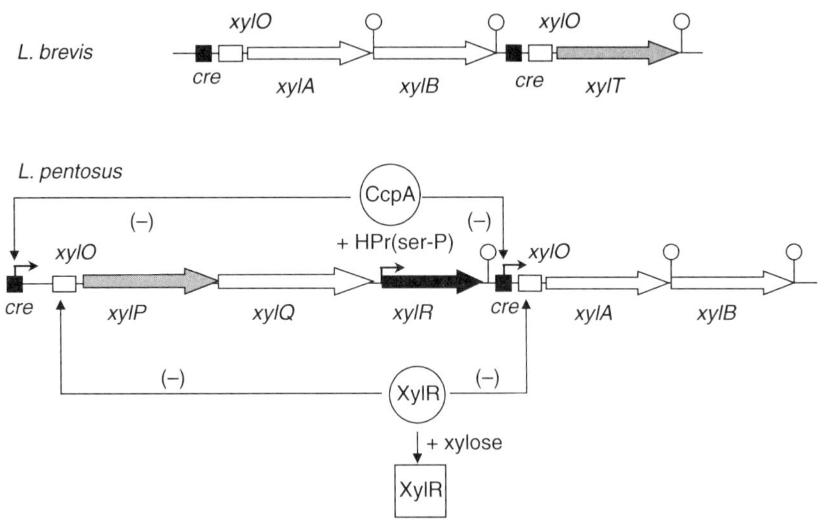

Figure 6.6. Regulation of *L. pentosus xyl* regulon by the repressor XylR and by the global regulator CcpA. The *xyl* locus of *L. brevis* is also depicted with the location of the putative regulatory elements.

monitored from the reduction of 2,6-dichlorophenol-indophenol at 600 nm. The uptake of isoprimeverose was stimulated by the presence of the non-oxidizable methyl-isoprimeverose on the trans-side of the membrane, indicating that exchange transport is faster than unidirectional downhill uptake. Unlike other members of the galactoside-pentoside-hexuronide family, XylP does not transport monosaccharides (xylose) but requires a glycosidic linkage at the anomeric carbon position. Consistent with a proton motive force-driven mechanism, the uptake was stimulated by a membrane potential (inside negative relative to outside) and inhibited by a pH gradient (inside acidic relative to outside) (Heuberger et al., 2001).

The xylose formed by the activity of the α-xylosidase (XylQ) on isoprimeverose is further catabolized into xylulose-5-phosphate (X5P) by xylose isomerase and xylulose kinase, encoded by the distal genes of the *xyl* regulon, *xylA* and *xylB*. The expression of the *xylPQ* and *xylAB* operons is regulated at the transcriptional level by the activity of the repressor protein encoded by *xylR* (Lokman et al., 1997). The *xylR* gene is transcribed as a single gene from its own constitutive promoter, or can be induced 10-fold together with the *xylPQ* genes from the P_{xylP} promoter. Transcription analysis showed that deletion of the *xylR* gene resulted in a xylose-independent expression of the *xylPQ* and *xylAB* genes. The repression mediated by XylR takes place after the binding of the repressor to highly conserved operator sequences (*xylO*) located between the transcription start site of the *xylA* or *xylP* promoters and the start codon of these genes.

In *L. brevis*, the *xyl* regulon does not comprise the *xylPQ* genes found in *L. pentosus* (Bor et al., 1992; Chaillou et al., 1998a). Instead, a gene encoding a xylose H^+-symporter (XylT) similar to that of *E. coli, B. megaterium*, and to the xylose Na^+-symporter of *Tetragenococcus halophila* was found downstream of the *xylB* gene. The arrangement of the *xyl* genes in *L. brevis* also showed striking similarities with that of *B. megaterium* and *T. halophila* (Schmiedel et al., 1997; Takeda et al., 1998). Surprisingly, no *xylR* gene is located upstream of the *xylAB* operon in *L. brevis*. However, Southern hybridization experiments performed with the *L. pentosus xylR* gene as a probe, revealed the existence of a *xylR* homologue in *L. brevis* that is not located together with the *xylABT* locus. The existence of a functional XylR in *L. brevis* was further suggested by the presence of *xylO* sequences upstream of *xylA* and *xylT*, and by the requirement of D-xylose for the induction of D-xylose isomerase, D-xylulose kinase, and D-xylose transport activities (Chaillou et al., 1998a). The transcriptional regulation of the *L. brevis xyl* genes has not been studied in detail but putative promoters and other regulatory elements could be detected in front of *xylA* and of *xylT* suggesting the presence of two transcriptional units.

The mechanism by which the repressor XylR regulates the *xylAB* operon in Gram-positive bacteria has been extensively studied, and is now well established. An operator, *xylO* has been identified downstream of the *xylAB* promoter site in all Gram-positive organisms studied, and complex formation between *xylO* and XylR was demonstrated in *Bacillus* spp. by gel mobility-shift experiments and DNA-footprinting studies (Gärtner et al., 1992; Sizemore et al., 1992; Scheler and Hillen, 1994). The *xylO* sequence is an inverted repeat (IR) of 27 bp. Each repeat consists of two XylR binding sites, O_L and O_R, which are spaced by 4 bp and which contribute to the efficient regulation *in vivo* (Dahl et al., 1994). The alignment shown in Figure 6.7 indicates that the *xylO* sequences detected in the promoter regions of *L. pentosus xylAB, xylPQ* genes and *L. brevis xylAB, xylT* genes display similarities to the consensus *xylO* established for *Bacillus* species, although the consensus sequence of the putative overlapping operators may differ slightly between the two genera.

In *L. pentosus*, expression of the *xyl* genes is subject to glucose-mediated CR. Putative *cre* sequences which were detected overlapping −35 or −10 elements of two xylose-inducible promoters, first suggested that the glucose effect could proceed through transcription regulation via the CcpA pathway. Indeed, further analysis demonstrated that the glucose-mediated CR of the *xylPQ* and *xylAB* operons was relieved upon *ccpA* disruption (Lokman et al., 1997; Chaillou et al., 1998b). In *L. brevis*, xylose isomerase and xylulose kinase activities were reduced 4-fold and the xylose transport activity 6-fold, when glucose was added to the growth medium in addition to xylose. The presence of a CcpA-mediated CR is further suggested by the presence of putative *cre* sites in the *xylA* and *xylT* promoter regions (Table 6.5). Nevertheless, the CcpA homologue of *L. brevis* remains to be identified to fully establish its role in the regulation of the *xyl* genes.

Unlike *L. brevis, L. pentosus* does not transport xylose via proton symport. In this organism, xylose is taken up by a mechanism of facilitated diffusion via a non xylose-specific transporter, which was characterized as the EII^{Man} complex. Evidence for such an a specific transport of xylose stems from the observation that several $2DG^R$ mutants, inactive in the EII^{Man} complex, are unable to transport xylose (Chaillou et al., 1999, 2000).

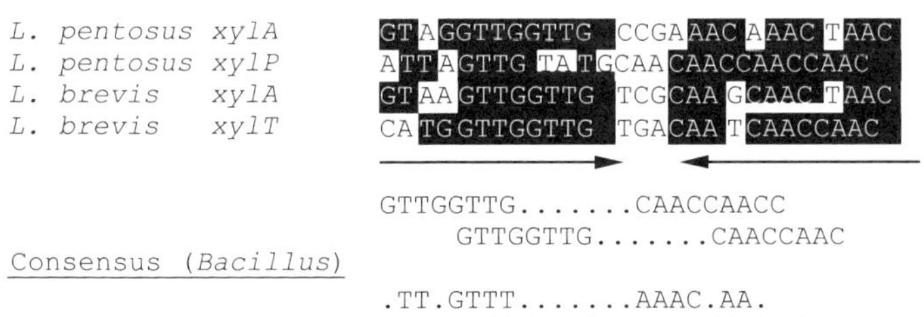

Figure 6.7. Alignment of *xylO* sequences characterized in lactobacilli and comparison of the deduced consensus with that obtained with *Bacillus* species.

Genetics of Ribose Metabolism

The genes responsible for ribose utilization in *L. sakei* have been cloned and partially characterized (Stentz and Zagorec, 1999). The *rbs* gene cluster comprises four genes in the order *rbsUDKR*, encoding, respectively, two proteins with a putative transport activity (RbsU and RbsD), ribose kinase (RbsK), and a repressor protein (RbsR). This structure of the operon is thus different from that in the *E. coli* or *B. subtilis rbs* operon since no gene encoding the RbsA, RbsB, and RbsC subunits of the ribose ABC-transporter were found in *L. sakei*. The *rbsUDK* genes are transcribed as a monocistronic unit, whose expression is induced by the presence of ribose in the medium, whereas *rbsR* is presumably expressed constitutively from its own promoter. Deletion of *rbsR* was shown to lead to constitutive expression of the *rbsUDK* operon. RbsR is thus believed to bind to a DNA target in the promoter region of the *rbsUDK* operon. The sequence of the RbsR binding site is not yet known. Nevertheless, the similarity between the *L. sakei* repressor protein and the *E. coli* RbsR protein suggests a common mechanism of repression between the two organisms.

Transcription analysis of *rbsUDK* in a *rbsR* mutant grown on various carbon sources revealed that this operon is not subject to glucose-mediated CR at the transcriptional level. On the other hand, growth on ribose is 2-fold increased in a *ptsI* mutant which suggests that the PTS is regulating ribose utilization in *L. sakei*. The level of transcription of *rbsUDK* in the *ptsI* mutant is similar to that found for wild-type bacteria. Therefore, the regulation mediated by the PTS does not take place at the level of transcription. In contrast, ribose transport activity and ribose ATP-dependent phosphorylation activity were increased about 2-fold in the *ptsI* mutant compared to that of wild-type bacteria. These observations are consistent with an increased growth rate of the *ptsI* mutant on ribose, and they strongly indicate that the PTS regulates ribose utilization via allosteric control of the ribose transport and/or ribose kinase activities. However, the precise mechanism of this regulation remains to be established.

General Part of the Phosphoketolase Pathway

Fermentation of pentoses like xylose, ribose, and arabinose can be divided in two parts: a specific part, in which pentoses are taken up and converted by sugar-specific enzymes into X5P, and a general part in which further metabolism of X5P follows the PKP. Xpk is the central enzyme of the PKP. In the presence of inorganic phosphate, the enzyme converts X5P into glyceraldehyde-3-P and acetyl-P. The gene encoding XpkA from *L. pentosus* has been cloned and sequenced. *xpkA* encodes a protein of 788 amino acids with a calculated mass of 88,705 Da. Most of the residues involved in correct binding of the cofactor thiamin pyrophosphate (TPP) that are conserved in transketolase, pyruvate decarboxylase, and pyruvate oxidase, were also conserved at a similar position in XpkA, implying a similar TPP binding fold for XpkA. An *xpkA* knockout mutant of *L. pentosus* had lost XpkA activity and was not able to grow on energy sources that are fermented via the PKP, indicating that X5P metabolism requires a functional phosphoketolase. Expression of *xpkA* in *L. pentosus* was induced by sugars that are fermented via the PKP and was subject to CR mediated by CcpA and by the mannose PTS (Posthuma et al., 2002a).

Acetyl-phosphate that is formed by the action of Xpk is converted into acetate by acetate kinase, while glyceraldehyde-3-phosphate is metabolized into lactate by glycolytic enzymes (Kandler, 1983). The acetate kinase gene has been cloned and sequenced for several species: *L. pentosus* (Posthuma et al., unpublished observations), *L. sanfranciscensis* (Knorr et al., 2001), and *L. sakei* (Stentz and Zagores, 1999; Dudez et al., 2002). *L. sakei* has two genes, situated at almost opposite location on the chromosome. It is not known whether they are both functional. It should be noted that *Lc. lactis* also showed the presence of two putative acetate kinase genes. An *ackA* knockout mutant of *L. pentosus* lacked acetate kinase activity and was unable to grow on energy sources that are fermented via the PKP, indicating that *ackA* is the only gene encoding a functional acetate kinase in *L. pentosus*. Northern blot analysis revealed that *ackA* is transcribed into monocistronic mRNA. Acetate kinase activity in *L. pentosus* was comparable during growth on fructose, gluconate, ribose, xylose, or arabinose, but 3-fold lower during growth on glucose. In mutants of *L. pentosus* deficient in CcpA or mannose PTS activity, repression of *ackA* expression was relieved during growth on glucose, indicating that *ackA* expression is negatively controlled by CcpA and the mannose PTS (Posthuma et al., unpublished observations).

Genetics of Sorbose Metabolism

Sequence analysis of the genes encoding L-sorbose metabolism of *L. casei* ATCC 393 revealed seven complete genes and a partial open reading frame transcribed as two units. The deduced amino acid sequences of the first transcriptional unit (*sorRE*) showed high similarity to the transcriptional regulator and the L-sorbose-1-phosphate reductase of the sorbose (*sor*) operon from *Klebsiella pneumoniae*. The other genes are transcribed as one unit (*sorFABCDG*) in opposite direction to *sorRE*. The deduced peptide sequence of *sorF* showed homology with the D-sorbitol-6-phosphate dehydrogenase encoded in the *sor* operon from *K. pneumoniae* and *sorABCD* to components of the mannose phosphotransferase system (PTS) family but especially to domains EIIA, EIIB, EIIC, and EIID of the phosphoenolpyruvate-dependent L-sorbose PTS from *K. pneumoniae*. Finally, the deduced amino acid sequence of a truncated gene (*sorG*) located downstream of *sorD* presented high similarity with ketose-1,6-bisphosphate aldolases. Results of studies on enzyme activities and transcriptional analysis revealed that the two gene clusters, *sorRE* and *sorFABCDG*, are induced by L-sorbose and subject to CR by D-glucose. CR is mediated by components of the PTS elements and by CcpA. Sugar uptake assays in *L. casei* wild-type and *sorBC* mutant strains indicated that L-sorbose is taken up by L-sorbose-specific enzyme II. Results of growth analysis of those strains and a *man sorBC* double mutant suggested that L-sorbose is probably also transported by the D-mannose PTS (Yebra et al., 2000).

Stress Response

Bacteria and cells from eukaryotic organisms that are exposed to stress conditions react by synthesizing a particular set of proteins to protect the organism against the adverse effects of the environmental change. In *E. coli*, for example, certain genes are induced in response to DNA damage (SOS response), radicals and hydrogen peroxide (OxyR system), and heat shock (HS; Demple and Amabile-Cuevas, 1991; Farr and Kogoma, 1991; Parsell and Lindquist, 1993; Walker, 1996). In contrast to other stress responses observed during the exponential phase of growth which are rather specific, HS responses are implicated in several stress conditions such as a sudden HS, oxygen, high salt, alkaline conditions or ethanol (Lindquist, 1991). Many of the heat shock proteins (HSP) are highly conserved in all organisms. A study of the regulation of expression of stress response genes is not only of scientific interest as the mode of expression is rather uncommon, but is also of great economic importance. The outcome of fermentation processes depends on a balanced control of numerous parameters. When bacteria are exposed to stress conditions such as oxygen, this may lead to unwanted effects, for example, the formation of hydrogen peroxide, rancidity or color changes, or with other stress conditions, lysis of the bacteria.

Proteins whose synthesis is induced by HS and other stress conditions include ATP-dependent chaperones and proteases. Chaperones are involved in many steps of protein synthesis preventing protein degradation, aggregation, and improper folding (Georgopoulos and Welch, 1993). The principal HSPs studied are GroEL (HSP60), DnaK (HSP70), and ClpB (HSP100). ClpB belongs to the Clp ATPase family, which consists of two groups of proteins with two and one ATP binding domain, respectively (Schirmer et al., 1996; Derre et al., 1999b). The regulation of induction of stress genes, in particular that of HS genes, has been investigated in detail for *E. coli*. Transcription of the *E. coli* HS regulon comprising more than 20 genes is dependent on two RNA polymerase subunits, σ^{32} and σ^{E} (Bukau, 1993). In contrast to *E. coli*, the HS response in *B. subtilis* involves at least three different classes of heat-inducible genes. These classes are distinguished by different regulation mechanisms (Hecker et al., 1996). Expression of class I genes, which encode chaperones like GroEL and DnaK that function in association with GroES, is dependent on σ^{A}-dependent promoters and the highly conserved CIRCE element, which is the binding site for the HcrA repressor (Zuber and Schumann, 1994; Yuan and Wong, 1995; Mogk et al., 1997). It appears that *Lactobacillus* is endowed with similar stress response mechanisms as described for *Bacillus* and *E. coli*. In a response to a change in acidity, the HSPs GroES, GroEL, and DnaK from *L. delbrueckii* subsp. *bulgaricus* were found to be induced (Lim et al., 2000). In *L. helveticus* and *L. johnsonii groEL* and *groES* genes and in *L. sakei*, the HS genes *hrcA, groE, dnaK*, and *dnaJ* have been identified and sequenced (GenBank AJ006274; Broadbent et al., 1998; Schmidt et al., 1999; Walker et al., 1999). The dnaK gene region of *L. sakei* consists of four HS genes with the organization *hrcA–grpE–dnaK–dnaJ*. Northern hybridization analysis revealed that the transcription of the genes is induced by HS as well as by salt (6%) or ethanol (10%) stress. The transcription start sites of the *dnaK* operon varied with the applied stress condition. A regulatory CIRCE element was identified located between the transcription and translation start site. The kinetics of transcriptional induction in *L. sakei* LTH681 by heat shocking of *gusA* that was transcriptionally fused to the promoter region including CIRCE was identical to that of the *dnaK* operon confirming the involvement of the CIRCE element in regulation of gene expression (Schmidt et al., 1999).

Analysis of the *groESL* promoter region from *L. johnsonii* revealed three transcription initiation sites, as well as three sets of IRs positioned between the transcription and translation start sites. Two of the three IR sets bore significant homology to the CIRCE elements. Northern analysis and primer extension revealed that multiple temperature-sensitive promoters preceded the *groESL* chaperone operon, suggesting that stress protein production in *L. johnsonii* is strongly regulated (Walker et al., 1999).

Class II genes that are induced by HS and other general stress conditions are dependent on the σ^{B} subunit. Class III genes, which include, for example, the Clp ATP-proteases (Msadek et al., 1994, 1998; Gerth et al., 1996, 1998) are negatively regulated by a repressor, CtsR, which is the product of the first gene of the *clpC* operon (Derre et al., 1999b). The CtsR repressor specifically binds to a nucleotide sequence (operator) present in *clp* and other HS genes in several Gram-positive bacteria, including the *clpE* gene of

L. sakei (Derre et al., 1999a). Two cold shock protein (CS proteins) genes have been characterized in *L. plantarum* (Mayo et al., 1997). They display strong conservation with the Csp family of CS proteins found in *E. coli* and *B. subtilis*, thought to be involved in gene expression and possibly acting as RNA chaperones (increasing RNA life time when cell division is seriously reduced).

FNR

Another potential global regulatory system in *Lactobacillus* sensing the redox state of the cell was suggested based on the observation that *L. casei* harbors a gene, *flp*, formerly called *orfX* and located on the distal end of the *trp* operon (Natori et al., 1990), encoding an FNR-like protein (FLP). FLP is the first example of a CRP–FNR family protein in Gram-positive bacteria (Irvine and Guest, 1993; Gostick et al., 1998). In *E. coli* FNR is a regulator for FNR and CRP regulates the expression of target genes in response to anaerobiosis and availability of carbon sources. When expressed in *E. coli*, FLP could not complement a deficiency in either FNR or CRP. In line with this observation, FLP was found to interact with two, nonidentical sequences in the *melR* region of *E. coli*, which are different from the classical FNR- and CRP binding sites. A putative FLP consensus sequence (CA/CTGA-N_4-TCAG/TG) was defined based on DNA gel retardation assays. FLP from *L. casei* is a homodimeric protein in which each subunit can form an intramolecular disulfide bond. Site-specific DNA binding was abolished by reduction of the intrasubunit disulfide bonds of FLP, providing the basis for a novel redox-mediated transcriptional switch. Expression in *E. coli* of the *lacZ* operon which was placed under the control of a semi-synthetic promoter containing an FLP-binding site was 70% repressed by FLP under aerobic conditions but only 16% under anaerobic conditions. Repression was abolished with a mutant FLP that could not form an intramolecular disulfide bridge (Gostick et al., 1998).

Catalase

Most lactic acid bacteria are aerotolerant and have inducible oxidative stress responses to deal with the resulting superoxide anion (O_2^-) and H_2O_2 (Condon, 1987; Sanders et al., 1995; Rallu et al., 1996). Many species of *Lactobacillus* lack the enzyme catalase but use superoxide dismutase and high concentrations of Mn^{2+} to deal with oxygen radicals. H_2O_2 can be decomposed by induction of NADH peroxidase. In the species that contain catalase activity, two types of enzyme can be distinguished. One group of enzymes, the true catalases, are active when hematin is added. A second group of enzymes are the so-called non-heme catalases, or pseudocatalases or manganese catalases. The gene, *katA*, encoding the true catalase of *L. sakei* LTH677, has been cloned and characterized (Knauf et al., 1992). In wild-type *L. sakei* LTH677 and recombinant *L. casei* or *L. curvatus* strains carrying a *katA*-bearing plasmid, expression of the *katA* gene was induced when the culture was shifted from anaerobic to aerobic conditions or when H_2O_2 was added to an anaerobic culture. The increase in catalase activity was accompanied by an increase in *katA* mRNA, which was regulated at the level of transcription initiation. The site of transcription initiation was found to be the same (67 nt before the start of the *katA* reading frame) in cells grown anaerobically and in bacteria that were cultivated in the presence of H_2O_2 or were grown with aeration. A stem-loop structure was found 32 nt downstream from the transcription start point. This sequence showed some similarity to the consensus sequence of potential binding sites for FNR homologues (Spiro and Guest, 1990; Spiro, 1994). A small putative regulatory sequence of at least 25 bp was identified upstream of the −35 promoter sequence. This sequence may be the target site for an activator protein, as was inferred from competition experiments with plasmid encoded copies of the *katA* promoter region (Hertel et al., 1998).

Antimicrobials

Many bacteria including several species of lactobacilli produce antimicrobial peptides called bacteriocins that are secreted into the medium. In a number of these species, as for example, *L. plantarum* C11 and *L. sakei* LTH673, the synthesis of bacteriocin is arrested when the cultures are extremely diluted (Diep et al., 1995; Eijsink et al., 1996). The explanation for this phenomenon is that expression of the genes involved in bacteriocin production is induced by peptides (IP). Our understanding of how these complex systems are controlled was considerably increased by the pioneering work of Nes and coworkers. This topic will be reviewed by Nes in Chapter 8. In summary, the following picture has emerged. Production of sakacin-P in *L. sakei* and of plantaricin-A in *L. plantarum* is controlled by an auto-induction system, different from that of nisin in *Lc. lactis*, in that in *L. sakei* the induction is not exerted by the bacteriocin itself but rather by a peptide pheromone that senses the cell density. These IPs are short amphiphilic peptides that resemble bacteriocins but have no bacteriocin activity (Eijsink et al., 1996). The IP is thought to interact with a histidine kinase that is part of a two-component signal transduction pathway, resulting in autophosphorylation of the kinase. Subsequently, the phosphate residue is transferred to the response regulator that specifically binds to promoters of the bacteriocin regulon, to activate the promoters (Brurberg et al., 1997). The response regulator binds to characteristic repeats found in the −80 to −40 regions of *spp* operon. The promoters controlling bacteriocin operons are strictly regulated, and their activity is increased more than 1,000-fold upon activation. Constitutive expression for the regulatory and transport operons is driven, at least in part, by promoters upstream of the −80 to −40 regions. The results reveal how promoters involved in quorum sensing-based regulation of bacteriocin production in *Lactobacillus* differ in strength and timing of their activity (Risoen et al., 2000).

Conclusions

The economical importance of lactobacilli for food fermentation processes and the potential use of these organisms as probiotics and delivery vehicles for targeting biologically active compounds to the mucosa have greatly stimulated research on these organisms. The past decade has seen an increased interest in the genetics of lactobacilli in particular, reflected by a sharp increase in the number of publications on this subject. Considering that the first report on electro-transformation of lactobacilli dates from 1987, the acquired knowledge on how to manipulate these organisms is impressive.

The structure of regulatory elements, in particular, promoters, translation initiation elements, and secretion signals in lactobacilli, has now been firmly established. The knowledge about these regulatory sequences has been instrumental in designing expression and secretion vectors with which heterologous proteins can be efficiently expressed, secreted, and anchored to the surface of lactobacilli. Expression and secretion vectors developed at TNO have been used successfully in EC projects by different partners to express foreign antigens or enzymes in different *Lactobacillus* species.

Studies on regulation of gene expression in lactobacilli have been largely confined so far to sugar metabolism, amino acid metabolism, and stress response. The regulatory circuit which in *B. subtilis* transfers signals derived from the transport and metabolism of rapidly metabolizable carbon sources to that of other carbon sources, and which involves the repressor CcpA as well as one of the elements of the PTS, HPr, has also been elucidated in different *Lactobacillus* species. A small number of differences were observed, yet the mechanisms are largely the same in the two genera. Although less extensively studied, some progress has also been made regarding the regulation of expression of amino acid biosynthetic or catabolizing genes, and stress response genes. It appears that mechanisms that are operating in *Bacillus* and *Lactococcus* also exist in lactobacilli. By studying the differences that were found, we may get a better insight in the mechanisms of gene expression in lactobacilli.

Despite the obviously considerable progress that has been made, our knowledge on gene expression in lactobacilli lags behind that of the paradigm lactic acid bacterium, *Lactococcus*. Recent developments in genomics, proteomics, and DNA chip technology are, however, expected to result in dramatic changes in knowledge acquisition in these areas in the near future. The nucleotide sequence of the *Lc. lactis* genome has been published (Bolotin et al., 1999) while sequence determination of the genome of *L. acidophilus, L. delbrueckii, L. plantarum*, and *L. sakei* is advanced or even complete. Once the complete genome sequences are available, we will be in a position to determine the function of all individual genes and to exploit that information for a detailed analysis of the regulatory mechanisms. These technological developments, which mark a revolution in biology, are expected to have a great impact on industrial applications of lactobacilli, not only for their traditional market, the food industry, but also for applications in public and animal health. The future of lactobacilli appears a shining one.

Acknowledgments

The research carried out in the author's laboratory (P.H.P) was, in part, supported by financial contributions from the EC (BIO-CT-96-0380 and BIO-CT-96-0542). We thank J. Steele for permission to include in this article unpublished promoter sequences.

References

Abe, K., and Uchiba, K. (1989). Correlation between depression of catabolite control of xylose metabolism and a defect in the phosphoenolpyruvate: mannose phosphotransferase system in *Pediococcus halophilus*. *Journal of Bacteriology* 171: 1793–1800.

Adachi, S. (1992). Lactic acid bacteria and the control of tumours. In: B. J. B. Wood (Ed.), *The lactic acid bacteria: Volume 1 The lactic acid bacteria in health and disease* (pp. 233–261). London and New York: Elsevier Applied Science.

Alpert, C.-A., and Chassy, B. M. (1990a). Molecular cloning and DNA sequence of *lacE*, the gene encoding the lactose-specific enzyme II of the phosphotransferase system of *Lactobacillus casei*. Evidence that a cysteine residue is essential for sugar phosphorylation. *Journal of Biological Chemistry* 265: 22561–22568.

Alpert, C.-A., and Chassy, B. M. (1990b). Molecular cloning and nucleotide sequence of the factor III^{Lac} gene of *Lactobacillus casei*. *Gene* 62: 277–288.

Alpert, C.-A., and Siebers, U. (1997). The *lac* operon of *Lactobacillus casei* contains *lacT*, a gene coding for a protein of the BglG family of transcriptional antiterminators. *Journal of Bacteriology* 179: 1555–1562.

Alvarez, M. A., Herrero, M., and Suarez, J. E. (1998). The site-specific recombination system of the *Lactobacillus* species bacteriophage A2 integrates in Gram-positive and Gram-negative bacteria. *Virology* 250: 185–193.

Arsenijevic, S., and Topisirovic, L. (2000). Molecular analysis of mutated *Lactobacillus acidophilus* promoter-like sequence P15. *Canadian Journal of Microbiology* 46: 938–945.

Auvray, F., Coddeville, M., Ritzenthaler, P., and Dupont, L. (1997). Plasmid integration in a wide range of bacteria mediated by the integrase of *Lactobacillus delbrueckii* bacteriophage mv4. *Journal of Bacteriology* 179: 1837–1845.

Bettenbrock, K., Sieber, U., Ehrenreich, P., and Alpert, C.-A. (1999). *Lactobacillus casei* 64H contains a phosphoenolpyruvate dependent phosphotransferase system for uptake of galactose, as confirmed by analysis of *ptsH* and different *gal* mutants. *Journal of Bacteriology* 181: 225–230.

Bhowmik, T., Fernandez, L., and Steele, J. L. (1993). Gene replacement in *Lactobacillus helveticus*. *Journal of Bacteriology* 175: 6341–6344.

Bolotin, A., Mauger, S., Malarme, K., Ehrlich, S. D., and Sorokin, A. (1999). Low-redundancy sequencing of the entire *Lactococcus lactis* IL1403 genome. *Antonie van Leeuwenhoek* 76: 27–76.

Boot, H. J., Kolen, C. P., Andreadaki, F. J., Leer, R. J., and Pouwels, P. H. (1996). The *Lactobacillus acidophilus* S-layer protein gene expression site comprises two consensus promoter sequences, one of which directs transcription of stable mRNA. *Journal of Bacteriology* 178: 5388–5394.

Bor, Y. C., Moraes, C., Lee, S. P., Crosby, W. L., Sinskey, A. J., and Batt, C. A. (1992). Cloning and sequencing the *Lactobacillus brevis* gene encoding xylose isomerase. *Gene* 114: 127–132.

Bourassa, S., Gauthier, L., Giguère, R., and Vadeboncoeur, C. (1990). A III^{Man} protein is involved in the transport of glucose, mannose and fructose by oral streptococci. *Oral Microbiology and Immunology* 5: 288–297.

Bringel, F., Frey, L., Boivin, S., and Hubert, J. C. (1997). Arginine biosynthesis and regulation in *Lactobacillus plantarum*: The *carA* gene and the *argCJBDF* cluster are divergently transcribed. *Journal of Bacteriology* 179: 2697–2706.

Broadbent, J. R., Oberg, C. J., and Wei, L. (1998). Characterization of the *Lactobacillus helveticus groESL* operon. *Research Microbiology* 149: 247–253.

Brurberg, M. B., Haandrikman, A. J., Leenhouts, K. J., Venema, G., and Nes, I. F. (1994). Expression of a chitinase gene from *Serratia marcescens* in *Lactococcus lactis* and *Lactobacillus plantarum*. *Applied Microbiology and Biotechnology* 42: 108–115.

Brurberg, M. B., Nes, I. F., and Eijsink, V. G. (1997). Pheromone-induced production of antimicrobial peptides in *Lactobacillus*. *Molecular Microbiology* 26: 347–360.

Brown, J. A., Barne, K. A., Minchin S. D. and Busky, S. J. W. (1997). In F. Eckstein and D. M. J. Lilley (Eds.), *Nucleic acids and molecular biology* Vol. 11 (pp. 41–52). Berlin, Germany: Springer Verlag.

Bukau, B. (1993). Regulation of the *Escherichia coli* heat-shock response. *Molecular Microbiology* 9: 671–680.

Chaillou, S., Bor, Y.-C., Batt, C. A., Postma, P. W., and Pouwels, P. H. (1998a). Molecular cloning and functional expression in *Lactobacillus plantarum* of *xylT* encoding the D-xylose-H^+ symporter of *Lactobacillus brevis*. *Applied and Environmental Microbiology* 64: 4720–4728.

Chaillou, S., Postma, P. W., and Pouwels, P. H. (2001). Contribution of the phosphoenolpyruvate : mannose phosphotransferase system to carbon catabolite repression in *Lactobacillus pentosus*. *Microbiology* 147: 671–679.

Chaillou, S., Lokman, B. C., Leer, R. J., Posthuma, C., Postma, P. W., and Pouwels, P. H. (1998b). Cloning, sequence analysis, and characterization of the genes involved in isoprimeverose metabolism in *Lactobacillus pentosus*. *Journal of Bacteriology* 180: 2312–2320.

Chaillou, S., Postma, P. W., and Pouwels, P. H. (1998c). Functional expression in *Lactobacillus plantarum* of *xylP* encoding the isoprimeverose transporter of *Lactobacillus pentosus*. *Journal of Bacteriology* 180: 4011–4014.

Chaillou, S., Pouwels, P. H., and Postma, P. W. (1999). Transport of D-xylose in *Lactobacillus pentosus*, *Lactobacillus casei* and *Lactobacillus plantarum*: Evidence for a mechanism of facilitated diffusion via the phospho-enolpyruvate:mannose phosphotransferase system. *Journal of Bacteriology* 181: 921–931.

Champomier-Verges, M. C., Zuniga, M., Morel-Deville, F., Perez-Martinez, G., and Zagorec, M. (1999). Relationship between arginine degradation, pH and survival in *Lactobacillus sakei*. *FEMS Microbiological Letters* 180: 297–304.

Chassy, B. M., Gibson, E. V., and Giuffrida, A. (1978). Evidence for plasmid associated lactose metabolism in *Lactobacilli casei* subsp. *casei*. *Current Microbiology* 1: 141–144.

Condon, S. (1987). Responses of lactic acid bacteria to oxygen. *FEMS Microbiological Reviews* 46: 269–280.

Cunin, R., Glansdorff, N., Pierard, A., and Stalon, V. (1986). Biosynthesis and metabolism of arginine in bacteria. *Microbiological Reviews* 50: 314–352.

Dahl, M. K., Degenkolb, J., and Hillen, W. (1994). Transcription of the *xyl* operon is controlled in *Bacillus subtilis* by tandem overlapping operators spaced by four base-pairs. *Journal of Molecular Biology* 243: 413–424.

David, S., Stevens, H., Van Riel, M., and De Vos, W. M. (1992). *Leuconostoc lactis* β-galactosidase is encoded by two translationally coupled genes. *Journal of Bacteriology* 174: 4475–4481.

De Ruyter, P. G., Kuipers, O. P., and de Vos, W. M. (1996). Controlled gene expression systems for *Lactococcus lactis* with the food-grade inducer nisin. *Applied and Environmental Microbiology* 62: 3662–3667.

Demple, B., and Amabile-Cuevas, C. F. (1991). Redox redux: The control of oxidative stress responses. *Cell* 67: 837–839.

De Roos, N. M., and Katan, M. B. (2000). Effects of probiotic bacteria on diarrhea, lipid metabolism, and carcinogenesis: A review of papers published between 1988 and 1998. *American Journal of Clinical Nutrition* 71: 405–411.

Derre, I., Rapoport, G., Devine, K., Rose, M., and Msadek, T. (1999a). ClpE, a novel type of HSP100 ATPase, is part of the CtsR heat shock regulon of *Bacillus subtilis*. *Molecular Microbiology* 32: 581–594.

Derre, I., Rapoport, G., and Msadek, T. (1999b). CtsR, a novel regulator of stress and heat shock response, controls *clp* and molecular chaperone gene expression in Gram-positive bacteria. *Molecular Microbiology* 31: 117–131.

Deutscher, J., Rizer, J., Fischer, C., Galinier, A., Saier, M. H., Jr., and Steinmetz, M. (1994). Loss of protein kinase-catalyzed phosphorylation of HPr, a phosphocarrier protein of the phosphotransferase system, by mutation of the *ptsH* gene confers catabolite repression resistance to several catabolic genes of *B. subtilis*. *Journal of Bacteriology* 176: 3336–3344.

Deutscher, J., Fischer, C., Charrier, V., Lindner, C., Darbon, E., and Dossonet, V. (1997). Regulation of carbon metabolism in Gram-positive bacteria by protein phosphorylation. *Folia Microbiology* 42: 171–178.

Deutscher, J., Küster, E., Bergstedt, U., Charrier, V., and Hillen, W. (1995). Protein kinase-dependent HPr/CcpA interaction links glycolytic activity to carbon catabolite repression in Gram-positive bacteria. *Molecular Microbiology* 15: 1049–1053.

Deutscher, J., Galinier, A., and Martin-Verstraete, I. (2001). Carbohydrate uptake and metabolism. In: A. I. Sonenshein, J. A. Hoch, and R. Losick (Eds.), *Bacillus subtilis and its closests relatives: From genes to cells* (pp. 137–158). Washington, DC: American Society for Microbiology.

Dicks, L., Du Plessis, E., Dellaglio, F., and Lauer, E. (1996). Reclassification of *Lactobacillus casei* subsp. *casei* ATCC 393 and *Lactobacillus rhamnosus* ATCC 15820 as *Lactobacillus zeae* nom. rev.; Description of ATCC 334 as the neotype of *L. casei* subsp. *casei*, and rejection of the name *Lactobacillus paracasei*. *International Journal Systematic Bacteriology* 46: 337–340.

Diep, D. B., Havarstein, L. S., and Nes, I. F. (1995). A bacteriocin-like peptide induces bacteriocin synthesis in *Lactobacillus plantarum* C11. *Molecular Microbiology* 18: 631–639.

Djordjevic, G. M., Tchieu, J. H., and Saier, M. H. Jr. (2001). Genes involved in control of galactose uptake in *Lactobacillus brevis* and reconstitution of the regulatory system in *Bacillus subtilis*. *Journal of Bacteriology* 183: 3224–3236.

Dossonet, V., Monedero, V., Zagorec, M., Galinier, A., Perez-Martinez, G., and Deutscher, J. (2000). Phosphorylation of HPr by the bifunctional HPr Kinase/P-ser-HPr phosphatase from *Lactobacillus casei* controls catabolite repression and inducer exclusion but not inducer expulsion. *Journal of Bacteriology* 182: 2582–2590.

Dudez, A. M., Chaillou, S., Hissler, L., Stentz, Champonier-Verges, M. C., Alpert, C. A., and Zagorez, M. (2002). Physical and genetic map of the *Lactobacillus sakei* 23K chromosome. *Microbiology* 148: 421–431.

Dupont, L., Boizet-Bonhoure, B., Coddeville, M., Auvray, F., and Ritzenthaler, P. (1995). Characterization of genetic elements required for site-specific integration of *Lactobacillus delbrueckii* subsp. *bulgaricus* bacteriophage mv4 and construction of an integration-proficient vector for *Lactobacillus plantarum*. *Journal of Bacteriology* 177: 586–595.

Eijsink, V. G., Brurberg, M. B., Middelhoven, P. H., and Nes, I. F. (1996). Induction of bacteriocin production in *Lactobacillus sake* by a secreted peptide. *Journal of Bacteriology* 178: 2232–2237.

Elagoz, A., Abdi, A., Hubert, J. C., and Kammerer, B. (1996). Structure and organisation of the pyrimidine biosynthesis pathway genes in *Lactobacillus plantarum*: A PCR strategy for sequencing without cloning. *Gene* 182: 37–43.

Erni, B., Zanolari, B., and Kocher, H. P. (1989). Mannose permease of *Escherichia coli*. Domain structure and function of the phosphorylating subunit. *Journal of Biological Chemistry* 264: 18733–18741.

Farr, S. B., and Kogoma, T. (1991). Oxidative stress responses in *Escherichia coli* and *Salmonella typhimurium*. *Microbiological Reviews* 55: 561–585.

Ferain, T., Garmyn, D., Bernard, N., Hols, P., and Delcour, J. (1994). *Lactobacillus plantarum ldhL* gene: Overexpression and deletion. *Journal of Bacteriology* 176: 596–601.

Ferain, T., Hobbs, J. N., Jr., Richardson, J., Bernard, N., Garmyn, D., Hols, P., Allen, N. E., and Delcour, J. (1996a). Knockout of the two *ldh* genes has a major impact on peptidoglycan precursor synthesis in *Lactobacillus plantarum*. *Journal of Bacteriology* 178: 5431–5437.

Ferain, T., Schanck, A. N., and Delcour, J. (1996b). 13C nuclear magnetic resonance analysis of glucose and citrate end products in an *ldhL-ldhD* double-knockout strain of *Lactobacillus plantarum*. *Journal of Bacteriology* 178: 7311–7315.

Fieulaine, S., Morera, S., Poncet, S., Monedero, V., Gueguen-Chaignon, V., Galinier, A., Janin, J., Deutscher, J., and Nessler, S. (2001). X-ray structure of HPr kinase: A bacterial protein kinase with a P-loop nucleotide-binding domain. *EMBO Journal* 20: 3917–3927.

Fons, M., Hege, T., Ladire, M., Raibaud, P., Ducluzeau, R., and Maguin, E. (1997). Isolation and characterization of a plasmid from *Lactobacillus fermentum* conferring erythromycin resistance. *Plasmid* 37: 199–203.

Fremaux, C., De Antoni, G. L., Raya, R. R., and Klaenhammer, T. R. (1993). Genetic organization and sequence of the region encoding integrative functions from *Lactobacillus gasseri* temperate bacteriophage phi *adh*. *Gene* 126: 61–66.

Fujita, Y., Miwa, Y., Galinier, A., and Deutscher, J. (1995). Specific recognition of the *Bacillus subtilis gnt cis*-acting catabolite-responsive element by a protein complex formed between CcpA and seryl-phosphorylated HPr. *Molecular Microbiology* 17: 953–960.

Galinier, A., Kravanja, M., Engelmann, R., Hengsterberg, W., Kilhoffer, M.-C., Deutscher, J., and Haiech, J. (1998). New protein kinase and protein phosphatase families mediate signal transduction in bacterial catabolite repression. *Proceedings of the National Academy of Sciences USA* 95: 1823–1828.

Garrigues, C., Loubiere, P., Lindley, N. D., and Cocaign-Bousquet, M. (1997). Control of the shift from homolactic acid to mixed-acid fermentation in *Lactococcus lactis*: Predominant role of the NADH/NAD+ ratio. *Journal of Bacteriology* 179: 5282–5287.

Gärtner, D., Degenkolb, J., Allmansberger, R., and Hillen, W. (1992). Regulation of the *Bacillus subtilis* W23 xylose utilization operon: Interaction of the Xyl repressor with the *xyl* operator and the inducer xylose. *Molecular General Genetics* 232: 415–422.

Gauthier, L., Bourassa, S., Brochu, D., and Vadeboncoeur, C. (1990). Control of sugar utilization in oral streptococci. Properties of phenotypically distinct 2-deoxyglucose-resistant mutants of *Streptococcus salivarius*. *Oral Microbiology and Immunology* 5: 352–359.

Georgopoulos, C., and Welch, W. J. (1993). Role of the major heat shock proteins as molecular chaperones. *Annual Review of Cellular Biology* 9: 601–634.

Germond, J. E., Lapierre, L., Delley, M., and Mollet, B. (1993). Novel IS element (ISL3) located next to the *Lactobacillus bulgaricus lacZ* gene. *FEMS Microbiological Reviews* 12: Abstract P10 A13.

Gerth, U., Kruger, E., Derre, I., Msadek, T., and Hecker, M. (1998). Stress induction of the *Bacillus subtilis clpP* gene encoding a homologue of the proteolytic component of the Clp protease and the involvement of ClpP and ClpX in stress tolerance. *Molecular Microbiology* 28: 787–802.

Gerth, U., Wipat, A., Harwood, C. R., Carter, N., Emmerson, P. T., and Hecker, M. (1996). Sequence and transcriptional analysis of *clpX*, a class-III heat-shock gene of *Bacillus subtilis*. *Gene* 181: 77–83.

Giraud, C., and Cuny, G. (1991). Molecular characterization of the alpha-1amylase genes of *lactobacillus plantarium Ale* and *Lactobacillus amylorous* reveals an unusual 3′ end structure with direct tandem repeats and suggests a common evolutionary origin. *Gene* 198: 149–157.

Gold, R. S., Meagher, M. M., Tong, S., Hutkins, R. W., and Conway, T. (1996). Cloning and expression of the *Zymomonas mobilis* "production of ethanol" genes in *Lactobacillus casei*. *Current Microbiology* 33: 256–260.

Gory, L., Montel, M. C., and Zagorec, M. (2001). Use of green fluorescent protein to monitor *L. sakei* in fermented meat products. *FEMS Microbiology Letters* 194: 127–133.

Gosalbes, M. J., Esteban, C. D., Galan, J. L., and Perez-Martinez, G. (2000). Integrative food-grade expression system based on the lactose regulon of *Lactobacillus casei*. *Applied and Environmental Microbiology* 66: 4822–4828.

Gosalbes, M. J., Esteban, C. D., and Perez-Martinez, G. (2002). *In vivo* effect of mutations in the antiterminator LacT in *Lactobacillus casei*. *Microbiology* 148: 695–702.

Gosalbes, M. J., Monedero, V., Alpert, C. A., and Perez-Martinez, G. (1997). Establishing a model to study the regulation of the lactose operon in *Lactobacillus casei*. *FEMS Microbiological Letters* 148: 83–89.

Gostick, D. O., Green, J., Irvine, A. S., Gasson, M. J., and Guest, J. R. (1998). A novel regulatory switch mediated by the FNR-like protein of *Lactobacillus casei. Microbiology* 144: 705–717.

Grangette, C., Muller-Alouf, H., Goudercourt, D., Geoffroy, M. C., Turneer, M., and Mercenier, A. (2001). Mucosal immune responses and protection against tetanus toxin after intranasal immunization with recombinant *Lactobacillus plantarum. Infection and Immununity* 69: 1547–1553.

Grundy, J. J., Rollins, S. M., and Henkin, T. M. (1994). Interaction between the acceptor end of tRNA and the T box stimulates antitermination in the Bacillus subtilis tyrS gene: A new role the discriminator case. *Journal of Bacteriology* 176: 4518–4526.

Havenith, C. E. G., Seegers, J. F. M. L., and Pouwels, P. H. (2002). Gut-associated lactobacilli for oral immunisation. *Food Research International* 35: 151–163.

Hecker, M., Schumann, W., and Volker, U. (1996). Heat-shock and general stress response in *Bacillus subtilis. Molecular Microbiology* 19: 417–428.

Hellendoorn, M., de Jong, A., Buist, G., Venema, G., and Kok, J. (1999). Regulation of components of the proteolytic system. *Abstracts from the sixth symposium on lactic acid bacteria*. The Netherlands: Veldhoven.

Hertel, C., Schmidt, G., Fischer, M., Oellers, K., and Hammes, W. P. (1998). Oxygen-dependent regulation of the expression of the catalase gene *katA* of *Lactobacillus sakei* LTH677. *Applied and Environmental Microbiology* 64: 1359–1365.

Heuberger, E. H., Smits, E., and Poolman, B. (2001). Xyloside transport by XylP, a member of the galactoside-pentoside-hexuronide family. *Journal of Biological Chemistry* 276: 34465–34472.

Hols, P., Slos, P., Dutot, P., Reymund, J., Chabot, P., Delplace, B., Delcour, J., and Mercenier, A. (1997). Efficient secretion of the model antigen M6-gp41E in *Lactobacillus plantarum* NCIMB 8826. *Microbiology* 143(Pt 8): 2733–2741.

Hueck, C., Kraus, A., and Hillen, W. (1994). Sequence of *ccpA* and two downstream *Bacillus megaterium* genes with homology to the *motAB* operon from *Bacillus subtilis. Gene* 143: 147–148.

Irvine, A. S., and Guest, J. R. (1993). *Lactobacillus casei* contains a member of the CRP-FNR family. *Nucleic Acids Research* 21: 753.

Jones, B. E., Dossonet, V., Küster, E., Hillen, W., Deutscher, J., and Klevit, R. E. (1997). Binding of the catabolite repressor protein CcpA to its DNA target is regulated by phosphorylation of its corepressor HPr. *Journal of Biological Chemistry* 272: 26530–26535.

Kanatani, K., Tahara, T., Oshimura, M., Sano, K., and Umezawa, C. (1995). Identification of the replication region of *Lactobacillus acidophilus* plasmid pLA103. *FEMS Microbiological Letters* 133: 127–130.

Kandler, O. (1983). Carbohydrate metabolism in lactic acid bacteria. *Antonie van Leeuwenhoek* 49: 209–224.

Kim, J. H., Voskuil, M. I., and Chambliss, G. H. (1998). NADP, corepressor for the *Bacillus* catabolite control protein CcpA. *Proceedings of the National Academy of Sciences USA* 95(16): 9590–9595.

Klaenhammer, T. R. (1988). Bacteriocins of lactic acid bacteria. *Biochimie* 70: 337–349.

Knauf, H. J., Vogel, R. F., and Hammes, W. P. (1992). Cloning, sequence, and phenotypic expression of *katA*, which encodes the catalase of *Lactobacillus sake* LTH677. *Applied and Environmental Microbiology* 58: 832–839.

Knorr, R., Ehrmann, M. A., and Vogel, R. F. (2001). Cloning, expression, and characterization of acetate kinase from *Lactobacillus sanfranciscensis. Microbiology Research* 156: 267–277.

Kok, J. (1996). Inducible gene expression and environmentally regulated genes in lactic acid bacteria. *Antonie van Leeuwenhoek* 70: 129–145.

Kunji, E. R., Mierau, I., Hagting, A., Poolman, B., and Konings, W. N. (1996). The proteolytic systems of lactic acid bacteria. *Antonie van Leeuwenhoek* 70: 187–221.

Langella, P., le Loir, Y., Ehrlich, S. D., and Gruss, A. (1993). Efficient plasmid mobilization by pIP501 in *Lactococcus lactis* subsp. *Lactis. Journal of Bacteriology* 175: 5806–5813.

Lapointe, R., Frenette, M., and Vadeboncoeur, C. (1993). Altered expression of several genes in III_L^{man}-defective mutants of *Streptococcus salivarius* demonstrated by two-dimensional gel electrophoresis of cytoplasmic proteins. *Research Microbiology* 144: 305–316.

Lauret, R., Morel-Deville, F., Berthier, F., Champonier-Verges, M., Postma, P. W., Ehrlich, S. D., and Zagorec, M. (1996). Carbohydrate utilization in *Lactobacillus sake. Applied and Environmental Microbiology* 62: 1922–1927.

Leloup, L., Ehrlich, S. D., Zagorec, M., and Morel-Deville, F. (1997). Single-crossover integration in the *Lactobacillus sake* chromosome and insertional inactivation of the *ptsI* and *lacL* genes. *Applied and Environmental Microbiology* 63: 2117–2123.

Leong-Morgenthaler, P., Zwahlen, M. C., and Hottinger, H. (1991). Lactose metabolism in *Lactobacillus bulgaricus*: Analysis of the primary structure and expression of the genes involved. *Journal of Bacteriology* 173: 1951–1957.

Lim, E. M., Ehrlich, S. D., and Maguin, E. (2000). Identification of stress-inducible proteins in *Lactobacillus delbrueckii* subsp. *bulgaricus*. *Electrophoresis* 21: 2557–2561.

Lin, M. Y., Harlander, S., and Savaiano, D. (1996). Construction of an integrative food-grade cloning vector for *Lactobacillus acidophilus*. *Applied Microbiology and Biotechnology* 45: 484–489.

Lindquist, S. (1991). Heat shock proteins and stress tolerance in microorganisms. *Current Opinion Genetic Developments* 2: 748–755.

Lokman, B. C., Heerikhuisen, M., Leer, R. J., van den Broek, A., Borsboom, Y., Chaillou, S., Postma, P. W., and Pouwels, P. H. (1997). Regulation of expression of the *Lactobacillus pentosus xylAB* operon. *Journal of Bacteriology* 179: 5391–5397.

Lokman, B. C., Leer, R. J., van Sorge, R., and Pouwels, P. H. (1994). Promoter analysis and transcriptional regulation of *Lactobacillus pentosus* genes involved in xylose catabolism. *Molecular and General Genetics* 245: 117–125.

Lokman, B. C., van Santen, P., Verdoes, J. C., Kruse, J., Leer, R. J., Posno, M., and Pouwels, P. H. (1991). Organization and characterization of three genes involved in D-xylose catabolism in *Lactobacillus pentosus*. *Molecular and General Genetics* 230: 161–169.

Maassen, C. B. M., Laman, J. D., Heijne den Bak-Glashouwer, M. J., Tielen, F. J., van Holten-Neelen, J. C. P. A., Hoogteijling, L., Antonissen, C., Leer, R. L., Pouwels, P. H., Boersma, W. J. A., and Shaw, D. M. (1999). Instruments for oral disease-intervention strategies: Recombinant *Lactobacillus casei* expressing tetanus toxin fragment C for vaccination or myelin proteins for oral tolerance induction in multiple sclerosis. *Vaccine* 17: 2117–2128.

Mahr, K., Hillen, W., and Titgemeyer, F. (2000). Carbon catabolite repression in *Lactobacillus pentosus*: Analysis of the *ccpA* region. *Applied and Environmental Microbiology* 66: 277–283.

Malleret, C., Lauret, R., Ehrlich, S. D., Morel-Deville, F., and Zagorec, M. (1998). Disruption of the sole *ldhL* gene in *Lactobacillus sakei* prevents the production of both L- and D-lactate. *Microbiology* 144: 3327–3333.

Manca de Nadra, M. C., Nadra, C. A., and Pesce de Ruiz Holgado, A. (1986). Arginine metabolism in *Lactobacillus leichmannii*. *Current Microbiology* 13: 155–158.

Marasco, R., Muscariello, L., Varcamonti, M., De Felice, M., and Sacco, M. (1998). Expression of the *bglH* gene of *Lactobacillus plantarum* is controlled by carbon catabolite repression. *Journal of Bacteriology* 180: 3400–3404.

Martin, M. C., Alonso, J. C., Suarez, J. E., and Alvarez, M. A. (2000). Generation of food-grade recombinant lactic acid bacterium strains by site-specific recombination. *Applied and Environmental Microbiology* 66: 2599–2604

Mayo, B., Derzelle, S., Fernandez, M., Leonard, C., Ferain, T., Hols, P., Suarez, J. E., and Delcour, J. (1997). Cloning and characterization of *cspL* and *cspP*, two cold-inducible genes from *Lactobacillus plantarum*. *Journal of Bacteriology* 179: 3039–3042.

Mayo, B., Gonzalez, B., Arca, P., and Suarez, J. E. (1994). Cloning and expression of the plasmid encoded beta-D-galactosidase gene from a *Lactobacillus plantarum* strain of dairy origin. *FEMS Microbiological Letters* 122: 145–151.

McCracken, A., and Timms, P. (1999). Efficiency of transcription from promoter sequence variants in lactobacillus is both strain and context dependent. *Journal of Bacteriology* 181: 6569–6572.

Mercenier, A., Pouwels, P. H., and Chassy, B. M. (1994). Genetic engineering of lactobacilli, *Leuconostoc* and *Streptococcus thermophilus*. In: M. J. Gasson and W. M. de Vos (Eds.), *Genetics and biotechnology of lactic acid bacteria* (pp. 252–293). Blackie, UK: Chapman and Hall.

Mercenier, A. (1999). Lactic acid bacteria as live vaccines. In: *Probiotics: A critical review* (pp. 113–127). Wymondham, UK: Horizon Scientific press.

Mercenier, A., Muller-Alouf, H., and Grangette, C. (2000). Lactic acid bacteria as live vaccines. *Current Issues Molecular Biology* 2: 17–25.

Mogk, A., Homuth, G., Scholz, C., Kim, L., Schmid, F. X., and Schumann, W. (1997). The GroE chaperonin machine is a major modulator of the CIRCE heat shock regulon of *Bacillus subtilis*. *EMBO Journal* 16: 4579–4590.

Monedero, V., Gosalbes, M. J., and Perez-Martinez, G. (1997). Catabolite repression in *Lactobacillus casei* ATCC 393 is mediated by CcpA. *Journal of Bacteriology* 179: 6657–6664.

Monedero V., Poncet, S., Mijakovic, I., Fieulaine, S., Dossonnet, V., Martin-Verstraete, I., Nessler, S., and Deutsche, J. (2001). Mutations lowering the phosphatase activity of HPr kinase/phosphatase switch off carbon metabolism. *EMBO Journal* 20: 3928–3937.

Montel, M. C., and Champomier, M. C. (1987). Arginine catabolism in *Lactobacillus sake* isolated from meat. *Applied and Environmental Microbiology* 53: 2683–2685.

Moreno, M. S., Schneider, B. L., Maile, R. R., Weyler, W., and Saier, M. H. Jr. (2001). Catabolite repression mediated by the CcpA protein in *Bacillus subtilis*: Novel modes of regulation revealed by whole-genome analyses. *Molecular Microbiology* 39: 1366–1381.

Morishita, T., Deguchi, Y., Yajima, M., Sakurai, T., and Yura, T. (1981). Multiple nutritional requirements of lactobacilli: Genetic lesions affecting amino acid biosynthetic pathways. *Journal of Bacteriology* 148: 64–71.

Morishita, T., Fukada, T., Shirota, M., and Yura, T. (1974). Genetic basis of nutritional requirements in *Lactobacillus casei*. *Journal of Bacteriology* 120: 1078–1084.

Msadek, T., Dartois, V., Kunst, F., Herbaud, M. L., Denizot, F., and Rapoport, G. (1998). ClpP of *Bacillus subtilis* is required for competence development, motility, degradative enzyme synthesis, growth at high temperature and sporulation. *Molecular Microbiology* 27: 899–914.

Msadek, T., Kunst, F., and Rapoport, G. (1994). MecB of *Bacillus subtilis*, a member of the ClpC ATPase family, is a pleiotropic regulator controlling competence gene expression and growth at high temperature. *Proceedings of the National Academy of Sciences USA* 91: 5788–5792.

Muscariello, L., Marasco, R., De Felice, M., and Sacco, M. (2001). The functional *ccpA* Ggne is required for carbon catabolite repression in *Lactobacillus plantarum*. *Applied and Environmental Microbiology* 67: 903–2907.

Natori, Y., Kano, Y., and Imamoto, F. (1990). Nucleotide sequences and genomic constitution of five tryptophan genes of *Lactobacillus casei*. *Journal of Biochemistry (Tokyo)* 107: 248–255.

Nicoloff, H., Hubert, J. C., and Bringel, F. (2000). In *Lactobacillus plantarum*, carbamoyl phosphate is synthesized by two carbamoyl-phosphate synthetases (CPS): Carbon dioxide differentiates the arginine-repressed from the pyrimidine-regulated CPS. *Journal of Bacteriology* 182: 3416–3422.

Obst, M., Meding, E. R., Vogel, R. F., and Hammes, W. P. (1995). Two genes encoding the beta-galactosidase of *Lactobacillus sake*. *Microbiology* 141: 3059–3066.

Oppenheim, D. S., and Yanofsky, C. (1980). Translational coupling during expression of the tryptophan operon of *Escherichia coli*. *Genetics* 95: 785–795.

Parsell, D. A., and Lindquist, S. (1993). The function of heat-shock proteins in stress tolerance: Degradation and reactivation of damaged proteins. *Annual Review of Genetics* 27: 437–496.

Pavan, S., Hols, P., Delcour, J., Geoffroy, M. C., Grangette, C., Kleerebezem, M., and Mercenier, A. (2000). Adaptation of the nisin-controlled expression system in *Lactobacillus plantarum*: A tool to study *in vivo* biological effects. *Applied and Environmental Microbiology* 66: 4427–4432.

Poolman, B., Driessen, A. J., and Konings, W. N. (1987). Regulation of arginine–ornithine exchange and the arginine deiminase pathway in *Streptococcus lactis*. *Journal of Bacteriology* 169: 5597–5604.

Poolman, B., Knol, J., Mollet, B., Niewenhuis, B., and Sulter, G. (1995). Regulation of bacterial sugar-H^+ symport by phosphoenolpyruvate-dependent phosphotransferase enzyme I/HPr-mediated phosphorylation. *Proceedings of the National Academy of Sciences USA* 92: 778–782.

Porter, E. V., and Chassy, B. M. (1988). Nucleotide sequence of the β-D-phospho-galactoside galactohydrolase gene of *Lactobacillus casei*: Comparison to analogous *pbg* genes of other Gram-positive organisms. *Gene* 62: 263–276.

Posthuma, C. C., Bader, R., Engelmann, R., Postma, P. W., Hengstenberg, W., and Pouwels, P. H. (2002a). Expression of the xylulose 5-phosphate phosphoketolase gene, *xpk*A, from *Lactobacillus pentosus* MD363 is induced by sugars that are fermented via the phosphoketolase pathway and is repressed by glucose mediated by CcpA and the mannose phosphoenolpyruvate phosphotransferase system. *Applied and Environmental Microbiology* 68: 831–837.

Posthuma, C. C. Bader, R., Postma, P. W., and Pouwels, P. H. (in press). Expression of the acetate kinase gene of *Lactobacillus pentosus* is regulated by carbon catabolite repression mediated by CcpA. *Microbiology*.

Postma, P. W., Lengeler, J. W., and Jacobson, G. R. (1993). Phosphoenolpyruvate:carbohydrate phosphotransferase systems of bacteria. *Microbiological Reviews* 57: 543–594.

Pouwels, P. H., and Leer, R. J. (1993). Genetics of lactobacilli: Plasmids and gene expression. *Antonie van Leeuwenhoek* 64: 85–107.

Pouwels, P. H., Leer, R. J., and Boersma, W. J. (1996). The potential of *Lactobacillus* as a carrier for oral immunization: Development and preliminary characterization of vector systems for targeted delivery of antigens. *Journal of Biotechnology* 44: 183–192.

Pouwels, P. H., Leer, R. J., Shaw, M., Heijne den Bak-Glashouwer, M. J., Tielen, F. D., Smit, E., Martinez, B., Jore, J., and Conway, P. L. (1998). Lactic acid bacteria as antigen delivery vehicles for oral immunization purposes. *International Journal of Food Microbiology* 41: 155–167.

Pouwels, P. H., and Leunissen, J. A. (1994). Divergence in codon usage of *Lactobacillus* species. *Nucleic Acids Research* 22: 929–936.

Pouwels, P. H., Vriesema, A., Martinez, B., Tielen, F. J., Seegers, J. F. M. L., Leer, R. J., and Smit, E. (2000). Lactobacilli as vehicles for targeting antigens to mucosal tissues by surface expression of foreign antigens. *Methods in Enzymology*, 336: 369–389.

Pridmore, D., Stefanova, T., and Mollet, B. (1994). Cryptic plasmids from *Lactobacillus helveticus* and their evolutionary relationship. *FEMS Microbiological Letters* 124: 301–305.

Rallu, F., Gruss, A., and Maguin, E. (1996). *Lactococcus lactis* and stress. *Antonie van Leeuwenhoek* 70: 243–251.

Raya, R. R., Fremaux, C., De Antoni, G. L., and Klaenhammer, T. R. (1992). Site-specific integration of the temperate bacteriophage phi *adh* into the *Lactobacillus gasseri* chromosome and molecular characterization of the phage (*attP*) and bacterial (*attB*) attachment sites. *Journal of Bacteriology* 174: 5584–5592.

Reizer, J., Hoischen, C., Titgemeyer, F., Rivolta, C., Rabus, R., Stülke, J., Karamat, D., Saier, M. H., Jr., and Hillen, W. (1998). A novel protein kinase that controls carbon catabolite repression in bacteria. *Molecular Microbiology* 27: 1157–1169.

Risoen, P. A., Brurberg, M. B., Eijsink, V. G., and Nes, I. F. (2000). Functional analysis of promoters involved in quorum sensing-based regulation of bacteriocin production in *Lactobacillus*. *Molecular Microbiology* 37: 619–628.

Rossi, F., Rudella, A., Marzotto, M., and Dellaglio, F. (2001). Vector-free cloning of a bacterial endo-1,4-beta-glucanase in *Lactobacillus plantarum* and its effect on the acidifying activity in silage: Use of recombinant cellulolytic *Lactobacillus plantarum* as silage inoculant. *Antonie van Leeuwenhoek* 80: 139–147.

Roy, D. G., Klaenhammer, T. R., and Hassan, H. M. (1993). Cloning and expression of the manganese superoxide dismutase gene of *Escherichia coli* in *Lactococcus lactis* and *Lactobacillus gasseri*. *Molecular and General Genetics* 239: 33–40.

Rush, C., Hafner, L., and Timms, P. (1997). Protein A as a fusion partner for the expression of heterologous proteins in *Lactobacillus*. *Applied Microbiological Biotechnology* 47: 537–542.

Russell, W. M., and Klaenhammer, T. R. (2001). Efficient system for directed integration into the *Lactobacillus acidophilus* and *Lactobacillus gasseri* chromosomes via homologous recombination. *Applied and Environmental Microbiology* 67: 4361–4364.

Sanders, J. W., Leenhouts, K. J., Haandrikman, A. J., Venema, G., and Kok, J. (1995). Stress response in *Lactococcus lactis*: Cloning, expression analysis, and mutation of the lactococcal superoxide dismutase gene. *Journal of Bacteriology* 177: 5254–5260.

Savijoki, K., Kahala, M., and Palva, A. (1997). High level heterologous protein production in *Lactococcus* and *Lactobacillus* using a new secretion system based on the *Lactobacillus brevis* S-layer signals. *Gene* 186: 255–262.

Scheler, A., and Hillen, W. (1994). Regulation of xylose utilization in *Bacillus licheniformis*: Xyl repressor-*xyl*-operator interaction studied by DNA modification protection and interference. *Molecular Microbiology* 13: 505–512.

Schick, J., Weber, B., Klein, J. R., and Henrich, B. (1999). PepR1, a CcpA-like transcription regulator of *Lactobacillus delbruckii* ssp. *lactis*. *Microbiology* 145: 3147–3154.

Schirmer, E. C., Glover, J. R., Singer, M. A., and Lindquist, S. (1996). HSP100/Clp proteins: A common mechanism explains diverse functions. *Trends in Biochemical Science* 21: 289–296.

Schmidt, B. F., Adams, R. M., Requadt, C., Power, S., and Mainzer, S. E. (1989). Expression and nucleotide sequence of the *Lactobacillus bulgaricus* β-galactosidase gene cloned in *Escherichia coli*. *Journal of Bacteriology* 171: 625–635.

Schmidt, G., Hertel, C., and Hammes, W. P. (1999). Molecular characterisation of the *dnaK* operon of *Lactobacillus sakei* LTH681. *Systematic and Applied Microbiology* 22: 321–328.

Schmiedel, D., Kintrup, M., Küster, E., and Hillen, W. (1997). Regulation of expression, genetic organization and substrate specificity of xylose uptake in *Bacillus megaterium*. *Molecular Microbiology* 23: 1053–1062.

Serror, P., Sasaki, T., Ehrlich, S. D., and Maguin, E. (2002). Electrotransformation of *Lactobacillus delbrueckii* subsp. *bulgaricus* and *L. delbrueckii* subsp. *lactis* with various plasmids. *Applied and Environmental Microbiology* 68: 46–52.

Shaw, D. M., Gaerthé, B., Leer, R. J., van der Stap, J. G. M. M., Smittenaar, C., Heijne-den Bak-Glashouwer, M.-J., Tielen, F. J., and Pouwels, P. H. (2000). Engineering the microflora to vaccinate the mucosa: Serum immunoglobulin G responses and activated draining cervical lymph nodes following mucosal application of tetanus toxin fragment C-expressing lactobacilli. *Immunology* 100: 510–518.

Shimizu-Kadota, M. (2001). A method to maintain introduced DNA sequences stably and safely on the bacterial chromosome: Application of prophage integration and subsequent designed excision. *Journal of Biotechnology* 89: 73–79.

Simpson, C. L., and Russell, R. R. B. (1998). Identification of a homolog of CcpA catabolite repressor protein in *Streptococcus mutans*. *Infection and Immunity* 66: 2085–2092.

Sizemore, C., Wieland, B., Götz, F., and Hillen, W. (1992). Regulation of *Staphylococcus xylosus* xylose utilization genes at the molecular level. *Journal of Bacteriology* 174: 3042–3048.

Sleytr, U. B., and Messner, P. (1983). Crystalline surface layers on bacteria. *Annual Review of Microbiology* 37: 311–339.

Spiro, S. (1994). The FNR family of transcriptional regulators. *Antonie van Leeuwenhoek* 66: 23–36.

Spiro, S., and Guest, J. R. (1990). FNR and its role in oxygen-regulated gene expression in *Escherichia coli*. *FEMS Microbiological Reviews* 6: 399–428.

Stentz, R., Lauret, R., Ehrlich, S. D., Morel-Deville, F., and Zagorec, M. (1997). Molecular cloning and analysis of the *ptsHI* operon in *Lactobacillus sake*. *Applied and Environmental Microbiology* 63: 2111–2116.

Stentz, R., and Zagorec, M. (1999). Ribose utilization in *Lactobacillus sakei*: Analysis of the regulation of the *rbs* operon and putative involvement of a new transporter. *Journal of Molecular and Microbiological Biotechnology* 1: 165–173.

Stentz, R., Loizel, C., Malleret, C., and Zagorec, M. (2000). Development of genetic tools for *Lactobacillus sakei*: Disruption of the beta-galactosidase gene and use of *lacZ* as a reporter gene to study regulation of the putative copper ATPase, AtkB. *Applied and Environmental Microbiology* 66: 4272–4278.

Stucky, K., Klein, J. R., Schüller, A., Matern, H., Henrich, B., and Plapp, R. (1995). Cloning and DNA sequence analysis of *pepQ*, a prolidase gene from *Lactobacillus delbrueckii* subsp. *lactis* DSM7290 and partial characterization of its product. *Molecular General Genetics* 247: 494–500.

Stucky, K., Schick, J., Klein, J. B., Henrich, B., and Plapp, R. (1996). Characterization of *pepR1*, a gene coding for a potential transcriptional regulator of *Lactobacillus delbrueckii* subsp. *lactis* DSL7290. *FEMS Microbiological Letters* 136: 63–69.

Stülke, J., Arnaud, M., Rapoport, G., and Martin-Verstraete, I. (1998). PRD—a protein domain involved in PTS-dependent induction and carbon catabolite repression of catabolic operons in bacteria. *Molecular Microbiology* 28: 865–874.

Takeda, Y., Takase, K., Yamato, I., and Abe, K. (1998). Sequencing and characterization of the *xyl* operon of a Gram-positive bacterium, *Tetragenococcus halophila*. *Applied and Environmental Microbiology* 64: 2513–2519.

Tannock, G. W., Luchansky, J. B., Miller, L., Connell, H., Thode-Andersen, S., Mercer, A. A., and Klaenhammer, T. R. (1994). Molecular characterization of a plasmid-borne (pGT633) erythromycin resistance determinant (*ermGT*) from *Lactobacillus reuteri* 100–63. *Plasmid* 31: 60–71.

Thompson, J. (1987). Regulation of sugar transport and metabolism in lactic acid bacteria. *FEMS Microbiological Reviews* 46: 221–231.

Thompson, J. K., McConville, K. J., Nicholson, C., and Collins, M. A. (2001). DNA cloning in *Lactobacillus helveticus* by the exconjugation of recombinant mob-containing plasmid constructs from strains of transformable lactic acid bacteria. *Plasmid* 46: 188–201.

Tonon, T., Bourdineaud, J. P., and Lonvaud-Funel, A. (2001). The *arcABC* gene cluster encoding the arginine deiminase pathway of *Oenococcus oeni*, and arginine induction of a CRP-like gene. *Research Microbiology* 152: 653–661.

Vandevoorde, L., Vande Woestyne, M., Bruyneel, B., Christiaens, H., and Verstraete, W. (1992). Critical factors governing the competitive behaviour of lactic acid bacteria in mixed cultures. In: B. J. B. Wood (Ed.), *The lactic acid bacteria: Volume 1 The lactic acid bacteria in health and disease* (pp. 447–475). London and New York: Elsevier Applied Science.

Veyrat, A., Gosalbes, M. J., and Perez-Martinez, G. (1996). *Lactobacillus curvatus* has a glucose transport system homologous to the mannose family of phosphoenolpyruvate-dependent phosphotransferase systems. *Microbiology* 142: 3469–3477.

Veyrat, A., Monedero, V., and Perez-Martinez, G. (1994). Glucose transport by the phosphoenolpyruvate : mannose phosphotransferase system in *Lactobacillus casei* ATCC 393 and its role in carbon catabolite repression *Microbiology* 140: 1141–1149.

Viana, R., Monedero, V., Dossonnet, V., Vadeboncoeur, C., Perez-Martinez, G., and Deutscher, J. (2000). Enzyme I and HPr from *Lactobacillus casei*: Their role in sugar transport, carbon catabolite repression and inducer exclusion. *Molecular Microbiology* 36: 570–584.

Voskuil, M. I., and Chambliss, G. H. (1998). The −16 region of *Bacillus subtilis* and other gram-positive bacterial promoters. *Nucleic Acids Research* 26: 3584–3590.

Walker, D. C., Aoyama, K., and Klaenhammer, T. R. (1996). Electrotransformation of *Lactobacillus acidophilus* group A1. *FEMS Microbiological Letters* 138: 233–237.

Walker, G. C. (1996). The SOS response of *Escherichia coli*. In F. C. Neidhardt (Ed.), Escherichia coli *and* salmonella: *Cellular and molecular biology* (2nd ed., pp. 1400–1416). Washington, DC: American Society for Microbiology.

Walker, D. C., Girgis, H. S., and Klaenhammer, T. R. (1999). The *groESL* chaperone operon of *L. johnsonii*. *Applied and Environmental Microbiology* 65: 3033–3041.

Wanker, E., Leer, R. J., Pouwels, P. H., and Schwab, H. (1995). Expression of *Bacillus subtilis* levanase gene in *Lactobacillus plantarum* and *Lactobacillus casei*. *Applied Microbiology and Biotechnology* 43: 297–303.

Weickert, J., and Adhya, S. (1992). A family of bacterial regulators homologous to Gal and Lac repressors. *Journal of Biological Chemistry* 267: 15869–15874.

Wells, J. M., Robinson, K., Chamberlain, L. M., Schofield, K. M., and Le Page, R. W. F. (1996). Lactic acid bacteria as vaccine delivery vehicles. *Antonie van Leeuwenhoek*, 70: 317–330.

Ye, J. J. (1996). Regulation of carbohydrate transport in *Lactococcus* and *Lactobacillus*. *Research Microbiology* 147: 523–527.

Ye, J. J., Neal, J. W., Cui, X., Reizer, J., and Saier, M. H. (1994a). Regulation of the glucose : H^+ symporter by metabolite-activated ATP-dependent phosphorylation of HPr in *Lactobacillus brevis*. *Journal of Bacteriology* 176: 3484–3492.

Ye, J. J., and Saier, M. H. J. (1995a). Allosteric regulation of the glucose : H^+ symporter of *Lactobacillus brevis*: Cooperative binding of glucose and HPr(Ser-P). *Journal of Bacteriology* 177: 1900–1902.

Ye, J. J., and Saier, M. H. J. (1995b). Cooperative binding of lactose and HPr(Ser-P) to the lactose : H^+ permease of *Lactobacillus brevis*. *Proceedings of the National Academy of Sciences USA* 92: 417–421.

Ye, Y.-Y., Cui, J., and Saier, M. H. J. (1994c). ATP-dependent phosphorylation of serine-46 in the phosphocarrier protein HPr regulates lactose/H^+ symport in *Lactobacillus brevis*. *Proceedings of the National Academy of Sciences USA* 91: 3102–3106.

Yebra, M. J., Veyrat, A., Santos, M. A., and Perez-Martinez, G. (2000). Genetics of L-sorbose transport and metabolism in *Lactobacillus casei*. *Journal of Bacteriology* 182: 155–163.

Yuan, G., and Wong, S. L. (1995). Regulation of *groE* expression in *Bacillus subtilis*: The involvement of the sigma A-like promoter and the roles of the inverted repeat sequence (CIRCE). *Journal of Bacteriology* 177: 5427–5433.

Zuber, U., and Schumann, W. (1994). CIRCE, a novel heat shock element involved in regulation of heat shock operon *dnaK* of *Bacillus subtilis*. *Journal of Bacteriology* 176: 1359–1363.

Zuniga, M., Champomier-Verges, M., Zagorec, M., and Perez-Martinez, G. (1998). Structural and functional analysis of the gene cluster encoding the enzymes of the arginine deiminase pathway of *Lactobacillus sakei*. *Journal of Bacteriology* 180: 4154–4159.

7

Genetics of Proteolysis in *Lactococcus lactis*

Jan Kok and Girbe Buist

Summary

Genetic and biochemical research over the past 15 years on milk protein degradation by *Lactococcus lactis* has resulted in a detailed picture of how casein is broken down into its sub-fragments and used for cellular growth. Starting with the action of an extracellular but cell-wall-located proteinase, milk protein is degraded into oligopeptides that are internalized by a specialized and essential oligopeptide permease (Opp) system. Without Opp, cells of *Lc. lactis* cannot grow in milk. Notwithstanding this, the organism has two uptake systems for the internalization of di- and tripeptides. Once inside, a host of intracellular peptidases degrade the oligopeptides into smaller peptides and amino acids that are needed for cell growth. Both general aminopeptidases and more specialized enzymes are involved in this degradation process, as are a number of oligopeptidases. Most of the genes of the components making up the casein degradation pathway have been cloned and sequenced and most of these have been targeted by insertional mutagenesis to allow for an analysis of the function and importance of the components in the pathway. The casein degradation route has been engineered in various ways by the overexpression or stabilization of certain genes, by deleting genes, by mutating enzyme specificities or by expressing heterologous proteolytic enzymes in *Lc. lactis*. In a number of cases, the modified strains have been used in (small-scale) cheese trials to assess the effects of the changes on the organoleptic quality of the fermentation product. More recently the regulation of the various genes in response to the growth phase of the cells and to medium composition has been studied. Even more recent is the discovery, through the determination of the nucleotide sequence of the chromosome of a widely studied laboratory strain of *Lc. lactis*, of a number of additional proteinase genes not yet described in this organism. It is no exaggeration to claim that the caseinolytic pathway of *Lc. lactis* is the

Jan Kok and Girbe Buist • Department of Genetics, Groningen Biomolecular Sciences and Biotechnology Institute (GBB), University of Groningen, PO Box 14, 9750 AA Haren, The Netherlands; e-mail: kokj@biol.rug.nl

best studied of the protein degradation pathways of micro-organisms. This chapter deals with the unravelling of the intricacies of this industrially important catabolic route.

Introduction

Lc. lactis is the main component of the starter cultures used for cheese making. It is either present in these starter cultures as a mixture of defined single strains or in a largely uncharacterized mixture with a number of other lactic acid bacteria (LAB). As such it plays a very important role in human nutrition worldwide. The main activity of *Lc. lactis* during milk fermentation is the conversion of lactose to lactic acid, which results in the lowering of the pH in the product. A very important factor that determines the ultimate quality of the end product is the speed with which this acidification takes place in the early stages of the fermentation process. Acidification in the first stages of milk fermentation should be fast and, consequently, the bacteria have to grow quickly. *Lc. lactis* is an amino acid auxotroph that needs an extracellular source of essential amino acids (Chopin, 1993). However, the amount of free amino acids and small peptides in fresh milk is too low to allow for the fast growth rates needed for good cheese production. As the milk proteins α_{S1}- and β-casein are the major sources of sequestered amino acids in milk (Thomas and Pritchard, 1987; Juillard et al., 1995b), *Lc. lactis* is fully dependent on a proteolytic system that can liberate these amino acids from casein. Apart from allowing rapid growth of the bacteria to cell densities needed for good quality cheese production, the proteolytic breakdown by *Lc. lactis* of casein is an important parameter in cheese flavor development. Breakdown products of casein are either flavors or flavor precursors that undergo further chemical and/or enzymatic conversion to the typical flavor compounds that are highly appreciated by the consumer and make cheese not only a healthy product but also one that adds to the enjoyment of life.

It is this central role that casein breakdown plays in the industrial process of cheese making that spurred a huge research effort to unravel the intricacies of the pathway. Especially during the last 15 years a vast amount of data has been gathered concerning the components that make up the caseinolytic pathway in *Lc. lactis*. Table 7.1 gives a list of the proteins and enzymes that will be described in this review. Most of the enzymes and proteins that take part in the process of liberating peptides from casein, the uptake of these peptides and their intercellular degradation to free amino acids have been characterized to considerable detail biochemically as well as genetically. In fact, the development of tools for the genetic analysis of these bacteria has contributed considerably to the understanding of this industrially important metabolic pathway. The pathway of casein degradation by *Lc. lactis* is the best understood of the proteolytic pathways in bacteria and the finesses of this system are the point of focus of this review. Due to space limitation, and because the proteolytic pathway of *Lc. lactis* can be seen as the paradigm for proteolysis in other LAB, the knowledge obtained more on casein breakdown by various species of Lactobacilli and *Streptococcus thermophilus* will not be dealt with. Several activities that have been described in Lactococcus have also been detected in Lactobacillus species and *Strep. thermophilus* and the reader is referred to an excellent review on this subject published by Christensen et al. on the Sixth Symposium on Lactic Acid Bacteria, held in the Netherlands in September 1999 (Christensen et al., 1999). Only those enzymes that are unique to Lactobacillus and have been expressed in *Lc. lactis* will be discussed here as to their effect on altering the peptidase make-up of *Lc. lactis*.

Table 7.1. Components of the Proteolytic System of *Lc. lactis*

Enzymes	Name	MW (KD)[e]	Structure[a]	Substrate[b]	Class[f]	Reference
Proteinases	PrtP	200		Extracellular proteins	S	Kok, 1990
	HtrA	42		Exported proteins, pro-peptides	S	Poquet et al., 2000
	ClpP	22	Complex[d]	Misfolded proteins	S	Frees and Ingmer, 1999
	DnaK	69	Complex[d]	Misfolded proteins		Arnau et al., 1996
	NisP	75		Nisin precursor	S	Van der Meer et al., 1993
	LagD	80		Pre-lactococcin	C	Havarstein et al., 1995
	LcnC	80		Pre-lactococcin	C	Franke et al., 1999
	PedD	80		Pre-pediocin	C	Venema et al., 1995
Transporters	Aac[c]			Specific amino acids		Bolotin et al., 1999
	DtpT	51		Hydrophilic di- and tripeptides		Hagting et al., 1994
	DtpP			Hydrophobic di- and tripeptides		Foucaud et al., 1995
	Opp	~200 kDa Complex[d]	Complex[d]	Peptides of 4 to up to 18 amino acid residues		Tynkkynen et al., 1993
Endopeptidases	PepF1	70	1		M	Monnet et al., 1994
	PepF2	70				Nardi et al., 1997
	PepO1	71.5	1		M	Mierau et al., 1993
	PepO2	71.8				Hellendoorn et al., 1999
Aminopeptidases	PepN	95	1	X↓(X)n	M	Van Alen-Boerrigter et al., 1991
	PepC	50	6	X↓(X)n	C	Chapot-Chartier et al., 1993
	PepT	46	2	X↓X-X	M	Mierau et al., 1994
	PepV	49	2	X↓X	M	Hellendoorn et al., 1997
Pro-specific peptidases	PepX	88	2	X-Pro↓(X)n	S	Mayo et al., 1991
	PepQ	40	1	X↓Pro	M	Hellendoorn et al., 1999
	PepP	46	1	X↓Pro-(X)n	M	Matos et al., 1998
Special task peptidases	PepA	38	3/6	Glu↓X	M	l'Anson et al., 1995
	Pcp	23		Pyr–Glu↓X	C	Buist et al., 1999
Signal peptidase	LspL	17		Signal peptides of lipoproteins	A	Genbank ref. U63724

[a]Quaternary structure: 1, monomer; 2, dimer; 3, trimer; 6, hexamer.
[b]Cleavage sites are indicated by arrows; for details on the actual nature of X, see text.
[c]Amino acid transporters. No classification has been made.
[d]Opp consists of the proteins OppA. B, C, D, and F; ClpP and DnaK form active complexes with their respective chaperones (see text).
[e]Deduced from the nucleotide sequences.
[f]S, serine peptidase; M, metallo peptidase; C, cysteine peptidase; A, aspartic proteinase.

Proteinases

The first step in casein degradation by *Lc. lactis* is performed by the extracellular proteinase PrtP, which because of its importance in cellular growth as well as the performance of the starter in cheese production, has been the prime subject of many investigations during the last twenty years or so. These analyses were biochemical, enzymological as well as immunological, and genetic in nature and, together, have given a quite complete picture of what is happening in the first stage of the protein breakdown pathway of *Lc. lactis*.

General Characteristics of PrtP

The mature proteinase PrtP of *Lc. lactis* is a large cell-surface-located enzyme. C-terminally truncated active forms of 135–190 kDa can be isolated upon incubation of cells in a Ca^{2+}-free buffer, which leads to the loss of weakly bound Ca- ions and exposure of a site susceptible to autoproteolysis (Exterkate and Alting, 1999; for a review, see Exterkate, 1995). C-terminally truncated forms of the enzyme have also been made by genetic techniques, and proteinase variants with deletions of up to at least the last 130 amino acid residues are active and are secreted into the medium (Kok et al., 1988; see below). PrtP is a typical serine proteinase and is inhibited by PMSF and DFP, while Ca^{2+} ions stabilize the enzyme and, at high concentrations, are inhibitory.

β-Casein Degradation and Proteinase Classification

Different ways of classifying lactococcal proteinases have been proposed in the past (for reviews, see Kok, 1990; Kok and de Vos, 1994) but classification on the basis of their caseinolytic specificity has received most attention, mostly because it is reliable and rapid. The substrate specificity of lactococcal proteinases is a major factor in determining the nature of the casein degradation products. These degradation products, in turn, determine the growth of the organism in milk and, ultimately, contribute to flavor development in cheese. Thus, many studies deal with the caseinolytic specificity of the lactococcal proteinases. The PrtPs of strains Wg2 and SK11 represent two extremes in proteinase cleavage specificity as defined by their degradation patterns of α_{S1}-, β-, and κ-casein (Visser et al., 1986). The PrtP of strain Wg2 exhibits PI-type cleavage specificity (PrtPI), while that of strain SK11 is a PIII-type enzyme (PrtPIII). PrtPI-type enzymes preferentially cleave β-casein and hardly cleave α_{s1}- and κ-casein, while PrtPIII degrades α_{S1}-, κ-, and β-casein with a specificity different from that of PrtPI (Visser et al., 1986; Bockelmann et al., 1989).

In an extensive study, the action of proteinases from 16 different *Lc. lactis* strains was tested on the model substrate α_{S1}-CN(f1-23), allowing a refinement of the lactococcal proteinase classification and the definition of seven specificity groups (Exterkate et al., 1993). It is clear from these studies, combined with the genetic data (see below), that minor changes in the amino acid sequence of the various natural PrtP variants are the cause of the small differences in the casein breakdown specificity between the enzymes.

By liquid chromatography combined with Edman degradation and/or amino acid composition analysis of purified peptides a rough first indication of *in vitro* casein hydrolysis by purified proteinases was obtained (Monnet et al., 1986, 1989, 1992; Visser et al., 1988, 1991; Reid et al., 1991a,b). In these studies, the focus was mainly on the larger fragments produced. A thorough investigation of β-casein degradation by purified PrtPI from *Lc. lactis* Wg2 was performed using liquid chromatography in combination with on-line ion-spray mass spectrometry (Juillard et al., 1995a). More than 95% of the produced fragments were recovered in this study, which revealed that PrtPI degrades β-casein into over 100 different oligopeptides ranging in size from 4 to up to 30 amino acid residues. Eighteen of the oligopeptides were 4–8 residues in size and contained all 20 amino acids. Amino acids (except traces of Phe) and di- and tripeptides were not produced at detectable levels. As was observed in earlier studies, most of the peptides produced originate from the C-terminus of β-casein.

The degradation into major products of α_{S1}-, and κ-casein has been investigated for several enzymes but either HPLC analysis or SDS-PAGE has identified only major products (Reid et al., 1991a, 1994; Monnet et al., 1992; Visser et al., 1994). A large number of small oligopeptides were found as a result of cleavage by the enzymes at both identical and unique bonds.

The lactococcal proteinase PrtP appears from all of the studies cited above to be an enzyme with very broad substrate specificity and, although certain bonds in casein seem to be preferentially hydrolyzed, a clear consensus cleavage site cannot be defined. This may be in part caused by the enzyme itself but may also be due to the fact that in all studies the natural substrate caseins were used. These proteins are highly flexible in solution with many solvent accessible sites (Holt and Sawyer, 1988).

Genetics of PrtP

Early observation of instability of the proteolytic phenotype in *Lc. lactis* can be explained now by the fact that in many strains, but not all (Nissen-Meyer et al., 1992), the gene for the proteinase *prtP* is located on plasmids (for reviews, see McKay, 1983; Kok and Venema, 1988). The *prtP* genes of several lactococcal strains have been cloned, sequenced, and analyzed (Kok et al., 1985, 1988; Kiwaki et al., 1989; Vos et al., 1989a). The genetic analyses revealed that the primary *prtP* translation products of strains Wg2 and NCDO763 are 1902 amino acid residues and, thus, are much larger than the active mature enzymes isolated from cells. The primary product of the *prtP* gene of strain SK11 is even larger (1962 residues) as it contains a 60-amino-acid-duplication in the C-terminus. The proteinases are initially produced as pre–pro-enzymes with a 33-amino-acids-signal sequence followed by 154 amino acids that constitute the pro-region. They are post-translationally shortened to the mature, active form. Upstream of all *prtP* genes sequenced so far, a gene is present that specifies a 33 kDa PrtP maturation protein, PrtM (Haandrikman et al., 1989; Vos et al., 1989b). PrtM is a lipoprotein that, after glyceride-fatty-acid-modification of the Cys22 residue and cleavage by signal peptidase II, is anchored to the cell membrane (Haandrikman et al., 1991). Recently, we have cloned and sequenced the gene for this peptidase and have shown that it is the only activity present in *Lc. lactis* MG1363 capable of processing PrtM (unpublished results). PrtM is homologous to PrsA of *B. subtilis* (Jacobs et al., 1993) and to PpiC, the peptidyl–propyl *cis/trans* isomerase of *E. coli* (for a review, see Rudd et al., 1995). Cells carrying an intact copy of *prtP* but lacking *prtM* produce an inactive proteinase that is larger than when *prtM* is present (de Vos et al., 1991; Haandrikman et al., 1991). PrtM is believed to play a role as an extracellular chaperone, inducing the pro-proteinase to adopt a conformation in which it is able to autoproteolytically cleave off the pro-region (for a review, see Kok, 1990).

The three lactococcal proteinases mentioned above are over 98% identical and, through amino acid sequence alignments, were shown to belong to the subtilases, a superfamily of subtilisin-like proteinases (Kok et al., 1988; Vos et al., 1989a; Siezen and Leunissen, 1997).

The regions around the amino acid residues constituting the active site (Asp30, His94, and Ser433) are especially well conserved, as is the essential Asn196 of the oxyanion hole. The substrate binding regions identified in the subtilases are also conserved (Kok et al., 1988; Vos et al., 1989a; Siezen et al., 1991, 1993). The PrtPI and PrtPIII enzymes produced by the strains Wg2 and SK11, respectively, differ in only 44 of the over 1900 amino acid residues. These differences, then, should determine the observed differences in the caseinolytic specificities of the two proteinases. By constructing hybrids of the PrtPI and PrtPIII enzymes, the differences between the two proteinases could be limited to only a few amino acid substitutions located mostly in the substrate binding cleft (Vos et al., 1991). Engineering of single or multiple residues confirmed that major changes occur as a result of small variations in the substrate binding region of PrtP (Siezen et al., 1993; Bruinenberg et al., 1994).

PrtP Is a Multi-Domain Enzyme

PrtP and a number of cell-envelope proteinases of other LAB have been compared by multiple sequence alignment, secondary structure prediction, and data base homology searches (Siezen, 1999). PrtP appears to have a modular, multi-domain structure (see Figure 7.1). The N-terminus contains the pre–pro domain involved in secretion and activation (see above) and the active site domain with a dispensable so-called I domain of 130–150 residues of unknown function. The first of two large middle domains of unknown function may be involved in the regulation of proteolytic activity and/or specificity of the

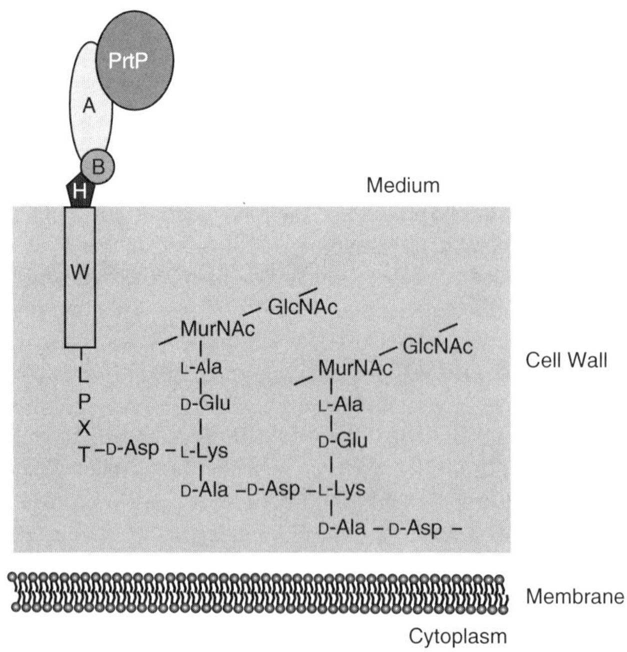

Figure 7.1. Schematic presentation of the sorting of the extracellular lactococcal proteinase PrtP after cleavage of the C-terminal LPXTG motif in the extreme C-terminal of the protein. PrtP is indicated in blocks symbolizing the different domains, as defined by Siezen (1999). The active mature proteinase is shown, devoid of its pre–pro region: W, cell wall anchor domain; H, helical spacer domain; A, B, middle domains A and B, respectively; PrtP, proteinase domain with active site region and (not indicated) insert domain. Only part of the peptidoglycan is enlarged: GlcNac, *N*-acetyl-glucosamine; MurNac, *N*-acetyl-muramic acid.

catalytic domain, while the second domain probably contains a Ca-binding site and may play a role in stabilization of the catalytic domain. The C-terminal part of PrtP consists of a helical spacer domain that may function in positioning the more N-terminal domains away from the cell surface, a hydrophilic Gly/Thr/Asp-rich cell wall spacer or attachment domain that may span the peptidoglycan layer, and, lastly, a cell wall anchor domain. The cell wall spacer domain is duplicated in PrtPIII of *Lc. lactis* SK11 suggesting that this proteinase may be placed further outward of the cell. The cell wall anchor domain of PrtP contains the pentapeptide LPXTG that is conserved among surface proteins of Gram-positive bacteria, followed by a hydrophobic putative membrane spanning α-helix and a small charged tail (Haandrikman et al., 1989; Vos et al., 1989a; Navarre and Schneewind, 1994). In analogy to the events in the other Gram-positive examples, the LPXTG sorting signal of PrtP is thought to be cleaved after translocation between the Thr and Gly residues. Subsequently, an amide-bond is formed between the carboxyl group of the Thr and the amino acid(s) of the peptide cross-bridge of the peptidoglycan (Navarre and Schneewind, 1994). Recently, the gene encoding the sortase SrtA of *Staphylococcus aureus*, a transpeptidase that performs this coupling reaction, has been cloned and sequenced (Sarkis et al., 1999). Proper cell wall sorting also seems to occur in *Lc. lactis* and a number of other LAB, as was evidenced by the cell wall anchoring of the *Strep. pyogenes* M6 protein in these organisms (Piard et al., 1997). As a consequence of the above it can now be understood that, upon removal of the C-terminus of PrtP by autoproteolysis or by genetic means, the truncated proteinase is secreted into the medium (Kok et al., 1988).

Other Proteinases in *Lc. lactis*

Apart from the "caseinase" PrtP, several other proteinases have been identified in *Lc. lactis*, either as enzyme activities or on the basis of homologies with known proteinases. Especially in the last category, a number of new putative activities have been discovered in the genome of *Lc. lactis* IL1403. As these will and cannot be treated here in detail, the reader is referred to the paper by Bolotin et al. (1999) describing the annotated diagnostic nucleotide sequence of the chromosome of this lactococcal strain. The proteinases to be described now have more general (stress-related) functions in protein turnover and recycling of native proteins, or are very specific enzymes needed for the maturation of bacteriocins and do not play a (major) role in casein utilization.

HtrA

Until recently, PrtP and NisP were thought to be the only extracellular lactococcal proteinases. The degradation of various secreted fusion proteins from a PrtP-negative strain of *Lc. lactis* pointed to the existence of another extracellular proteinase (Poquet et al., 2000). Using the conserved domains of the HtrA protease family an HtrA/DegP homologue was identified in the genome sequence of IL1403 (Poquet et al., 2000). The lactococcal HtrA homologue of 408 amino acid residues is a typical HtrA trypsin-like serine proteinase containing the Ser, His, and Asp catalytic triad. HtrA is predicted to be a membrane-bound enzyme with most of the protein, including the active site, exposed to the cell surface. An *htrA* insertion mutant is thermo-sensitive for growth, which is consistent with a role in heat shock response and in survival at high temperatures. Degradation of several secreted proteins and of cell-surface-associated fusion proteins consisting of the *S. aureus* nuclease and lactococcal export signals, as normally observed in an *Lc. lactis* wild-type strain, was completely abolished in the *htrA* mutant. Degradation of the fusion proteins occurred only at the cell surface. The HtrA protein is also involved in pro-peptide processing and maturation of *S. aureus* nuclease and in cleavage of the C-terminal repeats of the cell-surface-located lactococcal autolysin AcmA. In conclusion, HtrA is a unique housekeeping surface proteinase of *Lc. lactis*, which degrades fusion proteins and cell-surface-located or secreted misfolded proteins (Poquet et al., 2000).

The milk protein β-casein is a good substrate for the *E. coli* HtrA homologues DegP and DegQ (Waller and Saver, 1996). Degradation of partly unfolded β-casein was recently shown to be temperature dependent while this was not the case for fully unfolded β-casein (Kim et al., 1999). These data suggest that the lactococcal HtrA protein may also be involved in the release of peptides from milk protein. If this would be the case, HtrA is not capable of releasing enough peptides for nutrition, as PrtP-minus strains do not grow in milk (see above). Nevertheless, HtrA activity could lead to production of specific (flavor) peptides.

Clp

In a general response to stress, prokaryotic and eukaryotic cells synthesize a complex of chaperones and proteinases known as the Clp complex (*c*aseino*l*ytic *p*rotease; Katayama et al., 1988). The chaperones assist in the proper (re)folding or assembly of proteins, while the proteinases degrade the proteins that cannot be refolded. In *E. coli*, the ClpP proteinase can associate with specific chaperones to form the Clp proteolytic complex. By itself, ClpP has only peptidase activity, but when it is associated with other proteins of the Clp family, the resulting complex has serine proteinase activity (Maurizi et al., 1990). Isolation of a protein induced 3-fold at pH 5 identified the lactococcal homologue of *E. coli* ClpP (Frees and Ingmer, 1999). Lactococcal *clpP* expression was also induced by heat and by the t-RNA analogue puromycin. Induction was at the translational level. A disruption mutant was more sensitive to heat and puromycin and synthesized elevated levels of DnaK, GroEL, GroES, and Hsp-85 at 30°C. Recently the genes for the Clp proteins B, C, and E have been cloned from *Lc. lactis* MG1363 (Ingmer et al., 1999). All proteins contain two conserved ATP binding domains. Based on phylogenetic analyses, ClpE was placed into a new Clp family (ClpE). Transcription of *clpB* and *clpE* is induced tenfold by heat shock, while that of *clpC* is only moderately induced. Single mutants of *clpB*, *clpC*, or *clpE* were as tolerant of heat and salt as the wild type. While the *clpE* mutant was more sensitive to puromycin, an antibiotic which causes premature termination of translation resulting in the synthesis of truncated, randomly folded proteins, both *clpB* and *clpC* strains were slightly more resistant to the antibiotic. It was proposed (Ingmer et al., 1999) that ClpE recognizes truncated or partly folded proteins leading to subsequent degradation by the ClpP protease. This would agree with the notion that a *clpP* mutant is also sensitive to puromycin. The lactococcal *clpA* homologue *clpL* is located on a transposon (Huang et al., 1993) and seems not to be present in all lactococcal strains (Coward et al., 1995). All of these data indicate that *Lc. lactis* also produces intracellular proteinases specifically involved in the degradation of misfolded proteins.

DnaK

DnaK is the bacterial member of the widespread, highly conserved Hsp70 family of 70 kDa heat-shock-induced chaperone proteins. *E. coli* DnaK cooperates with DnaJ and GrpE in a chaperone complex that plays an important role in the folding of nascent protein chains under normal growth conditions, and in the refolding of proteins after thermal damage. The DnaK/DnaJ/GrpE complex participates in ATP-dependent proteolysis in the cell (for reviews see Bukau, 1993; Gross, 1996; Mayhew and Hartl, 1996). The genes for the chaperones DnaK, DnaJ, GrpE, GroEL, and GroES have all been identified in *Lc. lactis*. Also, the response to heat shock of *Lc. lactis* was shown to be similar to that of other bacteria. The temporal induction patterns suggest that the heat shock proteins of *Lc. lactis* are part of more than one induction class. DnaK, GroEL, and GroES are also induced during salt stress (Whitaker and Batt, 1991; Arnau et al., 1996; Kilstrup et al., 1997). An *Lc. lactis dnaK* mutant was temperature sensitive for growth and contained elevated levels of other heat shock proteins at 30°C (Koch et al., 1998). From the available data it seems reasonable to assume that a functional heat-shock-induced proteolytic DnaK/DnaJ/GrpE complex is also operative in *Lc. lactis*.

Proteinases Involved in Bacteriocin Maturation

Nisin is a modified antimicrobial peptide produced by a limited number of strains of *Lc. lactis* (see Chapter 8). The bacteriocin is encoded by a large operon, *nisABTCIPRKFEG* of which the sixth gene encodes an extracellular endopeptidase, NisP, involved in the cleavage of the nisin precursor molecule into its active form (van der Meer et al., 1993). NisP belongs to the subtilase family of serine proteinases and is initially produced as a pre–pro-protein of 682 amino acid residues. Deletion of *nisP* from the nisin gene cluster resulted in the secretion of a fully modified, inactive precursor with the leader sequence still attached to the N-terminus. NisP is specifically needed for nisin processing and is not necessary for growth in milk. No data are available about its possible contribution to casein degradation.

The proteins LcnC, LagD, and PedD are all examples of ATP-binding cassette (ABC) transporters (Higgins, 1992). They are large integral membrane proteins and aid in conjunction with so-called accessory proteins in the secretion of linear unmodified (Class II) bacteriocins produced by certain strains of LAB (Havarstein et al., 1995; Venema et al., 1995; Franke et al., 1999) Apart from having a transporter function, the proteins carry an enlargement at their N-termini that is not present in other ABC transporters. This domain in the three transporters has been shown to be involved in the processing and activation of the inactive precursor forms of their respective bacteriocins. A His-tagged truncated form of LagD comprising the first 150 amino acids of the protein was able to cleave bacteriocin precursor *in vitro* (Havarstein et al., 1995). Pre-bacteriocin processing was observed *in vivo* in *E. coli* (using a truncated form of PedD encompassing the first 172 amino acids) as well as in *Lc. lactis* (expressing the 164-amino-acids N-terminus of LcnC). In both cases, the active bacteriocin remained inside the cell (Venema et al., 1995; Franke et al., 1999). Processing entails the cleavage of a conserved leader peptide from the N-terminus of the bacteriocin precursor. The leader peptide and processing site, with a conserved glycine doublet at positions −1 and −2, do not follow the rules of von Heijne (1983) for signal peptides required for *sec*-dependent protein export, which fits the above finding of a dedicated pathway of bacteriocin secretion. The N-termini of the bacteriocin transporters share two conserved motifs, one of which contained a conserved cysteine. Replacement of that Cys residue by Ala completely destroyed leader-specific proteolytic cleavage. Thus, LcnC, LagD, and PedD were placed in a new family of cysteine proteinases (Havarstein et al., 1995).

Peptide Uptake Systems of *Lc. lactis*

As we have seen above, the products from casein degradation by PrtP are oligopeptides with a size from 4 to up to at least 30 amino acid residues. Apart from traces of Phe, amino acids are not produced from β-casein. Also, free amino acids are found in only minor amounts in fresh milk. Nevertheless, when confronted with amino acids (for instance, in a chemically defined medium [CDM]), lactococci can internalize them using an array of at least 10 different amino acid transport systems with a high specificity for structurally similar amino acids (for an extensive review, see Konings et al., 1989). Studies of peptide transport across the cytoplasmic membrane of *Lc. lactis* have revealed that the organism possesses at least three distinct peptide transporters, which will be discussed now.

Uptake of Di- and Tripeptides

Di- and tripeptides are transported across the cytoplasmic membrane of *Lc. lactis* by two distinct systems.

Relatively hydrophilic peptide substrates are internalized via a proton motive force-driven transport mechanism of which the gene, *dtpT*, has been cloned via complementation of an *E. coli proC* mutant (Smid et al., 1989; Hagting et al., 1994). DtpT catalyses the uptake of di- and tripeptides in symport with a proton(s) and belongs to the widely distributed peptide transport family (PTR), examples of which are found in other microorganisms, in plants, as well as in rat and human intestines (Steiner et al., 1995). A detailed kinetic analysis of lactococcal DtpT revealed that, for high-affinity interaction with DtpT, the peptides need to have free amino and carboxyl termini, *trans*-peptide bonds, and the residues should be in the L-configuration (Fang et al., 2000). Peptides longer than three residues do not interact with DtpT, making the transporter more restrictive in its substrate recognition than the eukaryotic homologues.

The presence of a second di- and tripeptide transport system in *Lc. lactis* was discovered using a mutant devoid of Opp (the oligopeptide transport system; see below) and DtpT (Foucaud et al., 1995). The specificity of this system (DtpP) partially overlaps that of DtpT. DtpP preferentially transports di- and tripeptides that are composed of hydrophobic (branched-chain amino acid) residues, while DtpT has a higher specificity for more hydrophilic and charged peptides. Like DtpT, DtpP does not transport amino acids or oligopeptides. The toxic peptide analogue L-phenylalanyl-β-chloro-L-alanine (FCA) was used to isolate a DtpP-negative (FCA^R) mutant in a strain that already lacked DtpT. The *dtpT dtpP* double mutant had completely lost all di- and tripeptide transport activity (Foucaud et al., 1995). Inhibition of dtpP by *o*-vanadate indicates that ATP or a related energy-rich phosphorylated intermediate drives DtpP.

Uptake of Peptides Larger than Three Amino Acid Residues

Oligopeptides are taken up by *Lc. lactis* via an ATP-driven transport system (Kunji et al., 1993). The genes encoding this transport system (Opp, for oligopeptide permease) have been cloned and sequenced (Tynkkynen et al., 1993). Opp is encoded by an operon of five genes (*oppDFBCA*) that is immediately followed by the gene for an oligopeptidase, *pepO* (see below). The five *opp* genes encode proteins that are typical for binding protein-dependent transport systems and the permease belongs to the ABC superfamily as defined by Higgins (1992). OppA is a membrane-bound peptide-binding lipoprotein that, like prtM, has been shown to be processed by LspL, the lactococcal signal peptidase II (our unpublished results). It serves as a receptor protein that delivers the oligopeptides to the membrane-bound translocator complex constituted by the other proteins OppB, OppC, OppD, and OppF. OppB and OppC are highly hydrophobic, contain six putative membrane-spanning α-helices each, and probably form the channel that facilitates the translocation of the oligopeptides across the cytoplasmic membrane. OppD and OppF show homology to the ATP-binding protein (domains) of the ABC superfamily and, most likely, couple ATP hydrolysis to the transport process. The Opp system of *Lc. lactis* can transport oligopeptides containing 4 to up to at least 18 amino acid residues with little specificity for particular side chains (Tynkkynen et al., 1993; Detmers et al., 1998). In a strain overproducing OppA eightfold, the rate of uptake of bradykinin (Arg–Pro–Pro–Gly–Phe–Ser–Pro–Phe–Arg) increased only 40% indicating that transport of this peptide is not greatly rate-determined by OppA activity (Picon et al., 2000). Kinetic analysis of peptide binding to OppA revealed a direct relationship between the oligopeptide dissociation constant and the length of the peptide. These results and data from analyses of pre-steady-state kinetics of binding suggest that the slow dissociation rate constants for the larger peptides are rate determining in the translocation of the peptide across the cytoplasmic membrane (Lanfermeijer et al., 1999). Transport of oligopeptides by Opp is proposed to take place via four kinetically distinguishable steps: (a) binding of the peptide to the binding protein OppA; (b) docking of the OppA-peptide complex to the membrane complex OppBC(DF); (c) donation of the oligopeptide to the membrane complex; and (d) translocation of the peptide across the membrane (Lanfermeijer et al., 1999). In conclusion, the rate of transport of oligopeptides in *Lc. lactis* seems to be determined to a large extent by the donation of the peptides from the OppA protein to the translocator complex.

Peptidases of *Lc. lactis*

Lc. lactis does not produce extracellular peptidases that play a major direct role in casein breakdown, apart from the proteinase PrtP, an endopeptidase by definition. The casein breakdown products liberated by PrtP and internalized by Opp are degraded in the cytoplasm by an array of different peptidases. The full peptidase complement of *Lc. lactis* of over 12 enzymes, as we shall see below, can be sub-divided into two major groups according to their hydrolytic activity. The endopeptidases degrade their substrate from within the peptide while the aminopeptidases liberate either one or two amino acids from a free N-terminus of a peptide. Enzymes that degrade peptides from their C-terminus (carboxypeptidases) have not been described in *Lc. lactis*, although such enzymes are present: a homologue of *B. subtilis* DacA, a very specific enzyme with d-alanyl-d-alanine carboxypeptidase activity, was identified in the genome sequence of *Lc. lactis* IL1403 (Bolotin et al., 1999). A good deal of information concerning peptidases of *Lc. lactis* had been gathered by biochemical means halfway through the 1980s, but the cloning and further analysis of peptidase genes and their products in the ensuing years have rapidly expanded our knowledge of peptidolysis. The latter developments will be discussed below.

Endopeptidases

As we have seen above, the Opp system internalizes the casein-derived oligopeptides produced by PrtP. Interestingly, the *opp* operon specifying this transporter is followed by a gene for an oligopeptidase, PepO (Mierau et al., 1993). The gene for PepO was cloned using an antibody raised against the purified enzyme. PepO is a 71.5 kDa protein that shows 37% overall similarity to mammalian neutral endopeptidase (enkephalinase; EC 3.4.24.11). A stretch of 42 amino acids of higher similarity (72% identity) contains the His-Glu-Xxx-Xxx-Glu motif characteristic of zinc-dependent metallopeptidases as well as the putative active site of the enzyme. A gene for an enzyme with 88% amino acid sequence identity to PepO has been identified in *Lc. lactis* and was named PepO2. PepO2 is slightly larger than PepO and can be visualized as a slightly slower migrating protein band in Western blot analysis using polyclonal antibodies raised against PepO (Hellendoorn et al., 1999).

The genes of two other oligopeptidases, PepF1 and PepF2, have been cloned and sequenced. One of the genes, formerly named *pepF* and later renamed *pepF1* (Monnet et al., 1994; Nardi et al., 1997) is located on the 55-kb lactose/proteinase plasmid of *Lc. lactis* subsp. *cremoris* NCDO763. It is also present in the chromosome of *Lc. lactis* subsp. *lactis* IL1403. Subsequently, from biochemical and genetic evidence it was inferred that a second PepF-like enzyme was present in the strain under study. The gene was cloned and sequenced and coined *pepF2*. PepF1 and PepF2 are 84% identical. The identity is especially high in the region comprising the zinc-binding motif (91% identity in a stretch of 45 amino acids) and in an area in which both proteins show homology with creatine and arginine kinase. Not only are the proteins very similar, also their genes are 80% identical. The fact that *pepF2* on the chromosome of strain NCDO763 and the chromosomal copy of *pepF1* in strain IL1403 are 80% identical agrees with the divergence observed between genes of the two subspecies *cremoris* and *lactis* (Godon et al., 1992). The fact that the chromosomal gene in strain IL1403 (*pepF1*) is almost identical to *pepF1* on the plasmid gene in strain NCDO763 suggests a recent transfer of the genes between the two subspecies. Although the mechanism of transfer is not known, the presence of two different IS elements upstream and downstream of *pepF1* on the plasmid of NCDO763 is suggestive of IS-directed mobilization of *pepF1* from the chromosome to the plasmid. Subsequently, the gene could have been transferred to different strains such as NCDO763, as the lactose/proteinase plasmid of this strain is conjugative (Gasson, 1990).

Exopeptidases

Exopeptidases are enzymes that degrade a peptide substrate from its extremities. Carboxypeptidases have not been reported in *Lc. lactis* so far, leaving the aminopeptidases, which hydrolyze (oligo)peptides from a free amino terminus, to be discussed here. Over 10 different enzyme activities have been described in the literature and several thorough investigations of the biochemical properties of the various enzymes have been published (for reviews covering this subject, see Kok, 1990; Pritchard and Coolbear, 1993; Kok and de Vos, 1994; Kunji et al., 1996a). In what follows an overview will be given with an emphasis on the genetic characterization of the peptidase genes. For more details on the biochemistry of the enzymes, the reader is referred to the original literature that can also be found in the reviews cited above. The aminopeptidases will be treated in two major but rather arbitrary subgroups, namely the general aminopeptidases of which most, but not all, have broad substrate specificity and the proline-specific peptidases.

General Aminopeptidases

General aminopeptidases are common in *Lc. lactis* and were among the first enzymes to be examined in the species. Most of the general aminopeptidases have a broad substrate specificity: they degrade amino acyl-*para*-nitroanilide labelled substrates and a wide variety of di-, tri-, tetra-, and/or oligopeptides. Most of the enzymes are metalloenzymes and are inhibited by EDTA.

Aminopeptidase N. The genes encoding the aminopeptidases N from *Lc. lactis* subsp. *cremoris* strains MG1363 and Wg2 have been cloned and sequenced and shown to differ in only a few nucleotides (van Alen-Boerrigter et al., 1991; Strøman, 1992; Tan et al., 1992). *Lc. lactis* PepN belongs to a family of eukaryotic and bacterial zinc-metalloenzymes (EC 3.4.11.2) that includes aminopeptidase N from human, rat, rabbit, pig, mouse, and *E. coli*. A stretch of 750 residues in the C-terminus shows 27% identity with mammalian aminopeptidase N. Multiple sequence alignments revealed six regions in *Lc. lactis* PepN with significantly higher sequence similarity to the mammalian enzymes. In addition, one of these regions in rat aminopeptidase N (corresponding to amino acids 281–301 in PepN of *Lc. lactis*) shows homology with the active site and an essential Zn-ion binding site of thermolysin, a zinc-dependent neutral proteinase.

The deduced molecular weight of PepN of 95.368 is in good agreement with the experimentally determined value of 95.000 (Tan and Konings, 1990; Tan et al., 1992). PepN is most probably active as a monomer and the homology with thermolysin agrees with the observation that PepN is irreversibly inactivated by EDTA and, thus, should be classified as a metallopeptidase. PepN has a very broad substrate specificity, liberating the N-terminal amino acid from di- and tripeptides as well as larger oligopeptides. As we shall see below, PepN plays a major role in the degradation of bitter peptides that can occur during the cheese making process.

Aminopeptidase C. Aminopeptidase C (PepC) is a thiol aminopeptidase and the enzyme from *Lc. lactis* was the first prokaryotic protein of this class to be characterized and cloned (Neviani et al., 1989; Chapot-Chartier et al., 1993). The enzyme is inhibited by the sulfhydryl-group inhibitors iodoacetamide, *N*-ethylmaleimide and *p*-chloromercuric benzoic acid. Biochemical and preliminary X-ray crystallography data show that PepC is a hexameric protein composed of identical subunits of 436 amino acid residues (Neviani et al., 1989; Mistou et al., 1994). PepC is a strict aminopeptidase with a broad substrate specificity: it accepts all residues except Pro in the N-terminal position, hydrolyses β-NA and *p*-nitroanilide substituted amino acids and liberates N-terminal amino acids from peptides and proteins (Neviani et al., 1989; Mistou and Gripon, 1998).

The gene encoding PepC of *Lc. lactis* subsp. *cremoris* AM2 has been sequenced (Chapot-Chartier et al., 1993). PepC shows homology with cysteine proteinases such as papain, aleurin, and cathepsin B and H in only two regions encompassing the active site residues. A region of 16 amino acids in PepC contains the active site Cys residue (Cys25 of papain) and a Gln residue that is conserved in papain. A second region of 35 amino acids in PepC contains properly spaced equivalents of the catalytic site residues Asn-175, Trp-177, and His-159 of papain. The highest similarity was observed between PepC and eukaryotic bleomycin hydrolases, and on the basis of sequence similarities as well as common biochemical and enzymatic properties, they were placed in a new family of thiol aminopeptidases among the cysteine peptidases (Chapot-Chartier et al., 1994b). Structural model comparisons between PepC and yeast bleomycin hydrolase suggested that the C-terminus of PepC partially occupies the active site cleft (Mata et al., 1997, 1999). By deleting the four C-terminal residues (Gly432–Ala433–Leu434–Ala435) the aminopeptidase specificity was completely abolished. The truncated form of PepC (PepCΔ432–435) possesses an extended substrate binding site that can accommodate four residues at each side of the bond to be cleaved and, in contrast to full-length PepC, is sensitive to the thiolpeptidase inhibitors leupeptin and E64. Thus, PepCΔ432–435 has properties of an endopeptidase from the papain family (Mata et al., 1997, 1999).

Narrow Specificity Aminopeptidases. Two narrow spectrum aminopeptidases have been described in *Lc. lactis*. Aminopeptidase A (PepA) is a metallopeptidase highly specific for glutamyl and aspartyl residues on the N-terminal of di- and tripeptides and of larger peptides (Exterkate and de Veer, 1987; Niven, 1991; Bacon et al., 1994). The N-terminal sequence of purified PepA was used to clone the gene using degenerate primers (l'Anson et al., 1995). The deduced product contained 353 amino acid residues (molecular weight 38.1 kDa) and is apparently active as a trimer of 130.000 molecular weight, although this point is still not fully solved (Exterkate and de Veer, 1987; Niven, 1991; Baankreis, 1992). PepA has 30% identity in a stretch of 294 amino acids with an endoglucanase of *Clostridium thermocellum* (l'Anson et al., 1995).

Pyrrolidone carboxyl peptidase (Pcp) is able to cleave off pyroglutamyl residues from the N-terminus of peptides and has been partly purified from *Lc. lactis* (Exterkate, 1977; Baankreis, 1992). Measuring Pcp activity in cell-free extracts using L-pyroglutamyl *p*-nitroanilide as the substrate is hindered by the presence in lactococcal strains of an amidase activity that degrades this substrate (Buist et al., unpublished results). The gene encoding Pcp has been cloned and sequenced from *Lc. lactis* MG1363 using degenerate primers based on the known amino acid sequences of Pcp from *B. subtilis* and *Strep. pneumoniae* (Buist et al., 1999). The gene has an unusually high G + C content (46.8% vs. 35.4% for the *Lc. lactis* average). The presence of an IS element upstream of *pcp* in several strains of *Lc. lactis*, together with the occurrence of repeated DNA sequences in the immediate vicinity of the gene that are widespread among lactococci, are suggestive of horizontal transfer of *pcp* into *Lc. lactis*. Notwithstanding this, *pcp* is not present in all strains of *Lc. lactis*, as was shown by Southern blot analyses, and is not or only very poorly expressed in *Lc. lactis* MG1363 and other strains, as evidenced by Western blotting using antibodies directed against Pcp from *Strep. pyogenes*. Active Pcp was obtained in *E. coli* and *Lc. lactis* by placing the gene under the control of inducible promoters (Buist et al., 1999). Pcp of *Lc. lactis* shows high sequence similarity to the Pcps of other microorganisms and a number of amino acid residues that have been shown to be essential for catalytic activity (Cys-144, His-166) and stability (Glu-81, Asp-89, Asp-94) of Pcp from *Pseudomonas fluorescens* are all conserved in the lactococcal enzyme. *Lc. lactis* Pcp has a deduced molecular size of 23.135 kDa and may be active as a multimer (Exterkate, 1977; Baankreis, 1992), although the biochemical data are conflicting in this respect. X-ray studies of Pcp from *B. amyloliquefaciens* and *Thermococcus litoralis* have shown that these two enzymes are homo-tetramers (Odagaki et al., 1999; Singleton et al., 1999). Pcps constitute a new class of cysteine proteinases.

Dipeptidases

Broad-specificity dipeptide hydrolysing activities have been described in and purified to homogeneity from several strains of *Lc. lactis* (Hwang et al., 1981, 1982; van Boven et al., 1988). The gene for a dipeptidase from *Lc. lactis* MG1363, PepV, has been cloned by complementation of a peptidase-negative *E. coli* strain (Hellendoorn et al., 1997). PepV was expressed in *E. coli* as a 50 kDa protein that reacted with monoclonal antibodies directed against the dipeptidase from strain Wg2 (Laan et al., 1996) and was catalytically active. It hydrolyzed a broad range of dipeptides but no tri-, tetra-, or larger oligopeptides. Dipeptides with Pro, His, Gly, or Glu as the N-terminal amino acid, or dipeptides with Pro in the second position are not degraded (van Boven et al., 1988). PepV is a metallopeptidase that is severely inhibited by EDTA and 1,10-phenanthroline. The deduced molecular size of PepV, 52 kDa (472 amino acid residues), is in accordance with that determined for the purified protein (49 kDa). The enzyme is most probably active as a monomer. PepV showed highest sequence similarity with the carnosinase PepV of *Lb. delbrueckii* subsp. *lactis* DSM7290 and, accordingly, was also able to degrade β-alanyl-leucine (carnosine). Both PepVs have 45.7% identical and 12.3% similar amino acids (Hellendoorn et al., 1997). Two signature sequences of the ArgE/*DapE*/ACY1/CPG2/*YscS* family of proteins are present in both PepVs. The first sequence contains a conserved His residue possibly involved in metal ion binding while the second sequence contains a number of conserved charged residues. Alignment with DapE of *E. coli* and *Haemophilus influenzae* only revealed two additional stretches of high sequence similarity, the significance of which is unknown to date.

Tripeptidases

The tripeptidase PepT from *Lc. lactis* has been purified to homogeniety (Bosman et al., 1990; Bacon et al., 1993). The gene specifying PepT from *Lc. lactis* MG1363 has been cloned by reverse genetics using the N-terminal amino acid sequence of the purified tripeptidase from *Lc. lactis* subsp. *cremoris* Wg2 (Mierau et al., 1994). PepT is a protein with a deduced molecular size of 46 kDa (413 amino acid residues), which is somewhat smaller than that determined biochemically (52 kDa). Lactococcal PepT is highly similar to PepT from *Salmonella typhimurium*, especially in three regions in which both enzymes show similarity to carboxypeptidase G of *Pseudomonas putida* and which are thought to be involved in metal binding and/or are important in catalysis or protein structure.

PepT is a metalloenzyme reversibly inactivated by EDTA and inhibited to some extent also by Cu^{2+} and the reducing agents DTT and β-mercaptoethanol. Sulfhydryl group reagents stimulate the enzyme approximately 2-fold. A wide range of substrates is hydrolyzed by PepT but the enzyme has a strict requirement for tripeptides: di-, tetra-, or larger oligopeptides are not degraded. Tripeptides with Pro in the N-terminal or C-terminal position are hydrolyzed but they are not degraded when Pro is present in the middle position.

Proline-Specific Peptidases

The high proline content of caseins would limit the efficiency of the proteolytic system of *Lc. lactis* in liberating free amino acids if it did not contain specific peptidases that can deal with proline-containing peptides. The general aminopeptidases described above do not hydrolyze beyond the Pro-residue of Pro-containing peptides liberated from casein through the action of the lactococcal proteinase PrtP. To hydrolyze proline-rich oligopeptides requires the activity of proline-specific peptidases. Several of these have been purified from *Lc. lactis* and their genes have been cloned, sequenced, and further characterized.

X-Prolyl Dipeptidyl Aminopeptidase. As is clear from the name of the enzyme, X-prolyl dipeptidyl aminopeptidase (PepX) liberates dipeptides of the structure Xxx–Pro from the amino terminus of peptides. The rate of hydrolysis depends on the nature of the amino acids surrounding the Pro residue. The enzyme has also been reported to liberate Xxx–Ala dipeptides from a larger substrate and to hydrolyse Pro–Pro–$(Xxx)_n$ but not, or only slightly, hydrolyze Xxx–Pro–Pro. It was also shown to liberate the N-terminal Tyr-Gly dipeptide from Met-enkephaline (Kiefer-Partsch et al., 1989; Zevaco et al., 1990; Booth et al., 1990a; Lloyd and Pritchard, 1991; Mayo et al., 1993).

PepX is a serine-peptidase and is severely inhibited by PMSF and DFP. It has been isolated from a number of lactococcal strains. The *pepX* genes from two strains of

Lc. lactis subsp. *cremoris* have been cloned and sequenced (Mayo et al., 1991; Nardi et al., 1991). The deduced PepX enzymes were almost identical: they differed in only 7 of the 763 amino acid residues two of which are, moreover, conserved amino acid replacements. When the *pepX* genes were introduced in the heterologous hosts *B. subtilis* and *E. coli*, two bacterial species that do not normally produce this enzyme, PepX expression was evidenced by the degradation of the chromogenic substrate Gly–Pro–β–NA. The deduced molecular size of PepX (88 kDa) agrees with that reported under denaturing conditions (85–89 kDa; Zevaco et al., 1990; Kiefer-Partsch et al., 1989, respectively). Under native conditions the enzyme behaves as a dimer. The nucleotide sequences of the *pepX* genes of a number of different organisms, including several LAB, have been determined and the deduced amino acid sequences reveal that the enzymes only show homology amongst themselves.

Prolidase. The Xxx–Pro dipeptides liberated from oligopeptides by the action of PepX are substrates for prolidase (PepQ). PepQ has been purified from *Lc. lactis*, is severely inhibited by the metal chelators EDTA and 1,10-phenanthroline, and by DTT and *N*-ethyl-maleimide. Enzyme activity of EDTA-treated PepQ could only be recovered by the addition of Co^{2+} ions. The molecular size of the prolidase was approximately 42 kDa (Kaminogawa et al., 1984; Booth et al., 1990b). A range of Xxx–Pro dipeptides (except Gly–Pro) is hydrolyzed, as are Pro–Val, Pro–Ala, Pro–Pro, and a number of di- and tripeptides lacking Pro residues. The *pepQ* gene has been cloned and sequenced from *Lc. lactis* MG1363 (Hellendoorn et al., 1999). The deduced enzyme (362 amino acid residues with a predicted molecular size of 39.9 kDa) was highly similar to the (deduced) amino acid sequences of all known prolidases to date (Hellendoorn et al., 1999). The PROSITE signature of aminopeptidase P and proline dipeptidase is present in PepQ of *Lc. lactis*, as are five putative Co^{2+}-binding sites also present in the other prolidases. Like all *pepQ* genes cloned to date from various organisms, *pepQ* of *Lc. lactis* is also in a back to back orientation with *ccpA* (see Figure 7.2). CcpA is involved in carbon catabolite repression in Gram-positive bacteria (for reviews, see Hueck and Hillen, 1995; Monedero et al., 1997; Luesink et al., 1998; Schick et al., 1999). The CcpA homologue PepR1 of *Lb. delbrueckii* subsp. *lactis* strain DSM7290 is also encoded by a gene upstream of and in opposite orientation to *pepQ*. PepR1 enhanced transcription of the Lactobacillus *pepQ* promoter in *E. coli* twofold only when a 14-bp *cre*-like element, situated 16 nucleotides upstream of *pepQ*, was intact. *cre* is the binding site for CcpA, an interaction that is enhanced by Hpr(Ser-P) (Deutscher et al., 1995) and binding of the complex affects transcription of the downstream genes. PerR1 specifically interacted with the *pepQ* promoter fragment and with promoter fragments of the *pepX, pepI*, and *brnQ* genes, all of which contained *cre*-like elements (Schick et al., 1999). Also in *Lc. lactis*, CcpA negatively affects the expression of PepQ, albeit that the effect is minor (Hellendoorn et al., unpublished). These results point to an intriguing possibility of a link between carbon and nitrogen metabolism.

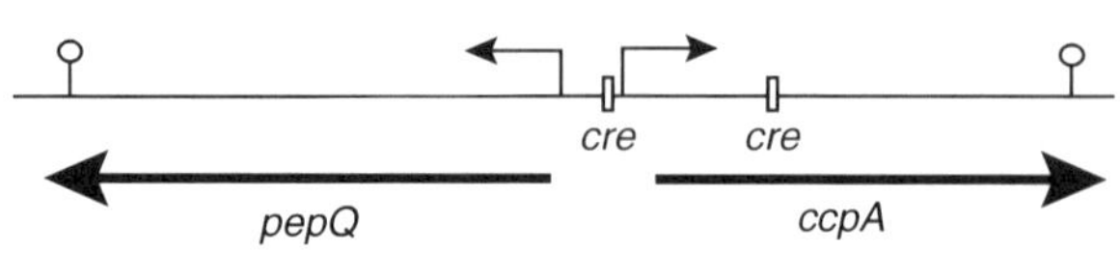

Figure 7.2. Map of the *ccpA–pepQ* region of *Lc. lactis*. The position and direction of the promoters (arrows), putative *cre*-elements, and terminators (lollipops) are indicated.

Aminopeptidase P. An aminopeptidase liberating the N-terminal amino acid from a peptide when the second residue is a proline was described in *Lc. lactis* (Mars and Monnet, 1995). This enzyme, PepP, which preferentially cleaves Xxx–Pro–Pro–$(Xxx)_n$ peptides, was relatively active on tripeptides and on oligopeptides with up to nine amino acid residues, but did not hydrolyze dipeptides. The optimal substrate size is near five residues. The *pepP* gene was cloned by reverse genetics and sequenced (Matos et al., 1998). The deduced molecular mass of PepP of 46 kDa was in accordance with that determined on the purified protein by SDS PAGE and gelfiltration (43 kDa), indicating that PepP is active as a monomer. PepP displays significant homology with other aminopeptidases P, with a number of prolidases and with methionine aminopeptidases, all of which belong to the M24 family of metallo-peptidases. The Asp-210, Asp-221, His-281, Glu-315, and Glu-329 residues are potential metal ligands of *Lc. lactis* PepP. Indeed, PepP was clearly identified as a metalloenzyme as it was severely inhibited by EDTA and *o*-phenanthroline, while Mn^{2+} and Co^{2+} restored inhibition by EDTA (Mars and Monnet, 1995). Lactococcal PepP liberates the N-terminal Met residue from Met–Pro–Pro–Gly–Phe and is proposed, like PepP from *E. coli*, to play a role in the maturation of specific nascent proteins. While the *pepP* gene was shown to exist in many strains of *Lc. lactis* by Southern hybridization, no signal was obtained with *Strep. thermophilus* and a number of different species of Lactobacillus.

Prolinase and Proline Iminopeptidase. Proline iminopeptidase activity (cleavage of N-terminal Pro residues from (oligo)peptides) and prolinase activity (specific for Pro–Xxx dipeptides) are less strictly separable than they may seem on the basis of these definitions and their activities may overlap. A proline iminopeptidase activity has been described in *Lc. lactis* that hydrolyzes a range of di- and tripeptides carrying Pro as the N-terminal amino acid but does not degrade longer peptides or dipeptides of the structure Xxx–Pro (Baankreis and Exterkate, 1991). The enzyme is severely inhibited by EDTA and DTT and has a molecular size of approximately 50 kDa on SDS PAGE. The gene encoding this enzyme has not been identified. A true prolinase activity has not been described in *Lc. lactis*.

The Physiological Role of the Components of the Proteolytic System

One of the reasons why the knowledge of the proteolytic system of *Lc. lactis* is much more advanced than that of other LAB is the availability of efficient techniques to genetically manipulate the organism (see elsewhere in this volume). In particular, the development of methods to make single and double cross-over integration mutants has contributed considerably to our understanding of the pathway of casein degradation, the various components involved, the order in which they participate and the importance of each of them in the process.

The Proteinase and the Peptide Uptake Systems

As we have seen above, the extracellular proteinase of *Lc. lactis* is the key enzyme in the proteolytic degradation of caseins. The enzyme performs the first step in the cascade, degrading the milk protein into oligopeptides that are substrates for the Opp system. The pivotal role of the proteinase in the pathway is clear from the fact that proteinase-deficient lactococci cannot effectively grow in milk: they only reach cell densities of 5–25% (depending on the quality of the milk) of that of the wild-type strains. The growth problem is alleviated when a source of amino acids or peptides (casein hydrolysate) is added.

Apparently, milk protein is the major source of amino acids in milk for these multiple amino acid auxotrophs (Thomas and Pritchard, 1987; Juillard et al., 1995b).

Oligopeptide uptake is a crucial step in the proteolytic pathway; in fact we know now that Opp is the only peptide transporter that is essential during growth of *Lc. lactis* in milk. A mutant expressing a functional proteinase but in which the gene for the binding protein, *oppA*, has been insertionally inactivated, is unable to grow in milk (Tynkkynen et al., 1993). Other data have underpinned this observation: first, the proteinase only releases peptides of more than four residues from (β)-casein (Juillard et al., 1995a). Second, as also indicated above, *Lc. lactis* does not produce extracellular peptidases. Third, amino acid accumulation does not occur in proteinase expressing cells in which Opp has been inactivated, while this is not the case in cells with a mutation in the di- and tripeptide transporter DtpT. Inactivation of DtpT has no effect on growth in milk (Kunji et al., 1995). The fact that Opp-defective proteinase-producing cells do not grow in milk and that the *opp* mutation blocks amino acid accumulation provides compelling evidence for the notion that *Lc. lactis* does not produce extracellular peptidases involved in casein utilization (apart from the cell-wall-bound proteinase PrtP).

The Peptidases

The genetic information on the peptidase genes of *Lc. lactis* has been used to construct single as well as multiple peptidase mutants by targeted disruption or deletion strategies. It has become the standard to mutate a peptidase gene once its nucleotide sequence is known and to assess the effect of the mutation on cellular growth under various conditions and, most importantly, in milk. These studies have revealed that no single peptidase is essential for growth of *Lc. lactis* in milk. Lactococcal mutants lacking either PepX, PepT, PepO, PepO2, PepF1, PepF2, PepC, PepN, PepA, PepV, or PepQ are not or only slightly affected in their ability to grow in milk (Mayo et al., 1993; Mierau et al., 1993, 1994; Monnet et al., 1994; l'Anson et al., 1995; Erra-Pujada et al., 1995; Hellendoorn et al., 1999). Apparently, the activity of each of these peptidases is taken over by one or more of the remaining enzymes, or the cell is provided with essential amino acids via a peptide degradation route that is not touched by the mutation. Also, it is still possible that certain peptidases described above are, in fact, not involved in casein degradation at all. For instance, an alternative role for PepF has been proposed in (intracellular) protein maturation (see above).

To assess the function of the various peptidases in the growth of *Lc. lactis* in milk is a formidable task. First, milk is a very complex medium that, due to the activity of the cells, is constantly changing with respect to (peptide) composition. Second, many peptidases exist inside the cell that, as we have just discussed, may have overlapping specificities. To enable a detailed analysis of the peptide breakdown pathway, two avenues were taken to reduce this complexity (Mierau et al., 1996; Kunji et al., 1996b). Medium complexity was reduced by using a CDM to which peptides and/or amino acids could be added. In addition, a genetic approach was taken to abolish peptidase activities by successively mutating their chromosomal genes using a food-grade gene replacement strategy (Leenhouts et al., 1996). In this way, single, double, triple, quadruple, and quintuple mutants have been made in which a combination of the genes for PepX, PepT, PepO, PepC, and PepN had been deleted (Mierau et al., 1996). The growth of all of these mutants in a rich medium (M17) or in CDM with all twenty amino acids was not affected. In milk, however, an increase in the number of *pep* mutations resulted in a decrease in the growth rate. Except for the fourfold and fivefold mutants, the final cell densities reached in milk stay more or less the same. Ultimately, the fivefold mutant *pepXpepTpepOpepCpepN* (expressing a functional proteinase) grows more then tenfold slower in milk than the proteinase-positive wild-type strain. These results show that the peptidase mutations in themselves are not detrimental to the lactococcal cell and that casein-derived peptides can still be hydrolyzed, but at a lower rate (Mierau et al., 1996). The intracellular amino acids pool was much lower in the slowest growing mutants (*pepXpepTpepCpepN; pepXpepTpepOpepCpepN*) than that in the wild type, while they accumulated peptides intracellularly, providing direct evidence for the functioning of lactococcal peptidases in hydrolysis of casein.

By growing the mutants in CDM, in which of the twenty amino acids the essential amino acid leucine was replaced by a leucine-containing peptide, it was possible for the first time to assess the role of individual peptidases in the degradation of specific peptides *in vivo* (Kunji et al., 1996a). In some cases, one or only a limited set of peptidases is able to degrade a certain peptide: PepT or PepN degrade Leu–Gly–Gly, while Ala–Pro–Leu is mainly degraded by PepX. The tetrapeptide Gly–Leu–Gly–Leu is hydrolyzed by PepN or, if *pepN* is mutated, by PepC in combination with PepT. Removal of PepN together with either of the other two enzymes precludes the cells from growing on the tetrapeptide showing that, apart from these three enzymes, no other peptidases are present in the cell which can degrade this substrate (Kunji et al., 1996b). The presence of a second PepO-like enzyme was also indicated by these growth experiments: the 5-fold mutant *pepXpepTpepOpepCpepN* still grows on Tyr–Gly–Gly–Phe–Leu (a PepO substrate). This was later confirmed by the cloning of the gene for this enzyme, PepO2 (see above; Hellendoorn et al., 1999).

The fact that several multiple peptidase mutants cannot utilize certain peptides and accumulate them intracellularly, together with the observation that peptide transport mutants do not accumulate peptides, settles an old debate in the literature as to how peptides are internalized. These studies prove that peptides are taken up intact and, only when they are inside the cell, are taken apart (Kunji et al., 1996b).

Regulation of the Caseinolytic Pathway

Relatively few studies have been done regarding the regulation of the components of the protein breakdown pathway and these will be discussed below. With most of the genes of the pathway cloned and sequenced now, proteolytic pathway regulation will be the focus of (near) future intensified research. In some cases, putative regulator genes have been identified in the vicinity of proteolytic genes but for most of these their involvement in regulation of the expression of the proteolytic component, let alone in the entire pathway, still has to be examined. For those components of the pathway that are not easily measurable (due to, for instance, high background, overlapping activities), the nucleotide sequences allow making fusions with genes of easily assessable reporter enzymes to measure activities of promoters under various growth conditions. Also, genetic techniques will enable to identify and isolate possible proteolytic gene or proteolytic pathway regulators.

Early on, it was observed that proteinase production in a number of lactococcal strains is inhibited when the growth medium is rich in peptides, for example, contains casitone, a tryptic digest of casein (Exterkate, 1985; Laan et al., 1993). Addition of the dipeptide Leu–Pro to a CDM inhibited PrtP synthesis, and the presence of a palindromic sequence involving the *prtP* and *prtM* promoters was speculated to play a role in the phenomenon (Laan et al., 1993). This was later substantiated by fusing both *prt* promoters of the PrtPIII proteinase of *Lc. lactis* strain SK11 to the *gusA* gene encoding the reporter enzyme β-glucuronidase and measuring medium-dependent gene expression directly (Marugg et al., 1995). Both *prtP* and *prtM* are controlled in a similar way and at the transcriptional level. Expression was highest in media containing low amounts of peptides. Addition of Pro-Leu or Leu-Pro lowered the expression level of the *prtP :: gusA* fusion. Expression of *prtP :: gusA* in strains lacking the di- and tripeptide transporter DtpT was not down-regulated by peptides, indicating that the internal concentration of small (di–tri)peptides or the amino acids derived thereof are important in the regulation of proteinase production (Marugg et al., 1995). A deletion analysis of the *prt* promoter region revealed that a 90-bp region encompassing the transcription start sites of both *prtP* and *prtM* retained full promoter activity and was subject to normal regulation (Marugg et al., 1996). Specific disruptions of the inverted repeat present in this region, while only marginally influencing promoter activity, led to derepression of the expression of the *prtP* and *prtM* promoters in media with a high peptide concentration. It was speculated that this palindromic region in the intergenic region between *prtP* and *prtM* might be involved in the recognition or binding of a repressor protein, and that specific dipeptides may directly or indirectly act as effectors of this regulator (Marugg et al., 1996).

The expression of all peptide transport systems of *Lc. lactis* is also affected by the medium composition. Expression of DtpP (Foucaud et al., 1995), DtpT (Kunji et al., 1996a) and OppA (Detmers et al., 1998; Hellendoorn et al., 1999) are increased approximately 3-, 5-, and 10-fold when cells are grown in CDM with amino acids instead of complex M17 broth. OppA expression is repressed more than 20-fold when Leu–Pro or Pro–Leu were added to the growth medium (Hellendoorn et al., unpublished results).

The expression of PepX and PepN in *Lc. lactis* MG1363 was shown to be regulated in a way similar to that of PrtP: highest specific enzyme activity levels were observed in milk while the levels decreased at increasing casitone (peptide) concentrations in whey permeate medium. The effects were most pronounced for PepN. The lowest levels (2- to 5-fold lower than those in milk for PepX and PepN, respectively) were found in the peptide-rich M17 medium (Meijer et al., 1996). In contrast to PrtP expression, medium-dependent PepN and PepX regulation appeared to be strain dependent as the activity levels of both enzymes in SK1128, a derivative of *Lc. lactis* subsp. *cremoris* SK11, were not significantly influenced by the peptide content of the medium (Meijer et al., 1996).

Expression of luciferase reporter gene fusions to the promoters of *pepA, pepN, pepC, pepX, pepQ, pepT, pepM, pepP, pepDA1*, to the four endopeptidase promoters and to that of *prtP* was examined in different media. Five of the fusions (those to the promoters of *pepC, pepN, pepO1, pepO2*, and *prtP*) were reported to be more active in CDM with amino acids than in CDM plus casitone or M17 (Guédon et al., 1999). From these studies it is clear that exogenous amino acids and peptides regulate the expression of several of the components of the proteolytic system of *Lc. Lactis*. The actual player(s) involved in the signalling and regulation remain(s) to be elucidated.

Engineering of the Casein Breakdown Pathway

During cheese making, proteolysis of milk protein is due to the action of the rennet, of the indigenous milk proteinases, and of the starter proteinases added to the cheese milk. The proteolytic enzymes produced by the starter bacteria hydrolyze these casein-derived peptides into smaller peptides and amino acids. These small peptides and amino acids contribute directly, or only after chemical or enzymatic conversion to volatile compounds, to the organoleptic quality of the cheese (Rank et al., 1985; Nath, 1992; Visser, 1993; Christensen et al., 1999; Weimer et al., 1999). The availability of the genes of components of the proteolytic system and of strains mutated in various steps in the pathway enables a completely new analysis of cheese flavor development, to target the important steps with the ultimate aim of influencing and steering the process. Several approaches have been taken to enhance or change the complex pathway of casein degradation by *Lc. lactis*. As discussed above the simplest intervention always undertaken is to make single- or double-cross-over mutants of any newly discovered gene of a component of the system, in order to assess its importance in casein breakdown (for instance, by growing the mutant in milk). In addition, overexpression of homologous as well as heterologous genes has been attempted, both on resident plasmids and by stably integrating the genes in the chromosome. The recent development of food-grade cloning systems for *Lc. lactis* has made it possible to construct strains containing only lactococcal DNA, adding a new dimension to starter culture engineering with the ultimate aim to use the strains in the dairy industry.

Analysis of Mutants for Cheese Flavor Development

Cheeses made with proteinase-deficient starter cultures develop little or no flavor (Stadhouders et al., 1988; Law et al., 1993; Exterkate and Alting, 1995). PepN- and PepX-deficient mutants have been analyzed in Gouda cheese making experiments. A starter strain mixture containing 90% of a *pepN* mutant clearly produced "bitter" reinforcing the notion that PepN is an important debittering enzyme (see below). Cheese made with a mixed starter containing a high concentration of a *pepX* strain in the starter suffered from a general decrease in organoleptic quality (Baankreis, 1992).

Engineering and Stabilization of Proteinase Production

Early studies already revealed that the first step in casein degradation performed by PrtP is a relatively unstable trait due to the location of *prtP* on plasmids in many lactococcal strains (for reviews, see McKay, 1983; Kok, 1990; Kok and de Vos, 1994). One way to intervene with the proteolytic system was to stabilize proteolysis by PrtP. This was done by integrating the *prtP* and *prtM* genes into the chromosome of the proteinase-negative strain MG1363 (Leenhouts et al., 1991; Law et al., 1992). In both cases the elevated copy numbers caused by gene amplification resulted in an increase in the rate of casein degradation. Proteinase overproduction was also achieved by placing the *prtP* and *prtM* genes on plasmids with elevated copy numbers or by placing the genes in an operon structure under the control of a promoter stronger than the original *prt* promoters (Bruinenberg et al., 1992; Van der Vossen et al., 1992). Two other examples of altering proteolysis, namely by protein engineering, have already been discussed above: by swapping domains between the proteinases PrtPI and PrtPIII, hybrid proteinases with new specificities were created (Vos et al., 1991), while the deletion of the C-terminal 4 residues of PepC resulted in altered peptidase specificity (Mata et al., 1999). None of these new enzymes have been tested yet in (pilot-scale) cheese trials in order to investigate their effect on cheese flavor development.

Overproduction of Homologous Proteolytic Enzymes in *Lc. lactis*

Aminopeptidase N was the first homologous intracellular peptidase to be overexpressed in *Lc. lactis*. Cloning of *pepN* on a multicopy plasmid resulted in a 20-fold increase in lysyl-aminopeptidase activity that corresponded to several percent of total protein (van Alen-Boerrigter et al., 1991). Although PepN is a debittering enzyme that degrades hydrophobic peptides in a "bitter" tryptic digest of β-casein (Tan et al., 1993), Cheddar cheeses produced with two different lactococcal strains containing the *pepN* plasmid did not have improved body, texture, or flavor characteristics (McGarry et al., 1994). PepN was functionally overproduced to up to 47% of total intracellular protein by using a nisin-inducible gene expression vector system (de Ruyter et al., 1996; see elsewhere in this volume). In a mixed culture containing an equal amount of cells overexpressing PepN and cells overexpressing the lysin and holin proteins of the lactococcal bacteriophage ϕUS3 involved in cell wall degradation, production and release of PepN could be enhanced simultaneously (de Ruyter et al., 1997). The *pepN* overexpression vector was made food-grade by replacing its chloramphenicol resistance gene by *lacF*, which should allow high-level, food-grade, controlled overproduction of PepN and many other (proteolytic) enzymes (de Ruyter et al., 1996, 1997).

The genes for PepN, PepC, PepV, PepO, PepT, and PepX of *Lc. lactis* were overexpressed using the food-grade plasmid pFG1 that utilizes a nonsense suppressor gene (*supB*), encoding a lactococcal $tRNA^{Gln}$, as a selectable marker. The host strain is an *Lc. lactis* mutant unable to grow without added purines as it has a nonsense mutation in one of the genes for purine biosynthesis. It is, thus, unable to grow in milk without the *supB* plasmid, as milk does not contain purines (Dickely et al., 1995). All peptidases were overproduced several-fold (Strøman et al., 1998). Four of the vectors (encoding PepN, PepC, PepO, and PepV) were introduced in a lactose- and proteinase-positive derivative of *Lc. lactis* MG1363 and subjected to pilot-scale Cheddar cheese trials (200 *L* scale). Cheese composition (content of moisture, fat, salts, and protein), cheese microbiology, contaminating non-starter LAB, and pH were analyzed (Strøman et al., 1998). Two different trained sensoric panels assessed cheese organoleptic quality. Only after 4 and 6 months of storage were statistically significant differences observed between the various cheeses (see Figure 7.3). Bitter flavor was significantly reduced while flavor preference was increased only in those strains overproducing the general aminopeptidases PepN and PepC.

The results using pFG1 are obscured by the fact that this vector is very unstable in industrial strains and causes severe growth inhibition and reduced acidification rates.

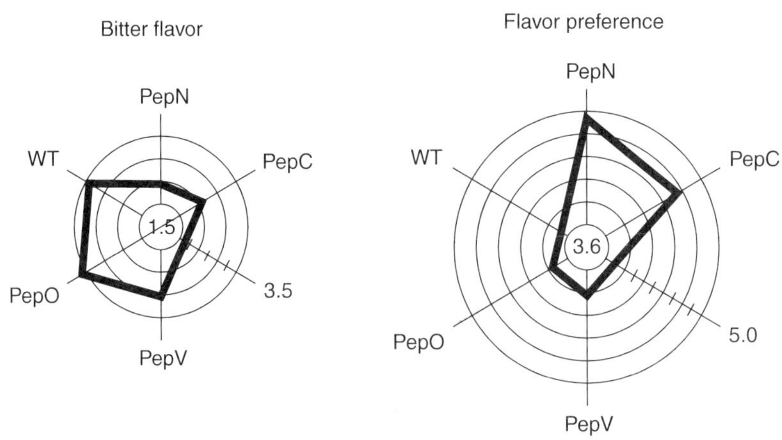

Figure 7.3. Sensoric evaluation of Cheddar cheeses manufactured with *Lc. lactis* strain MG1363 (Lac^+, Prt^+) overproducing either PepN, PepC, PepO, or PepV. Scores for bitter flavor (1.5–3.5) and flavor preference (3.4–4.8) are indicated in the figure (adapted from Strøman et al., 1998).

An improved version of the system was made by replacing the ochre suppressor gene *supB* by an amber suppressor (*supD*). *supD* encodes an altered $tRNA^{Ser}$ and suppresses only amber stop codons, which are present in only 10% of the lactococcal genes (Sørensen et al., 2000). Suppressible pyrimidine auxotrophs of industrial strains carrying plasmid pGF200 grew perfectly well in milk with high acidification rates and 8- to 20-fold increased expression of lysine aminopeptidase activity was obtained. No data are yet available on the performance of the strains under industrial-scale fermentation conditions.

Expression of Heterologous Proteolytic Enzymes in *Lc. lactis*

The first heterologous proteolytic activity expressed in *Lc. lactis* was the neutral protease, NprE, of *B. subtilis* (Van de Guchte et al., 1990). The *nprE* gene was cloned on a multicopy plasmid downstream of a strong lactococcal promoter and active proteinase was secreted from the recombinant strain. When two different strains containing the recombinant plasmid were used in cheese making accelerated proteolysis was observed (McGarry et al., 1994).

Bovine plasmin, the predominant serine proteinase in milk and an enzyme shown to accelerate cheese ripening, has been expressed in *Lc. lactis* (Arnau et al., 1997). The proteinase was secreted using the secretion signal sequence of the lactococcal extracellular protein Usp45 and was biologically active. Production of active plasmin led to physiological stress resulting in cell lysis. The highest production was obtained when the protein was produced intracellularly. Production of full-length plasmin resulted in deletion formation and it was concluded that plasmin could only be produced in low amounts in *Lc. lactis* (Arnau et al., 1997).

Several peptidases from other LAB have been expressed in *Lc. lactis*. Some of these peptidases represent activities that are not naturally present in *Lc. lactis*, providing an opportunity to assess whether the newly acquired activity might have a favorable effect on dairy characteristics of the strains.

Introduction of the *pepN* gene from *Lb. helveticus* on a plasmid enhanced the aminopeptidase activity of *Lc. lactis* more than 180-fold. In a 6 month old Cheddar cheese made with a mixed culture containing the lactococcal strain producing *Lactobacillus* PepN, a 1,000-fold greater aminopeptidase activity was obtained and elevated levels of amino acids and small peptides were detected. The increased free amino acid pool did not result in accelerated flavor development, however (Christensen et al., 1995a,b). Using the strong gene expression signals of the *Lb. brevis* surface layer protein A gene (*slpA*), the *pepN* gene of *Lb. helveticus* was expressed in *Lc. lactis, Lb. plantarum*, and *Lb. gasseri*, increasing the specific aminopeptidase activity 10-, 290-, and 30-fold, respectively (Kahala and Palva, 1999).

Other Lactobacillus-derived peptidases have been expressed in *Lc. lactis* using the nisin-inducible gene expression system (see elsewhere in this volume). The *Lb. delbrueckii* subsp. *lactis pepI* (proline iminopeptidase), *pepL* (prolinase), *pepW* (endopeptidase), and *pepG* (endopeptidase) genes, for which no counterparts are present in *Lc. lactis*, and the gene encoding *pepQ* (prolidase) were translationally fused to the *nisA* promoter. The constructs were introduced in the fivefold peptidase mutant of *Lc. lactis* (*pepXpepTpepOpepCpepN*) in which the genes *nisK* and *nisR* had been integrated in the chromosome to allow for nisin-induced gene expression (Wegmann et al., 1999). Although identical transcription and translation signals were used, expression levels of the various peptidases varied considerably. The highest expression was obtained for *pepW, pepG*, and *pepI*. Activity for all peptidases could be detected in cell extracts, although only *pepL* and *pepG* expression resulted in the release of peptides as a source of essential amino acids needed for growth. Expression of each of the five peptidases resulted in peptidase-specific changes in the intracellular amino acid pool. Induction of *pepG* or *pepW* resulted in accelerated growth in milk of the 5-fold peptidase mutant.

The gene encoding the proline iminopeptidase (Pip) of *Propionibacterium shermanii* was also cloned in *Lc. lactis* (Leenhouts et al., 1998). Pip is responsible for the typical sweet flavor of Swiss-type cheeses. High expression was obtained by placing the gene under control of a strong constitutive lactococcal promoter on a plasmid. *In trans* expression of the plasmid replication protein was required to maintain the plasmid. This stability problem was overcome by integrating *pip* into the chromosome using a food-grade integration system based on sucrose selection. A clear but non-linear gene dosage effect was observed in strains carrying multiple copies of the integrated gene. The highest activities in the recombinant *Lc. lactis* strains were 3- to 4-fold higher than those in *P. shermanii*.

A Connection between Proteolysis and Autolysis

Autolysis, the lysis caused by the cell's own cell wall hydrolases, has from early days on been proposed to play a role in cheese flavor development (Hansen, 1941; Law et al., 1974; Bie and Sjöström, 1975a,b). The importance of lysis in flavor development can, in the light of what has been presented above, now be understood as the release of the intracellular peptidase complement as well as amino acid convertases of the lactococcal starter strains. High cell wall lytic activity was correlated with prominent release of intracellular peptidase activity and with an increase in the amino nitrogen in cheese, although a fine balance between autolyzed and intact cells may be important (Chapot-Chartier et al., 1994a; Crow et al., 1995). Several strategies have been employed to increase lysis with the aim of liberating the intracellular flavor generating enzymes. First off, the availability of genes specifying cell wall hydrolysing enzymes and (inducible) gene expression signals (see elsewhere in this volume) have been used to devise genetic constructs with which it is possible to induce lysis of starter cultures by external stimulus (Kuipers et al., 1997; Nauta et al., 1997; see elsewhere in this volume). Induction of prophages, provided that it is done under well controlled conditions, could be another means to induce lysis of a culture that, however, may not be easily and reliably applied under industrial-scale conditions. Addition of a cocktail of bacteriocins to a starter culture also resulted in the lysis of the strain with release of intracellular proteins (Ross et al., 1999). This system has been successfully implemented in the form of a triple-strain mixture, in which one strain produces (and is resistant to) the bacteriocin, the other bacteriocin-resistant strain is a rapid acid producer, while the third strain, the sacrificial strain, is bacteriocin sensitive, lyses rapidly, and releases its intracellular enzyme complement in the cheese matrix.

The gene for the enzyme responsible for autolysis in *Lc. lactis, acmA*, has been cloned, sequenced and deleted from the chromosome (Buist et al., 1995). Unlike the wild-type strain, its AcmA-negative counterpart did not autolyze during the stationary phase and did not release intracellular proteins. These studies showed that autolysis is, indeed, an important factor in intracellular peptidase release in wild-type starter strains, especially during the stationary phase, when cell wall synthesis is shut down while the cell wall hydrolase is still active. An indirect but important link between autolysis, proteolysis and, thus, possibly cheese flavor development was recently uncovered with the observation that the lactococcal proteinase PrtP degrades AcmA. The extent to which the autolysin is hydrolysed is dependent on the specificity of the proteinase: PrtPI is more aggressive in this respect than PrtPIII. Consequently, a strain producing PrtPIII lyses to a greater extent with concomitant greater release of intracellular peptidase activity (Buist et al., 1998). In conclusion, to manipulate proteinase for better casein degradation specificity may not be as straightforward if one has to also take into account the activity of the engineered proteinase on the autolysin.

Considering the importance of PrtP in the production of the oligopeptides that are needed for the intracellular enzymes to "work on" and produce the flavor (precursors) it should not be surprising that Prt-negative starters produce little flavor. However, this notion would be too simple if it would suggest merely overproducing proteinase to accelerate cheese ripening. First, proteinases of certain specificity (PI-type, see above) are known to produce bitter peptides from casein, notably the C-terminal proline-rich part of β-casein. In other words, "bitter" could develop in cheese as a consequence of proteinase activity if the ensuing peptidase complement of the starter insufficiently copes with bitter peptide production. Second, as discussed above, the effect on autolysis has to be taken into account.

Conclusions

The last 15 to 20 years of the previous century have seen a tremendous increase in our knowledge of the pathway of casein breakdown by *Lc. lactis*. This has been accomplished in a relatively short period of time through combined physiology, biochemistry, and genetic studies and, currently, the proteolytic system of *Lc. lactis* is the best-known protein breakdown pathway in prokaryotes and a paradigm for the other LAB. We are at the brink of being able to apply this knowledge in a meaningful way to the benefit of both the dairy product producer and the consumer, provided that we are able to deal with the important issues of the use of genetically modified (micro)organisms in foods. Nevertheless, even if the industrial application may still be quite far ahead, the use of genetic techniques to answer fundamental questions regarding proteolysis by *Lc. lactis* has been very valuable already and will remain so in the (near) future. We now know the main players in the field, the order in which they appear to do their job, and their importance in the game (see Figure 7.4). The proteinase PrtP kicks off by degrading casein into oligopeptides that are tackled by the Opp. The proteinase produces a large range of different oligopeptides, which differ considerably in size and amino acid composition and the OppA protein is fully geared toward "Venus fly-trapping" quite a large number of these oligopeptides with high affinity and passing them on to the translocator. Once inside the cell a host of different peptidases (aminopeptidases, oligopeptidases, and proline-specific peptidases) line up to chop the various internalized oligopeptides into smaller ones and into amino acids. By using single and multiple peptidase knock-out mutants the specific role of some of the peptidases in the break down of certain peptides could be examined, both *in vitro* as well as *in vivo*; it is expected that we will see more of the molecular details of the intracellular peptide degradation pathway along similar research lines in the near future.

Somewhat disappointingly perhaps (as it seems more exciting to work on an "important" enzyme, that is, one which kills the cell when removed), none of the peptidases appeared to be essential for *Lc. lactis* when it was growing in milk. In the case of *Lc. lactis*, however, the fact that the peptidases are not essential has important and enticing practical applications. It allowed assessment of the importance of some of the enzymes already important in flavor formation under actual (pilot) cheese making conditions. Similar studies

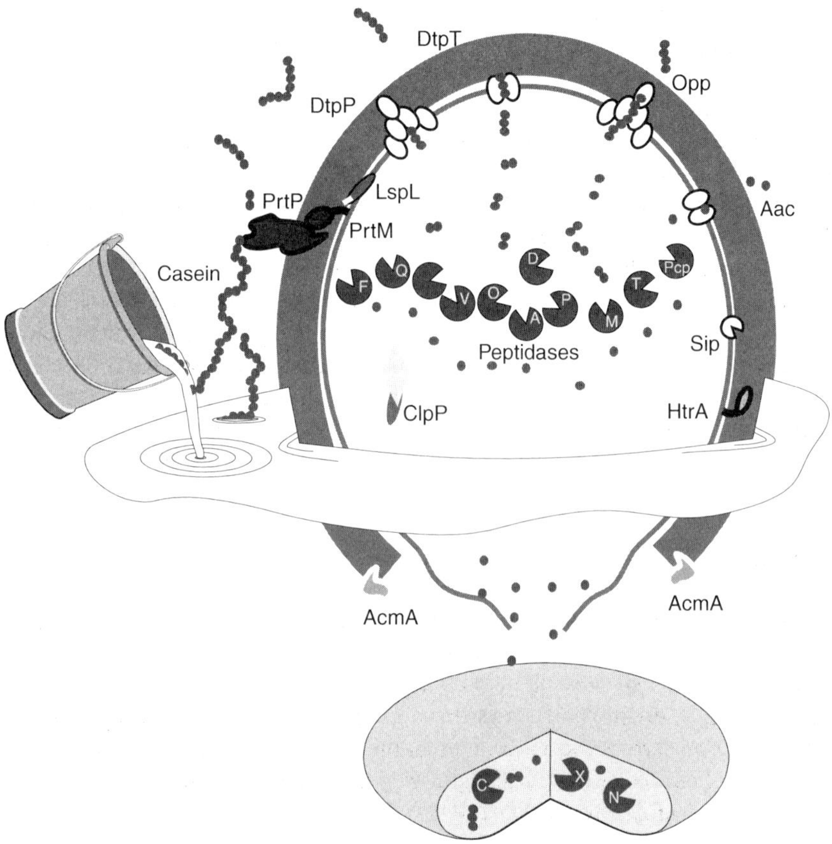

Figure 7.4. Artist impression of the known components of the *Lc. lactis* proteolytic pathway. A cell in milk is shown while it is lysing due to the action of its autolysin AcmA, to underpin the events going on during cheese ripening. In principle, all intracellular proteins are released in this process but here only PepC, PepN, and PepX are shown in the cheese matrix as these activities have been implicated in cheese flavor development. For abbreviations used to indicate the various proteins/enzymes: see the text.

are currently being performed with other peptidase mutants and their outcome will soon give a good deal more information as to the effect of a certain (combination of) peptidase mutations on flavor development in milk fermentations or, equally, in other food-related processes. This should allow workers to decide which peptidases to remove or to overproduce in order to change flavor patterns. The reciprocity of this approach is illustrated by the observation that cheeses made with a *pepN* mutant develop bitterness, while significantly lower bitterness scores were recorded when PepN was overproduced. Overproduction of heterologous proteolytic enzymes has been used to modulate specific intracellular amino acid pools, and equipping *Lc. lactis* with novel enzymatic activities, is very possible with all the (inducible) gene expression vectors at hand. Novel developments are expected soon, but, to use the strains in an actual dairy product and to put it out on the market may take a great deal of time and effort to accomplish due to current strict regulations.

These are exciting times for molecular (micro)biologists and for industrialists alike: with the publishing of the annotation of the first nucleotide sequence of the entire chromosome of a lactic acid bacterium, that of *Lc. lactis* subsp. *lactis* strain IL1403 (Bolotin et al., 1999), a more complete picture of the proteolytic pathway is expected to emerge. By analyzing all open reading frames (genes) present in this genome we should now be able to target enzymes or proteins that have gone undetected so far. PepM (methioninepeptidase) and another dipeptidase (pepDA, a homologue of the *Lactobacillus* enzyme) have been detected recently, for instance (P. Renault, pers. comm.). Also, it opens up a completely new way of analyzing proteolysis and regulation of the proteolytic pathway. It allows us to apply DNA micro-array techniques to *Lc. lactis* and analyze at the same time all the genes of the organism under specific growth conditions or in certain mutant strains. Such a genome-wide analysis of gene expression, coupled to high-throughput whole-cell protein analysis, will be implemented soon in *Lc. lactis* and is expected to advance our in-depth knowledge of the working of this industrially important organism tremendously in the coming decade (for a short review on this subject, see Kuipers et al., 1999). No doubt we will see a lot of progress in the field of proteolysis by *Lc. lactis*, both with regard to understanding its importance and function under industrial conditions as well as the more fundamental aspects.

Note Added in Proof

During processing of the manuscript the following important information became available: A fully annotated sequence of the *L. lactis* IL 1403 genome has been published (Bolotin et al., *Genome Res.* 11: 731–753). The signal controlling casitone-dependent repression of proteolysis is the intracellular pool of branched-chain amino acids (Guedon et al., *J. Bacteriol.* 183: 3614–3622). CodY senses this signal and has been pinpointed as an important (central) regulator (repressor) of the proteolytic pathway (Guedon et al., *Mol. Microbiol.* 40: 1227–1239). CodY was shown to repress transcription of *prtP* and *prtM* and to bind to the intergenic region between *prtP* and *prtM* (Gajic, 2003, Thesis University of Groningen, The Netherlands). Expression in lactococcal cells of PrtP with a duplicated cell wall domain, or of a heterologous protein containing this duplication, resulted in cell sedimentation due to protein–protein interaction between the duplicated domains (Gajic, 2003, Thesis University of Groningen, The Netherlands).

Acknowledgments

We are grateful to our colleagues for sharing results prior to publication. Part of this work was supported by a grant from the European Union (BIO-4-96-0016; BIO-4-CT-98-4396).

References

Arnau, J., Hjerl-Hansen, E., and Israelsen, H. (1997). Heterologous gene expression of bovine plasmin in *Lactococcus lactis*. *Applied Microbiology and Biotechnology* 48: 331–338.

Arnau, J., Sørensen, K. I., Appel, K. F., Vogensen, F. K., and Hammer, K. (1996). Analysis of heat shock gene expression in *Lactococcus lactis* MG1363. *Microbiology* 142: 1685–1691.

Baankreis, R. (1992). The role of lactococcal peptidases in cheese ripening. Ph.D. thesis. University of Amsterdam, The Netherlands.

Baankreis, R., and Exterkate, F. A. (1991). Characterization of a peptidase from *Lactococcus lactis* ssp. *cremoris* HP that hydrolyses di- and tripeptides containing proline or hydrophobic residues as the aminoterminal amino acid. *Systematic and Applied Microbiology* 14: 317–323.

Bacon, C. L., Jennings, P. V., Fhaoláin, I. N., and O'Cuinn, G. (1994). Purification and characterization of an aminopeptidase A from cytoplasm of *Lactococcus lactis* subsp. *cremoris* AM2. *International Dairy Journal* 4: 503–519.

Bacon, C. L., Wilkinson, M., Jennings, P. V., Fhaoláin, I. N., and O'Cuinn, G. (1993). Purification and characterization of an aminotripeptidase from cytoplasm of *Lactococcus lactis* subsp. *cremoris* AM2. *International Dairy Journal* 3: 163–177.

Bie, R., and Sjöström, G. (1975a). Autolytic properties of some lactic acid bacteria used in cheese production. Part I: Material and methods. *Milchwissenschaft* 30: 653–657.

Bie, R., and Sjöström, G. (1975b). Autolytic properties of some lactic acid bacteria used in cheese production. Part II: Experiments with fluid substrates and cheese. *Milchwissenschaft* 30: 739–747.

Bockelmann, W., Monnet, V., Geis, A., Teuber, M., and Gripon, J.-C. (1989). Comparison of cell wall proteinases from *Lactococcus lactis* subsp. *cremoris* AC1 and *Lactococcus lactis* subsp. *lactis* NCDO 763. *Applied Microbiology and Biotechnology* 31: 278–282.

Bolotin, A., Mauger, S., Malarme, K., Ehrlich, S. D., and Sorokin, A. (1999). Low-redundancy sequencing of the entire *Lactococcus lactis* IL1403 genome. *Antonie van Leeuwenhoek* 76: 27–76.

Booth, M., Fhaoláin, I. N., Jennings, P. V., and O'Cuinn, G. (1990a). Purification and characterization of a post-proline dipeptidyl aminopeptidase from *Streptococcus cremoris* AM2. *Journal of Dairy Research* 57: 89–99.

Booth, M., Jennings, V., Fhaoláin, I. N., and O'Cuinn, G. (1990b). Prolidase activity of *Lactococcus lactis* subsp. *cremoris* AM2: partial purification and characterization. *Journal of Dairy Research* 57: 245–254.

Bosman, B. W., Tan, P. S. T., and Konings, W. N. (1990). Purification and characterization of a tripeptidase from *Lactococcus lactis* subsp. *cremoris* Wg2. *Applied and Environmental Microbiology* 56: 1839–1843.

Bruinenberg, P. G., de Vos, W. M., and Siezen, R. J. (1994). Prevention of C-terminal autoprocessing of *Lactococcus lactis* SK11 cell-envelope proteinase by engineering of an essential surface loop. *Biochemical Journal* 302: 957–963.

Bruinenberg, P. G., Vos, P., and de Vos, W. M. (1992). Proteinase overproduction in *Lactococcus lactis* strains: regulation and effect on growth and acidification in milk. *Applied and Environmental Microbiology* 58: 78–84.

Buist, G., Kok, J., Leenhouts, K. J., Drabowska, M., Venema, G., and Haandrikman, A. J. (1995). Molecular cloning and nucleotide sequence of the gene encoding the major peptidoglycan hydrolase of *Lactococcus lactis*, a muramidase needed for cell separation. *Journal of Bacteriology* 177: 1554–1563.

Buist, G., Benus, G., Haandrikman, A., Venema, G., and Kok, J. (1999). Pyrrolidone carboxyl peptidase of *Lactococcus lactis* MG1363. *Sixth Symposium on Lactic Acid Bacteria*, Book of abstracts, K32.

Buist, G., Venema, G., and Kok, J. (1998). Autolysis of *Lactococcus lactis* is influenced by proteolysis. *Journal of Bacteriology* 180: 5947–5953.

Bukau, B. (1993). Regulation of the *Escherichia coli* heat-shock response. *Molecular Microbiology* 9: 671–680.

Chapot-Chartier, M.-P., Deniel, C., Rousseau, M., Vassal, L., and Gripon, J.-C. (1994a). Autolysis of two strains of *Lactococcus lactis* during cheese ripening. *International Dairy Journal* 4: 251–269.

Chapot-Chartier, M.-P., Nardi, M., Chopin, M.-C., Chopin, A., and Gripon, J.-C. (1993). Cloning and sequencing of *pepC*, a cysteine aminopeptidase gene from *Lactococcus lactis* subsp. *cremoris* AM2. *Applied and Environmental Microbiology* 59: 330–333.

Chapot-Chartier, M.-P., Rul, F., Nardi, M., and Gripon, J.-C. (1994b). Gene cloning and characterization of PepC, a cysteine aminopeptidase from *Streptococcus thermophilus*, with sequence similarity to the eukaryotic bleomycin hydrolase. *European Journal of Biochemistry* 224: 497–506.

Christensen, J. E., Lin, D.-L., Palva, A., and Steele, J. L. (1995a). Sequence analysis, distribution and expression of an aminopeptidase N-encoding gene from *Lactobacillus helveticus* CNRZ32. *Gene* 155: 89–93.

Christensen, J. E., Johnson, M. E., and Steele, J. L. (1995b). Production of cheddar cheese using a *Lactococcus lactis* ssp. *cremoris* SK11 derivative with enhanced aminopeptidase activity. *International Dairy Journal* 5: 367–379.

Christensen, J. E., Dudley, E. G., Pederson, J. A., and Steele, J. (1999). Peptidases and amino acids catabolism in lactic acid bacteria. *Antonie van Leeuwenhoek* 76: 217–246.

Chopin, A. (1993). Organization and regulation of genes for amino acid biosynthesis in lactic acid bacteria. *FEMS Microbiological Reviews* 12: 21–38.

Coward, C., Le Page, R. W. F., and Wells, J. M. (1995). Lon and Clp-like ATP-dependent proteases of *Lactococcus lactis*, pp. 481–486. In: J. J. Ferretti, M. S. Gilmore, T. R. Klaenhammer, and F. Brown (Eds.), *Genetics of Streptococci, Enterococci and Lactococci. Developments in biological standardization*. Basel: Karger.

Crow, V. L., Coolbear, T., Gopal, P. K., Martley, F. G., Mckay, L. L., and Riepe, H. (1995). The role of autolysis of lactic acid bacteria in the ripening of cheese. *International Dairy Journal* 5: 855–875.

De Ruyter, P. G. G. A., Kuipers, O. P., and de Vos, W. M. (1996). Controlled gene expression systems for *Lactococcus lactis* with the food-grade inducer nisin. *Applied and Environmental Microbiology* 62: 3662–3667.

De Ruyter, P. G. G. A., Kuipers, O. P., Meijer, W. C., and de Vos, W. M. (1997). Food-grade controlled lysis of *Lactococcus lactis* for accelerated cheese ripening. *Nature Biotechnology* 15: 976–979.

Detmers, F. J. M., Kunji, E. R. S., Lanfermeijer, F. C., Poolman, B., and Konings, W. N. (1998). Kinetics and specificity of peptide uptake by the oligopeptide transport system of *Lactococcus lactis*. *Biochemistry* 37: 16671–16679.

Deutscher, J., Küster, E., Bergstedt, U., Charrier, V., and Hillen, W. (1995). Protein kinase-dependent HPr/CcpA interaction links glycolytic activity to carbon catabolite repression in Gram-positive bacteria. *Molecular Microbiology* 15: 1049–1053.

de Vos, W. M., Boerigter, I., Vos, P., Bruinenberg, P., and Siezen, R. J. (1991). Production, processing, and engineering of the *Lactococcus lactis* SK11 proteinase. In: G. M. Dunny, P. P. Cleary, and L. L. McKay (Eds.), *Genetics and molecular biology of Streptococci, Lactococci and Enterococci* (pp. 115–119). Washington, DC: American Society for Microbiology.

Dickely, R., Nilsson, D., Hansen, E. B., and Johansen, E. (1995). Isolation of *Lactococcus lactis* nonsense suppressors and construction of a food-grade cloning vector. *Molecular Microbiology* 15: 839–847.

Erra-Pujada, M., Mistou, M. Y., and Gripon, J.-C. (1995). Construction et étude d'une souche de *Lactococcus lactis* don't le gène *pepC* n'est plus fonctionnel. *7ème Colloque du Club des Bactéries Lactiques*, poster p. 8.

Exterkate, F. A. (1995). The lactococcal cell envelope proteinases: differences, calcium-binding effects and role in cheese ripening. *International Dairy Journal* 5: 995–1018.

Exterkate, F. A. (1985). A dual directed control of cell wall proteinase production in *S. cremoris* AM1: A possible mechanism of regulation during growth in milk. *Journal of Dairy Science* 68: 562–571.

Exterkate, F. A. (1977). Pyrrolidone carboxylyl peptidase in *Streptococcus cremoris*: Dependence on an interaction with membrane components. *Journal of Bacteriology* 129: 1281–1288.

Exterkate, F. A., and Alting, A. C. (1999). Role of calcium in activity and stability of the *Lactococcus lactis* cell envelope proteinase. *Applied and Environmental Microbiology* 65: 1390–1396.

Exterkate, F. A., and Alting, A. C. (1995). The role of starter peptidases in the initial proteolytic events leading to amino acids in Gouda cheese. *International Journal of Dairy Science* 5: 15–28.

Exterkate, F. A., Alting, A. C., and Bruinenberg, P. G. (1993). Diversity of cell envelope proteinase specificity among strains of *Lactococcus lactis* and its relationship to charge characteristics of the substrate-binding region. *Applied and Environmental Microbiology* 59: 3640–3647.

Exterkate, F. A., and De Veer, G. J. C. M. (1987). Purification and some properties of a membrane-bound aminopeptidase A from *Streptococcus cremoris*. *Applied and Environmental Microbiology* 53: 577–583.

Fang, G., Konings, W. N., and Poolman, B. (2000). Kinetics and substrate specificity of membrane-reconstituted peptide transporter DtpT of *Lactococcus lactis*. *Journal of Bacteriology* 182: 2530–2535.

Foucaud, C., Kunji, E. R. S., Hagting, A., Richard, J., Konings, W. N., Desmazeaud, M., and Poolman, B. (1995). Specificity of peptide transport systems in *Lactococcus lactis*: evidence for a third system which transports hydrophobic di- and tripeptides. *Journal of Bacteriology* 177: 4652–4657.

Franke, C. M., Tiemersma, J., Venema, G., and Kok, J. (1999). Membrane topology of the lactococcal bacteriocin ATP-binding cassette transporter protein LcnC. Involvement of LcnC in lactococcin a maturation. *Journal of Biological Chemistry* 274: 8484–8490.

Frees, D., and Ingmer, H. (1999). Clp participates in the degradation of misfolded protein in *Lactococcus lactis*. *Molecular Microbiology* 31: 79–87.

Gasson, M. J. (1990). *In vivo* genetic systems in lactic acid bacteria. *FEMS Microbiological Reviews* 87: 43–60.

Godon, J.-J., Delorme, C., Ehrlich, S. D., and Renault, P. (1992). Divergence of genomic sequences between *Lactococcus lactis* subsp. *lactis* and *Lactococcus lactis* subsp. *cremoris*. *Applied and Environmental Microbiology* 58: 4045–4047.

Gross, C. A. (1996). Function and regulation of the heat shock proteins. In: F. C. Neidhardt, R. Curtiss III, J. L. Ingraham, E. C. C. Lin, K. B. Low, B. Magasanik, W. S. Reznikoff, M. Riley, M. Schaechter, and H. E. Umbarger (Eds.), Escherichia coli *and* Salmonella: *cellular and molecular biology* (pp. 1382–1399 2nd ed.). Washington, DC: ASM Press.

Guédon, E., Renault, P., Ehrlich, S. D., and Delorme, C. (1999). Environmental and genetic factors affecting the expression of peptidase genes in lactococci. *Sixth Symposium on Lactic Acid Bacteria*, Book of abstracts, K34.

Haandrikman, A. J., Kok, J., Laan, H., Soemitro, S., Ledeboer, A. M., Konings, W. N., and Venema, G. (1989). Identification of a gene required for maturation of an extracellular lactococcal proteinase. *Journal of Bacteriology* 171: 2789–2794.

Haandrikman, A. J., Kok, J., and Venema, G. (1991). Lactococcal proteinase maturation protein PrtM is a lipoprotein. *Journal of Bacteriology* 173: 4517–4525.

Hagting, A., Kunji, E. R. S., Leenhouts, K. J., Poolman, B., and Konings, W. N. (1994). The di- and tripeptide transport protein of *Lactococcus lactis*. *Journal of Biological Chemistry* 269: 11391–11399.

Hansen, P. A. (1941). A study in cheese ripening. The influence of autolysed cells of *Streptococcus cremoris* and *Streptococcus lactis* on the development of *Lactobacillus casei*. *Journal of Dairy Science* 24: 969–976.

Havarstein, L. S., Diep, D. B., and Nes, I. F. (1995). A family of bacteriocin ABC transporters carry out proteolytic processing of their substrates concomitant with export. *Molecular Microbiology* 16: 229–240.

Hellendoorn, M., De Jong, A., Buist, G., Venema, G., and Kok, J. (1999). Regulation of components of the proteolytic system. *Sixth Symposium on Lactic Acid Bacteria*, Book of abstracts, K33.

Hellendoorn, M. A., Franke-Fayard, B. M. D., Mierau, I., Venema, G., and Kok, J. (1997). Cloning and analysis of the *pepV* dipeptidase gene of *Lactococcus lactis* MG1363. *Journal of Bacteriology*. 179: 3410–3415.

Higgins, C. F. (1992). ABC transporters: from microorganisms to man. *Annual Review of Cell and Developmental Biology* 8: 67–113.

Holt, C., and Sawyer, L. (1988). Primary and predicted secondary structures of the caseins in relation to their biological function. *Protein Engineer* 2: 251–259.

Huang, D. C., Huang, X. F., Novel, G., and Novel, M. (1993). Two genes present on a transposon-like structure in *Lactococcus lactis* are involved in a Clp-family proteolytic activity. *Molecular Microbiology* 7: 957–965.

Hueck, C. J., and Hillen, W. (1995). Catabolite repression in *Bacillus subtilis*: A global regulatory mechanism for the Gram-positive bacteria? *Molecular Microbiology* 15: 395–401.

Hwang, I.-K., Kaminogawa, S., and Yamauchi, K. (1981). Purification and properties of a dipeptidase from *Streptococcus cremoris*. *Agricultural and Biological Chemistry* 45: 159–165.

Hwang, I.-K., Kaminogawa, S., and Yamauchi, K. (1982). Kinetic properties of a dipeptidase from *Streptococcus cremoris*. *Agricultural and Biological Chemistry* 46: 3049–3053.

Ingmer, H., Vogensen, F. K., Hammer, K., and Kilstrup, M. (1999). Disruption and analysis of the *clpB, clpC* and *clpE* genes in *Lactococcus lactis*: ClpE, a new Clp family in Gram-Positive bacteria. *Journal of Bacteriology* 181: 2075–2083.

Jacobs, M., Andersen, J. B., Kontinen, V., and Sarvas, M. (1993). *Bacillus subtilis* PrsA is required *in vivo* as an extracytoplasmic chaperone for secretion of active enzymes synthesized either with of without prosequences. *Molecular Microbiology* 8: 957–966.

Juillard, V., Laan, H., Kunji, E. R. S., Jeronimus-Stratingh, C. M., Bruins, A. P., and Konings, W. N. (1995a). The extracellular P_I-type proteinase of *Lactococcus lactis* hydrolyzes beta-casein into more than one hundred different oligopeptides. *Journal of Bacteriology* 177: 3472–3478.

Juillard, V., Le Bars, D., Kunji, E. R. S., Konings, W. N., Gripon, J.-C., and Richard, J. (1995b). Oligopeptides are the main source of nitrogen for *Lactococcus lactis* during growth in milk. *Applied and Environmental Microbiology* 61: 3024–3030.

Kahala, M., and Palva, A. (1999). The expression signals of the *Lactococcus brevis slpA* gene direct efficient heterologous protein production in lactic acid bacteria. *Applied Microbiology and Biotechnology* 51: 71–78.

Kaminogawa, S., Azuma, N., Hwang, I. K., Suzuki, Y., and Yamauchi, K. (1984). Isolation and characterization of a prolidase from *Streptococcus cremoris* H61. *Agricultural and Biological Chemistry* 48: 3035–3040.

Katayama, Y., Gottesman, S., Pumphrey, J., Rudikoff, S., Clark, W. P., and Maurizi, M. R. (1988). The two-component, ATP-dependent Clp protease of *Escherichia coli*. Purification, cloning and mutational analysis of the ATP binding component. *Journal of Biological Chemistry* 263: 15226–15236.

Kilstrup, M., Jacobsen, S., Hammer, K., and Vogensen, F. K. (1997). Induction of heat shock proteins DnaK, GroEL, and GroES by salt stress in *Lactococcus lactis*. *Applied and Environmental Microbiology* 63: 1826–1837.

Kiefer-Partsch, B., Bockelmann, W., Geis, A., and Teuber, M. (1989). Purification of an X-prolyl-dipeptidyl aminopeptidase from the cell wall proteolytic system of *Lactococcus lactis* subsp. *cremoris*. *Applied Microbiology and Biotechnology* 31: 75–78.

Kim, K. I., Park, S. C., Kang, S. H., Cheong, G. W., and Chung, C. H. (1999). Selective degradation of unfolded proteins by the self-compartmentalizing HtrA protease, a periplasmic heat shock protein in *Escherichia coli*. *Journal of Molecular Biology* 294: 1363–1374.

Kiwaki, M., Ikemura, H., Shimizu-Kadota, M., and Hirashima, A. (1989). Molecular characterization of a cell wall associated proteinase gene of *Streptococcus lactis* NCDO763. *Molecular Microbiology* 3: 359–369.

Koch, B., Kilstrup, M., Vogensen, F. K., and Hammer, K. (1998). Induced levels of heat shock proteins in a *dnaK* mutant of *Lactococcus lactis*. *Journal of Bacteriology* 180: 3873–3881.

Kok, J. (1990). Genetics of the proteolytic system of lactic acid bacteria. *FEMS Microbiological Reviews* 87: 15–41.

Kok, J., and de Vos, W. M. (1994). The proteolytic system of lactic acid bacteria. In: M. Gasson and W. De Vos (Eds.), *Genetics and biotechnology of lactic acid bacteria* (pp. 169–210). London, England: Blackie and Professional.

Kok, J., Leenhouts, K. J., Haandrikman, A. J., Ledeboer, A. M., and Venema, G. (1988). Nucleotide sequence of the cell wall proteinase gene of *Streptococcus cremoris* Wg2. *Applied and Environmental Microbiology* 54: 231–238.

Kok, J., Van Dijl, J. M., van der Vossen, J. M. B. M., and Venema, G. (1985). Cloning and expression of a *Streptococcus cremoris* proteinase gene in *Bacillus subtilis* and *Streptococcus lactis*. *Applied and Environmental Microbiology* 50: 94–101.

Kok, J., and Venema, G. (1988). Genetics of proteinases in lactic acid bacteria. *Biochimie* 70: 475–488.

Konings, W. N., Poolman, B., and Driessen, A. J. M. (1989). Bioenergetics and solute transport in lactococci. *CRC Critical Reviews in Microbiology* 16: 419–476.

Kuipers, O. P., De Jong, A., Holsappel, S., Bron, S., Kok, J., and Hamoen, L. W. (1999). DNA-micro-arrays and food-biotechnology. *Antonie van Leeuwenhoek* 76: 353–355.

Kuipers, O. P., De Ruyter, P. G. G. A., Kleerebezem, M., and De Vos, W. M. (1997). Controlled overproduction of proteins by lactic acid bacteria. *Trends in Biotechnology* 15: 135–140.

Kunji, E. R. S., Hagting, A., De Vries, C. J., Juillard, V., Haandrikman, A. J., Poolman, B., and Konings, W. N. (1995). Transport of β-casein-derived peptides by the oligopeptide transport system is a crucial step in the proteolytic pathway of *Lactococcus lactis*. *Journal of Biological Chemistry* 270: 1569–1574.

Kunji, E. R. S., Mierau, I., Hagting, A., Poolman, B., and Konings, W. N. (1996a). The proteolytic systems of lactic acid bacteria. *Antonie van Leeuwenhoek* 70: 187–221.

Kunji, E. R. S., Mierau, I., Poolman, B., Konings, W. N., Venema, G., and Kok, J. (1996b). The fate of peptides in peptidase mutants of *Lactococcus lactis*. *Molecular Microbiology* 21: 123–131.

Kunji, E. R. S., Smid, E. J., Plapp, R., Poolman, B., and Konings, W. N. (1993). Di- , tripeptides and oligopeptides are taken up via distinct transport mechanisms in *Lactococcus lactis*. *Journal of Bacteriology* 175: 2052–2059.

Laan, H., Bolhuis, H., Poolman, B., Abee, T., and Konings, W. N. (1993). Regulation of proteinase synthesis in *Lactococcus lactis*. *Acta Biotechnology* 13: 95–101.

Laan, H., Haverkort, R. E., De Leij, L., and Konings, W. N. (1996). Detection and localisation of lactococcal peptidases with monoclonal antibodies. *Journal of Dairy Research* 63: 245–256.

Lanfermeijer, F. C., Picon, A., Konings, W. N., and Poolman, B. (1999). Kinetics and consequences of binding of nona- and dodecapeptides to the oligopeptide binding protein (OppA) of *Lactococcus lactis*. *Biochemistry* 38: 14440–14450.

l'Anson, K. J., Movahedi, S., Griffin, H. G., Gasson, M. J., and Mulholland, F. (1995). A non-essential glutamyl aminopeptidase is required for optimal growth of *Lactococcus lactis* MG1363 in milk. *Microbiology* 141: 2873–2881.

Law, J., Fitzgerald, G. R., Uniacke-Lowe, T., Daly, C., and Fox, P. F. (1993). The contribution of lactococcal starter proteinases to proteolysis in Cheddar cheese. *Journal of Dairy Science* 76: 2455–2467.

Law, B. A., Sharpe, M. E., and Reiter, B. (1974). The release of intracellular dipeptidase from starter streptococci during Cheddar cheese ripening. *Journal of Dairy Research* 41: 137–146.

Law, J., Vos, P., Hayes, F., Daly, C., de Vos, W. M., and Fitzgerald, G. F. (1992). Cloning and partial sequencing of the proteinase gene complex from *Lactococcus lactis* subsp. *lactis* UC317. *Journal of General Microbiology* 138: 1–10.

Leenhouts, K., Bolhuis, A., Boot, J., Deutz, I., Toonen, M., Venema, G., Kok, J., and Ledeboer, A. (1998). Cloning, expression, and chromosomal stabilization of the *Propionibacterium shermanii* proline iminopeptidase gene (*pip*) for food-grade application in *Lactococcus lactis*. *Applied and Environmental Microbiology* 64: 4736–4742.

Leenhouts, K. J., Buist, G., Bolhuis, A., Ten Berge, A., Kiel, J., Mierau, I., Dabrowska, M., Venema, G., and Kok, J. (1996). A general system for generating unlabelled gene replacements in the bacterial chromosome. *Molecular & General Genetics* 253: 217–224.

Leenhouts, K., Gietema, J., Kok, J., and Venema, G. (1991). Chromosomal stabilization of the proteinase genes in *Lactococcus lactis*. *Applied and Environmental Microbiology* 57: 2568–2575.

Lloyd, R. J., and Pritchard, G. G. (1991). Characterization of X-prolyl dipeptidyl aminopeptidase from *Lactococcus lactis* ssp. *lactis* H1. *Journal of General Microbiology* 137: 49–56.

Luesink, E. J., Van Herpen, R. E. M. A., Grossiord, B. P., Kuipers, O. P., and de Vos, W. M. (1998). Transcriptional activation of the glycolytic *las* operon and catabolite repression of the *gal* operon in *Lactococcus lactis* are mediated by the catabolite control protein CcpA. *Molecular Microbiology* 30: 789–798.

Mars, I., and Monnet, V. (1995). An aminopeptidase P from *Lactococcus lactis* with original specificity. *Biochimica et Biophysica Acta* 1243: 209–215.

Marugg, J. D., Meijer, W. C., Van Kranenburg, R., Laverman, P., Bruinenberg, P. G., and de Vos, W. M. (1995). Medium-dependent regulation of proteinase gene expression in *Lactococcus lactis*: control of transcription initiation by specific dipeptides. *Journal of Bacteriology* 177: 2982–2989.

Marugg, J. D., Van Kranenburg, R., Laverman, P., Rutten, G. A. M., and de Vos, W. M. (1996). Identical transcriptional control of the divergently transcribed *prtP* and *prtM* genes that are required for proteinase production in *Lactococcus lactis* SK11. *Journal of Bacteriology* 178: 1525–1531.

Mata, L., Erra-Pujada, M., Gripon, J.-C., and Mistou, M.-Y. (1997). Experimental evidence for the essential role of the C-terminal residue in the strict aminopeptidase activity of the thiol aminopeptidase PepC, a bacterial bleomycin hydrolase. *Biochemical Journal* 328: 343–347.

Mata, L., Gripon, J.-C., and Mistou, M.-Y. (1999). Deletion of the four C-terminal residues of PepC converts an aminopeptidase into an oligopeptidase. *Protein Engineering* 12: 681–686.

Matos, J., Nardi, M., Kumura, H., and Monnet, V. (1998). Genetic characterization of *pepP*, which encodes an aminopeptidase P whose deficiency does not affect *Lactococcus lactis* growth in milk, unlike deficiency of the X-prolyl dipeptidyl aminopeptidase. *Applied and Environmental Microbiology* 64: 4591–4595.

Maurizi, M. R., Clark, W., Kim, S. H., and Gottesman, S. (1990). ClpP represents a unique family of serine proteases. *Journal of Biological Chemistry* 265: 12546–12552.

Mayhew, M., and Hartl, F.-U. (1996). Molecular chaperone proteins. In: F. C. Neidhardt, R. Curtiss III, J. L. Ingraham, E. C. C. Lin, K. B. Low, B. Magasanik, W. S. Reznikoff, M. Riley, M. Schaechter, and H. E. Umbarger (Eds.), Escherichia coli *and* Salmonella: *cellular and molecular biology* (pp. 922–937, 2nd ed.). Washington, DC: ASM Press.

Mayo, B., Kok, J., Bockelmann, W., Haandrikman, A., Leenhouts, K. J., and Venema, G. (1993). The effect of X-prolyl dipeptidyl aminopeptidase deficiency in *Lactococcus lactis*. *Applied and Environmental Microbiology* 59: 2049–2055.

Mayo, B., Kok, J., Venema, K., Bockelmann, W., Teuber, M., Reinke, H., and Venema, G. (1991). Molecular cloning and sequence analysis of the X-prolyl dipeptidyl aminopeptidase gene from *Lactococcus lactis* subsp. *cremoris*. *Applied and Environmental Microbiology* 57: 38–44.

McGarry, A., Law, J., Coffey, A., Daly, C., Fox, P. F., and Fitzgerald, G. F. (1994). Effect of genetically modifying the lactococcal proteolytic system on ripening and flavor development in Cheddar cheese. *Applied and Environmental Microbiology* 60: 4226–4233.

McKay, L. L. (1983). Functional properties of plasmids in lactic streptococci. *Antonie van Leeuwenhoek* 49: 259–274.

Meijer, W. C., Marugg, J. D., and Hugenholtz, J. (1996). Regulation of proteolytic enzyme activity in *Lactococcus lactis*. *Applied and Environmental Microbiology* 62: 156–161.

Mierau, I., Haandrikman, A. J., Velterop, O., Tan, P. S. T., Leenhouts, K. L., Konings, W. N., Venema, G., and Kok, J. (1994). Tripeptidase gene (*pept*) of *Lactococcus lactis*: molecular cloning and nucleotide sequencing of *pepT* and construction of a chromosomal deletion mutant. *Journal of Bacteriology* 176: 2854–2861.

Mierau, I., Kunji, E. R. S., Leenhouts, K. J., Hellendoorn, M. A., Haandrikman, A. J., Poolman, B., Konings, W. N., Venema, G., and Kok, J. (1996). Multiple-peptidase mutants of *Lactococcus lactis* are severely impaired in their ability to grow in milk. *Journal of Bacteriology* 178: 2794–2803.

Mierau, I., Tan, P. S. T., Haandrikman, A. J., Kok, J., Leenhouts, K. J., Konings, W. N., and Venema, G. (1993). Cloning and sequencing of the gene for a lactococcal endopeptidase, an enzyme with sequence similarity to mammalian enkephalinase. *Journal of Bacteriology* 175: 2087–2096.

Mistou, M.-Y., and Gripon, J.-C. (1998). Catalytic properties of the cysteine aminopeptidase PepC, a bacterial bleomycin hydrolase. *Biochimica et Biophysica Acta* 3: 63–70.

Mistou, M.-Y., Rigolet, P., Chapot-Chartier, M.-P., Nardi, M., Gripon, J.-C., and Brunie, S. (1994). Crystallization and preliminary X-ray analysis of PepC, a thiol aminopeptidase from *Lactococcus lactis* homologous to bleomycin hydrolase. *Journal of Molecular Biology* 237: 160–162.

Monedero, V., Gosalbes, M. J., and Perez-Martinez, G. (1997). Catabolite repression in *Lactobacillus casei* ATCC 393 is mediated by CcpA. *Journal of Bacteriology* 179: 6657–6664.

Monnet, V., Bockelmann, W., Gripon, J.-C., and Teuber, M. (1989). Comparison of cell wall proteinases from *Lactococcus lactis* subsp. *cremoris* AC1 and *Lactococcus lactis* subsp. *lactis* NCDO 763. *Applied Microbiology and Biotechnology* 31: 112–118.

Monnet, V., Le Bars, D., and Gripon, J.-C. (1986). Specificity of a cell wall proteinase from *Streptococcus lactis* NCDO 763 towards bovine β-casein. *FEMS Microbiological Letters* 36: 127–131.

Monnet, V., Ley, J. P., and Gonzalez, S. (1992). Substrate specificity of the cell envelope-located proteinase of *Lactococcus lactis* subsp. *lactis* NCDO 763. *International Journal of Biochemistry* 24: 707–718.

Monnet, V., Nardi, M., Chopin, A., Chopin, M.-C., and Gripon, J.-C. (1994). Biochemical and genetic characterization of PepF, an oligopeptidase from *Lactococcus lactis. Journal of Biological Chemistry* 269: 32070–32076.

Nardi, M., Chopin, M.-C., Chopin, A., CALS, M.-M., and Gripon, J.-C. (1991). Cloning and DNA sequence analysis of an X-prolyl dipeptidyl peptidase gene from *Lactococcus lactis* subsp. *lactis* NCDO 763. *Applied and Environmental Microbiology* 57: 45–50.

Nardi, M., Renault, P., and Monnet, V. (1997). Duplication of the *pepF* gene and shuffling DNA fragments on the lactose plasmid of *Lactococcus lactis. Journal of Bacteriology* 13: 4164–4171.

Nath, K. R. (1992). Cheese. In: *Dairy science and technology handbook* (pp. 161–255). New York: VCH Publishers, Inc.

Navarre, W. W., and Schneewind, O. (1994). Proteolytic cleavage and cell wall anchoring at the LPXTG motif of surface proteins in Gram-positive bacteria. *Molecular Microbiology* 14: 115–121.

Nauta, A., Van Den Burg, B., Karsens, H., Venema, G., and Kok, J. (1997). Design of thermolabile bacteriophage repressor mutants by comparative molecular modelling. *Nature Biotechnology* 15: 980–983.

Neviani, E., Boquien, C. Y., Monnet, V., Phan Thanh, L., and Gripon, J.-C. (1989). Purification and characterization of an aminopeptidase from *Lactococcus lactis* ssp. *cremoris* AM2. *Applied and Environmental Microbiology* 55: 2308–2314.

Nissen-Meyer, J., Lillehaug, D., and Nes, I. F. (1992). The plasmid-encoded lactococcal envelope-associated proteinase is encoded by a chromosomal gene in *Lactococcus lactis* subsp. *cremoris* BC101. *Applied and Environmental Microbiology* 58: 750–753.

Niven, G. W. (1991). Purification and properties of aminopeptidase A from *Lactococcus lactis* subsp. *lactis* NCDO 712. *Journal of General Microbiology* 137: 1207–1212.

Odagaki, Y., Hayashi, A., Okada, K., Hirotsu, K., Kabashima, T., Ito, K., Yoshimoto, T., Tsuru, D., Sato, M., and Clardy, J. (1999). The crystal structure of pyroglutamyl peptidase I from *Bacillus amyloliquefaciens* reveals a new structure for a cysteine protease. *Structure* 7: 399–411.

Piard, J.-C., Hautefort, I., Fischetti, V. A., Ehrlich, S. D., Fons, M., and Gruss, A. (1997). Cell wall anchoring of the *Streptococcus pyogenes* M6 protein in various lactic acid bacteria. *Journal of Bacteriology* 179: 3068–3072.

Picon, A., Kunji, E. R. S., Lanfermeijer, F. C., Konings, W. N., and Poolman, B. (2000). Specificity mutants of the binding protein of the oligopeptide transport system of *Lactococcus lactis. Journal of Bacteriology* 182: 1600–1608.

Poquet, I., Saint, V., Seznec, E., Simoes, N., Bolotin, A., and Gruss, A. (2000). HtrA is the unique surface housekeeping protease in *Lactococcus lactis* and is required for natural protein processing. *Molecular Microbiology* 35: 1042–1051.

Pritchard, G. G., and Coolbear, T. (1993). The physiology and biochemistry of the proteolytic system in lactic acid bacteria. *FEMS Microbiological Reviews* 12: 179–206.

Rank, T. C., Grappin, R., and Olson, N. F. (1985). Secondary proteolysis of cheese during ripening: A review. *Journal of Dairy Science* 68: 801–805.

Reid, J. R., Coolbear, T., Pillidge, C. J., and Pritchard, G. G. (1994). Specificity of hydrolysis of bovine κ-casein by cell envelope-associated proteinases from *Lactococcus lactis* strains. *Applied and Environmental Microbiology* 60: 801–806.

Reid, J. R., Ng, K. H., Moore, C. H., Coolbear, T., and Pritchard, G. G. (1991b). Comparison of bovine β-casein hydrolysis by P_I and P_{III}-type proteinases from *Lactococcus lactis* subsp. *cremoris. Applied Microbiology and Biotechnology* 36: 344–351.

Reid, J. R., Moore C. H., Midwinter, G. G., and Pritchard, G. G. (1991a). Action of a cell wall proteinase from *Lactococcus lactis* subsp. *cremoris* SK11 on bovine α_{s1}-casein. *Applied Microbiology and Biotechnology* 35: 222–227.

Ross, R. P., Galvin, M., Mcauliffe, O., Morgan, S. M., Ryan, M. P., Twomey, D. P., Meaney, W. J., and Hill, C. (1999). Developing applications for lactococcal bacteriocins. *Antonie van Leeuwenhoek* 76: 337–346.

Rudd, K. E., Sofia, J. H., Koonin, E. V., Plunkett G. III, Lazar, S., and Rouviere, P. E. (1995). A new family of peptidyl-prolyl isomerases. *Trends in Biochemical Sciences* 20: 12–14.

Sarkis, K. M., Liu, G., Ton-That, H., and Schneewind, O. (1999). *Staphylococcus aureus* sortase, an enzyme that anchors surface proteins to the cell wall. *Nature* 285: 760–763.

Schick, J., Weber, B., Klein, J. R., and Henrich, B. (1999). PepR1, a CcpA-like transcription regulator of *Lactobacillus delbrueckii* subsp. *lactis. Microbiology* 145: 3147–3154.

Siezen, R. J. (1999). Multi-domain, cell-envelope proteinases of lactic acid bacteria. *Antonie van Leeuwenhoek* 76: 139–155.
Siezen, R. J., Bruinenberg, P. G., Vos, P., van Alen-Boerrigter, I. J., Nijhuis, M., Alting, A. C., Exterkate, F. A., and de Vos, W. M. (1993). Engineering of the substrate binding region of the subtilisin-like, cell envelope proteinase of *Lactococcus lactis. Protein Engineering* 6: 927–937.
Siezen, R. J., and Leunissen, J. A. M. (1997). Subtilases: the superfamily of subtilisin-like serine proteases. *Protein Science* 6: 501–523.
Siezen, R. J., de Vos, W. M., Leunissen, J. A. M., and Dijkstra, B. W. (1991). Homology modelling and protein engineering strategy of subtilases, the family of subtilisin-like proteinases. *Protein Engineering* 4: 719–737.
Singleton, M. R., Isupov, M. N., and Littlechild, J. A. (1999). X-ray structure of pyrrolidone carboxyl peptidase from the hyperthermophilic archaeon *Thermococcus litoralis. Structure* 7: 237–244.
Smid, E. J., Driessen, A. J., and Konings, W. N. (1989). Mechanism and energetics of dipeptide transport in membrane vesicles of *Lactococcus lactis. Journal of Bacteriology* 171: 292–298.
Sørensen, K. I., Larsen, R., Kibenich, A., Junge, M. P., and Johansen, E. (2000). A food-grade system for industrial strains of *Lactococcus lactis. Applied and Environmental Microbiology* 66: 1253–1258.
Stadhouders, J., Toepoel, L., and Wouters, J. T. M. (1988). Cheese making with prt^- and prt^+ variants of N-streptococci and their mixtures. Phage sensitivity, proteolysis and flavour development during ripening. *Netherlands Milk Dairy Journal* 42: 183–193.
Steiner, H. Y., Naider, F., and Becker, J. M. (1995). The PTR family: a new group of peptide transporters. *Molecular Microbiology* 16: 825–834.
Strøman, P., Williams, D., Behrndt, H., and Johansen, E. (1998). Starter cultures with genetically modified peptidase activity for production of cheese. Proceedings, 1st Int. Symposium on Enzymatic Protein Processing, Noordwijkerhout, The Netherlands.
Strøman, P. (1992). Sequence of a gene (*lap*) encoding a 95.3-kDa aminopeptidase from *Lactococcus lactis* ssp. *cremoris* Wg2. *Gene* 113: 107–112.
Tan, P. S. T., van Alen-Boerrigter, I. J., Poolman, B., Siezen, R. J., de Vos, W. M., and Konings, W. N. (1992). Characterization of the *Lactococcus lactis pepN* gene encoding an aminopeptidase homologous to mammalian aminopeptidase N. *FEBS Letters* 306: 9–16.
Tan, P. S. T., and Konings, W. N. (1990). Purification and characterization of an aminopeptidase from *Lactococcus lactis* ssp. *cremoris* Wg2. *Applied and Environmental Microbiology* 56: 526–532.
Tan, P. S. T., Van Kessel, T. A. J. M., Van De Veerdonk, F. L. M., Zuurendonk, P. F., Bruins, A. P., and Konings, W. N. (1993). Degradation and debittering of a tryptic digest from beta-casein by aminopeptidase N from *Lactococcus lactis* subsp. *cremoris* Wg2. *Applied and Environmental Microbiology* 59: 1430–1436.
Thomas, T. D., and Pritchard, G. G. (1987). Proteolytic enzymes of dairy starter cultures. *FEMS Microbiological Reviews* 46: 245–268.
Tynkkynen, S., Buist, G., Kunji, E., Kok, J., Poolman, B., Venema, G., and Haandrikman, A. (1993). Genetic and biochemical characterization of the oligopeptide transport system of *Lactococcus lactis. Journal of Bacteriology* 175: 7523–7532.
van Alen-Boerrigter, I. J., Baankreis, R., and de Vos, W. M. (1991). Characterization and overexpression of the *Lactococcus lactis pepN* gene and localization of its product, aminopeptidase N. *Applied and Environmental Microbiology* 57: 2555–2561.
van Boven, A., Tan, P. S. T., and Konings, W. N. (1988). Purification and characterization of a dipeptidase from *Streptococcus cremoris* Wg2. *Applied and Environmental Microbiology* 54: 43–49.
van De Guchte, M., Kodde, J., Van der Vossen, J. M. B. M., KOK, J., and Venema, G. (1990). Heterologous gene expression in *Lactococcus lactis* subsp. *lactis*: Synthesis, secretion, and processing of the *Bacillus subtilis* neutral protease. *Applied and Environmental Microbiology* 56: 2606–2611.
van Der Meer, J. R., Polman, J., Beerthuyzen, M. M., Siezen, R. J., Kuipers, O. P., and de Vos, W. M. (1993). Characterization of the *Lactococcus lactis* nisin A operon genes *nisP*, encoding a subtilisin-like serine protease involved in precursor processing, and *nisR*, encoding a regulatory protein involved in nisin biosynthesis. *Journal of Bacteriology* 175: 2578–2588.
van der Vossen, J. M. B. M., Kodde, J., Haandrikman, A. J., Venema, G., and Kok, J. (1992). Characterization of transcription initiation and termination signals of the proteinase genes of *Lactococcus lactis* Wg2 and enhancement of proteolysis in *L. lactis. Applied and Environmental Microbiology* 58: 3142–3149.
Venema, K., Kok, J., Marugg, J. D., Toonen, M. Y., Ledeboer, A. M., Venema, G., and Chikindas, M. L. (1995). Functional analysis of the pediocin operon of *Pediococcus acidilactici* PAC1.0: PedB is the immunity protein and PedD is the precursor processing enzyme. *Molecular Microbiology* 17: 515–522.

Visser, S. (1993). Proteolytic enzymes and their relation to cheese ripening and flavor: An overview. *Journal of Dairy Science* 76: 329–350.

Visser, S., Exterkate, F. A., Slangen, K. J., and De Veer, G. J. C. M. (1986). Comparative study of the action of cell wall proteinases from various strains of *Streptococcus cremoris* on bovine α_s1- β- and κ-casein. *Applied and Environmental Microbiology* 52: 1162.

Visser, S., Robben, A. J. P. M., and Slangen, C. J. (1991). Specificity of a cell-envelope-located proteinase (P_{III}-type) from *Lactococcus lactis* subsp. *cremoris* AM1 in its action on bovine β-casein. *Applied Microbiology and Biotechnology* 35: 477–483.

Visser, S., Slangen, C. J., Exterkate, F. A., and De Veer, G. J. C. M. (1988). Action of a cell wall proteinase (P_I) from Streptococcus cremoris HP on bovine β-casein. *Applied Microbiology and Biotechnology* 29: 61–66.

Visser, S., Slangen, C. J., Robben, A. J. P. M., Van Dongen, W. D., Heerma, W., and Haverkamp, J. (1994). Action of a cell-envelope proteinase (CEP_{III}-type) from *Lactococcus lactis* subsp. *cremoris* AM1 on bovine β-casein. *Applied Microbiology and Biotechnology* 41: 644–651.

Von Heijne, G. (1983). Pattern of amino acids near signal-sequence cleavage sites. *European Journal of Biochemistry* 133: 17–21.

Vos, P., Boerrigter, I. J., Buist, G., Haandrikman, A. J., Nijhuis, M., De Reuver, M. B., Siezen, R. J., Venema, G., de Vos, W. M., and Kok, J. (1991). Engineering of the *Lactococcus lactis* proteinase by construction of hybrid enzymes. *Protein Engineering* 4: 479–484.

Vos, P., Simons, G., Siezen, R. J., and De Vos, W. M. (1989a). Primary structure and organization of the gene for a prokaryotic cell-envelope-located serine proteinase. *Journal of Biological Chemistry* 264: 13579–13585.

Vos, P., Van Asseldonk, M., Van Jeveren, F., Siezen, R. J., Simons, G., and De Vos, W. M. (1989b). A maturation protein is essential for the production of active forms of *Lactococcus lactis* SK11 serine proteinase located in or secreted from the cell envelope. *Journal of Bacteriology* 171: 2795–2802.

Waller, P. R. H., and Sauer, R. T. (1996). Characterization of *degQ* and *degS, Escherichia coli* genes encoding homologs of the DegP protease. *Journal of Bacteriology* 178: 1146–1153.

Wegmann, U., Klein, J. R., Drumm, I., Kuipers, O. P., and Henrich, B. (1999). Introduction of peptidase genes from *Lactobacillus delbrueckii* subsp. *lactis* into *Lactococcus lactis* and controlled expression. *Applied and Environmental Microbiology* 65: 4729–4733.

Weimer, B., Seefeldt, K., and Dias, B. (1999). Sulfur metabolism in bacteria associated with cheese. *Antonie van Leeuwenhoek* 76: 247–261.

Whitaker, R. D., and Batt, C. A. (1991). Characterization of the heat shock response in *Lactococcus lactis* subsp. *lactis*. *Applied and Environmental Microbiology* 57: 1408–1412.

Zevaco, C., Monnet, V., and Gripon, J.-C. (1990). Intracellular X-prolyl dipeptidyl peptidase from *Lactococcus lactis* ssp. *lactis*: Purification and properties. *Journal of Applied Bacteriology* 68: 357–366.

8

Genetics of Bacteriocin Production in Lactic Acid Bacteria

Morten Skaugen, Luis M. Cintas, and Ingolf F. Nes

Introduction

Peptides with antimicrobial activity are widely distributed in nature and are produced by a wide range of mammals, birds, insects, plants, and microorganisms (Cammue et al., 1994; Sahl, 1994; Nissen-Meyer and Nes, 1997; Boman, 2000). Ribosomally synthesized antimicrobial peptides in bacteria are generally referred to as bacteriocins, and are produced by numerous Gram-positive and Gram-negative bacteria (Klaenhammer, 1993; Nes et al., 1996; Nissen-Meyer and Nes, 1997). Most bacteriocins from Gram-negative bacteria are proteins larger than 20 kDa. Notable exceptions to this general rule are colicin V, the microcins from *Escherichia coli/Klebsiella pneumoniae*, and haemocin from *Haemophilus influenzae* (Håvarstein et al., 1994; Murley et al., 1997, 1998, Blond et al., 1999; Lagos et al., 1999; Rodriguez et al., 1999), which resemble the peptide-bacteriocins (usually smaller than 60 amino acids) produced by lactic acid bacteria (LAB).

Whereas the production of antimicrobial peptides is usually constitutive in higher eukaryotes, it is regulated in lower eukaryotes. The eukaryotic peptides are involved in processes such as the immune response to bacterial infection, and are often referred to as being part of the innate immune response system. In prokaryotes, antimicrobial peptides provide the producer with a competitive advantage for nutrition in the surroundings. Despite differences in their primary structures, antimicrobial peptides are, with few exceptions, cationic and often amphiphilic, reflecting their ability to kill target cells by permeabilizing

Morten Skaugen • Laboratory of Microbial Gene Technology, Department of Chemistry and Biotechnology, Agricultural University of Norway, Norway **Luis M. Cintas** • Departamento de Nutrición y Bromotología III, Facultad de Veterinaria, Universidad Complutense de Madrid, 28040-Madrid, Spain **Ingolf F. Nes** • Laboratory of Microbial Gene Technology, Department of Chemistry and Biotechnology, Agricultural University of Norway, Norway; e-mail: Ingolf.Nes@ikb.nlh.no

the cell membrane (Hancock and Chapple, 1999). Bacteriocinogenic strains are very common in a number of LAB species and, primarily due to their application potential as biopreservatives in food and feed, the LAB bacteriocins have been subjected to extensive research in recent years.

Classification of Bacteriocins from Lactic Acid Bacteria

Based on biochemical and genetic features, the bacteriocins from LAB may be categorized into two major classes: (I) the lantibiotics, and (II) the non-lantibiotics, or heat stable, non-modified bacteriocins. With few exceptions (the type B lantibiotics, see below) Class I and II bacteriocins kill sensitive cells by permeabilizing the cytoplasmic membrane. A few bacteriocins may be grouped into a third class consisting of heat-labile bacteriocins larger than 30 kDa (Klaenhammer, 1993; Nes et al., 1996). Because of their abundance and application in industrial processes, bacteriocins belonging to the first two classes are the most thoroughly studied. An overview of the LAB bacteriocin classes is given in Table 8.1.

The most prominent member of the Class I bacteriocins is nisin, which is produced by various strains of *Lactococcus lactis*. Nisin exhibits a broad inhibitory spectrum compared to most other LAB bacteriocins, and is bactericidal towards a wide range of Gram-positive bacteria, including *Staphylococcus aureus, Listeria monocytogenes*, and most LAB (Abee et al., 1995; Delves-Broughton et al., 1996). In addition, nisin prevents spore outgrowth and is bactericidal towards vegetative cells of *Bacillus* and *Clostridium* ssp. The production and regulation of nisin has been thoroughly studied for many years, and this bacteriocin has achieved commercial status as an important food additive (Delves-Broughton et al., 1996), in particular because of its antimicrobial effect against *Clostridium* species in processed cheeses, dairy products, and canned foods.

The Class II (non-lantibiotic) bacteriocins is a heterogeneous group of bacteriocins which nevertheless have a number of features in common: they are all small (<10 kDa), heat stable peptides with a high content of small amino acids such as glycine. They are generally highly cationic and possess a hydrophobic and/or amphiphilic region, which correlates with their activity on membranes (Abee et al., 1995; Moll et al., 1999). The Class II bacteriocins may be further subdivided into at least two subclasses (Klaenhammer, 1993; Nes et al., 1996): Class IIa bacteriocins, which are produced by a wide variety of *Pediococcus, Lactobacillus, Leuconostoc*, and *Enterococcus* strains, have in common a strong anti-*Listeria* activity, and the peptides show a high degree of sequence conservation (38–80% sequence identity on the amino acid level), particularly in the N-terminal part of

Table 8.1. Classification of LAB Bacteriocins

Main Category	Subcategory
Class I—lantibiotics	*Type A*, elongated molecules *Type B*, globular molecules
Class II—nonmodified, heat-stable bacteriocins	*Subclass 1* (Class IIa): Pediocin-like bacteriocins *Subclass 2* (Class IIb): two-peptide bacteriocins *Subclass 3*: Other bacteriocins
Class III—large, heat-labile bacteriocins	

the peptides (Aymerich et al., 1996). Class IIa is also known as the pediocin family, which refers to the most thoroughly studied and first discovered bacteriocin of the subgroup, pediocin PA-1 (Henderson et al., 1992; Marugg et al., 1992; Motlagh et al., 1992; Nieto Lozano et al., 1992). Class IIb consists of bacteriocins whose activity depends on the complementary action of two peptides (van Belkum et al., 1991; Nissen-Meyer et al., 1992; Jimenez-Diaz et al., 1995; Diep et al., 1996; Anderssen et al., 1998).

In most cases, the primary translation product of all Class II bacteriocin genes is a non-active pre-peptide that includes an N-terminal leader sequence of the double-glycine type (Holo et al., 1991). The leader sequence is subsequently removed by the ABC transporter involved in the secretion process (Håvarstein et al., 1994, 1995a). It has recently become apparent, however, that some of the Class II peptides have a *sec*-dependent leader rather than the ubiquitous double-Gly sequence (Worobo et al., 1994; Leer et al., 1995; Cintas et al., 1997). The *sec*-dependent bacteriocins are otherwise indistinguishable from the ABC transporter-dependent bacteriocins, and are consequently not put into a sub-class of their own.

The few Class III bacteriocins from LAB that have been characterized seem to inhibit sensitive bacteria by other mechanisms than the membrane-disruption activity associated with ClassI and II bacteriocins. It has, for instance, been shown that enterolysin A from *Enterococcus faecalis* specifically cleaves the stem peptide of the peptidoglycan of sensitive bacteria, generating a free NH_2-Glu (Nilsen et al., 2002). Another example is constituted by lactococcin 972, which was recently shown to act by interfering with septum formation in sensitive lactococci (Martinez et al., 2000).

Lantibiotics

The lantibiotics (Schnell et al., 1988) constitute a group of low molecular weight antimicrobial peptides produced—apparently exclusively—by Gram-positive bacteria. The main distinguishing feature of the lantibiotics is the presence of the "cyclic" residues lanthionine and/or methyl-lanthionine, which are introduced through a sequence of post-translational modification reactions apparently unique to these peptides (see below). Most members also contain one or both of the α,β di-dehydro amino acids dehydroalanine (Dha) or dehydrobutyrine (Dhb), which are generated by the dehydration of specific serine and threonine residues, respectively, in the pre-peptide (Jack et al., 1998). In addition, some lantibiotics contain other modified residues, for example, D-alanines (lactocin S [Skaugen et al., 1994] and lacticin 3147 [Ryan et al., 1999]) or S-aminovinyl cysteine (e.g., epidermin [Allgaier et al., 1986] and mutacin 1140 [Hillman et al., 1998]), which are also introduced post-translationally by dedicated enzymes encoded in the lantibiotic gene clusters (see below). The subdivision of lantibiotics into type A and B molecules was introduced (Jung, 1991) to account for major structural and functional differences among the peptides. However, as the original criteria for the subdivision was based on a limited selection of related peptides, a significant number of the lantibiotics, which have since been characterized, may seem to fit both groups poorly. In spite of this, most workers in the field still adhere to a somewhat simplified version of the original categorization: type B lantibiotics have reasonably well defined, globular structures and a range of different molecular targets, whereas type A lantibiotics are more elongated, flexible molecules acting by permeabilizing the cytoplasmic membrane of sensitive cells. All known type A lantibiotics are synthesized by species belonging to the low-G + C branch of the Gram-positive bacteria (see Table 8.2). The majority of type B producers are found within the high-G + C branch. None of the LAB

Table 8.2. Type A Lantibiotic Pre-Peptide Sequences

Lantibiotic	Leader Peptide	Pro-Peptide Domain	Producer Organism	Reference
Type AI				
NisinA	MSTKDFNLDLVSVSKKDSGASPR	ITSISLCTPGCKTGALMGCNMKTATCHCSIHVSK	*Lc. lactis*	Buchman et al., 1988
Nisin Z	MSTKDFNLDLVSVSKKDSGASPR	ITSISLCTPGCKTGALMGCNMKTATCNCSIHVSK	*Lc. lactis*	Mulders et al., 1991
Subtilin	MSKFDDFDLDVVKVSKQDSKITPQ	WKSESLCTPGCVTGALQTCFLQTLTCNCKISK	*Bacillus subtilis*	Banerjee and Hansen, 1988
Ericin S	MSKFDDFDLDVVKVSKQDSKITPQ	WKSESVCTPGCVTGVLQTCFLQTITCNCHISK	*Bacillus subtilis*	Stein et al., 2002
Ericin A	MTNMSKFDDFDLDVVKVSKQDSKITPQ	VLSKSLCTPGCITGPLQTCYLCFPTFAKC	*Bacillus subtilis*	Stein et al., 2002
Pep5	MKNNKNLFDLEIKKETSQNTDELEPQ	TAGPAIRASVKQCQKTLKATRLFTVSCKGKNGCK	*S. epidermidis*	Kaletta et al., 1989
Epicidin 280	MENKKDLFDLEIKKDNMENNNELEAQ	SLGPAIKATRQVCPKATRFVTVSCKKSDCQ	*S. epidermidis*	Heidrich et al.,1998
Epilancin K7	MNNSLFDLNLNKGVETQKSDLEPQ	SASVLKTSIKVSKKYCKGVTLTCGCNITGGK	*S. epidermidis*	van de Kamp et al., 1995
Streptin	MNNTIKDFDLDLKTNKKDTATPY	VGSRYLCTPGSCWKLVCFTTTVK	*Strep. pyogenes*	Karaya et al., 2001
Epidermin	MEAVKEKNDLFNLDVKVNAKESNDSGAEPR	IASKFICTPGCAKTGSFNSYCC	*S. epidermidis*	Schnell et al., 1988
Gallidermin	MEAVKEKNELFDLDVKVNAKESNDSGAEPR	IASKFLCTPGCAKTGSFNSYCC	*S. gallinarum*	Schnell et al., 1989
Mutacin 1140	MSNTQLLEVLGTETFDVQEDLFAFDTTDTTIVASNDDPDTR	FKSWSLCTPGCARTGSFNSYCC	*Strep. mutans*	Hillman et al., 1998
Mutacin III	MSNTQLLEVLGTETFDVQEDLFAFDTTDTTIVASNDDPDTR	FKSWSLCTPGCARTGSFNSYCC	*Strep. mutans*	Qi et al., 1999b
Lactocin S	MKTEKKVLDELSLHASAKMGARDVESSMNAD	STPVLASVAVSMELLPTASVLYSDVAGCFKYSAKHHC	*L. sakei*	Skaugen et al., 1994
Type AII				
Lacticin 481	MKEQNSFNLLQEVTESELDLILGA	KGGSGVIHTISHECNMNSWQFVFTCCS	*Lc. lactis*	Piard et al., 1993b
Bacteriocin J46[a]	MKEQNSFNLLQEVTESELDLILGA	KGGSGVIHTISHEVIYNSWNFVFTCCS	*Lc. lactis*	Huot et al., 1996
Butyrivibriocin OR79	MNKELNALTNPIDEKELEQILGG	GNGVIKTISHECHMNTWQFIFTCCS	*Butyrivibrio fibrisolvens*	Kalmokoff et al., 1999

Streptococcin A-FF22	MEKNNEVINSIQEVSLEELDQIIGA	GKNGVFKTISHECHLNTWAFLATCCS	*Strep. pyogenes*	(Hynes et al., 1993)
Variacin	MTNAFQALDEVTDAELDAILGG	GSGVIPTISHECHMNSFQFVFTCCS	*Micrococcus varians*	(Pridmore et al., 1996)
Nukacin	MENSKVMKDIEVANLLEEVQEDELNEVLGA	KKKSGVIPTVSHDCHMNSFQFVFTCCS		(Sashihara et al., 2000)
Mutacin II	MNKLNSVAVVSLNEVSDSELDTILGG	NRWWQGVVPTVSYECRMNSWQHVFTCC	*Strep. mutans*	(Woodruff et al., 1998)
Ruminococcin A	MRNDVLTLTNPMEEKELEQILGG	GNGVLKTISHECNMNTWQFLFTCC	*Ruminococcus gnavus*	(Dabard et al., 2001)
Salivaricin	MNAMKNSKDILNNAIEEVSEKELMEVACG	KRGSGWIATITDDCPNSVFVCC	*Strep. salivarius*	(Ross et al., 1993)
Sublancin 168	MEKLFKEVKLEELENQKGS	GLGKAQCAALWLQCASGGTIGCGGGAVACQNYRQFCR	*Bacillus subtilis*	(Paik et al., 1998)
Lacticin 3147 A1	MKNEIETQPVTWLEEVSDQNFDEDVFGA	CSTNTFSLSDYWGNNGAWCTLTHECMAWCK	*Lc. lactis*	(Dougherty et al., 1998)
Staphylococcin C55 α	MKSSFLEKDIEEQVTWFEEVSEQEFDDDIFGA	CSTNTFSLSDYWGNKGNWCTATHECMSWCK	*S. aureus*	(Navaratna et al., 1999)
Lacticin 3147 A2	MKEKNMKKNDTIELQLGKYLEDDMIELAEGDESHGG	TTPATPAISILSAYISTNTCPTTKCTRAC	*Lc. lactis*	(Dougherty et al., 1998)
Staphylococcin C55 β	MKNELGKFLEENELELGKFSESDMLEITDDEVYAA	GTPLALLGGAATGVIGYISNQTCPTTACTRAC	*S. aureus*	(Navaratna et al., 1999)
Plantaricin W α	MKISKIEAQARKDFFKKIDTNSNLLNVNGA	KCKWWNISCDLGNNGHVCTLSHECQVSCN	*L. plantarum*	(Holo et al., 2001)
Plantaricin W β	MTKTSRRKNAIANYLEPVDEKSINESFGAGDPEAR	SGIPCTIGAAVAASIAVCPTTKCSKRCGKRKK	*L. plantarum*	(Holo et al., 2001)
Cytolysin, CylL1	MENLSVVPSFEELSVEEMEAIQGS	GDVQAETTPVCAVAATAAASSAACGWVGGGIFTGVTVVVSLKHC	*E. faecalis*	(Gilmore et al., 1994)
Cytolysin, CylL2	MLNKENQENYYSNKLELVGPSFEELSLEEMEAIQGS	GDVQAETTPACFTIGLGVGALFSAKFC	*E. faecalis*	(Gilmore et al., 1994)

[a]This bacteriocin is reported not to contain any modified residues.

lantibiotics belong to the type B group, which will therefore not be discussed further in what follows.

As is the case for the majority of the non-modified low molecular weight bacteriocins, the production of lantibiotics includes the proteolytic separation of a leader peptide from the modified, active moiety. In some systems, the leader peptide, which is not modified, is important for one or more aspects (i.e., modification, processing, and export) of lantibiotic maturation (van der Meer et al., 1994; Neis et al., 1997; van den Hooven et al., 1997). The sequence and processing features of lantibiotic leader peptides provide the basis for a recently proposed subdivision of type A lantibiotics (de Vos et al., 1995): The leader peptides of the AI category, which include the "classical" lantibiotics like nisin, subtilin, epidermin, and Pep5, are moderately conserved, and are cleaved by a dedicated serine proteinase—LanP (Siezen et al., 1996)—of the subtilase type. The leader peptides of the lantibiotics belonging to the AII category are more closely interrelated, and have the "double-Gly" processing sites (Håvarstein et al., 1995a; Håvarstein et al., 1994), which dominate among the type II bacteriocins. As will be discussed further in the next section (Class II LAB bacteriocins) of this chapter, pre-peptides of the double-Gly variety are recognized and cleaved by the integral proteolytic activity of a subgroup of the ABC transporter family.

Like the Class II LAB bacteriocins, the type A lantibiotics include members whose activities depend on two distinct peptides, encoded by separate genes in the gene clusters. Three two-peptide lantibiotic systems have been characterized: cytolysin (Ike et al., 1990; Gilmore et al., 1994), lacticin 3147 (Dougherty et al., 1998; McAuliffe et al., 1998; Ryan et al., 1999), and staphylococcin C55 (Navaratna et al., 1998; Navaratna et al., 1999), which are produced by strains of *E. faecalis, Lc. lactis*, and *Staphylococcus aureus*, respectively. Using the above criteria, all the two-peptide lantibiotics belong to the AII class.

A substantial fraction of all known type A lantibiotics (Table 8.2) are produced by strains belonging to the genera *Lactococcus, Lactobacillus, Carnobacterium, Streptococcus*, or *Enterococcus*, but, as few bacterial groups have been subject to more intense scientific scrutiny over the past two decades than the LAB, the apparent overrepresentation may be temporary. Regardless of this possible bias, however, a significant part of what constitute the current views of molecular diversity, biosynthesis, biological activities, immunity, and gene regulation originates from studies of lantibiotics produced by LAB. For general, in-depth discussions of lantibiotic biosynthesis, biological activities, and immunity, the reader is referred to recent reviews covering these topics in detail (de Vos et al., 1995; Jack et al., 1995; Moll et al., 1996, 1999; Jack et al., 1998; Sahl and Bierbaum, 1998).

Biological Activities

The lantibiotics constitute group I in the current classification system of bacteriocins produced by LAB (Klaenhammer, 1993). Although obviously distinct from the other LAB bacteriocins by a number of criteria, the lantibiotics share some characteristics with the unmodified, low molecular weight bacteriocins (Class II, see next section). The most conspicuous of the shared features is probably the general mechanism of antimicrobial activity, which in both cases is the formation of transient pores in the cytoplasmic membrane of sensitive cells (for a recent review, see Moll et al., 1999). For type A lantibiotics the efficacy of pore formation is influenced by the components of the proton motif force, $\Delta\Psi$ and ΔpH (Benz et al., 1991; Sahl, 1991; Moll et al., 1996, 1999). The pores, which vary in both size and duration, allow the efflux of amino acids, nucleotides, and other solutes from the target cell, resulting in a rapid arrest of essential cellular processes and, consequently, cell death (Jack et al., 1998). The molecular architecture of the pores and the precise mechanism by which they are formed is not known for any lantibiotic. However, a number of reports on the interaction of nisin with artificial membranes has resulted in the so-called wedge model for pore formation, which could apply to other type A lantibiotics as well (Figure 8.1). According to this model, the binding of a sufficient number of lantibiotic molecules causes a local disturbance of the lipid dynamics. The subsequent co-insertion of lantibiotic and lantibiotic-bound phospholipids creates a nonspecific, wedge-shaped pore where the membrane surface is bent back on itself, rather than being penetrated by the lantibiotic (Moll et al., 1996, 1999).

Lantibiotics like nisin and Pep5 have MIC values in the low nanomolar range, yet the concentration of bacteriocin applied in artificial membrane systems has to be raised by orders of magnitude for the pore-forming activity to be observed. In the case of nisin and the staphylococcal epidermin, a recently discovered molecular interaction between the lantibiotic and the cytoplasmic membrane of target cells offers an explanation for this discrepancy and, more importantly, identifies a specific factor that is essential in determining the sensitivity of bacteria towards a particular lantibiotic species (Brötz et al., 1998b; Breukink et al., 1999). The identified target cell molecule is lipid II, which is a universal, membrane-anchored cell wall precursor previously shown to be the molecular target for the cell wall synthesis inhibiting lantibiotic mersacidin (Brötz et al., 1995, 1997, 1998a).

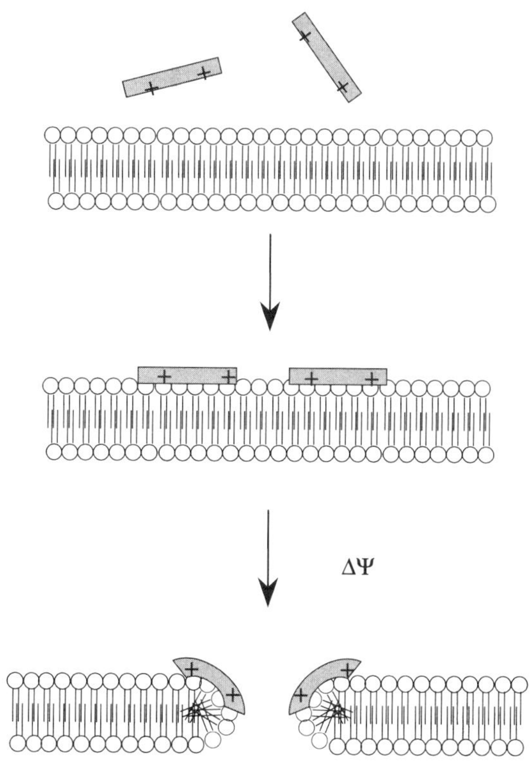

Figure 8.1. Wedge model (Moll et al., 1996) for pore formation by type A lantibiotics, according to the association of the amphiphilic, cationic lantibiotic molecules to the anionic membrane surface causes a high local peptide concentration and a disturbance of the lipid dynamics. In the presence of a $\Delta\Psi$ above threshold level, the formation of a pore is induced.

Rather than challenging the notion of lethal pore forming, however, it has been proposed that lipid II serves as a molecular "docking" for the lantibiotic at the cell surface, thus lowering the critical concentration for pore formation (Brötz et al., 1998b). That the "pore-promoting" interaction with lipid II is not a feature shared by all type A lantibiotics, is demonstrated by the fact that the concentration required for pore formation by Pep5 and epilancin K7 is unaffected by the inclusion of lipid II in artificial membrane systems. This observation points to the interesting possibility that other lantibiotics may interact with other kinds of docking molecules, which thereby function as major factors in defining the range of inhibition for this group of antimicrobial peptides.

Biosynthesis

Like the type II bacteriocins, the biosynthesis of lantibiotics proceeds via normal ribosomal assembly of a pre-peptide. The pre-lantibiotics subsequently undergo a sequence of modification reactions prior to processing and export from the producer cell. Although there is some variability among the lantibiotics with respect to both the degree and the nature of the amino acid modifications, they have in common the presence of (2S, 6R)-*meso*-lanthionine (Lan) and/or (2S,3S,6R)-3-methyllanthionine (MeLan) residues, which gives the molecules a polycyclic structure through intrachain sulfide bridges. Also common is the presence of the α,β-didehydroamino acids Dha and/or Dhb, which are formed through the dehydration of serine and threonine residues, respectively, and which serve as precursors for Lan and MeLan. The proteins LanB and LanC, both of which are encoded by the nisin cluster and related systems, and LanM, which is encoded by the lactocin S and type AII systems' gene clusters, are proteins apparently occurring exclusively in lantibiotic gene clusters, and for a number of years these proteins have been the prime modification enzyme candidates. Although there is little experimental support for this assumption, a role for LanC in thioether-bridge formation has been indicated by the analysis of peptides secreted by mutants in the Pep5 system (Meyer et al., 1995). More recently, it was demonstrated that overexpression of *nis*B in a nisin producing strain significantly reduced the fraction of a partially dehydrated form of nisin (Ser33) in bacteriocin preparations, thus providing the first direct evidence for the involvement of a LanB protein in the modification of lantibiotics (Karakas Sen et al., 1999). Although the LanM proteins, which share some conserved motifs with LanC (Siezen et al., 1996), have been shown to be essential for lantibiotic production in several cases (Gilmore et al., 1994; Rince et al., 1994; Skaugen et al., 1997), there is presently no direct evidence that this class of proteins is involved in lantibiotic modification. The gene cluster specifying the production of the two-peptide lantibiotic lacticin 3147 contains two M genes (Dougherty et al., 1998), as is probably the case in the related system staphylococcin C55 also (Navaratna et al., 1999). The significance of expressing two *lan*M homologues is presently not known.

Other modifications may be particular for one peptide or a subgroup of the lantibiotics. Notable examples of such modified residues are the D-alanines identified in mature lactocin S and, more recently, in lacticin 3147 (Skaugen et al., 1994; Ryan et al., 1999). The protein responsible for the proposed Dha reduction leading to the introduction of the D-configured residues has not been formally identified in either case. Analysis of lactocin S negative mutants has, however, indicated a gene encoding a flavodoxin-like protein, LasN, as a candidate Dha reductase (Skaugen, unpublished observations). Although clearly speculative at this point, the absence of a *las*N-homologue in the lacticin 3147 cluster suggests the possibility of convergent evolution of this particular feature, that is, that the genes encoding the Dha reductase in the two systems may have evolved from two distinct ancestor genes.

In early studies of nisin and subtilin studies it was demonstrated that the NisB/SpaB proteins are membrane-associated in the producer cells, and it was proposed that the post-translational steps in lantibiotic biosynthesis—at least in the case of these particular lantibiotic species—take place at the cytoplasmic membrane (Engelke et al., 1992; Gutowski-Eckel et al., 1994). The results of yeast two-hybrid (Fields and Song, 1989; Chien et al., 1991) experiments carried out with components involved in subtilin (SpaS/SpaB/SpaC/SpT) and nisin (NisA/NisB/NisC/NisT) production has provided support for the notion of a membrane-associated, multienzyme synthetase complex for both of these lantibiotics (Siegers et al., 1996; Kiesau et al., 1997). Whether similar complexes are involved in the biosynthesis of other lantibiotics as well remains to be determined.

Export and Processing

Unlike the Class II LAB bacteriocins, there are no known exceptions to the rule that export of the mature lantibiotic is carried out by a member of the ABC transporter protein family (Higgins et al., 1986; Higgins, 1992; Fath and Kolter, 1993). In all cases, the transporter (LanT) is of the single-protein type, that is, both the ATP binding and the transmembrane domains are present on the same polypeptide. As mentioned above, however, some of the lantibiotic exporters belong to the bi-functional (transport and pre-peptide processing, see next section) group of proteins, which dominate among the group II bacteriocins, while the remaining lantibiotics are exported by a subclass of ABC transporters lacking the proteolytic function. Both the ABC transporter subgroups involved in lantibiotic export constitute distinct clusters (cluster 10 and 0, respectively) in a recent phylogenetic analysis of this large protein family (Saurin et al., 1999). The producers of epicidin 280 (Heidrich et al., 1998) and epidermin (Peschel et al., 1997) both lack a dedicated transporter enzyme, and LanT-mutants of the Pep5 producing strains still secrete substantial amounts (10–30% of wild-type level) of active peptide (Meyer et al., 1995). In these cases, which may be peculiar to the *Staphylococcus* strains under study (but see heterologous complementation in the lacticin 481 system, below), it is assumed that some chromosomally encoded, broad-specificity transporter substitutes for the cognate lantibiotic export enzyme.

In the cases where processing is not carried out by LanT, leader peptide cleavage is dependent on the activity of a subtilase type serine protease, LanP. Although obviously belonging to the same protein family, the LanP proteins constitute a heterogeneous group of proteins: The proteolysis of pre-nisin is carried out extracellularly by the pre-pro protein NisP, which is a 682 residue protein remaining attached to the producer cell through a C-terminal lipid anchor domain (van der Meer et al., 1993). CylA (Segarra et al., 1991; Gilmore et al., 1994; Booth et al., 1996), which is required for the final proteolysis in the enterococcal two-peptide cytolysin system, is also an extracellular enzyme, but the protein lacks the C-terminal membrane anchor, as does the epidermin-associated leader peptidase, EpiP (Geißler et al., 1996). The cytolysin system is a special case with respect to proteolytic processing: the *cyl* gene cluster encodes a serine protease as well as a bifunctional LanT protein, suggesting that cytolysin maturation may involve two successive processing steps (Siezen et al., 1996). A third variety of the pre-lantibiotic processing serine proteases lacks the N-terminal secretion signal as well as the C-terminal extension, and therefore presumably cleaves the pre-lantibiotic intracellularly, prior to export of the mature peptide.

This type of processing enzymes is exemplified by LasP, which is a 266 residue protein encoded by the lactocin S gene cluster (Skaugen et al., 1997), and PepP, which is a slightly larger (285 aa) protein involved in Pep5 production (Meyer et al., 1995). The subtilin gene cluster contains neither a *lan*P nor a proteolytic *lan*T homologue (Klein and Entian, 1994). This situation is similar to the one discussed above concerning epidermin export inasmuch as the apparent lack of a dedicated protease in the subtilin system has led to the suggestion that this function may be performed by a broad-specificity host enzyme yet to be identified.

Producer Self-Protection (Immunity)

Although a number of genes involved in lantibiotic producer self protection, or immunity, have been identified during the past few years, the concept of lantibiotic immunity remains poorly defined in most cases. The genetic complexity of lantibiotic immunity varies between the different systems: in the case of nisin and subtilin, four genes have been shown to be involved, while systems like Pep5 and lacticin 3147 apparently depend on only one specific protein for self protection. The most common complement of immunity genes appears to be *lan*FEG (*lan*FE or FG in some clusters), which has been so designated because of a weak sequence similarity to genes involved in immunity to the *E.coli* bacteriocin microcin B17 (Garrido et al., 1988). By analogy to the microcin system, it has been proposed that the function of *lan*FEG, which probably encodes subunits of a multipartite ABC transporter, is to capture and translocate the lantibiotic out of harm's way. The analogy between lantibiotic and microcin B17 immunity is not perfect, as the molecular target of the latter is a cytoplasmic protein (DNA gyrase), and not the cell membrane. It is conceivable, therefore, that the function in immunity of this second lantibiotic transporter is to remove the lantibiotic from the membrane by ATP-driven *import* (for subsequent intracellular proteolytic degradation), rather than to externalize it. In the only published study addressing the issue, it is concluded that the direction of lantibiotic transport by the LanFEG pump is outwards (Otto et al., 1998), but this particular transporter (*epi*FEG, encoded by the epidermin cluster) may be a special case, since it also contributes to lantibiotic production (Peschel and Götz, 1996). As already indicated, the *lan*FEG unit is common amng the lantibiotics, and with the exception of Pep5, epicidin 280, cytolysin, and lactocin S, the unit, or a derivative thereof, is present in all completely sequenced lantibiotic gene clusters. The reported contribution to immunity, however, varies considerably (see also below): While the *lct*FEG genes appear to be the only genes involved in immunity to lacticin 481 (Rince et al., 1997), corresponding genes in other systems may contribute only partially to the immunity phenotype, as in the nisin cluster (Duan et al., 1996; Ra et al., 1999), or not at all, which was found in the case of lacticin 3147 (McAuliffe et al., 2000). In the nisin and subtilin systems, a fourth gene is involved in immunity. This gene, which has been termed *nis*I (Kuipers et al., 1993; Engelke et al., 1994) and *spa*I (Klein and Entian, 1994) in the nisin and subtilin clusters, respectively, encodes a lipoprotein in both cases, but there are no further similarities between NisI and SpaI.

In four cases lantibiotic immunity has been found to depend on the expression of only one gene. Two recent papers report on single-gene encoded self protection against the two-peptide lantibiotics cytolysin (Coburn et al., 1999) and lacticin 3147 (McAuliffe et al., 2000). CylI is a putatively membrane-associated protein of 327 residues, showing no significant similarities to other proteins in database searches. *cyl*I is situated immediately downstream of *cyl*A, and polar effects of Tn*917* mutations is offered as an explanation for the previously proposed role in immunity of the latter gene (Gilmore et al., 1996).

*ltn*I, which is part of the lacticin 3147 gene cluster, also encodes a protein likely to be associated with the membrane. However, LtnI is considerably smaller than CylI (116 instead of 327 residues), and the two proteins have no significant sequence similarity (McAuliffe et al., 2000). *ltn*I is located next to, and is co-transcribed with, two genes which are similar to the *lan*F and *lan*E genes discussed above. The inactivation of one or both of these genes, however, does not affect the immunity phenotype of the host (McAuliffe et al., 2000).

For Pep5, it was initially published that immunity required the expression of the pre-pep5 gene, *pepA*, as well as the suspected immunity gene, *pep*I (Reis and Sahl, 1991; Reis et al., 1994). It has later been demonstrated, however, that the expression of *pep*I alone is sufficient for full immunity to externally applied Pep5 (Pag et al., 1999). It has also been shown (Reis et al., 1994) that the 69 residue, hydrophobic protein PepI is loosely attached to the cytoplasmic membrane, but the mechanism by which PepI provides Pep5 immunity remains unclear. In another recent publication by the same group, lantibiotic cross-immunity was observed for the first time, by the demonstration of significant, reciprocal lantibiotic protection by the producers of Pep5 and a novel staphylococcal lantibiotic, epicidin 280 (Heidrich et al., 1998). A PepI homologue was identified in the epicidin gene cluster, and the sequence comparison of the two gene products highlighted conserved residues, some of which are shared by the non-lantibiotic divergicin immunity peptide, DviA (Worobo et al., 1995), as well as the 57 residue LasI (previously Orf57 [Skaugen et al., 1997]) in the lactocin S operon. As neither divergicin nor lactocin S share sequence similarity with Pep5/epicidin 280, these observations point to the interesting possibility of a new general mechanism of bacteriocin immunity.

Genetic Regulation of Lantibiotic Production

Lantibiotic production may be viewed as a complex process with only one apparent function, namely inhibiting the growth of competitors (which are likely to be related organisms) for a limited nutrition supply. It seems reasonable to assume that the ability to express such a complex trait in a regulated manner, that is, as a function of the status of some factor(s) in the cell's environment, would constitute an advantage that could be favored by natural selection. The growth-phase-dependent production of nisin and subtilin was recognized early on (Banerjee and Hansen, 1988; Buchman et al., 1988), and in both cases the genes that were involved in the regulation of bacteriocin production were identified only a few years later (Klein et al., 1993; Kuipers et al., 1993; van der Meer et al., 1993; Engelke et al., 1994). The identified genes encode the two components of a signal transduction system, which is employed by both prokaryotes and eukaryotes to regulate a wide variety of cellular activities in response to an environmental signal (Stock et al., 1995). This so-called two-component system, which is discussed in more detail in the next section of this chapter, employs a succession of phosphate-transfer reactions to transduce the external signal from a membrane-bound receptor (the histidine protein kinase, or HPK) to a cytoplasmic effector molecule (the response regulator, or RR). In the case of nisin and subtilin (among other bacteriocins, see below), the intracellular effect is the transcriptional stimulation of lantibiotic gene expression, and the external signal is the lantibiotic itself (Kuipers et al., 1995; Kleerebezem et al., 1999). As with the regulated Class II bacteriocins, the lantibiotic gene regulation by the HPK/RK system has been interpreted as an example of a quorum sensing mechanism (Kleerebezem et al., 1997b). The promoters which are recognized by the phosphorylated RR protein in the nisin and subtilin clusters have been analyzed (de Ruyter et al., 1996b; Kleerebezem et al., 1999), and have been shown to contain short direct repeats with a conserved spacing between repeats. In both cases, however, the repeats are shorter (5 bp) and the spacing narrower (6 bp) than those observed for the *Lactobacillus* regulated promoters discussed in the next section, and the position of the repeats with respect to the consensus promoter elements is also different (Kleerebezem et al., 1999).

The application potential of the nisin regulatory circuit was recognized relatively early on, and the system has in recent years been exploited for the controlled (over)expression of a wide variety of genes in *Lc. lactis* as well as in other Gram-positive bacteria (de Ruyter et al., 1996a; de Ruyter et al., 1997; Kleerebezem et al., 1997a, 1999; Kuipers et al., 1997; Eichenbaum et al., 1998; Lopez de Felipe et al., 1998). Recently, it was reported that transcription from at least one of the nisin-inducible promoters (the nisA promoter) could be induced in the absence of nisin (and the HPK/RR unit). The inducing agent was tentatively identified as galactose, and the maximum induction efficiency was approximately one order of magnitude lower than the nisin induced control (Chandrapati and O'Sullivan, 1999).

HPK- and RR-encoding genes have also been identified in the streptococcin A-FF22 cluster (McLaughlin et al., 1999), but have not yet been subjected to the analyses (i.e., mutation and complementation experiments) necessary to ascertain the function of these genes in bacteriocin gene regulation. It is also not known whether the input signal is the lantibiotic molecule, as in the nisin system, or some other stimulus. Also, with respect to regulation, the epidermin system is a special case: the expression of *epi* genes is dependent on transcriptional stimulation by EpiQ (Peschel et al., 1993), which is weakly similar to RRs like PhoB (Makino et al., 1986), but there is no gene encoding a HPK homologue present in the cluster. This leaves open the question of the nature of the signal as well as the mechanism of signal transduction in the case of epidermin gene regulation.

Recently, a different type of regulatory gene was identified in three different lantibiotic loci: the mutacin II (Chen et al., 1999; Qi et al., 1999a), mutacin III (Qi et al., 1999b), and lactocin S clusters (Skaugen and Nes, 2000) all contain a gene with weak, but significant sequence similarity to *rgg*, which encodes a positive regulator of the glucosyl transferase gene in *Strep. gordonii* (Sulavik et al., 1992; Sulavik and Clewell, 1996). The phenotype of mutants has been analyzed at the transcriptional level for both the mutacin II (Qi et al., 1999a) and lactocin S (Rawlinson et al., 2002; Skaugen et al., 2002) homologues, and in both cases the results are consistent with the notion that these genes encode transcriptional activators. It is not known, however, whether this stimulation is coupled to an environmental signal(s), or if there are additional factors involved in mutacin and lactocin S gene regulation.

A third type of regulatory gene is found in the lacticin 3147 cluster (Dougherty et al., 1998). *ltn*R encodes a 79 residue protein which belong to the Xre family (Wood et al., 1990) of transcriptional repressors. Although it has been demonstrated that *ltn*R mutants have no effect on the immunity phenotype of the host, the function of LtnR with respect to the expression of the lacticin 3147 genes is still unclear at present (McAuliffe et al., 2000).

In addition to the genes encoding the *trans*-acting regulatory factors discussed above, which may or may not be present in the lantibiotic clusters, a *cis*-acting element is involved in the modulation of lantibiotic gene expression in a number of cases. The *cis*-acting element is a short, palindromic sequence located in the non-coding region between the pre-bacteriocin gene (*lan*A) and the downstream gene. The palindromes resemble factor-independent transcriptional terminators, and it has been proposed that the sequences function as "leaky" terminators, allowing only a fraction of the initiated transcripts to be extended beyond the terminator into the downstream genes. The expected effect of such a "leaky" termination would be a differential expression (on the RNA level) of the "structural" and ancillary genes, which is precisely what has been observed in a number of cases (Banerjee and Hansen, 1988; Buchman et al., 1988; Augustin et al., 1992; Piard et al., 1993b; Skaugen et al., 1997). The palindromes may also have a stabilizing effect on the *lan*A-specific transcript by slowing down 3′–5′ exonucleolytic degradation. Except for the hairpin-formation potential, there are few similarities between the palindromes of the different lantibiotic systems, and the calculated energies of formation for the stem-loop structures vary considerably.

The apparent absence of (closely linked) regulatory genes in several of the characterized lantibiotic clusters (lacticin 481, Pep5, epicidin 280, cytolysin) suggests that the ability to regulate gene expression may be regarded as an "optional" trait. However, few of these systems have been studied in sufficient detail to exclude the possibility that the expression of lantibiotic genes is regulated by factors and mechanisms not yet identified.

Organization of Lantibiotic Gene Clusters

In all cases where sufficient sequence information is available, the pre-lantibiotic gene(s) (*lan*A) is closely associated with all the necessary accessory genes, forming tight gene clusters of varying complexity. The clusters may be located on plasmids, as in the case of, for example, lacticin 3147 (Dougherty et al., 1998), lacticin 481 (Piard et al., 1993a), and lactocin S (Mørtvedt and Nes, 1990), or in the chromosome, as in the case of most of the characterized nisin clusters (Horn et al., 1991; Steen et al., 1991; Rauch and de Vos, 1992; Ra et al., 1996). In addition to the nisin locus, which in most cases is located on a conjugative transposon (Horn et al., 1991; Rauch and de Vos, 1992; Rauch et al., 1994; Immonen et al., 1995; Siegers and Entian, 1995), the association of transposable elements (i.e., insertion sequences) with the bacteriocin gene clusters has been found also for the three other well characterized "true LAB" lantibiotics: lacticin 3147, lacticin 481, lactocin S (Rince et al., 1997; Skaugen et al., 1997; Dougherty et al., 1998; McLaughlin et al., 1999). It is not known whether the IS elements in the latter cases are involved in the mobility of the associated gene clusters.

Several lantibiotic gene clusters have now been completely sequenced and, although there are similarities, the clusters are surprisingly diverse. The observed heterogeneity is of course partly due to differences in the complexity of the biosynthesis/immunity phenotypes (e.g., additional modifications, one-protein versus multi-protein immunity, presence/absence of regulators). However, even after having corrected for this (expected) variation, there are few obvious organizational similarities between the different lantibiotic gene clusters: the number and relative orientation of transcription units may vary, as may the relative location of genes within transcription units. Some of this variability among lantibiotic gene clusters is illustrated in Figure 8.2, where the best characterized gene clusters involved in the production of LAB lantibiotics are presented.

Class II Bacteriocins

As has been pointed out on several occasions, the LAB producers of Class II bacteriocins need primarily four kind of genes; a gene encoding the (pre-) bacteriocin, two genes encoding the transporter function, and one encoding the immunity protein, which is required to protect the producer against its own bacteriocin. With few exceptions, these genes constitute one- or two-operon clusters, which may be located in the chromosome or

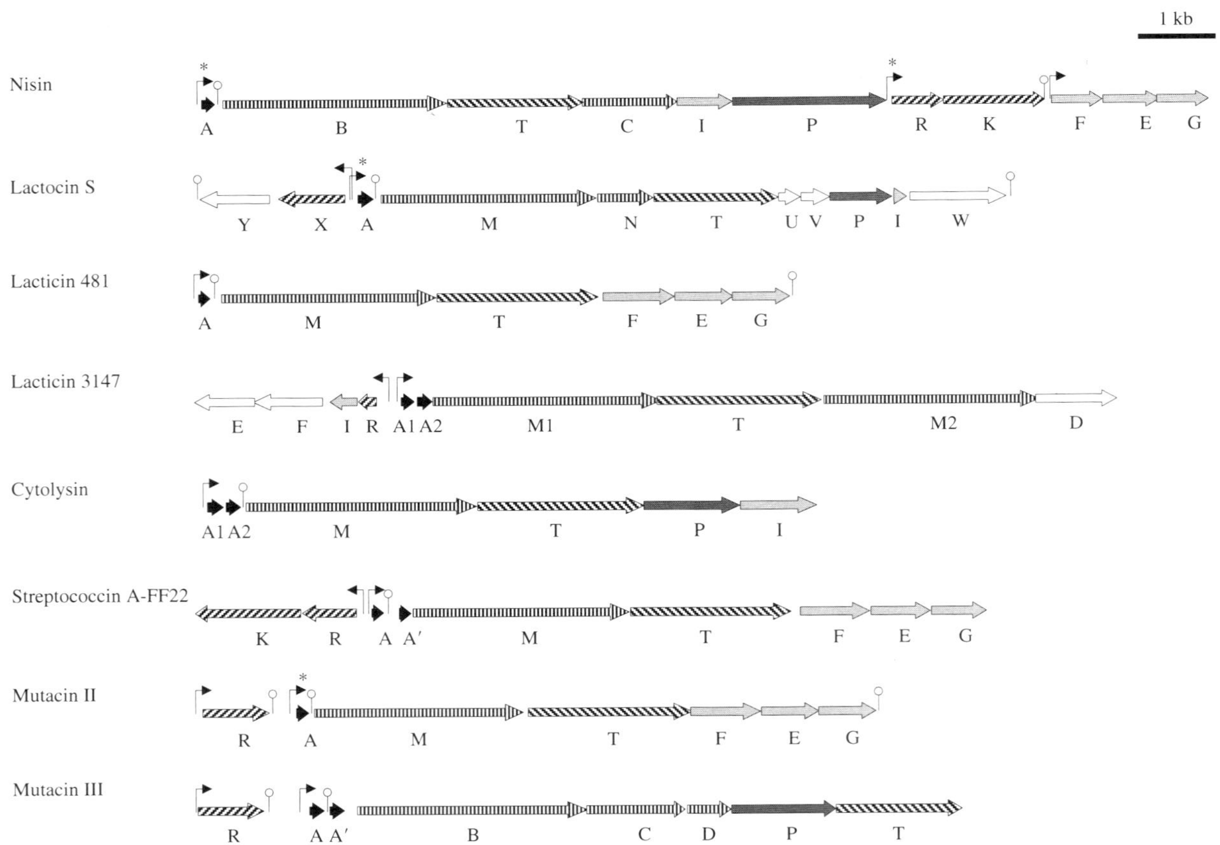

Figure 8.2. Organization of the gene clusters specifying the nisin, lactocin S, lacticin 481, and lacticin 3147 phenotypes. The enterococcal (cytolysin) and streptococcal (mutacin II and III, and streptococcin S-AFF22) gene clusters were included to illustrate the differences in organization and complexity observed between clusters from relatively closely related organisms. The pre-bacteriocin genes are represented by black arrows. The second pre-lantibiotic genes in the streptococcin and mutacin III (A′) clusters probably do not encode functional pre-bacteriocins. The hatched arrows represent the modification (vertical), bacteriocin export (including the bifunctional transporters; backward slanting), and regulatory genes (forward slanting). The shaded arrows represent immunity (light) and leader peptidase (heavy) genes. The unfilled arrows represent genes with no identified function. Promoters are depicted as thin arrows, and the regulated promoters are marked with asterisks. Transcription terminators are marked with ball-and-stick symbols. See text for details.

on plasmids (Nes et al., 1995, 1996). A feature that is becoming increasingly apparent is that multiple bacteriocins are often produced by a single bacterial strain. The genetic determinants for multiple bacteriocin production are usually gathered in clusters and the bacteriocins use the same transporter system while each of the bacteriocins does have its own dedicated immune protein.

The production of several Class II bacteriocins is regulated by a quorum sensing system. The regulatory systems are often referred to as three-component systems, and each includes a dedicated pheromone peptide (inducer), a histidin protein kinase (the sensor/receptor) and a RR (the effector). Despite the obvious similarities, this system is distinct from the regulatory circuit associated with nisin production, where the inducer is the bacteriocin itself. The inducer in all regulated Class II bacteriocin systems is encoded by a separate gene, and the peptide may, or may not, have an antimicrobial activity of its own.

The genetic organization and determinants of the various bacteriocin systems are in many ways similar, and the genes are often clustered and easily identified. Consequently, the following section will focus on the function of the different classes of genes involved, rather than the individual gene clusters or bacteriocin subclasses. A selection of typical Class II gene clusters is presented in Figure 8.3.

The Bacteriocin Gene(s)

The first two Class II bacteriocin operons to be characterized were those encoding lactococcin A and lactacin F (Holo et al., 1991; Muriana and Klaenhammer, 1991a,b; van Belkum et al., 1991). One of the important findings in these studies was the discovery of the N-terminal leader sequence, which was later termed the double-glycine leader (Håvarstein et al., 1994). These N-terminal extensions, which are between 15 and 30 residues long and have a few conserved amino acids separated by defined spacings, are cleaved C-terminal to the two conserved glycines. The consensus leader is (based on 43 sequences):

$$\mathbf{MK\ldots\ldots\ldots L_{70}\ S_{53}\text{-}K_{44}\ E_{70}\ L_{72}\text{--}I_{58}\text{--}G_{100}\ G_{90},}$$

where the numbers indicate the frequency of occurence for the amino acid in these positions. The proteolytic processing of the pre-bacteriocin is carried out by a domain of the dedicated ABC transporter (see below).

While most LAB bacteriocins are single molecules, it has been shown that some strains secrete two peptides, both of which are needed for full bacteriocin activity. In all known cases, the genes encoding the individual peptides of these so-called two-peptide bacteriocins (Table 8.3) are located next to each other in the gene cluster, and in the majority of the cases the bacteriocins are synthesized as pre-peptides with double-glycine leaders. The mature peptides are undistinguishable from the one-peptide bacteriocins except when it comes to antimicrobial activity. Interestingly, both the one-peptide and two-peptide bacteriocins depend on a single protein for immunity.

As mentioned above, some bacteriocins do not have an N-terminal extension of the double-glycin type. A few years ago, it was discovered that some Class II bacteriocins depend on the general secretory pathway for proteolytic activation and externalization (Leer et al., 1995; Worobo et al., 1995). Consequently, these peptides have a *sec*-type leader sequence rather than the double-glycine variety. Presently, only five LAB bacteriocins are known to use this system (Table 8.3). It has later been shown that an originally ABC transporter-dependent bacteriocin can be secreted by the general secretory system by

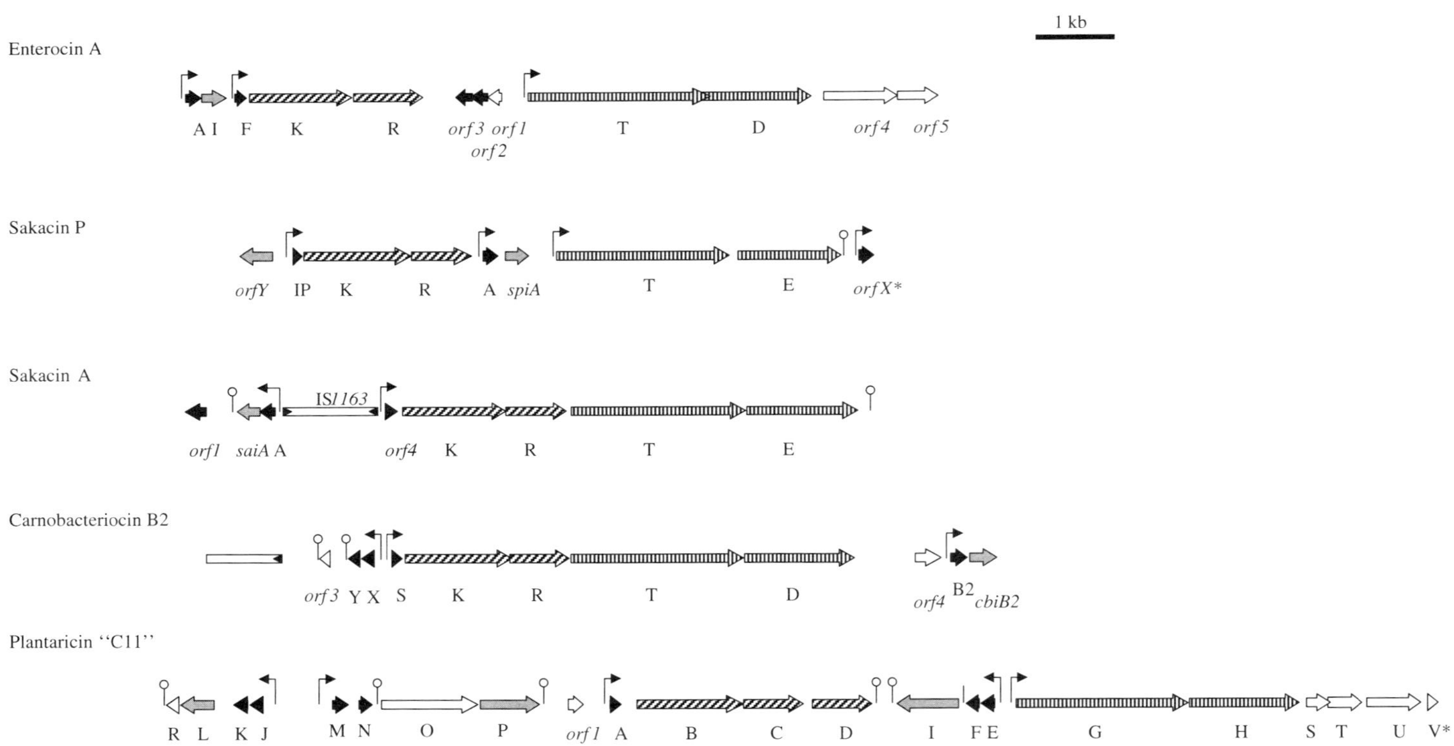

Figure 8.3. Organization of the gene clusters specifying bacteriocin production in *Enterococcus faecium* DPC1146 (O'Keeffe et al., 1999), *Lactobacillus sakei* LTH673 (Huhne et al., 1996; Brurberg et al., 1997), *L. sakei* Lb706 (Axelsson and Holck, 1995), *Carnobacterium piscicola* LV17 (Quadri et al., 1997; Saucier et al., 1997), and *Lactobacillus plantarum* C11 (Diep et al., 1996). The bacteriocin (and bacteriocin-like) and inducing genes are shown as black arrows, and the immunity (and immunity-like) genes as shaded arrows. The genes encoding the HPKs (K; B in *L. plantarum* C11) and RRs (R; C and D in *L. plantarum* C11) are shown as cross-hatched arrows, while the vertically hatched arrows represent the ABC transporter (T; G in *L. plantarum* C11) and accessory export (D,E, or H) genes. Regulated promoters and transcriptional terminators are represented by thin arrows and ball-and-stick symbols, repectively. The rectangles in the sakacin A (marked IS*1163*) and carnobacteriocin B2 clusters represent insertion sequences.

Table 8.3. Overview of Genetically and Biochemically Characterized Class II and III Bacteriocins[a]

Bacteriocin	Producer Organism	Reference(s)
Class II: One and two-peptide bacteriocins		
1. Non-subgrouped bacteriocins		
Lactococcin A	*Lc. lactis*	Holo et al., 1991; Morgan et al., 1995; van Belkum et al., 1991
Bovicin 255	*Strep.* spp.	Whitford et al., 2001
Thermophilin A	*Strep. thermophilus* ST134	Ward and Somkuti, 1995
Lactococcin B	*Lc. lactis*	Morgan et al., 1995; van Belkum et al., 1992
Diacetin B	*Lc. lactis* subsp. *diacetylactis* UL720	Ali et al., 1995
Carnobacteriocin A	*Carnobacterium piscicola* LV17A	Holck et al., 1994b;
Piscicolin 61	*Carnobacterium piscicola* LV61	Worobo et al., 1994
Lactobin A	*L. amylovorus* LMG P-13139	Contreras et al., 1997
Divergicin 750	*Carnobacterium divergens* 750	Holck et al., 1996
Enterocin B	*Enterococcus faecium* T136/C492	Casaus et al., 1997
Peptide A	*L. acidophilus* LF221	Bogovic-Matijasic et al., 1998
Peptide B	*L. acidophilus* LF221	Bogovic-Matijasic et al., 1998
Acidocin 8912	*L. acidophilus* TK8912	Kanatani et al., 1995b
Lactocin 705	*L. casei* CRL 705	Palacios et al., 1999
Leucocin B-TA33a	*Leuconostoc mesenteroides* TA33a	Papathanasopoulos et al., 1998
Gassericin B3	*L. gasseri* JCM 2124	Tahara et al., 1997
Brevicin 27	*L. brevis* SB27	Benoit et al., 1997
Plantaricin 1.25β	*L. plantarum* 1.25	Ehrmann et al., 2000
2. Cyclic peptide bacteriocins		
Acidocin 8912	*L. acidophilus* TK8912	Kawai et al., 1998a
Antimicrobial peptide AS-48	*E. faecalis*	Gonzalez et al., 2000
Gassericin A	*L. gasseri* LA39	Kawai et al., 1998b
3. Class IIa—antilisterial pediocin-like bacteriocins		
Leucocin A	*Leuconsostoc gelidum* UAL 187	Hastings et al., 1991;
Leucocin A-TA33a	*Leuconostoc mesenteroides* TA33a	Papathanasopoulos et al., 1998
Pediocin PA-1	*Pediococcus acidilactici* PAC 1.0	Henderson et al., 1992; Marugg
Pediocin AcH	*Pediococcus acidilactici* AcH	et al., 1992; Motlagh et al., 1992; Nieto Lozano et al., 1992
Sakacin P	*L. sakei* LTH674	Holck et al., 1994a; Huhne et al.,
Bavaricin A	*L. sakei* 674	1996; Larsen et al., 1993;
Sakacin 674	*L. bavaricus* MI104	Tichaczek et al., 1994
Curvacin A	*L. curvatus* LTH1174	Axelsson and Holck, 1995; Holck
Sakacin A	*L. sakei* Lb706	et al., 1992; Tichaczek et al., 1993
Mesenterocin Y105	*Leuconostoc mesenteroides* Y105	Fremaux et al., 1995; Hechard et al., 1992
Mesenterocin 52B	*Leuconostoc mesenteroides* FR52	Hechard et al., 1999;
Mesentericin B105	*Leuconostoc mesenteroides* Y105	Revol-Junelles et al., 1996
Carnobacteriocin B2	*Carnobacterium piscicola* LV17B	Quadri et al., 1994
Carnobacteriocin BM1/	*Carnobacterium piscicola* LV17B	Bhugaloo-Vial et al., 1996;
Piscicocin V1b	*Carnobacterium piscicola* V1	Quadri et al., 1994
Acidocin A	*L. acidophilus* TK9201	Kanatani et al., 1995a
Acidocin 8912,	*L. acidophilus* TK8912	Kanatani et al., 1995b
Enterocin A	*E. faecium* CTC492/T136 *E. faecium* DPC1146	Aymerich et al., 1996; Nilsen et al., 1998; O'Keeffe et al., 1999

(continued)

Table 8.3. (*continued*)

Bacteriocin	Producer Organism	Reference(s)
Bavaricin MN	*L. sakei* MN	Kaiser and Montville, 1996
Piscicolin 126	*Carnobacterium piscicola* JG126	Bhugaloo-Vial et al., 1996;
Piscicocin V1a	*Carnobacterium piscicola* V1	Jack et al., 1996
Mundticin	*E. mundtii* AT06	Bennik et al., 1998
Divercin V41	*Carnobacterium divergens* V41	Metivier et al., 1998
Enterocin CRL 35	*E. faecium* CRL 35	Farias et al., 1996
Leucocin B-Ta11a	*Leuconostoc carnosum* Ta11	Felix et al., 1994
Curvaticin FS47	*L. curvatus* FS47	Garver and Muriana, 1994
Carnocin CP5	*Carnobacterium piscicola* CP5	Herbin et al., 1997
Plantaricin C19	*L. plantarum* C19	Atrih et al., 2001
Bifidocin B	*Bifidobacterium bifidum* NCFB 1454	Yildirim et al., 1999
Leucocin c-TA33a	*Leuconostoc mesenteroides TA33a*	Papathanasopoulos et al., 1998
Lactococcin MMFII	*L. lactis* MMFII	Ferchichi et al., 2001
4. *sec*-dependent bacteriocins		
Acidocin B	*L. acidophilus* M46	Leer et al., 1995
Divergicin A	*Carnobacterium divergens* LV13	Worobo et al., 1995
Enterocin P	*E. faecium* P13	Cintas et al., 1997
Bacteriocin 31	*E. faecalis* 31	Tomita et al., 1996
Lactococcin 972	*L. lactis* IPLA 972	Martinez et al., 1999
5. Bacteriocins without leader sequence		
Enterocin L50	*E. faecium* L50	Cintas et al., 1998
Enterocin I	*E. faecium* 6T1a	Floriano et al., 1998
Enterocin Q	*E. faecium* L50	Cintas et al., 2000
6. Class IIb, two-peptide bacteriocins		
Lactococcin G (LcnGα and LcnG-β)	*L. lactis* LMG2081	Nissen-Meyer et al., 1992
Lactococcin M (LcnM and LcnN)	*L. lactis* 9B4,	van Belkum et al., 1991
Lactacin F (LafA and LafX)	*L. johnsonii* VPI11088	Allison et al., 1994
Thermophilin 13 (ThmA and ThmB)	*Strep. thermophilus* Sfi13	Marciset et al., 1997
Plantaricin S (PlsA and PlsB)	*L. plantarum* LCP010	Jimenez-Diaz et al., 1995; Stephens et al., 1998
Plantaricin EF (PlnE and PlnF)	*L. plantarum* C11	Anderssen et al., 1998; Diep et al., 1996
Plantaricin JK (PlnJ and PlnK)	*L. plantarum* C11	Anderssen et al., 1998; Diep et al., 1996
Leucocin H (α and β)	*Leuconostoc* ssp. MF215B	Blom et al., 1999
Enterocin 1071	*E. feacalis* FAIR-E309	Franz et al., 2002
ABP-118	*L. salivarius* UCC118	Flynn et al., 2002
Class III: High molecular weight protein bacteriocins		
Helveticin J	*L. helveticus* 481	Joerger and Klaenhammer, 1990
Enterolysin	*E. faecalis*	Nilsen et al., 2002

[a]Bacteriocins with identical amino acid sequences set together.

replacing the double-glycine leader with the *sec*-type leader (McCormick et al., 1996, 1999). This observation implies that the recognition signal for the secretion process is embedded in the leader sequences and not in the bacteriocin peptides. It has been speculated that the N-terminal sequence may render the peptide inactive, thereby protecting the producer cell until the active, processed bacteriocin is released to the surroundings.

A further complication of the concept of Class II bacteriocin production came with the discovery of enterocin L50, which was isolated from an *E. faecium* strain. The enterocin L50 activity was shown to depend on the presence of two almost identical (approximately 70% identity) peptides, and is therefore technically a two-peptide bacteriocin (Cintas et al., 1998). The subsequent cloning and sequencing of the enterocin L50 genes revealed the expected two enterocin peptide genes located next to each other in an operon-like structure. Surprisingly, however, no genes encoding immunity or transport could be found, despite extensive upstream and downstream sequencing. Perhaps, even more surprisingly, the two bacteriocin genes did not encode a leader sequence or signal peptide, that is, the isolated peptides were identical to the translation of the identified genes. Presently it is not known how the producer protects itself against this bacteriocin or how the peptides are secreted.

The Immunity Gene

In most cases, the immunity gene of Class II bacteriocins is located next to, and in the same operon as the pre-bacteriocin gene(s) (Figure 8.4), and the immunity protein is produced in high amounts (Holo et al., 1991; Nissen-Meyer et al., 1993; Quadri et al., 1995; Venema et al., 1995a,b). There are, however, exceptions to this organization: in both the enterocin B and the carnobacteriocin A clusters the pre-bacteriocin and immunity genes are transcribed in separate, oppositely oriented units (Franz et al., 1999, 2000). It should be noted that, although the immunity and bacteriocin genes reside in separate transcription units, they are not necessarily transcribed independently (Worobo et al., 1994; Casaus et al., 1997; Franz et al., 2000).

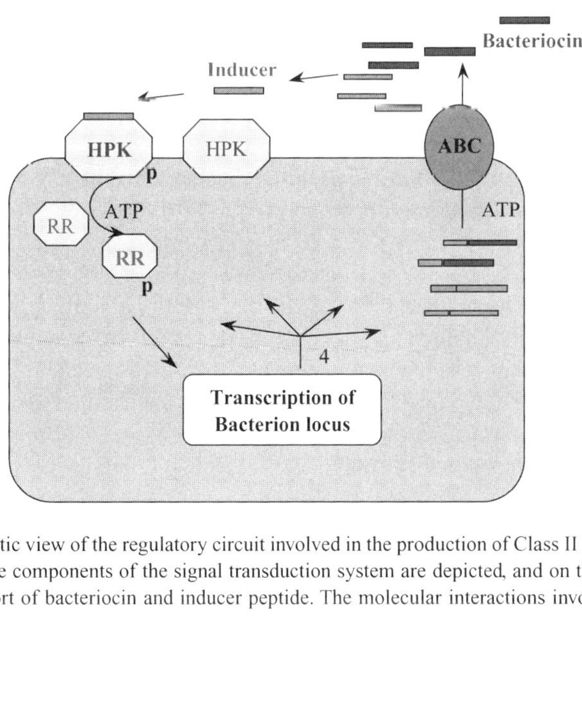

Figure 8.4. Schematic view of the regulatory circuit involved in the production of Class II LAB bacteriocins. On the left-hand side the components of the signal transduction system are depicted, and on the right-hand side the processing and export of bacteriocin and inducer peptide. The molecular interactions involved are explained in the text.

The immunity gene is expressed with no modification or processing, and the protein is located in the cytosolic fraction of the cell with a minor fraction associated with the membrane. When the immunity gene is cloned and expressed in a bacteriocin-susceptible bacterium, the latter is rendered resistant to the bacteriocin (Holo et al., 1991; Quadri et al., 1995; Allison and Klaenhammer, 1996). The immunity proteins identified so far are generally slightly hydrophobic, with pI values between 7 and 10, and a size range of 51–257 amino acids (Tichaczek et al., 1993; Diep et al., 1996).

The Transporter Genes

In the majority of cases (i.e., the double-glycine group), the production of Class II bacteriocins is dependent on the co-expression of two transporter genes. Both of these genes, which encode an ABC transporter and an accessory protein, are required for proper export and proteolytic activation of the bacteriocin. The ABC transporters involved in the production of double-glycine-type bacteriocins (including many lantibiotics, see above) have in common an N-terminal extension of approximately 150 amino acids, which is missing in other members of this large protein family (Stoddard et al., 1992; Håvarstein et al., 1995a). By the elegant work of Håvarstein and coworkers, who overexpressed a C-terminally truncated form of the lactococcin A transporter LcnC in *E. coli*, it was shown that the "extra" N-terminal domain is responsible for proteolytic processing of the pre-bacteriocin, thus demonstrating the bifunctionality of this and related ABC transporters (Håvarstein et al., 1995a). Although the function of the accessory protein is unclear at present, it has been shown to be essential for the secretion of bacteriocins (Venema et al., 1995a). Both the ABC transporter and the accessory protein (Franke et al., 1996) are integral membrane proteins, but the organization of the hypothetical export complex is not known.

Although bacteriocin-associated ABC transporters are often referred to as dedicated transporters, a single transporter can be involved in the transport of several peptides, as is the case with the lactococcins and the plantaricins (see Figure 8.4) (Diep et al., 1996; Quadri et al., 1997). In addition it has been demonstrated that secretion of one bacteriocin can be facilitated by the transport system of another bacteriocin (Allison et al., 1995a; van Belkum et al., 1997), and by other non-cognate transporters encoded by the host (Venema et al., 1996). As mentioned above, the latter phenomenon is also observed in some lantibiotic systems (Rince et al., 1994; Peschel et al., 1997; Heidrich et al., 1998).

Some variation has been observed as to the location of transport genes relative to the corresponding bacteriocin and immunity genes. The two transporter genes required for lactococcin A, B, and MN secretion are located on a separate operon some distance from the three bacteriocin operons, but the four operons are on the same plasmid. In the pediocin PA-1 cluster all four genes are organized in one transcriptional unit, whereas the two genes needed for secretion of sakacin A and the carnobacteriocins are located on an operon containing the three-component regulatory system as well (Axelsson et al., 1993; Quadri et al., 1997). It should also be noted that some transporter operons include several additional *orfs* with no known function (Diep et al., 1996).

The observation that, at least in some cases, the export and processing of bacteriocins can be relatively easily manipulated is very interesting, and holds promise for the engineering of bacteriocin-producing starter cultures (Allison et al., 1995a,b; McCormick et al., 1996, 1998, 1999). One could imagine, for instance, the future construction of a bacterial strain producing several unrelated bacteriocins, all of which are secreted and processed by the general secretory pathway of the producer.

The Regulation of Bacteriocin Synthesis

In many cases, bacteriocin production is an unstable trait. A common cause for this phenomenon is plasmid instability, as many bacteriocins are encoded by plasmid borne genes (Klaenhammer, 1993). The insertional inactivation of bacteriocin genes by endogenous insertion elements is another documented cause of the loss of the Bac^+ phenotype (Skaugen and Nes, 1994, 2000). Another kind of instability was found for *Lactobacillus plantarum* C11, where it was observed that the ability to produce bacteriocin was sometimes lost after diluting a liquid culture. The Bac^+ phenotype could be recovered, however, by supplementing the non-producer with spent broth from a producing culture (Diep et al., 1995). This key observation triggered a succession of experiments on C11 and other *Lactobacillus* strains, providing the current concept of the so-called three-component regulatory system involved in LAB bacteriocin production.

General Features of the HPK/RR Regulatory Systems

The general architecture of the bacterial HPK includes an N-terminal input domain with sensor function(s), which is located on the outside of the cytoplasmic membrane. This domain is coupled to a C-terminal transmitter module located on the cytoplasmic side, and the two domains are linked by two (or, occasionally, more [Island et al., 1992]) membrane-spanning segments (Parkinson and Kofoid, 1992; Stock et al., 1989, 1990, 1995, 2000). The primary structures of the sensor domains differ considerably, reflecting the vast range of chemical and physical stimuli detected. The site for autophosphorylation (ATP is the donor), which is crucial for signal transduction, is located at an absolutely conserved histidine residue N-terminal to the kinase domain, and in all cases studied so far a bimolecular reaction is involved, where one kinase catalyzes the phosphorylation of another kinase (Ninfa et al., 1993; Swanson et al., 1993; Wolfe and Stewart, 1993). The activation mechanism, thus, requires that the HPKs act as homodimers. The organizations of sequence motifs that are conserved amongst HPKs have also been identified in the HPK associated with bacteriocins production.

The second reaction in the phospho-relay is the transfer of phosphate from the HPK to the RR, which is also a two-domain protein: a highly conserved N-terminal receiver domain with aspartic acid residue serving as the phosphorylation site in all known RRs (Stock et al., 1990), and a far less conserved C-terminal output domain that executes the actual response. In the present context, the response is the activation of the promoters directing the transcription of pre-bacteriocin and associated genes. The genetic organization of the regulatory system of bacteriocin production and a schematic model of the events taking place in the regulatory circuit is shown in Figure 8.4.

The Pheromone

Until recently, the synthesis of peptide bacteriocins was thought to depend on the action of four genes (five genes for the two-peptide bacteriocins), encoding the necessary functions required for the production, processing, and secretion of the antimicrobial peptides. However, during DNA sequencing of bacteriocin operons it was found that regulatory genes were included in these gene clusters. The full significance of these findings was not comprehended until the peptide pheromones were identified. Amongst Class II bacteriocins, a specific peptide pheromone (Phe) was purified and shown to be needed for gene transcription and consequently for the translation. The peptide turned out to be a bacteriocin-like peptide and it was translated in a pre-form including a double-glycine leader just like the bacteriocins. Although the Phes shared many of the physico-chemical properties of the bacteriocins, the pheromones have low or no antimicrobial activity, and are generally shorter than the bacteriocins (the current range is between 19 and 26 residues). Another distinction between bacteriocins and their corresponding pheromones concerns the concentration range for observable biological activity: while the MIC values of most bacteriocins are in the nanomolar range, the minimum Phe concentration necessary for the activation of bacteriocin production ranges of 10^{-16} and 10^{-10} M, depending on the three-component system.

In addition to the pheromone from *L. plantarum* C11 (also termed PlnA, because of its bactericidal activity), Phe from other Class II bacteriocin producing LAB have been identified. These include Phe from *Lactobacillus sakei* LTH673 (Eijsink et al., 1996), Phe-LV17 from *Carnobacterium piscicola* LV17 (Quadri et al., 1997; Saucier et al., 1997), and Phe-492 from *E. faecium* CTC-492 (Nilsen et al., 1998). Orf4 from *L. sakei* Lb706 also appears to encode a Phe (Axelsson and Holck, 1995). The discovery of the three-component regulatory system of LAB bacteriocins also aided the identification of the competence factor pheromone of *Strep. pneumonia* (Håvarstein et al., 1995b).

The Histidine Protein Kinase

The HPK is located in the cytoplasmic membrane, where it serves as a receptor for the peptide pheromone. HPK is activated (autophosphorylated) by a specific interaction between its N-terminal domain and the incoming pheromone peptide. This interaction is very specific, thus preventing the pheromone of one regulatory system from activating the transcription of bacteriocin operons belonging to a different system.

The components of regulatory systems found in Class II bacteriocin producers are highly similar to systems that are involved in competence development and virulence (Diep et al., 1995; Pestova et al., 1996), and it has been proposed that, combined, they constitute a separate subfamily of two-component systems that respond to Phes in the external environment, presumably through an auto-induction system by quorum sensing (described below). The HPK of the competence regulatory system in *Strep. pneumonia* shows significant homology to the bacteriocin HPK with its 5–7 transmembrane segments. Experiments performed on closely related streptococci indicate that the strain specific part of the HPK lies in the N-terminus of the proteins and within the first 2–3 transmembrane segments (Håvarstein et al., 1996). Recently, the transmembrane topology of an HPK belonging to this subfamily was determined, showing that the histidine kinase AgrC from *S. aureus* contains five transmembrane helices (Lina et al., 1998).

Due to the high degree of similarity between the streptococcal systems and the regulatory systems for bacteriocin production in LAB, it seems likely that strain-specificity to Phes in LAB are located in the same domain. Recently, Brurberg et al. (1997) confirmed that induction of bacteriocin production in *Lactobacillus* is highly dependent on the addition of strain-specific Phe, and that the response relies on the specific interaction between the HPK and the Phe. In contrast to most known HPKs, which contain two segments spanning the cytoplasmic membrane (including the HPK of nisin), the N-terminal domains of the HPKs involved in regulation of competence, bacteriocin synthesis, and virulence are predicted to contain between five and seven membrane spanning segments (Pestova et al., 1996). As they appear to possess a similar topology, the described HPKs are believed to comprise a separate subfamily of proteins.

Response Regulators and Target Promoters

The final step in transducing the signal to its target, the regulated genes, is the binding of the activated phosphorylated RRs to the dedicated promoters. The RR gene is located immediately downstream of the HPK and pheromone genes, and the three genes constitute an operon. The LAB bacteriocin-associated RR genes have some sequence similarity to the pneumococcal RR genes. All known three-component regulatory systems have a single RR, with the exception of the plantaricin system. The two plantaricin regulators (PlnC and PlnD) are approximately 60% identical on the amino acid level (Axelsson and Holck, 1995; Diep et al., 1995). Recent studies indicate that both proteins function as dimers by binding to the promoter fragments containing direct repeats. Both the phosphorylated and non-phosphorylated forms of the plantaricin RRs bind to the promoters *in vitro*, but the phosphorylated forms bind stronger (Risøen et al., 1998).

The comparison of Class II bacteriocin promoters of different origin has revealed striking similarities, including the presence of conserved direct repeats just upstream of a weak nonconsensus −35 region. The 9–10 bp repeats are separated by 12–13 nucleotides (Nes et al., 1995; Diep et al., 1996; Risøen et al., 1998), indicating that transcriptional regulators bind to these genetic elements as dimers. The promoter elements contain normal −10 regions, and the most probable candidate for binding to the direct repeats is the RR of the three-component system. In a previous report, two RRs were shown to bind to DNA fragments containing such direct repeats. The data revealed that PlnCD from *L. plantarum* C11 could bind to their own adjacent promoter region preceding the three-component regulatory system (*plnABCD*), as well as to the promoter regions of two nearby operons containing bacteriocin and putative immunity genes (*plnEFI* and *plnJKLR*) and the transporter-encoding operon (*plnGHSTUV*).

The locus responsible for bacteriocin production in *L. plantarum* C11 comprises five operons that are all preceded by promoters containing regulatory elements resembling direct repeats (see Figure 8.4). The spacing between the repeats, as well as the presence of conserved nucleotides are crucial for the binding of dimer proteins. Recently, the functional analysis of promoters in the related sakacin P system was performed, using the promoterless chloramphenicol acetyl transferase (CAT) gene of the promoter screening vector pGKV210 (van der Vossen et al., 1987). These promoters are very similar to those found in the C11 cluster, and when constructs containing the promoters were transformed to *L. plantarum* C11, CAT activity was obtained by induction with Phe-C11 of Bac$^-$ cultures (Brurberg et al., 1997). The analysis of the promoters involved in regulation of sakacin P production confirmed that the promoter preceding the three-component system is leaky, while those in front of the structural bacteriocin genes are tightly regulated. With respect to the promoter preceding the transporter system, no differences were observed between induced and non-induced cells.

Induction of Bacteriocin Production

Two models have been proposed to explain how bacteriocin synthesis is induced. According to the quorum sensing model, the inducer (Phe) is constitutively expressed and secreted in low amounts and accumulates in the environment. When a threshold level of Phe, which is a measure of cell density, is reached, the regulatory circuit is engaged, which in turn leads to a burst in the expression of bacteriocin genes. The alternative model is similar, but postulates increased inducer gene transcription (triggered by some unidentified environmental signal) as the cause of Phe accumulation, rather than the constant, slow build-up to threshold level.

As indicated above, recent studies on bacteriocin regulation in *Lactobacillus* revealed that the promoter preceding the three-component regulatory system was leaky during non-induced conditions (Brurberg et al., 1997). The results indicate that the Phe is indeed produced constitutively at low levels, and at a certain point the accumulated Phe probably triggers an auto-induction loop resulting in the transcription of the genes involved in the production of bacteriocin(s). Although the latter observations are in agreement with the quorum sensing model, the model does not explain the puzzling phenomenon observed in *L. plantarum* C11, where cells rendered Bac^- by extreme dilution have to be presented with externally added Phe to reactivate the regulatory system (Diep et al., 1995). Although no specific factors other than the ones already mentioned has so far been implicated, the data do not exclude the possibility that additional factors do exist and play a role in the regulation of bacteriocin production in the LAB.

Concluding Remarks

During the past few years, tremendous progress has been made toward a better understanding of bacteriocin production, activity, and immunity in LAB. The emerging insights come from the identification and characterization of new bacteriocins as well as from the application and increasingly sophisticated analyses of the better-known systems. The potential application of bacteriocins and bacteriocinogenic strains in the manufacturing of food and feed has been one of the main driving forces (and an important source of funding) behind the rapid accumulation of information, and in a few cases (e.g., lacticin 3147) promising new bacteriocins have been put to the test in the manufacturing of food. However, as should be evident from the above presentation of this fast-growing field, there are still a number of issues that need continued attention in order to fully comprehend the molecular biology of bacteriocin production, which in our opinion is a general requirement for the future safe exploitation of this feature of the LAB.

References

Abee, T., Krockel, L., and Hill, C. (1995). Bacteriocins: Modes of action and potentials in food preservation and control of food poisoning. *International Journal of Food Microbiology* 28(2): 169–185.

Ali, D., Lacroix, C., Thuault, D., Bourgeois, C. M., and Simard, R. E. (1995). Characterization of diacetin B, a bacteriocin from *Lactococcus lactis* subsp. *lactis* bv. *diacetylactis* UL720. *Can J Microbiol* 41(9): 832–841.

Allgaier, H., Jung, G., Werner, R. G., Schneider, U., and Zähner, H. (1986). Epidermin: Sequencing of a heterodet tetracyclic 21-peptide amide antibiotic. *European Journal of Biochemistry* 160: 9–22.

Allison, G. E., Ahn, C., Stiles, M. E., and Klaenhammer, T. R. (1995a). Utilization of the leucocin A export system in *Leuconostoc gelidum* for production of a *Lactobacillus* bacteriocin. *FEMS Microbiology Letters* 131: 87–93.

Allison, G. E., Fremaux, C., and Klaenhammer, T. R. (1994). Expansion of bacteriocin activity and host range upon complementation of two peptides encoded within the lactacin F operon. *Journal of Bacteriology* 176(8): 2235–2241.

Allison, G. E., and Klaenhammer, T. R. (1996). Functional analysis of the gene encoding immunity to lactacin F, lafI, and its use as a *Lactobacillus*-specific, food-grade genetic marker. *Applied Environmental Microbiology* 62(12): 4450–4460.

Allison, G. E., Worobo, R. W., Stiles, M. E., and Klaenhammer, T. R. (1995b). Heterologous expression of the lactacin F peptides by *Carnobacterium piscicola* LV17. *Applied Environmental Microbiology* 61(4): 1371–1377.

Anderssen, E. L., Diep, D. B., Nes, I. F., Eijsink, V. G. H., and Nissen-Meyer, J. (1998). Antagonistic activity of *Lactobacillus plantarum* C11: Two new two-peptide bacteriocins, plantaricins EF and JK, and the induction factor plantaricin A. *Applied Environmental Microbiology* 64(6): 2269–2272.

Atrih, A., Rekhif, N., Moir, A. J., Lebrihi, A., and Lefebvre, G. (2001). Mode of action, purification and amino acid sequence of plantaricin C19, an anti-Listeria bacteriocin produced by *Lactobacillus plantarum* C19. *International Journal of Food Microbiology* 68(1–2): 93–104.

Augustin, J., Rosenstein, R., Wieland, B., Schneider, U., Schnell, N., Engelke, G., Entian, K.-D., and Götz, F. (1992). Genetic analysis of epidermin biosynthetic genes and epidermin-negative mutants of *Staphylococcus aureus*. *European Journal of Biochemistry* 204: 1149–1154.

Axelsson, L., and Holck, A. (1995). The genes involved in production and immunity to sakacin A, a bacteriocin from *Lactobacillus sake* Lb706. *Journal of Bacteriology* 177(8): 2125–2137.

Axelsson, L., Holck, A., Birkeland, S.-E., Aukrust, T., and Blom, H. (1993). Cloning and nucleotide sequence of a gene from *Lactobacillus sake* Lb706 necessary for sakacin A production and immunity. *Applied Environmental Microbiology* 59(9): 2868–2875.

Aymerich, T., Holo, H., Havarstein, L. S., Hugas, M., Garriga, M., and Nes, I. F. (1996). Biochemical and genetic characterization of enterocin A from *Enterococcus faecium*, a new antilisterial bacteriocin in the pediocin family of bacteriocins. *Applied Environmental Microbiology* 62(5): 1676–1682.

Banerjee, S., and Hansen, J. N. (1988). Structure and expresion of a gene encoding the precursor of subtilin, a small protein antibiotic. *J Biol Chem* 263(19): 9508–9514.

Bennik, M. H., Vanloo, B., Brasseur, R., Gorris, L. G., and Smid, E. J. (1998). A novel bacteriocin with a YGNGV motif from vegetable-associated *Enterococcus mundtii*: Full characterization and interaction with target organisms. *Biochimica et Biophysica ACTA* 1373(1): 47–58.

Benoit, V., Lebrihi, A., Milliere, J. B., and Lefebvre, G. (1997). Purification and partial amino acid sequence of brevicin 27, a bacteriocin produced by *Lactobacillus brevis* SB27. *Current Microbiology* 34(3): 173–179.

Benz, R., Jung G., and Sahl, H.-G. (1991). Mechanism of channel formation by lantibiotics in black lipid membranes. In: G. Jung and H.-G. Sahl (Eds.), *Nisin and novel lantibiotics* (pp. 359–372). Leiden: Escom.

Bhugaloo-Vial, P., Dousset, X., Metivier, A., Sorokine, O., Anglade, P., Boyaval, P., and Marion, D. (1996). Purification and amino acid sequences of piscicocins V1a and V1b, two class IIa bacteriocins secreted by *Carnobacterium piscicola* V1 that display significantly different levels of specific inhibitory activity. *Applied Environmental Microbiology* 62(12): 4410–4416.

Blom, H., Katla, T., Holck, A., Sletten, K., Axelsson, L., and Holo, H. (1999). Characterization, production, and purification of leucocin H, a two-peptide bacteriocin from Leuconostoc MF215B. *Current Microbiology* 39(1): 43–48.

Blond, A., Peduzzi, J., Goulard, C., Chiuchiolo, M. J., Barthelemy, M., Prigent, Y., Salomon, R. A., Farias, R. N., Moreno, F., and Rebuffat, S. (1999). The cyclic structure of microcin J25, a 21-residue peptide antibiotic from *Escherichia coli*. *European Journal of Biochemistry* 259(3): 747–755.

Bogovic-Matijasic, B., Rogelj, I., Nes, I. F., and Holo, H. (1998). Isolation and characterization of two bacteriocins of *Lactobacillus acidophilus* LF221. *Applied Microbiology and Biotechnology* 49(5): 606–612.

Boman, H. G. (2000). Innate immunity and the normal microflora. *Immunological Reviews* 173: 5–16.

Booth, M. C., Bogie, C. P., Sahl, H. G., Siezen, R. J., Hatter, K. L., and Gilmore, M. S. (1996). Structural analysis and proteolytic activation of *Enterococcus faecalis* cytolysin, a novel lantibiotic. *Molecular Microbiology* 21(6): 1175–1184.

Breukink, E., Wiedemann, I., van Kraaij, C., Kuipers, O. P., Sahl, H., and de Kruijff, B. (1999). Use of the cell wall precursor lipid II by a pore-forming peptide antibiotic. *Science* 286(5448): 2361–2364.

Brurberg, M. B., Nes, I. F., and Eijsink, V. G. H. (1997). Pheromone-induced production of antimicrobial peptides in *Lactobacillus*. *Molecular Microbiology* 26(2): 347–360.

Brötz, H., Bierbaum, G., Leopold, K., Reynolds, P. E., and Sahl, H.-G. (1998a). The lantibiotic mersacidin inhibits peptidoglycan synthesis by targeting lipid II. *Antimicrobial Agents and Chemotherapy* 42(1): 154–160.

Brötz, H., Bierbaum, G., Markus, A., Molito, E., and Sahl, H.-G. (1995). Mode of action of the lantibiotic mersacidin: Inhibition of peptidoglycan biosynthesis via a novel mechanism. *Antimicrobial Agents and Chemotherapy* 39(3): 714–719.

Brötz, H., Bierbaum, G., Reynolds, P. E., and Sahl, H.-G. (1997). The lantibiotic mersacidin inhibits peptidoglycan biosynthesis at the level of transglycosylation. *European Journal of Biochemistry* 246: 193–199.

Brötz, H., Josten, M., Wiedemann, I., Schneider, U., Gotz, F., Bierbaum, G., and Sahl, H. G. (1998b). Role of lipid-bound peptidoglycan precursors in the formation of pores by nisin, epidermin and other lantibiotics. *Molecular Microbiology* 30(2): 317–327.

Buchman, G. W., Banerjee, S., and Hansen, J. N. (1988). Structure, expression, and evolution of a gene encoding the precursor of nisin, a small protein antibiotic. *J Biol Chem* 263(31): 16260–16266.

Cammue, B. P., De Bolle, M. F., Schoofs, H. M., Terras, F. R., Thevissen, K., Osborn, R. W., Rees, S. B., and Broekaert, W. F. (1994). Gene-encoded antimicrobial peptides from plants. *Ciba Found Symp* 186: 91–101.

Casaus, P., Nilsen, T., Cintas, L. M., Nes, I. F., Hernández, P. E., and Holo, H. (1997). Enterocin B, a new bacteriocin from *Enterococcus faecium* T136 which can act synergistically with enterocin A. *Microbiology* 143: 2287–2294.

Chandrapati, S., and O'Sullivan, D. J. (1999). Nisin independent induction of the nisA promoter in Lactococcus *lactis* during growth in lactose or galactose. *FEMS Microbiology Letters* 170(1): 191–198.

Chen, P., Qi, F., Novak, J., and Caufield, P. W. (1999). The specific genes for lantibiotic mutacin II biosynthesis in Streptococcus mutans T8 are clustered and can be transferred en bloc. *Applied Environmental Microbiology* 65(3): 1356–1360.

Chien, C. T., Bartel, P. L., Sternglanz, R., and Fields, S. (1991). The two-hybrid system: a method to identify and clone genes for proteins that interact with a protein of interest. *Proceedings of the National Academy of Sciences of the United States of America* 88(21): 9578–9582.

Cintas, L. M., Casaus, P., Herranz, C., Havarstein, L. S., Holo, H., Hernandez, P. E., and Nes, I. F. (2000). Biochemical and genetic evidence that enterococcus faecium L50 produces enterocins L50A and L50B, the *sec*-dependent enterocin P, and a novel bacteriocin secreted without an N-terminal extension termed enterocin Q. *Journal of Bacteriology* 182(23): 6806–6814.

Cintas, L. M., Casaus, P., Holo, H., Hernandez, P. E., Nes, I. F., and Havarstein, L. S. (1998). Enterocins L50A and L50B, two novel bacteriocins from *Enterococcus faecium* L50, are related to staphylococcal hemolysins. *Journal of Bacteriology* 180(8): 1988–1994.

Cintas, L. M., Casaus, P., Håvarstein, L. S., Hernández, P. E., and Nes, I. F. (1997). Biochemical and genetic characterization of enterocin P, a novel *sec*-dependent bacteriocin from *Enterococcus faecium* P13 with a broad antimicrobial spectrum. *Applied Environmental Microbiology* 63(11): 4321–4330.

Coburn, P. S., Hancock, L. E., Booth, M. C., and Gilmore, M. S. (1999). A novel means of self-protection, unrelated to toxin activation, confers immunity to the bactericidal effects of the Enterococcus faecalis cytolysin. *Infection and Immunity* 67(7): 3339–3347.

Contreras, B. G., De Vuyst, L., Devreese, B., Busanyova, K., Raymaeckers, J., Bosman, F., Sablon, E., and Vandamme, E. J. (1997). Isolation, purification, and amino acid sequence of lactobin A, one of the two bacteriocins produced by Lactobacillus amylovorus LMG P-13139. *Applied Environmental Microbiology* 63(1): 13–20.

Dabard, J., Bridonneau, C., Phillipe, C., Anglade, P., Molle, D., Nardi, M., Ladire, M., Girardin, H., Marcille, F., Gomez, A., and Fons, M. (2001). Ruminococcin A, a new lantibiotic produced by a *Ruminococcus gnavus* strain isolated from human feces. *Applied Environmental Microbiology* 67(9): 4111–4118.

de Ruyter, P. G., Kuipers, O. P., and de Vos, W. M. (1996a). Controlled gene expression systems for *Lactococcus lactis* with the food-grade inducer nisin. *Applied Environmental Microbiology* 62(10): 3662–3667.

de Ruyter, P. G., Kuipers, O. P., Meijer, W. C., and de Vos, W. M. (1997). Food-grade controlled lysis of *Lactococcus lactis* for accelerated cheese ripening. *Nature Biotechnology* 15(10): 976–979.

de Ruyter, P. G. G. A., Kuipers, O. P., Beerthuyzen, M. M., van Alen-Boerrigter, I., and de Vos, W. M. (1996b). Functional analysis of promoters in the nisin gene cluster of *Lactococcus lactis*. *Journal of Bacteriology* 178(12): 3434–3439.

de Vos, W. M., Kuipers, O. P., van der Meer, J. R., and Siezen, R. J. (1995). Maturation pathway of nisin and other lantibiotics: Post-translationally modified antimicrobial peptides exported by Gram-positive bacteria. *Molecular Microbiology* 17(3): 427–437.

Delves-Broughton, J., Blackburn, P., Evans, R. J., and Hugenholtz, J. (1996). Applications of the bacteriocin, nisin. *Antonie van Leeuwenhoek* 69(2): 193–202.

Diep, D. B., Havarstein, L. S., and Nes, I. F. (1995). A bacteriocin-like peptide induces bacteriocin synthesis in *Lactobacillus plantarum* C11. *Molecular Microbiology* 18(4): 631–639.

Diep, D. B., Havarstein, L. S., and Nes, I. F. (1996). Characterization of the locus responsible for the bacteriocin production in *Lactobacillus plantarum* C11. *Journal of Bacteriology* 178(15): 4472–4483.

Dougherty, B. A., Hill, C., Weidman, J. F., Richardson, D. R., Venter, J. C., and Ross, R. P. (1998). Sequence and analysis of the 60 kb conjugative, bacteriocin-producing plasmid pMRC01 from *Lactococcus lactis* DPC3147. *Molecular Microbiology* 29(4): 1029–1038.

Duan, K., Harvey, M. L., Liu, C. Q., and Dunn, N. W. (1996). Identification and characterization of a mobilizing plasmid, pND300, in *Lactococcus lactis* M189 and its encoded nisin resistance determinant. *Journal of Applied Bacteriology* 81(5): 493–500.

Ehrmann, M. A., Remiger, A., Eijsink, V. G., and Vogel, R. F. (2000). A gene cluster encoding plantaricin 1.25beta and other bacteriocin-like peptides in *Lactobacillus plantarum* TMW1.25. *Biochimica et Biophysica ACTA* 1490(3): 355–361. bin/cas/tree/store/bbaexp/cas_sub/browse/browse.cgi?year=2000&volume=149 0&issue = 3&aid = 91357.

Eichenbaum, Z., Federle, M. J., Marra, D., de Vos, W. M., Kuipers, O. P., Kleerebezem, M., and Scott, J. R. (1998). Use of the lactococcal nisA promoter to regulate gene expression in Gram-positive bacteria: Comparison of induction level and promoter strength. *Applied Environmental Microbiology* 64(8): 2763–2769.

Eijsink, V. G., Brurberg, M. B., Middelhoven, P. H., and Nes, I. F. (1996). Induction of bacteriocin production in *Lactobacillus sake* by a secreted peptide. *Journal of Bacteriology* 178(8): 2232–2237.

Engelke, G., Gutowski-Eckel, Z., Hammelmann, M., and Entian, K. D. (1992). Biosynthesis of the lantibiotic nisin: Genomic organization and membrane localization of the NisB protein. *Applied Environmental Microbiology* 58(11): 3730–3743.

Engelke, G., Gutowski-Eckel, Z., Kiesau, P., Siegers, K., Hammelmann, M., and Entian, K. D. (1994). Regulation of nisin biosynthesis and immunity in *Lactococcus lactis* 6F3. *Applied Environmental Microbiology* 60(3): 814–825.

Farias, M. E., Farias, R. N., de Ruiz Holgado, A. P., and Sesma, F. (1996). Purification and N-terminal amino acid sequence of Enterocin CRL 35, a "pediocin-like" bacteriocin produced by *Enterococcus faecium* CRL 35. *Letters in Applied Microbiology* 22(6): 417–419.

Fath, M. J., and Kolter, R. (1993). ABC transporters: bacterial exporters. *Microbiology Review* 57(4): 995–1017.

Felix, J. V., Papathanasopoulos, M. A., Smith, A. A., von Holy, A., and Hastings, J. W. (1994). Characterization of leucocin B-Ta11a: A bacteriocin from *Leuconostoc carnosum* Ta11a isolated from meat. *Current Microbiology* 29(4): 207–212.

Ferchichi, M., Frere, J., Mabrouk, K., and Manai, M. (2001). Lactococcin MMFII, a novel class IIa bacteriocin produced by *Lactococcus lactis* MMFII, isolated from a Tunisian dairy product. *FEMS Microbiology Letters* 205(1): 49–55.

Fields, S., and Song, O. (1989). A novel genetic system to detect protein–protein interactions. *Nature* 340(6230): 245–246.

Floriano, B., Ruiz-Barba, J. L., and Jimenez-Diaz, R. (1998). Purification and genetic characterization of enterocin I from *Enterococcus faecium* 6T1a, a novel antilisterial plasmid-encoded bacteriocin which does not belong to the pediocin family of bacteriocins. *Applied Environmental Microbiology* 64(12): 4883–4890.

Flynn, S., van Sinderen, D., Thornton, G. M., Holo, H., Nes, I. F., and Collins, J. K. (2002). Characterization of the genetic locus responsible for the production of ABP-118, a novel bacteriocin produced by the probiotic bacterium *Lactobacillus salivarius* subsp. *salivarius* UCC118. *Microbiology* 148(Pt 4): 973–984.

Franke, C. M., Leenhouts, K. J., Haandrikman, A. J., Kok, J., Venema, G., and Venema, K. (1996). Topology of LcnD, a protein implicated in the transport of bacteriocins from *Lactococcus lactis*. *Journal of Bacteriology* 178(6): 1766–1769.

Franz, C. M., Grube, A., Herrmann, A., Abriouel, H., Starke, J., Lombardi, A., Tauscher, B., and Holzapfel, W. H. (2002). Biochemical and genetic characterization of the two-peptide bacteriocin enterocin 1071 produced by *Enterococcus faecalis* FAIR-E 309. *Applied Environmental Microbiology* 68(5): 2550–2554.

Franz, C. M., van Belkum, M. J., Worobo, R. W., Vederas, J. C., and Stiles, M. E. (2000). Characterization of the genetic locus responsible for production and immunity of carnobacteriocin A: The immunity gene confers cross-protection to enterocin B. *Microbiology* 146(Pt 3): 621–631.

Franz, C. M., Worobo, R. W., Quadri, L. E., Schillinger, U., Holzapfel, W. H., Vederas, J. C., and Stiles, M. E. (1999). Atypical genetic locus associated with constitutive production of enterocin B by *Enterococcus faecium* BFE 900. *Applied Environmental Microbiology* 65(5): 2170–2178.

Fremaux, C., Hechard, Y., and Cenatiempo, Y. (1995). Mesentericin Y105 gene clusters in *Leuconostoc mesenteroides* Y105. *Microbiology* 141(Pt 7): 1637–1645.

Garrido, M. d. C., Herrero, M., Kolter, R., and Moreno, F. (1988). The export of the DNA replication inhibitor microcin B17 provides immunity for the host cell. *EMBO Journal* 7(6): 1853–1862.

Garver, K. I., and Muriana, P. M. (1994). Purification and partial amino acid sequence of curvaticin FS47, a heat-stable bacteriocin produced by *Lactobacillus curvatus* FS47. *Applied Environmental Microbiology* 60(6): 2191–2195.

Geißler, S., Götz, F., and Kupke, T. (1996). Serine protease EpiP from *Staphylococcus epidermidis* catalyzes the processing of the epidermin precursor peptide. *Journal of Bacteriology* 178(1): 284–288.

Gilmore, M. S., Segarra, R. A., Booth, M. C., Bogie, C. P., Hall, L. R., and Clewell, D. B. (1994). Genetic structure of the Enterococcus faecalis plasmid pAD1-encoded cytolytic toxin system and its relationship to lantibiotic determinants. *Journal of Bacteriology* 176(23): 7335–7344.

Gilmore, M. S., Skaugen, M., and Nes, I. (1996). Enterococcus faecalis cytolysin and lactocin S of *Lactobacillus sake*. *Antonie van Leeuwenhoek* 69(2): 129–138.

Gonzalez, C., Langdon, G. M., Bruix, M., Galvez, A., Valdivia, E., Maqueda, M., and Rico, M. (2000). Bacteriocin AS-48, a microbial cyclic polypeptide structurally and functionally related to mammalian NK-lysin. *Proceedings of the National Academy of Sciences of the United States of America* 97(21): 11221–11226.

Gutowski-Eckel, Z., Klein, C., Siegers, K., Bohm, K., Hammelmann, M., and Entian, K. D. (1994). Growth phase-dependent regulation and membrane localization of SpaB, a protein involved in biosynthesis of the lantibiotic subtilin. *Applied Environmental Microbiology* 60(1): 1–11.

Hancock, R. E., and Chapple, D. S. (1999). Peptide antibiotics. *Antimicrobial Agents and Chemotherapy* 43(6): 1317–1323.

Hastings, J. W., Sailer, M., Johnson, K., Roy, K. L., Vederas, J. C., and Stiles, M. E. (1991). Characterization of leucocin A-AUL 187 and cloning of the bacteriocin gene from *Leuconostoc gelidum*. *Journal of Bacteriology* 173(23): 7491–7500.

Hechard, Y., Berjeaud, J. M., and Cenatiempo, Y. (1999). Characterization of the mesB gene and expression of bacteriocins by *Leuconostoc mesenteroides* Y105. *Current Microbiology* 39(5): 265–269.

Hechard, Y., Derijard, B., Letellier, F., and Cenatiempo, Y. (1992). Characterization and purification of mesentericin Y105, an anti-Listeria bacteriocin from *Leuconostoc mesenteroides*. *Journal of General Microbiology* 138(Pt 12): 2725–2731.

Heidrich, C., Pag, U., Josten, M., Metzger, J., Jack, R. W., Bierbaum, G., Jung, G., and Sahl, H. G. (1998). Isolation, characterization, and heterologous expression of the novel lantibiotic epicidin 280 and analysis of its biosynthetic gene cluster. *Applied Environmental Microbiology* 64(9): 3140–3146.

Henderson, J. T., Chopko, A. L., and van Wassenaar, P. D. (1992). Purification and primary structure of pediocin PA-1 produced by *Pediococcus acidilactici* PAC-1.0. *Arch Biochem Biophys* 295(1): 5–12.

Herbin, S., Mathieu, F., Brule, F., Branlant, C., Lefebvre, G., and Lebrihi, A. (1997). Characteristics and genetic determinants of bacteriocin activities produced by Carnobacterium piscicola CP5 isolated from cheese. *Current Microbiology* 35(6): 319–326.

Higgins, C. F. (1992). ABC transporters: from microorganisms to man. *Annual Review of Cell Biology* 8: 67–113.

Higgins, C. F., Hiles, I. D., Salmond, G. P., Gill, D. R., Downie, J. A., Evans, I. J., Holland, I. B., Gray, L., Buckel, S. D., Bell, A. W. et al. (1986). A family of related ATP-binding subunits coupled to many distinct biological processes in bacteria. *Nature* 323(6087): 448–450.

Hillman, J. D., Novak, J., Sagura, E., Gutierrez, J. A., Brooks, T. A., Crowley, P. J., Hess, M., Azizi, A., Leung, K., Cvitkovitch, D., and Bleiweis, A. S. (1998). Genetic and biochemical analysis of mutacin 1140, a lantibiotic from *Streptococcus mutans*. *Infection and Immunity* 66(6): 2743–2749.

Holck, A., Axelsson, L., Birkeland, S. E., Aukrust, T., and Blom, H. (1992). Purification and amino acid sequence of sakacin A, a bacteriocin from *Lactobacillus sake* Lb706. *Journal of General Microbiology* 138(Pt 12): 2715–2720.

Holck, A., Axelsson, L., Hühne, K., and Kröckel, L. (1994a). Purification and cloning of sakacin 674, a bacteriocin from *Lactobacillus sake* Lb674. *FEMS Microbiology Letters* 115: 143–150.

Holck, A., Axelsson, L., and Schillinger, U. (1996). Divergicin 750, a novel bacteriocin produced by *Carnobacterium divergens* 750. *FEMS Microbiology Letters* 136(2): 163–168.

Holck, A. L., Axelsson, L., and Schillinger, U. (1994b). Purification and cloning of piscicolin 61, a bacteriocin from *Carnobacterium piscicola* LV61. *Current Microbiology* 29(2): 63–68.

Holo, H., Jeknic, Z., Daeschel, M., Stevanovic, S., and Nes, I. F. (2001). Plantaricin W from *Lactobacillus plantarum* belongs to a new family of two-peptide lantibiotics. *Microbiology* 147(Pt 3): 643–651.

Holo, H., Nilssen, Ø., and Nes, I. F. (1991). Lactococcin A, a new bacteriocin from *Lactococcus lactis* subsp. *cremoris*: Isolation and characterization of the protein and its gene. *Journal of Bacteriology* 173(12): 3879–3887.

Horn, N., Swindell, S., Dodd, H., and Gasson, M. (1991). Nisin biosynthesis genes are encoded by a novel conjugative transposon. *Molecular and General Genetics* 228: 129–135.

Huhne, K., Axelsson, L., Holck, A., and Krockel, L. (1996). Analysis of the sakacin P gene cluster from *Lactobacillus sake* Lb674 and its expression in sakacin-negative Lb. sake strains. *Microbiology* 142(Pt 6): 1437–1448.

Huot, E., Meghrous, J., BarrenaGonzalez, C., and Petitdemange, H. (1996). Bacteriocin J46, a new bacteriocin produced by *Lactococcus lactis* subsp. *cremoris* J46: Isolation and characterization of the protein and its gene. Anaerobe 2(3): 137–145.

Hynes, W. L., Ferretti, J. J., and Tagg, J. R. (1993). Cloning of the gene encoding streptococcin A-FF22, a novel lantibiotic produced by *Streptococcus pyogenes*, and determination of its nucleotide sequence. *Applied Environmental Microbiology* 59(6): 1969–1971.

Håvarstein, L. S., Coomaraswamy, G., and Morrison, D. A. (1995b). An unmodified heptadecapeptide pheromone induces competence for genetic transformation in *Streptococcus pneumoniae*. *Proceedings of the National Academy of Sciences of the United States of America* 92(24): 11140–11144.

Håvarstein, L. S., Diep, D. B., and Nes, I. F. (1995a). A family of bacteriocin ABC transporters carry out proteolytic processing of their substrates concomitant with export. *Molecular Microbiology* 16(2): 229–240.

Håvarstein, L. S., Gaustad, P., Nes, I. F., and Morrison, D. A. (1996). Identification of the streptococcal competence-pheromone receptor. *Molecular Microbiology* 21(4): 863–869.

Håvarstein, L. S., Holo, H., and Nes, I. F. (1994). The leader peptide of colicin V shares consensus sequences with leader peptides that are common among peptide bacteriocins produced by Gram-positive bacteria. *Microbiology* 140: 2383–2389.

Ike, Y., Clewell, D. B., Segarra, R. A., and Gilmore, M. S. (1990). Genetic analysis of the pAD1 hemolysin/bacteriocin determinant in *Enterococcus faecalis*: Tn917 insertional mutagenesis and cloning. *Journal of Bacteriology* 172(1): 155–163.

Immonen, T., Ye, S., Ra, R., Qiao, M., Paulin, L., and Saris, P. E. (1995). The codon usage of the nisZ operon in *Lactococcus lactis* N8 suggests a non-lactococcal origin of the conjugative nisin-sucrose transposon. *DNA Sequence* 5(4): 203–218.

Island, M. D., Wei, B. Y., and Kadner, R. J. (1992). Structure and function of the uhp genes for the sugar phosphate transport system in *Escherichia coli* and *Salmonella typhimurium*. *Journal of Bacteriology* 174(9): 2754–2762.

Jack, R., Bierbaum, G., Heidrich, C., and Sahl, H. G. (1995). The genetics of lantibiotic biosynthesis. *Bioessays* 17(9): 793–802.

Jack, R. W., Bierbaum, G., and Sahl, H.-G. (1998). *Lantibiotics and related peptides*. Berlin, Heidelberg: Springer-Verlag.

Jack, R. W., Wan, J., Gordon, J., Harmark, K., Davidson, B. E., Hillier, A. J., Wettenhall, R. E., Hickey, M. W., and Coventry, M. J. (1996). Characterization of the chemical and antimicrobial properties of piscicolin 126, a bacteriocin produced by *Carnobacterium piscicola* JG126. *Applied Environmental Microbiology* 62(8): 2897–2903.

Jimenez-Diaz, R., Ruiz-Barba, J. L., Cathcart, D. P., Holo, H., Nes, I. F., Sletten, K. H., and Warner, P. J. (1995). Purification and partial amino acid sequence of plantaricin S, a bacteriocin produced by *Lactobacillus plantarum* LPCO10, the activity of which depends on the complementary action of two peptides. *Applied Environmental Microbiology* 61(12): 4459–4463.

Joerger, M. C., and Klaenhammer, T. R. (1990). Cloning, expression, and nucleotide sequence of the Lactobacillus helveticus 481 gene encoding the bacteriocin helveticin J. *Journal of Bacteriology* 172(11): 6339–6347.

Jung, G. (1991). Lantibiotics: A survey. In: G. Jung and H.-G. Sahl (Eds.), *Nisin and novel lantibiotics* (pp. 1–34). Leiden: ESCOM.

Kaiser, A. L., and Montville, T. J. (1996). Purification of the bacteriocin bavaricin MN and characterization of its mode of action against *Listeria monocytogenes* Scott A cells and lipid vesicles. *Applied Environmental Microbiology* 62(12): 4529–4535.

Kaletta, C., Entian, K.-D., Kellner, R., Jung, G., Reis, M., and Sahl, H.-G. (1989). Pep5, a new lantibiotic: structural gene isolation and prepeptide sequence. *Archives of Microbiology* 152: 16–19.

Kalmokoff, M. L., Lu, D., Whitford, M. F., and Teather, R. M. (1999). Evidence for production of a new lantibiotic (butyrivibriocin OR79A) by the ruminal anaerobe *Butyrivibrio fibrisolvens* OR79: characterization of the structural gene encoding butyrivibriocin OR79A. *Applied Environmental Microbiology* 65(5): 2128–2235.

Kanatani, K., Oshimura, M., and Sano, K. (1995a). Isolation and characterization of acidocin A and cloning of the bacteriocin gene from *Lactobacillus acidophilus*. *Applied Environmental Microbiology* 61(3): 1061–1067.

Kanatani, K., Tahara, T., Oshimura, M., Sano, K., and Umezawa, C. (1995b). Cloning and nucleotide sequence of the gene for acidocin 8912, a bacteriocin from *Lactobacillus acidophilus* TK8912. *Letters in Applied Microbiology* 21(6): 384–386.

Karakas Sen, A., Narbad, A., Horn, N., Dodd, H. M., Parr, A. J., Colquhoun, I., and Gasson, M. J. (1999). Post-translational modification of nisin. The involvement of NisB in the dehydration process. *European Journal of Biochemistry* 261(2): 524–532.

Karaya, K., Shimizu, T., and Taketo, A. (2001). New gene cluster for lantibiotic streptin possibly involved in streptolysin S formation. *J Biochem (Tokyo)* 129(5): 769–775.

Kawai, Y., Saito, T., Kitazawa, H., and Itoh, T. (1998a). Acidocin 8912, a bacteriocin from *Lactobacillus acidophilus* TK8912 linked at N- and C-terminal ends. *Bioscience, Biotechnology, and Biochemistry* 62(12): 2438–2440.

Kawai, Y., Saito, T., Suzuki, M., and Itoh, T. (1998b). Sequence analysis by cloning of the structural gene of gassericin A, a hydrophobic bacteriocin produced by *Lactobacillus gasseri* LA39. *Bioscience, Biotechnology, and Biochemistry* 62(5): 887–892.

Kiesau, P., Eikmanns, U., Gutowski-Eckel, Z., Weber, S., Hammelmann, M., and Entian, K.-D. (1997). Evidence for a multimeric subtilin synthetase complex. *Journal of Bacteriology* 179(5): 1475–1481.

Klaenhammer, T. R. (1993). Genetics of bacteriocins produced by lactic acid bacteria. *FEMS Microbiology Review* 12: 39–86.

Kleerebezem, M., Beerthuyzen, M. M., Vaughan, E. E., de Vos, W. M., and Kuipers, O. P. (1997a). Controlled gene expression systems for lactic acid bacteria: transferable nisin-inducible expression cassettes for *Lactococcus, Leuconostoc,* and *Lactobacillus* spp. *Applied Environmental Microbiology* 63(11): 4581–4584.

Kleerebezem, M., de Vos, W. M., and Kuipers, O. P. (1999). The lantibiotics nisin and subtilin act as extracellular regulators of their own biosynthesis. In: G. M. Dunny and S. C. Winans (Eds.), *Cell–cell signaling in bacteria* (pp. 159–174). Washington D.C.: ASM Press.

Kleerebezem, M., Quadri, L. E., Kuipers, O. P., and de Vos, W. M. (1997b). Quorum sensing by peptide pheromones and two-component signal-transduction systems in Gram-positive bacteria. *Molecular Microbiology* 24(5): 895–904.

Klein, C., and Entian, K. D. (1994). Genes involved in self-protection against the lantibiotic subtilin produced by *Bacillus subtilis* ATCC 6633. *Applied Environmental Microbiology* 60(8): 2793–2801.

Klein, C., Kaletta, C., and Entian, K. D. (1993). Biosynthesis of the lantibiotic subtilin is regulated by a histidine kinase/response regulator system. *Applied Environmental Microbiology* 59(1): 296–303.

Kuipers, O. P., Beerthuyzen, M. M., de Ruyter, P. G., Luesink, E. J., and de Vos, W. M. (1995). Autoregulation of nisin biosynthesis in *Lactococcus lactis* by signal transduction. *J Biol Chem* 270(45): 27299–27304.

Kuipers, O. P., Beerthuyzen, M. M., Siezen, R., and de Vos, W. M. (1993). Characterization of the nisin-gene cluster *nisABCTIPR* of *Lactococcus lactis*. Expression requirement of the *nisA* and *nisI* gene for producing immunity. *European Journal of Biochemistry* 216: 281–291.

Kuipers, O. P., de Ruyter, P. G. G. A., Kleerebezem, M., and de Vos, W. M. (1997). Controlled overproduction of proteins by lactic acid bacteria. *Trends in Biotechnology* 15: 135–140.

Lagos, R., Villanueva, J. E., and Monasterio, O. (1999). Identification and properties of the genes encoding microcin E492 and its immunity protein. *Journal of Bacteriology* 181(1): 212–217.

Larsen, A. G., Vogensen, F. K., and Josephsen, J. (1993). Antimicrobial activity of lactic acid bacteria isolated from sour doughs: Purification and characterization of bavaricin A, a bacteriocin produced by *Lactobacillus bavaricus* MI401. *Journal of Applied Bacteriology* 75(2): 113–122.

Leer, R. J., van der Vossen, J. M., van Giezen, M., van Noort, J. M., and Pouwels, P. H. (1995). Genetic analysis of acidocin B, a novel bacteriocin produced by *Lactobacillus acidophilus*. *Microbiology* 141(Pt 7): 1629–1635.

Lina, G., Jarraud, S., Ji, G., Greenland, T., Pedraza, A., Etienne, J., Novick, R. P., and Vandenesch, F. (1998). Transmembrane topology and histidine protein kinase activity of AgrC, the agr signal receptor in *Staphylococcus aureus*. *Molecular Microbiology* 28(3): 655–662.

Lopez de Felipe, F., Kleerebezem, M., de Vos, W. M., and Hugenholtz, J. (1998). Cofactor engineering: A novel approach to metabolic engineering in *Lactococcus lactis* by controlled expression of NADH oxidase. *Journal of Bacteriology* 180(15): 3804–3808.

Makino, K., Shinagawa, H., Amemura, M., and Nakata, A. (1986). Nucleotide sequence of the phoB gene, the positive regulatory gene for the phosphate regulon of *Escherichia coli* K-12. *J Mol Biol* 190(1): 37–44.

Marciset, O., Jeronimus-Stratingh, M. C., Beat, M., and Poolman, B. (1997). Thermophilin 13, a nontypical antilisterial poration complex bacteriocin, that functions without a receptor. *J Biol Chem* 272(22): 14277–14284.

Martinez, B., Fernandez, M., Suarez, J. E., and Rodriguez, A. (1999). Synthesis of lactococcin 972, a bacteriocin produced by *Lactococcus lactis* IPLA 972, depends on the expression of a plasmid-encoded bicistronic operon. *Microbiology* 145(Pt 11): 3155–3161.

Martinez, B., Rodriguez, A., and Suarez, J. E. (2000). Lactococcin 972, a bacteriocin that inhibits septum formation in lactococci. *Microbiology* 146(Pt 4): 949–955.

Marugg, J. D., Gonzalez, C. F., Kunka, B. S., Ledeboer, A. M., Pucci, M. J., Toonen, M. Y., Walker, S. A., Zoetmulder, L. C. M., and Vandenbergh, P. A. (1992). Cloning, expression, and nucleotide sequence of genes involved in production of pediocin PA-1, a bacteriocin from Pediococcus acidilactici PAC1.0. *Applied Environmental Microbiology* 58(8): 2360–2367.

McAuliffe, O., Hill, C., and Ross, R. P. (2000). Identification and overexpression of ltnl, a novel gene which confers immunity to the two-component lantibiotic lacticin 3147. *Microbiology* 146(Pt 1): 129–138.

McAuliffe, O., Ryan, M. P., Ross, R. P., Hill, C., Breeuwer, P., and Abee, T. (1998). Lacticin 3147, a broad-spectrum bacteriocin which selectively dissipates the membrane potential. *Applied Environmental Microbiology* 64(2): 439–445.

McCormick, J. K., Klaenhammer, T. R., and Stiles, M. E. (1999). Colicin V can be produced by lactic acid bacteria. *Letters in Applied Microbiology* 29(1): 37–41.

McCormick, J. K., Poon, A., Sailer, M., Gao, Y., Roy, K. L., McMullen, L. M., Vederas, J. C., Stiles, M. E., and Van Belkum, M. J. (1998). Genetic characterization and heterologous expression of brochocin-C, an antibotulinal, two-peptide bacteriocin produced by *Brochothrix campestris* ATCC 43754. *Applied Environmental Microbiology* 64(12): 4757–4766.

McCormick, J. K., Worobo, R. W., and Stiles, M. E. (1996). Expression of the antimicrobial peptide carnobacteriocin B2 by a signal peptide-dependent general secretory pathway. *Applied Environmental Microbiology* 62(11): 4095–4099.

McLaughlin, R. E., Ferretti, J. J., and Hynes, W. L. (1999). Nucleotide sequence of the streptococcin A-FF22 lantibiotic regulon: Model for production of the lantibiotic SA-FF22 by strains of *Streptococcus pyogenes*. *FEMS Microbiology Letters* 175(2): 171–177.

Metivier, A., Pilet, M. F., Dousset, X., Sorokine, O., Anglade, P., Zagorec, M., Piard, J. C., Marion, D., Cenatiempo, Y., and Fremaux, C. (1998). Divercin V41, a new bacteriocin with two disulphide bonds produced by *Carnobacterium divergens* V41: Primary structure and genomic organization. *Microbiology* 144(Pt 10): 2837–2844.

Meyer, C., Bierbaum, G., Heidrich, C., Reis, M., Süling, J., Iglesias-Wind, M. I., Kempter, C., Molitor, E., and Sahl, H.-G. (1995). Nucleotide sequence of the lantibiotic Pep5 biosynthetic gene cluster and functional analysis of PepP and PepC: Evidence for a role of PepC in thioether formation. *European Journal of Biochemistry* 232: 478–489.

Moll, G. N., Konings, W. N., and Driessen, A. J. (1999). Bacteriocins: Mechanism of membrane insertion and pore formation. *Antonie van Leeuwenhoek* 76(1–4): 185–198.

Moll, G. N., Roberts, G. C., Konings, W. N., and Driessen, A. J. (1996). Mechanism of lantibiotic-induced pore-formation. *Antonie van Leeuwenhoek* 69(2): 185–191.

Morgan, S., Ross, R. P., and Hill, C. (1995). Bacteriolytic activity caused by the presence of a novel lactococcal plasmid encoding lactococcins A, B, and M. *Applied Environmental Microbiology* 61(8): 2995–3001.

Motlagh, A. M., Bhunia, A. K., Szostek, F., Hansen, T. R., Johnson, M. C., and Ray, B. (1992). Nucleotide and amino acid sequence of pap-gene (pediocin AcH production) in *Pediococcus acidilactici* H. *Letters in Applied Microbiology* 15: 45–48.

Mulders, J. W. M., Boerrigter, I. J., Rollema, H. S., Siezen, R. J., and de Vos, W. M. (1991). Identification and characterization of the lantibiotic nisin Z, a natural nisin variant. *European Journal of Biochemistry* 201: 581–584.

Muriana, P. M., and Klaenhammer, T. R. (1991a). Cloning, phenotypic expression, and DNA sequence of the gene for lactacin F, an antimicrobial peptide produced by *Lactobacillus* spp. *Journal of Bacteriology* 173(5): 1779–1788.

Muriana, P. M., and Klaenhammer, T. R. (1991b). Purification and partial characterization of lactacin F, a bacteriocin produced by *Lactobacillus acidophilus* 11088. *Applied Environmental Microbiology* 57(1): 114–121.

Murley, Y. M., Edlind, T. D., Plett, P. A., and LiPuma, J. J. (1998). Cloning of the haemocin locus of *Haemophilus influenzae* type b and assessment of the role of haemocin in virulence. *Microbiology* 144: 2531–2538.

Murley, Y. M., Edlind, T. D., Pozsgay, J. M., and LiPuma, J. J. (1997). Cloning and characterization of the haemocin immunity gene of *Haemophilus influenzae*. *Journal of Bacteriology* 179(5): 1684–1689.

Mørtvedt, C. I., and Nes, I. F. (1990). Plasmid-associated bacteriocin production by a *Lactobacillus sake* strain. *Journal of General Microbiology* 136: 1601–1607.

Navaratna, M. A., Sahl, H. G., and Tagg, J. R. (1998). Two-component anti-*Staphylococcus aureus* lantibiotic activity produced by *Staphylococcus aureus* C55. *Applied Environmental Microbiology* 64(12): 4803–4808.

Navaratna, M. A., Sahl, H. G., and Tagg, J. R. (1999). Identification of genes encoding two-component lantibiotic production in *Staphylococcus aureus* C55 and other phage group II S. aureus strains and demonstration of an association with the exfoliative toxin B gene. *Infection and Immunity* 67(8): 4268–4271.

Neis, S., Bierbaum, G., Josten, M., Pag, U., Kempter, C., Jung, G., and Sahl, H.-G. (1997). Effect of leader peptide mutations on biosynthesis of the lantibiotic Pep5. *FEMS Microbiology Letters* 149: 249–255.

Nes, I. F., Diep, D. B., Håvarstein, L. S., Brurberg, M. B., Eijsink, V., and Holo, H. (1996). Biosynthesis of bacteriocins in lactic acid bacteria. *Antonie van Leeuwenhoek* 70: 113–128.

Nes, I. F., Havarstein, L. S., and Holo, H. (1995). Genetics of non-lantibiotic bacteriocins. *Developments in Biological Standardization* 85: 645–651.

Nieto Lozano, J. C., Meyer, J. N., Sletten, K., Pelaz, C., and Nes, I. F. (1992). Purification and amino acid sequence of a bacteriocin produced by *Pediococcus acidilactici*. *Journal of General Microbiology* 138(Pt 9): 1985–1990.

Nilsen, T., Nes, I. F., and Holo, H. (1998). An exported inducer peptide regulates bacteriocin production in *Enterococcus faecium* CTC492. *Journal of Bacteriology* 180(7): 1848–1854.

Nilsen, T., Nes, I. F., and Holo, H. (2002). Enterolysin A, a Novel Cell Wall Degrading Bacteriocin Secreted From *Enterococcus faecalis* LMG 2333. *Manuscript in preparation.*

Ninfa, E. G., Atkinson, M. R., Kamberov, E. S., and Ninfa, A. J. (1993). Mechanism of autophosphorylation of *Escherichia coli* nitrogen regulator II (NRII or NtrB): Trans-phosphorylation between subunits. *Journal of Bacteriology* 175(21): 7024–7032.

Nissen-Meyer, J., Holo, H., Håvarsyein, L. S., Sletten, K., and Nes, I. F. (1992). A novel bacteriocin whose activity depends on the complementary action of two peptides. *Journal of Bacteriology* 174(17): 5686–5692.

Nissen-Meyer, J., Håvarstein, L. S., Holo, H., and Nes, I. F. (1993). Association of the lactococcin A immunity factor with the cell membrane: Purification and characterization of the immunity factor. *Journal of General Microbiology* 139: 1503–1509.

Nissen-Meyer, J., and Nes, I. F. (1997). Ribosomally synthesized antimicrobial peptides: their function, structure, biogenesis, and mechanism of action. *Archives of Microbiology* 167(2–3): 67–77.

O'Keeffe, T., Hill, C., and Ross, R. P. (1999). Characterization and heterologous expression of the genes encoding enterocin a production, immunity, and regulation in Enterococcus faecium DPC1146. *Applied Environmental Microbiology* 65(4): 1506–1515.

Otto, M., Peschel, A., and Gotz, F. (1998). Producer self-protection against the lantibiotic epidermin by the ABC transporter EpiFEG of *Staphylococcus epidermidis* Tu3298. *FEMS Microbiology Letters* 166(2): 203–211.

Pag, U., Heidrich, C., Bierbaum, G., and Sahl, H. G. (1999). Molecular analysis of expression of the lantibiotic pep5 immunity phenotype. *Applied Environmental Microbiology* 65(2): 591–598.

Paik, S. H., Chakicherla, A., and Hansen, J. N. (1998). Identification and characterization of the structural and transporter genes for, and the chemical and biological properties of, sublancin 168, a novel lantibiotic produced by *Bacillus subtilis* 168. *J Biol Chem* 273(36): 23134–23142.

Palacios, J., Vignolo, G., Farias, M. E., de Ruiz Holgado, A. P., Oliver, G., and Sesma, F. (1999). Purification and amino acid sequence of lactocin 705, a bacteriocin produced by *Lactobacillus casei* CRL 705. *Microbiol Res* 154(2): 199–204.

Papathanasopoulos, M. A., Dykes, G. A., Revol-Junelles, A. M., Delfour, A., von Holy, A., and Hastings, J. W. (1998). Sequence and structural relationships of leucocins A-, B- and C-TA33a from *Leuconostoc mesenteroides* TA33a. *Microbiology* 144(Pt 5): 1343–1348.

Parkinson, J. S., and Kofoid, E. C. (1992). Communication modules in bacterial signaling proteins. *Annual Review of Genetics* 26: 71–112.

Peschel, A., Augustin, J., Kupke, T., Stevanovic, S., and Götz, F. (1993). Regulation of epidermin biosynthetic genes by EpiQ. *Molecular Microbiology* 9(1): 31–39.

Peschel, A., and Götz, F. (1996). Analysis of the *Staphylococcus epidermidis* genes *epiF*, *-E*, and *-G* involved in epidermin immunity. *Journal of Bacteriology* 178(2): 531–536.

Peschel, A., Schnell, N., Hille, M., Entian, K.-D., and Götz, F. (1997). Secretion of the lantibiotics epidermin and gallidermin: Sequence analysis of the genes gdmT and gdmH, their influence on epidermin production and their regulation by EpiQ. *Molecular and General Genetics* 254: 312–318.

Pestova, E. V., Håvarstein, L. S., and Morrison, D. A. (1996). Regulation of competence for genetic transformation in *Streptococcus pneumoniae* by an auto-induced peptide pheromone and a two-component regulatory system. *Molecular Microbiology* 21(4): 853–862.

Piard, J. C., Delorme, C., Novel, M., Desmazeaud, M., and Novel, G. (1993a). Conjugal transfer of the determinants for bacteriocin (lacticin 481) production and immunity in *Lactococcus lactis* subsp. *lactis* CNRZ 481. *FEMS Microbiology Letters* 112(3): 313–318.

Piard, J.-C., Kuipers, O. P., Rollema, H. S., Desmazeaud, M. J., and de Vos, W. M. (1993b). Structure, organization, and expression of the lct gene for lacticin 481, a novel lantibiotic produced by *Lactococcus lactis* CNRZ 481. *J Biol Chem* 268(22): 16361–16368.

Pridmore, D., Rekhif, N., Pittet, A.-C., Suri, B., and Mollet, B. (1996). Variacin, a new lanthionine-containing bacteriocin produced by *Micrococcus varians*: Comparison to lacticin 481 of Lactococcus lactis. *Applied Environmental Microbiology* 62(5): 1799–1802.

Qi, F., Chen, P., and Caufield, P. W. (1999a). Functional analyses of the promoters in the lantibiotic mutacin II biosynthetic locus in *Streptococcus mutans*. *Applied Environmental Microbiology* 65(2): 652–658.

Qi, F., Chen, P., and Caufield, P. W. (1999b). Purification of mutacin III from group III streptococcus mutans UA787 and genetic analyses of mutacin III biosynthesis genes. *Applied Environmental Microbiology* 65(9): 3880–3887.

Quadri, L. E., Kleerebezem, M., Kuipers, O. P., de Vos, W. M., Roy, K. L., Vederas, J. C., and Stiles, M. E. (1997). Characterization of a locus from *Carnobacterium piscicola* LV17B involved in bacteriocin production and immunity: Evidence for global inducer-mediated transcriptional regulation. *Journal of Bacteriology* 179(19): 6163–6171.

Quadri, L. E., Sailer, M., Roy, K. L., Vederas, J. C., and Stiles, M. E. (1994). Chemical and genetic characterization of bacteriocins produced by *Carnobacterium piscicola* LV17B. *J Biol Chem* 269(16): 12204–12211.

Quadri, L. N., Sailer, M., Terebiznik, M. R., Roy, K. L., Vederas, J. C., and Stiles, M. E. (1995). Characterization of the protein conferring immunity to the antimicrobial peptide carnobacteriocin B2 and expression of carnobacteriocins B2 and BM1. *Journal of Bacteriology* 177(5): 1144–1151.

Ra, R., Beerthuyzen, M. M., de Vos, W. M., Saris, P. E., and Kuipers, O. P. (1999). Effects of gene disruptions in the nisin gene cluster of *Lactococcus lactis* on nisin production and producer immunity. *Microbiology* 145(Pt 5): 1227–1233.

Ra, S. R., Qiao, M., Immonen, T., Pujana, I., and Saris, E. J. (1996). Genes responsible for nisin synthesis, regulation and immunity form a regulon of two operons and are induced by nisin in *Lactoccocus lactis* N8. *Microbiology* 142(Pt 5): 1281–1288.

Rauch, P. J., Beerthuyzen, M. M., and de Vos, W. M. (1994). Distribution and evolution of nisin–sucrose elements in *Lactococcus lactis*. *Applied Environmental Microbiology* 60(6): 1798–1804.

Rauch, P. J. G., and de Vos, W. M. (1992). Characterization of the novel nisin–sucrose conjugative transposon Tn5276 and its insertion in *Lactococcus lactis*. *Journal of Bacteriology* 174(4): 1280–1287.

Rawlinson, E. L. A., Nes, I. F., and Skaugen, M. (2002). LasX, a transcriptional activator of the lactocin S biosynthetic genes in *Lactobacillus sakei* L45, acts both as an activator and a repressor. *Biochimie* 84: 559–567.

Reis, M., Eschbach-Bludau, M., Iglesias-Wind, M. I., Kupke, T., and Sahl, H. G. (1994). Producer immunity towards the lantibiotic Pep5: Identification of the immunity gene pepI and localization and functional analysis of its gene product. *Applied Environmental Microbiology* 60(8): 2876–2883.

Reis, M., and Sahl, H.-G. (1991). Genetic analysis of the producer self-protection mechanism ("immunity") against Pep5. In: G. Jung and H. G. Sahl (Eds.), *Nisin and novel lantibiotics* (pp. 320–331). Leiden: ESCOM.

Revol-Junelles, A. M., Mathis, R., Krier, F., Fleury, Y., Delfour, A., and Lefebvre, G. (1996). *Leuconostoc mesenteroides* subsp. *mesenteroides* FR52 synthesizes two distinct bacteriocins. *Letters in Applied Microbiology* 23(2): 120–124.

Rince, A., Dufour, A., Le Pogam, S., Thuault, D., Bourgeois, C. M., and Le Pennec, J. P. (1994). Cloning, expression, and nucleotide sequence of genes involved in production of lactococcin DR, a bacteriocin from *Lactococcus lactis* subsp. *lactis*. *Applied Environmental Microbiology* 60(5): 1652–1657.

Rince, A., Dufour, A., Uguen, P., Le Pennec, J. P., and Haras, D. (1997). Characterization of the lacticin 481 operon: The *Lactococcus lactis* genes lctF, lctE, and lctG encode a putative ABC transporter involved in bacteriocin immunity. *Applied Environmental Microbiology* 63(11): 4252–4260.

Risøen, P. A., Håvarstein, L. S., Diep, D. B., and Nes, I. F. (1998). Identification of the DNA-binding sites for two response regulators involved in control of bacteriocin synthesis in *Lactobacillus plantarum* C11. *Molecular and General Genetics* 259: 224–232.

Rodriguez, F., Gaggero, C., and Lavina, M. (1999). The structural gene for microcin H47 encodes a peptide precursor with antibiotic activity. *Antimicrobial Agents and Chemotherapy* 43(9): 2176–2182.

Ross, K. F., Ronson, C. W., and Tagg, J. R. (1993). Isolation and characterization of the lantibiotic salivaricin A and its structural gene salA from *Streptococcus salivarius* 20P3. *Applied Environmental Microbiology* 59(7): 2014–2021.

Ryan, M. P., Jack, R. W., Josten, M., Sahl, H. G., Jung, G., Ross, R. P., and Hill, C. (1999). Extensive post-translational modification, including serine to D-alanine conversion, in the two-component lantibiotic, lacticin 3147. *J Biol Chem* 274(53): 37544–37550.

Sahl, H.-G. (1991). Pore formation by cationic lantibiotics. In: G. Jung and H.-G. Sahl (Eds.), *Nisin and novel lantibiotics* (pp. 347–358). Leiden: ESCOM.

Sahl, H. G. (1994). Gene-encoded antibiotics made in bacteria. *Ciba Found Symp* 186: 27–42.

Sahl, H. G., and Bierbaum, G. (1998). Lantibiotics: biosynthesis and biological activities of uniquely modified peptides from Gram-positive bacteria. *Annu Rev Microbiol* 52: 41–79.

Sashihara, T., Kimura, H., Higuchi, T., Adachi, A., Matsusaki, H., Sonomoto, K., and Ishizaki, A. (2000). A novel lantibiotic, nukacin ISK-1, of *Staphylococcus warneri* ISK-1: Cloning of the structural gene and identification of the structure. *Bioscience, Biotechnology, and Biochemistry* 64(11): 2420–2428.

Saucier, L., Paradkar, A. S., Frost, L. S., Jensen, S. E., and Stiles, M. E. (1997). Transcriptional analysis and regulation of carnobacteriocin production in *Carnobacterium piscicola* LV17. *Gene* 188(2): 271–277.

Saurin, W., Hofnung, M., and Dassa, E. (1999). Getting in or out: Early segregation between importers and exporters in the evolution of ATP-binding cassette (ABC) transporters. *Journal of Molecular Evolution* 48(1): 22–41.

Schnell, N., Entian, K. D., Schneider, U., Gotz, F., Zahner, H., Kellner, R., and Jung, G. (1988). Prepeptide sequence of epidermin, a ribosomally synthesized antibiotic with four sulphide-rings. *Nature* 333(6170): 276–278.

Schnell, N., Entian, K.-D., Götz, F., Hörner, T., Kellner, R., and Jung, G. (1989). Structural gene isolation and prepeptide sequence of gallidermin, a new lanthionine containing antibiotic. *FEMS Microbiology Letters* 58: 263–268.

Segarra, R. A., Booth, M. C., Morales, D. A., Huycke, M. M., and Gilmore, M. S. (1991). Molecular characterization of the *Enterococcus faecalis* cytolysin activator. *Infection and Immunity* 59(4): 1239–1246.

Siegers, K., and Entian, K. D. (1995). Genes involved in immunity to the lantibiotic nisin produced by *Lactococcus lactis* 6F3. *Applied Environmental Microbiology* 61(3): 1082–1089.

Siegers, K., Heinzmann, S., and Entian, K. D. (1996). Biosynthesis of lantibiotic nisin. Posttranslational modification of its prepeptide occurs at a multimeric membrane-associated lanthionine synthetase complex. *J Biol Chem* 271(21): 12294–12301.

Siezen, R. J., Kuipers, O. P., and de Vos, W. M. (1996). Comparison of lantibiotic gene clusters and encoded proteins. *Antonie van Leeuwenhoek* 69(2): 171–184.

Skaugen, M., Abildgaard, C. I. M., and Nes, I. F. (1997). Organization and expression of a gene cluster involved in the biosynthesis of the lantibiotic lactocin S. *Molecular and General Genetics* 253: 674–686.

Skaugen, M., Andersen, E. L., Christie, V. H., and Nes, I. F. (2002). Identification, characterization, and expression of a second, bicistronic, operon involved in the production of lactocin S in *Lactobacillus sakei* L45. *Applied Environmental Microbiology* 68(2): 720–727.

Skaugen, M., and Nes, I. F. (1994). Transposition in *Lactobacillus sake* and its abolition of lactocin S production by insertion of IS*1163*, a new member of the IS*3* family. *Applied Environmental Microbiology* 60(8): 2818–2825.

Skaugen, M., and Nes, I. F. (2000). Transposition in *Lactobacillus sakei*: Inactivation of a second lactocin S operon by the insertion of IS1520, a new member of the IS3 family of insertion sequences. *Microbiology* 146(Pt 5): 1163–1169.

Skaugen, M., Nissen-Meyer, J., Jung, G., Stefanovic, S., Sletten, K., Abildgaard, C. I. M., and Nes, I. F. (1994). *In vivo* conversion of L-Serine to D-Alanine in a ribosomally synthesized polypeptide. *J Biol Chem* 269(44): 27183–27185.

Steen, M. T., Chung, Y. J., and Hansen, J. N. (1991). Characterization of the nisin gene as part of a polycistronic operon in the chromosome of *Lactococcus lactis* ATCC 11454. *Applied Environmental Microbiology* 57(4): 1181–1188.

Stein, T., Borchert, S., Conrad, B., Feesche, J., Hofemeister, B., Hofemeister, J., and Entian, K. D. (2002). Two different lantibiotic-like peptides originate from the ericin gene cluster of *Bacillus subtilis* A1/3. *Journal of Bacteriology* 184(6): 1703–1711.

Stephens, S. K., Floriano, B., Cathcart, D. P., Bayley, S. A., Witt, V. F., Jimenez-Diaz, R., Warner, P. J., and Ruiz-Barba, J. L. (1998). Molecular analysis of the locus responsible for production of plantaricin S, a two-peptide bacteriocin produced by *Lactobacillus plantarum* LPCO10. *Applied Environmental Microbiology* 64(5): 1871–1877.

Stock, A. M., Robinson, V. L., and Goudreau, P. N. (2000). Two-component signal transduction. *Annu Rev Biochem* 69: 183–215.

Stock, A. M., Surette, M. G., Levit, M., and Park, P. (1995). Two-component signal transduction systems: Structure–function relationships and mechanism of catalysis. In: J. A. Hoch and T. J. Silhavy (Eds.), *Two-component signal transduction* (pp. 25–51). Washington, DC: ASM Press.

Stock, J. B., Ninfa, A. J., and Stock, A. M. (1989). Protein phosphorylation and regulation of adaptive responses in bacteria. *Microbiology Review* 53(4): 450–490.

Stock, J. B., Stock, A. M., and Mottonen, J. M. (1990). Signal transduction in bacteria. *Nature* 344(6265): 395–400.

Stoddard, G. W., Petzel, J. P., van Belkum, M. J., Kok, J., and McKay, L. L. (1992). Molecular analysis of the lactococcin A gene cluster from *Lactococcus lactis* subsp. *lactis* biovar. *diacetylactis* WM4. *Applied Environmental Microbiology* 58(6): 1952–1961.

Sulavik, M. C., Tardif, G., and Clewell, D. B. (1992). Identification of a gene, rgg, which regulates expression of glucosyltransferase and influences the Spp phenotype of *Streptococcus gordonii* challis. *Journal of Bacteriology* 174(11): 3577–3586.

Sulavik, M. S., and Clewell, D. B. (1996). Rgg is a positive transcriptional regulator of the *Streptococcus gordonii* gtfG gene. *Journal of Bacteriology* 178(19): 5826–5830.

Swanson, R. V., Schuster, S. C., and Simon, M. I. (1993). Expression of CheA fragments which define domains encoding kinase, phosphotransfer, and CheY binding activities. *Biochemistry* 32(30): 7623–7629.

Tahara, T., Yoshioka, S., Utsumi, R., and Kanatani, K. (1997). Isolation and partial characterization of bacteriocins produced by *Lactobacillus gasseri* JCM 2124. *FEMS Microbiology Letters* 148(1): 97–100.
Tichaczek, P. S., Vogel, R. F., and Hammes, W. P. (1993). Cloning and sequencing of curA encoding curvacin A, the bacteriocin produced by *Lactobacillus curvatus* LTH1174. *Archives of Microbiology* 160(4): 279–283.
Tichaczek, P. S., Vogel, R. F., and Hammes, W. P. (1994). Cloning and sequencing of sakP encoding sakacin P, the bacteriocin produced by *Lactobacillus sake* LTH 673. *Microbiology* 140(Pt 2): 361–367.
Tomita, H., Fujimoto, S., Tanimoto, K., and Ike, Y. (1996). Cloning and genetic organization of the bacteriocin 31 determinant encoded on the *Enterococcus faecalis* pheromone-responsive conjugative plasmid pYI17. *Journal of Bacteriology* 178(12): 3585–3593.
van Belkum, M. J., Hayema, B. J., Jeeninga, R. E., Kok, J., and Venema, G. (1991). Organization and nucleotide sequences of two lactococcal bacteriocin operons. *Applied Environmental Microbiology* 57(2): 492–498.
van Belkum, M. J., Kok, J., and Venema, G. (1992). Cloning, sequencing, and expression in *Escherichia coli* of lcnB, a third bacteriocin determinant from the lactococcal bacteriocin plasmid p9B4-6. *Applied Environmental Microbiology* 58(2): 572–577.
van Belkum, M. J., Worobo, R. W., and Stiles, M. E. (1997). Double-glycine-type leader peptides direct secretion of bacteriocins by ABC transporters: Colicin V secretion in *Lactococcus lactis*. *Molecular Microbiology* 23(6): 1293–1301.
van de Kamp, M., van den Hooven, H. W., Konings, R. N. H., Bierbaum, G., Sahl, H.-G., Kuipers, O. P., Siezen, R. J., de Vos, W. M., Hilbers, C. W., and van de Ven, F. J. M. (1995). Elucidation of the primary structure of the lantibiotic epilancin K7 from *Staphylococcus epidermidis* K7. Cloning and characterization of the epilancin-K7-encoding gene and NMR analysis of mature epilancin K7. *European Journal of Biochemistry* 230: 587–600.
van den Hooven, H. W., Rollema, H. S., Siezen, R. J., Hilbers, C. W., and Kuipers, O. P. (1997). Structural features of the final intermediate in the biosynthesis of the lantibiotic nisin. Influence of the leader peptide. *Biochemistry* 36(46): 14137–14145.
van der Meer, J. R., Polman, J., Beerthuyzen, M. M., Siezen, R. J., Kuipers, O. P., and de Vos, W. M. (1993). Characterization of the *Lactococcus lactis* nisin A operon Genes nisP, encoding a subtilisin-like derine protease involved in prescursor processing, and nisR, encoding a regulatory protein involved in nisin biosynthesis. *Journal of Bacteriology* 175(9): 2578–2588.
van der Meer, J. R., Rollema, H. S., Siezen, R. J., Beerthuyzen, M. M., Kuipers, O. P., and de Vos, W. M. (1994). Influence of amino acid substitutions in the nisin leader peptide on biosynthesis and secretion of nisin by *Lactococcus lactis*. *J Biol Chem* 269(5): 3555–3562.
van der Vossen, J. M. B. M., van der Lelie, D., and Venema, G. (1987). Isolation and characterization of *Streptococcus cremoris* Wg2-specific promoters. *Applied Environmental Microbiology* 53(10): 2452–2457.
Venema, K., Dost, M. H. R., Beun, P. A. H., Haandrikman, A. J., Venema, G., and Kok, J. (1996). The genes for secretion and maturation of lactococcins are located on the chromosome of *Lactococcus lactis* IL1403. *Applied Environmental Microbiology* 62(5): 1689–1692.
Venema, K., Kok, J., Marugg, J. D., Toonen, M. Y., Ledeboer, A. M., Venema, G., and Chikindas, M. L. (1995a). Functional analysis of the pediocin operon of *Pediococcus acidilactici* PAC1.0: PedB is the immunity protein and PedD is the precursor processing enzyme. *Molecular Microbiology* 17(3): 515–522.
Venema, K., Venema, G., and Kok, J. (1995b). Lactococcal bacteriocins: Mode of action and immunity. *Trends in Microbiology* 3(8): 299–304.
Ward, D. J., and Somkuti, G. A. (1995). Characterization of a bacteriocin produced by *Streptococcus thermophilus* ST134. *Applied Microbiology and Biotechnology* 43(2): 330–335.
Whitford, M. F., McPherson, M. A., Forster, R. J., and Teather, R. M. (2001). Identification of bacteriocin-like inhibitors from rumen *Streptococcus* spp. and isolation and characterization of bovicin 255. *Applied Environmental Microbiology* 67(2): 569–574.
Wolfe, A. J., and Stewart, R. C. (1993). The short form of the CheA protein restores kinase activity and chemotactic ability to kinase-deficient mutants. *Proceedings of the National Academy of Sciences of the United States of America* 90(4): 1518–1522.
Wood, H. E., Devine, K. M., and McConnell, D. J. (1990). Characterisation of a repressor gene (xre) and a temperature-sensitive allele from the *Bacillus subtilis* prophage, PBSX. *Gene* 96(1): 83–88.
Woodruff, W. A., Novak, J., and Caufield, P. W. (1998). Sequence analysis of *mutA* and *mutM* genes involved in the biosynthesis of the lantibiotic mutacin II in *Streptococcus mutans*. *Gene* 206: 37–43.
Worobo, R. W., Henkel, T., Sailer, M., Roy, K. L., Vederas, J. C., and Stiles, M. E. (1994). Characteristics and genetic determinant of a hydrophobic peptide bacteriocin, carnobacteriocin A, produced by *Carnobacterium piscicola* LV17A. *Microbiology* 140(Pt 3): 517–526.

Worobo, R. W., Van Belkum, M. J., Sailer, M., Roy, K. L., Vederas, J. C., and Stiles, M. E. (1995). A signal peptide secretion-dependent bacteriocin from *Carnobacterium divergens*. *Journal of Bacteriology* 177(11): 3143–3149.

Yildirim, Z., Winters, D. K., and Johnson, M. G. (1999). Purification, amino acid sequence and mode of action of bifidocin B produced by *Bifidobacterium bifidum* NCFB 1454. *Journal of Applied Microbiology* 86(1): 45–54.

9

Lactic Acid Bacteria as Mucosal Delivery Vehicles

Jerry M. Wells and Annick Mercenier

Introduction

The development of effective strategies for the delivery of vaccine antigens to the mucosal tissues has received considerable attention over the past decade (reviewed in Michalek et al., 1994; O'Hagan, 1994; Wells and Pozzi, 1997). The main advantage of this route of administration is that it has the potential to elicit local immune responses leading to the production of antigen-specific secretory immunoglobulin A (sIgA) as well as systemic immune responses. Other advantages include low cost, ease of administration and minimization of adverse effects.

Moreover, delivery systems that direct cytokines, enzymes and other biologically active molecules to the mucosal tissues are also needed to elicit potent local effects and avoid any deleterious effects of systemic administration.

This chapter provides an overview of the physiology and functioning of the mucosal immune system and reviews the approaches taken to develop harmless lactic acid bacteria (LAB) as mucosal delivery vehicles.

Mucosal Surfaces and the Mucosal Immune System

The mucosal surfaces of the airways, gastrointestinal (GI), and urogenital tracts of humans are estimated to have a surface area of about 400 m^2, an area almost the same size as two tennis courts (Brandtzaeg et al., 1999). The epithelium of the GI tract plays an essential role in the absorption of nutrients and constitutes an effective barrier to the luminal contents. This huge epithelial surface is permanently challenged by exogenous

Jerry M. Wells • Head of Bacterial Infection and Immunology, Institute of Food Research, Norwich Research Park, Norwich, UK, NR4 7UA; e-mail jerry.wells@bbsrc.ac.uk **Annick Mercenier** • Head of Department, Microbiology of Ecosystems, Institut Pasteur de Lille, 1, rue du Prof Calmette, BP245, 59019 Lille Cedex, France, Current address: Nestlé Research Centre, CH-1000 Lausanne 26, Switzerland; e-mail: annick.mercenier@rdls.nestle.com

substances, including numerous pathogenic microorganisms that initiate infection at specific mucosal niches. The highly complex intestinal ecosystem contains about 1×10^{14} bacteria belonging to hundreds of different species, although certain commensal species predominate (Moore and Holdeman, 1974). The endogenous microflora corresponds to one of the mechanisms that help to prevent colonization and invasion of the mucosal epithelium by pathogenic bacteria. The main protective effect is thought to be mediated by competitive exclusion and this is a key characteristic attributed to specific probiotic organisms. Specialized cells in the epithelium also produce thick layers of mucins that cover the generalized epithelium. Mucus limits direct access of luminal bacteria to the epithelium and promotes their removal through the peristaltic action of the intestinal tract. In addition, protection includes other non-specific defense mechanisms such as the rapid turnover of epithelial cells, and the acid and proteolytic nature of the environment play an important role as well. However, the main mechanism of protection at the mucosal surface is mediated by the secretion of locally formed immunologobulin A (IgA) across the epithelium and into the lumen. An average adult weighing 70 kg is estimated to produce about 4.5 g of sIgA (for a review, see Lamm, 1997) per day, representing approximately 60% of the total amount of immunoglobulin produced by the body in this period (Conley and Delacroix, 1987; Mestecky and McGhee, 1987). The local production of sIgA plays a key role in protection against infection by neutralizing viral infectivity and by preventing bacterial adherence (Taylor and Dimmock, 1985; Winner et al., 1991; Michetti et al., 1992). SIgA are also able to bind toxins, antigens and microorganisms in the lumen and prevent their contact with the mucosal epithelium (Kilian et al., 1988). In addition, recent studies have shown that IgA can neutralize viruses intra-cellularly during transport of IgA through epithelial cells (Mazanec et al., 1992).

The immunological events leading to the production of sIgA are initiated at so-called inductive sites in the mucosal epithelium, also commonly referred to as mucosal associated lymphoid tissue (MALT). The inductive sites in the GI tract are referred to as the gastrointestinal associated lymphoid tissue (GALT) and those in the bronchial and nasopharyngeal mucosa are named BALT and NALT, respectively. The MALT is centered on lymphoid follicles and aggregates of these follicles form the linguinal tonsils, adenoids in the nasopharynx, and the Peyer's patches (PPs) in the small intestine (Figure 9.1).

The PP is considered to be a good model for the physiology and function of the MALT and is common to many mammals. Indeed, most of our knowledge concerning the physiology and function of the mucosal immune system has come from studies of the PPs. They are aggregates of lymphoid follicles found in the submucosa of the small bowel (ileum) and colon. A PP typically contains numerous lymphoid follicles (around 100 in humans) and is covered by a specialized mucosal epithelial layer called the follicle-associated epithelium (FAE). The FAE contains microfold cells (M cells) interdigitating with adjacent enterocytes that serve as a gateway to the underlying immune system (Hathaway and Kraehenbuhl, 2000; Nicoletti, 2000). M cells are relatively devoid of lysosomes and, thus, substances taken up into vesicles by M cells are not degraded but instead are transported through the cell to the basolateral membrane. The basolateral membrane of M cells is often invaginated and in close proximity to lymphoid cells, so substances released by M cells will immediately contact B cells or professional antigen presenting cells (APCs) (Figure 9.2). Evidence that M cells can express MHC class II molecules and participate in signaling to lymphocytes by releasing IL-1, suggested that they might play an active role in the induction of mucosal immune responses in addition to transporting antigens across the lumen (Allan et al., 1993; Finzi et al., 1993; Pappo and Mahlman, 1993).

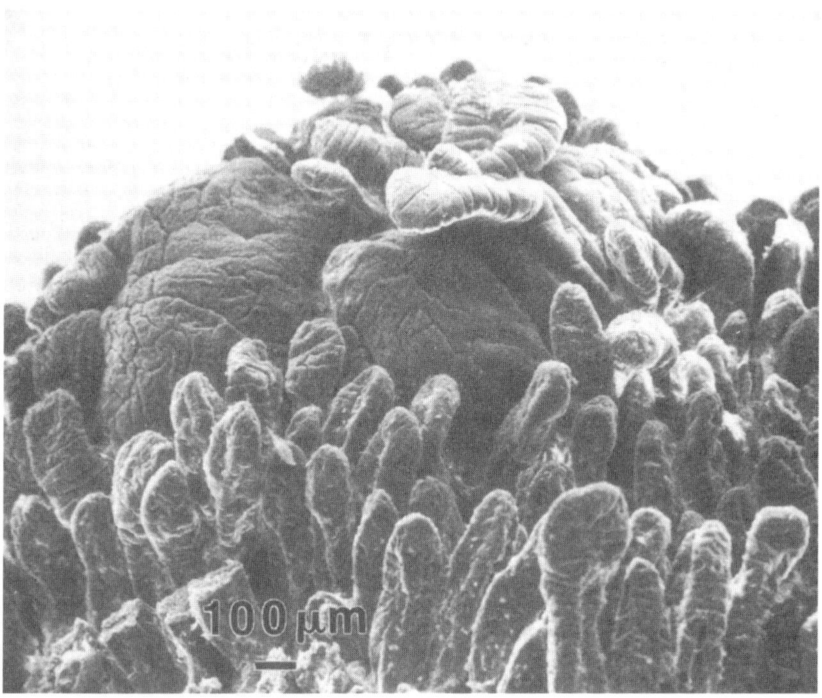

Figure 9.1A Scanning EM of Peyer's patch (PP) in the human small intestine. The dome shaped lymphoid nodule of the PP is seen among the villi of the intestinal epithelium. From *Gastroenterology* 66: 189–203, R.L. Owen, et al. "Epithelial Cell Specialization..." © 1974 American Gastroenterology Association.

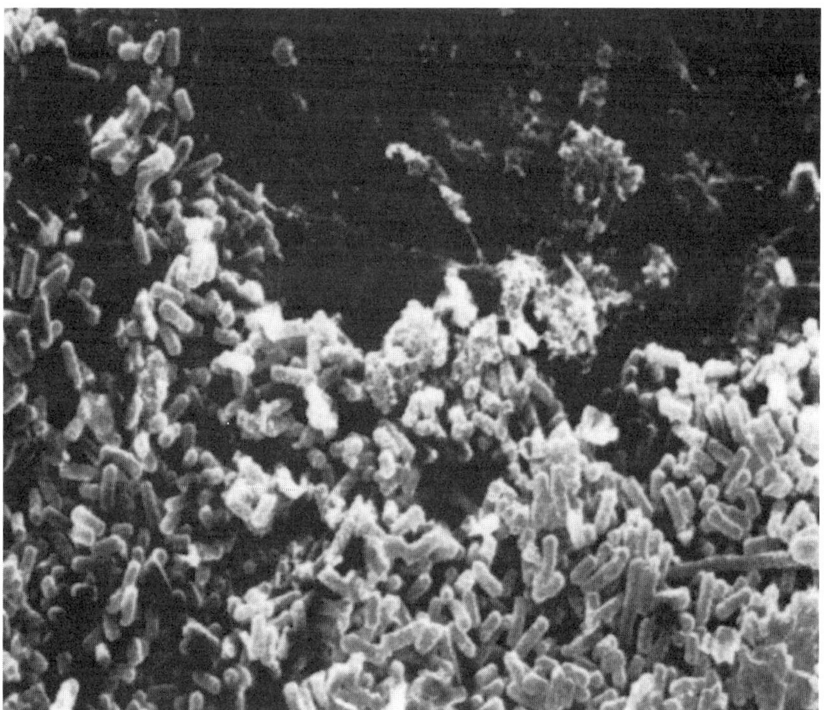

Figure 9.1B *L. fermentum* KLD cells associated with Peyer's patch tissue following a 20 minute incubation *in vitro*. There is decreased coverage of the Peyer's patch dome. Bar represents 10 μm. Image courtesy of L. Plant, University of New South Wales, Australia.

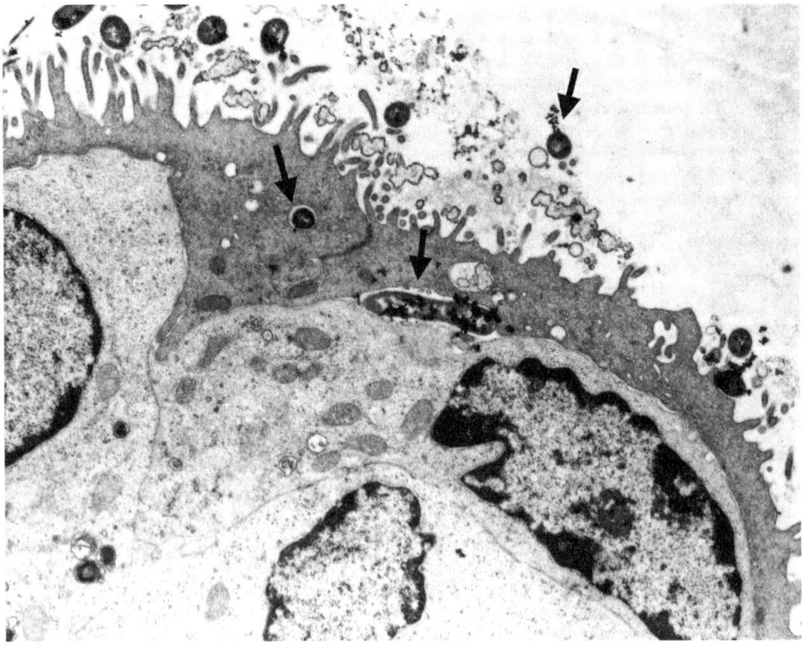

Figure 9.2 Uptake of tritium labelled *Vibrio cholerae* by rabbit M cells in the FAE covering the PP. Arrows indicate *Vibrios* in the extracellular lumen, inside vesicles within the M cell and at the basolateral membrane where they contact lymphocytes in the underlying lymphoid nodule.

For these reasons there has been considerable interest in presenting antigens to the mucosal immune system in association with substances taken up by M cells and in identifying receptors on M cells that could be used to target vaccines.

M cell mediated epithelial transport is naturally exploited by certain viruses and bacteria to gain entry into the body. *Salmonella*, for example, can bind to M cells and thereby gain entry to the MALT where they can invade and replicate inside macrophages (Jones et al., 1994).

Studies of cell populations in lymphoid follicles have shown that they contain B cells (IgM and IgD positive), CD4 + T "helper" cells, CD8 + T "cytotoxic" cells, and APCs such as macrophages and dendritic cells. It is thought that it is here in the lymphoid associated follicles that the immune response is initiated and that primed lymphoid cells are then disseminated around the body via the efferent lymphatics and bloodstream. Antigens transported by M cells can also enter the bloodstream via the draining lymphatics and thus encounter the lymphoid cells associated with the systemic immune system. Thus, mucosal transport of antigens can efficiently stimulate both the mucosal and systemic arms of the immune system. This is in contrast to administration of antigens by injection, where the mucosal immune system is generally inefficiently stimulated unless the site of injection is close to the draining lymphatic ducts of the MALT. Several studies have shown that mucosally derived lymphoid cells carry specific addressins that result in lymphocytes homing to the *lamina propria*, a region of connective tissue lying between the mucosal epithelium and *muscularis mucosa* (Stoolman, 1989; McGhee et al., 1992). The mechanism of lymphocyte homing supports the hypothesis that there is a common mucosal immune system that enables induction of an immune response at one site (e.g., GALT) to result in IgA production at distal mucosal surfaces. Some recent studies have indicated, however, that there may be further compartmentalization of the mucosal immune system and the specificity of lymphocyte homing may account for these observations (Bergmann and Waldman, 1988; Stoolman, 1989; Kantele et al., 1998).

The maturation of B cells to form polymeric IgA secreting plasma cells is thought to take place in the *lamina propria*. Polymeric IgA is transported across the epithelium via the polymeric IgA receptor in the basal membrane of the epithelial cells, and released into the lumen bound to the secretory component (Mestecky and McGhee, 1987; McGhee et al., 1992), thus, generating the so-called sIgA. Due to its structure, sIgA is more resistant than other forms of immunoglobulin to proteolytic degradation in the luminal milieu (Lamm, 1997).

It is well established that the mucosal immune system is relatively unresponsive to soluble proteins, presumably because responses to dietary antigens are not needed and in certain situations might indeed be detrimental. Immune responses to commensal bacteria are also relatively low or transient (Wold et al., 1989) but the exact mechanisms that enable the mucosal immune system to distinguish between pathogenic and commensal microorganisms are still poorly understood (see MacPherson et al., 2000). This topic is discussed further in Section 5 and detailed reviews of the literature can be found elsewhere (Autenrieth and Schmidt, 2000; Nagler-Anderson, 2000).

Bacterial Delivery Systems

Over the past decade a number of strategies for delivering antigens to the mucosal immune system have been investigated (Table 9.1). Among those, the use of recombinant bacteria as carrier systems has received particular attention, most vectors under development being derived from attenuated pathogenic bacteria such as *Salmonella, Listeria monocytogenes, Vibrio cholerae, Bordetella pertussis, Mycobacterium bovis* BCG, and so on (Michalek et al., 1994; Roberts et al., 1994; Giquel, 1995; Stahl et al., 1997; Locht, 2000). There is a huge body of literature on the use of attenuated *Salmonella* spp. as carriers for orally administered vaccines (recently reviewed in Levine et al., 1996; Sirard et al., 1999; Bumann et al., 2000). It has been conclusively shown that oral immunization with recombinant *Salmonella* can elicit IgA in mucosal secretions as well as serum antibodies to a variety of vaccine antigens from diverse sources. For this invasive pathogen, it is considered important to combine attenuating mutations at different loci in a single strain so as to decrease the chance of reversion by gene exchange and recombination. A full description of the development of attenuated *Salmonella* vaccine carriers can be found

Table 9.1. Delivery Systems for Mucosal Immunization

Liposomes
ISCOMS
Microparticles
Lectins
Cholera-toxin B subunit
Attenuated bacterial carriers (e.g., *Salmonella, Vibrio, Listeria, Bordetella*)
Non-pathogenic bacterial vectors (e.g., *Lactococcus lactis* and *Lactobacillus* spp.)
Attenuated viruses

elsewhere (Roberts et al., 1994). The great variation in the immunogenicity of the different attenuated strains has constituted a major problem since the generation of the initial mutants and it has indeed been difficult to reach the right balance between the level of attenuation (i.e., lack of disease symptoms) and immunogenicity (i.e., efficacy). Notably, the virulence of *S. typhi* mutant strains in humans could hardly be predicted with accuracy from the studies with *S. typhimurium* in a murine typhoid model. To date a limited combination of attenuating mutations have been found to be acceptable for use in human volunteers, but further improvements are required to increase the immunogenicity of heterologous antigens expressed in these *S. typhi* mutants (Bumann et al., 2000). The ultimate goal remains to produce a live vaccine that will elicit long-lived protective level immune responses against typhoid fever in adults after a single oral dose.

One major concern with the use of attenuated pathogens is that they may still be sufficiently virulent to cause disease in infants, the elderly, or partially immunocompromised individuals. In addition, immune responses against the bacterial vector itself can potentially interfere with efficient vaccination. For these reasons, attention has recently been given to the use of harmless commensal and food bacteria as delivery vehicles.

Lactic Acid Bacteria as Mucosal Delivery Vehicles

The choice of LAB as vaccine delivery vehicles is mainly based on the concept that they could be given orally in relatively large doses because of their non-pathogenic status. Indeed *Lactococcus lactis* and many species of *Lactobacillus* have a long history of safe consumption because of their use in food fermentation and preservation and they have a "generally regarded as safe" (GRAS) status within the food industry (Adams and Marteau, 1995). Certain species of the *Lactobacillus* genus are able to colonize the mucosal surfaces of the mouth, urogenital, and GI tracts of humans and animals, where they are thought to play a crucial role in maintaining a healthy microflora. The probiotic properties of certain strains of *Lactobacillus* species has been the basis of their use for lowering the incidence of urinary or digestive tract infections (Salminen et al., 1996; Guarner and Schaafsma, 1998; Reid, 2000). There are, however, a small number of reported cases of infections with dietary LAB but these have only occurred in severely immunocompromised individuals (Aguirre and Collins, 1993).

LAB offer additional advantages as potential mucosal delivery systems; the cell wall of these Gram-positive bacteria is devoid of lipopolysaccharide (LPS); most strains are quite acid resistant thus being well adapted to oral delivery; extensive fermentation know-how has been developed for these bacteria and the genetics of LAB has progressed considerably during the last two decades, so facilitating the construction of recombinant strains producing heterologous molecules. The use of LAB would, in addition, obviate the need to purify an antigen, thus reducing the cost of the vaccine.

The LAB are a diverse group of bacteria and the selection of model species and strains has been a critical step in the development of these bacteria as oral delivery vehicles. At the outset there were no indications of whether or not persisting/colonizing *Lactobacillus* or *Streptococcus* strains would be more efficiently recognized by the mucosal immune system than a non-colonizing bacterium such as *Lc. lactis*. It was anticipated that different species and strains of bacteria would also have inherently different characteristics as delivery systems, depending on factors such as their immunomodulatory properties, and the immune status of the host toward the carrier itself. In the past several years, a significant body of literature has now emerged on the use of LAB derived vaccines, largely as a consequence of the co-ordinated effort of several European laboratories and funding from the European Commission in two successive research networks (contracts BIO2-CT94-3055 and BIO4-CT96-0542; see Mercenier et al., 2000). Our current knowledge of the characteristics and properties of the three LAB systems being developed as mucosal delivery vehicles is summarized in the following sections.

Lactococcus lactis as Delivery Vehicle

Lc. lactis is a Gram-positive coccus (approx. 1 μm in diameter) that is widely used to produce cheese curds by the fermentation of milk. *Lc. lactis* is naturally auxotrophic for several amino acids and its natural environment is in milk and on the surfaces of plants and animals in the dairy environment.

Oral feeding experiments have indicated that *Lc. lactis* persists for less than 24 hr in the intestine of conventional mice. In contrast, this bacterium can colonize the digestive tract of germ-free mice (Gruzza et al., 1992), but the introduction of other microorganisms results in selective elimination of *Lc. lactis* (Gruzza et al., 1994). Studies involving the administration of recombinant *Lc. lactis* marked with the *gfp* fluorescent reporter gene to rats have shown that although lactococci are highly resistant to gastric acidity (90–98% survival) when included in feed, only 10–30% of the bacteria survived in the duodenum (Drouault et al., 1999). Using strains marked with a luciferase reporter gene (*luxA-luxB* of *Vibrio harveyi*) these authors demonstrated that metabolically active lactococci were nevertheless present in each compartment of the GI tract (Drouault et al., 1999). Similar experiments in mice with fluorescein isothiocyanate (FITC) labeled lactococci have shown that a proportion of the inoculum passes intact through the intestinal tract (Schofield, K., Lopez, M., and Wells, J. M., 1999, University of Cambridge, unpublished).

In Figure 9.3, fluorescently labeled lactococci can be seen in close proximity to the epithelium in the small bowel where antigens may be taken up across the PPs.

A limited number of experiments have analyzed the transit properties of *Lc. lactis* in humans. It was shown that after feeding healthy volunteers with 1×10^{11} c.f.u. on four consecutive days, only a small proportion of the original bacterial dose was recovered as viable organisms from the feces. A unique marker in the strain was followed by PCR and could be detected in the feces no longer than four days after cessation of feeding, indicating that the passage through the gut was only transient and actually similar to that of *Bacillus* spores used as passive transit markers (Klijn et al., 1995). More recently, Vesa et al. (2000) reported that *Lc. lactis* MG1363 was much more sensitive to the harsh conditions of the upper digestive tract than certain lactobacilli were. In view of its short persistence in the GI tract, *Lc. lactis* is expected to have only a limited capacity to replicate *in vivo* and, thus, to deliver antigens by secretion. As a consequence, attention has focused mainly on expressing antigens intra-cellularly in this bacterial vector, which might be considered as antigen synthesizing particles of the size taken up by M cells.

Lc. lactis can be efficiently transformed with recombinant DNA (Wells et al., 1993a) and genetic tools for expression in *Lc. lactis* are relatively well advanced (recently reviewed in de Vos, 1999). Both high level inducible and constitutive expression systems are available for production of antigens. Amongst others, a regulatable expression system based on nisin inducible activation of the *nisA* promoter has been widely used for the high level synthesis of heterologous proteins in this host. An alternative expression system has also been developed that utilizes the lactococcal lactose inducible lac promoter to regulate expression of T7 RNA polymerase. The nisin inducible system is more tightly regulated

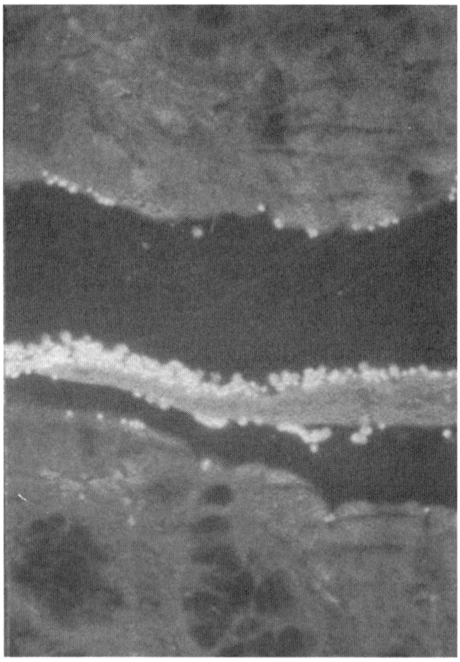

Figure 9.3 Fluorescently labelled *Lc. lactis* in contact with mucosal epithelium. Source: Schofield, K., Lopez, M., and Wells, J.M., 1999, University of Cambridge, U.K.

than the lactococcal T7 one and is therefore more suitable for the expression of genes that might have toxic effects or slow the normal growth of *Lc. lactis*. In addition, a series of constitutive expression vectors have been used extensively for the vaccine studies conducted by Wells et al. (1995); Robinson et al. (1997) and Steidler et al. (1998). The pTREX1 derivatives are based on a theta-replicating plasmid and have been found to be more structurally stable cloning vectors than those with a rolling circle replication mechanism. The pTREX1-derived vectors are also able to accommodate large inserts and are especially useful for the expression of operons (Wells and Schofield, 1996; Chamberlain et al., 1997).

Lactobacillus as a Delivery Vehicle

This genus is remarkably diverse and contains over 60 different species that differ widely in G + C content (G + C, 32–52%), metabolism, phenotypic properties, and distribution in nature. Some species are used for the preparation of fermented milk (e.g., yogurt, cheeses), vegetable, and meat products, while others are being developed for probiotic (e.g., health-promoting) applications. To date much attention has been focused on the commensal species of *Lactobacillus* that populate specific mucosal niches of humans and animals. Lactobacilli that have the capacity to persist in the body cavities have been viewed as health beneficial due to their competitive exclusion of harmful bacteria and additional properties such as stimulation or modulation of the immune system of the host (see below). It has been established that several *Lactobacillus* species or strains differ in their capacity to influence levels of various cytokines produced upon *in vitro* stimulation of human peripheral blood cells (Miettinen et al., 1998; Hessle et al., 1999; Müller-Alouf

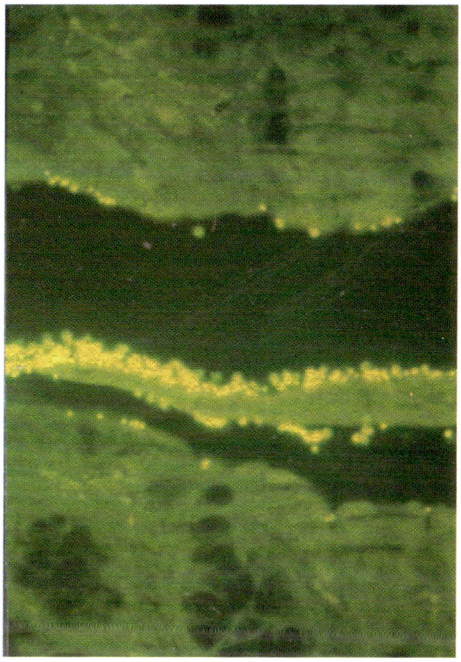

Figure 9.3 Fluorescently labelled *Lc. lactis* in contact with mucosal epithelium. Source: Schofield, K., Lopez, M., and Wells, J.M., 1999, University of Cambridge, U.K.

et al., 1999). These observations have recently been extended to *in vivo* analysis: seven *Lactobacillus* spp. were shown to induce a strain-dependent production of cytokine profiles in the gut of mice after oral administration. This aspect might have to be taken into account when selecting *Lactobacillus* strains for delivery of vaccines or induction of tolerance (Maassen et al., 2000).

In animal studies *Lb. casei* (ATCC 393), *Lb. paracasei* (LbTGS1.4; murine vaginal isolate), *Lb. fermentum* (KLD, human isolate), and *Lb. plantarum* (NCIMB 8826; human saliva isolate) have been found to persist in the GI tract and vagina of mice for over a week. The *Lb. plantarum* strain generally persisted somewhat longer than the three other lactobacilli, the transit time being in any case much longer than that observed for *Lc. lactis* (Mercenier et al., 1996).

A comparison of the survival rate and gut transit time of three non-recombinant chromosomally marked (Rif^R, Sm^R) strains of LAB has been performed in human volunteers. *Lb. fermentum* (strain KLD), *Lb. plantarum* (strain NCIMB 8826), and *Lc. lactis* (strain MG1363) were given orally to human volunteers as 150 g of fermented milk product. To enumerate the different species of bacteria, ileal fluid was aspirated by intestinal intubation. *Lb. plantarum* (7%) survived the stomach better than *Lc. lactis* and *Lb. fermentum* (0.5% and 1%, respectively) and was found in large numbers in the feces during the seven days ingestion period. However, none of the strains colonized the GI tract permanently. The authors considered that *Lb. plantarum* presented a promising survival/persistence profile as a candidate vaccine strain (Vesa et al., 2000). It is noteworthy that the pharmacokinetic profiles of these three strains in humans correlated well with the observations made in mice, which might, in this case at least, provide useful models for a preliminary estimation of the behavior of LAB strains in the GI tract. It should be stressed, however, that there is increasing evidence that colonization of a body cavity by a strain of *Lactobacillus* is both host- and tissue-specific and may also be influenced by environmental factors such as diet and age in experimental animals.

Because of the diversity of the *Lactobacillus* genus, the molecular tools needed to genetically manipulate lactobacilli tend to show a high degree of species and in some cases even strain specificity (Hols et al., 1997; Pouwels et al., 1998). Thus, methods for transformation, plasmids, and sequence elements required for gene expression may need to be specifically adapted to the strain under study (for reviews, see Pouwels and Leer, 1993; Klaenhammer, 1995; Rush et al., 1997; Kullen and Klaenhammer, 1999).

Most of the cloning vectors available for use in *Lactobacillus* have been derived from naturally occurring cryptic plasmids derived from lactobacilli or from *Lc. lactis* vectors containing the pSH71 or pWV01 replicon, most of which have a rolling circle replicative (RCR) mechanism. The broad host range theta-replicating pTREX series of plasmids developed by Wells et al. (1995) and Wells and Schofield (1996) for use in *Lc. lactis* have also been used for heterologous expression in *Lactobacillus* (Mercenier and Wells, unpublished). The pTREX vectors are generally more structurally stable than the RCR type plasmids but their poor segregational stability in the absence of antibiotic selection would be a disadvantage for their use with *Lactobacillus* spp.

Recent improvements to plasmid vectors and gene expression signals have mainly addressed structural stability and levels of heterologous protein expression in *Lactobacillus* spp. (see Pouwels et al., 1996, 1998; Mercenier et al., 2000). Even though strong or medium strength constitutive promoters have mostly been used so far for the production of antigens in lactobacilli (Pouwels et al., 1996, 1998; Hols et al., 1997; Rush et al., 1997; Kullen and Klaenhammer, 1999; Maassen et al., 1999; Grangette et al., 2001), a limited number of regulatable expression systems have also been developed for lactobacilli, such as those based on the α-amylase promoter from *Lb. amylovorus* or the nisin system from *Lc. Lactis* (see Pouwels et al., 1996; Kullen and Klaenhammer, 1999; Pavan et al., 2000). In the latter case it was necessary to integrate the nisin sensor and regulator genes into the chromosome of the *Lactobacillus* host strain. The optimized nisin inducible expression system developed in *Lactobacillus* was used to produce a variety of foreign proteins including the GFP marker (Geoffroy et al., 2000; Pavan et al., 2000). Fluorescent lactobacilli have been used to follow the interaction of bacteria with macrophages and to start analyzing their fate after local administration to mice.

Optimal cellular presentation of the immunogen may vary depending on factors such as its location in the bacteria, the choice of the carrier strain (i.e., persisting or non-persisting) and the fate of the bacterial carrier after administration to mice. Consequently, expression systems have been developed to direct the synthesis of the heterologous proteins to the cytoplasm, the external milieu, or the cell surface. Many expression constructs make use of endogenous secretion and cell wall attachment signals such as the prtP gene from *Lb. casei*, or the M6 system originally developed for *Strep. gordonii* (see section below; Pouwels et al., 1998; Maassen et al., 1999; Mercenier et al., 2000). Successful surface anchoring of the tetanus toxin fragment C has been reported leading to high exposure of the protein (≥1000 molecules per cell) as measured by FACSscan analysis (Maassen et al., 1999; Shaw et al., 2000).

A variety of integration systems are now available for use in *Lactobacillus* spp. that enable foreign genes to be inserted into the chromosome (see Martin et al., 2000; Mercenier et al., 2000). For example, an integration system has been developed that utilizes a non-replicative plasmid as a suicide vector and elements from a temperate bacteriophage to promote integration of the plasmid in the chromosal tRNAser gene without insertional inactivation (Dupont et al., 1995). Similarly Hols et al. (Hols P., Université Catholique de Louvain-la-Neuve, personal communication) have developed integration vectors that will insert either in the tRNAser or in the lactate dehydrogenase (L-ldh) locus of *Lb. plantarum*. Due to the existence of homologous sequences, excisants lacking all vector sequences including the antibiotic resistance marker, can be generated following a second spontaneous recombination event. Both of these systems have been used to construct candidate vaccine strains of *Lb. plantarum* expressing a chromosomally located antigen gene (see Mercenier et al., 2000).

Streptococcus gordonii as a Delivery Vehicle

Streptococcus gordonii, formerly classified as *Strep. sanguis*, is a normal constituent of the human oral cavity (Pozzi and Oggioni, 1994). The Challis strain has been used in several immunization studies and a single dose of 10^9 c.f.u. has been found to colonize the oral and vaginal mucosal cavities but not the GI tract of mice (Mercenier et al., 1996; Medaglini et al., 1997a; Pozzi et al., 1997). The number of mice that are colonized and the percentage of animals that remain colonized over time are dependent on the strain of mouse. For example, after a single oral inoculum of the *Strep. gordoni* Challis strain, 83% of Swiss CD1 mice were still colonized after two months whereas the percentage of colonized Balb/c mice was lower, around 20% (Pozzi et al., 1997). The Challis strain has been shown to colonize the vaginal mucosa of Balb/c mice for approximately 8 weeks with no need for a prior hormonal treatment as was described for lactobacilli (Dutot, 1996). Treatment of mice with antibiotics prior to inoculation does not influence rates of colonization or persistence time (Pozzi G., University of Siena, personal communication) and both recombinant and wild type strains colonize mice with equal efficiency (see e.g., Beninati et al., 2000).

The Challis strain is naturally competent and so homologous recombination and allelic exchange of genetic markers are relatively easier to accomplish in *Strep. gordonii* than in *Lactobacillus* spp. or *Lc. lactis*. The strategy for expressing foreign genes in *Strep. gordonii* is based on chromosomal integration of recombinant DNA. The main advantage of chromosomal integration is that it overcomes the structural or segregational instability observed with some host–vector systems, thus leading to stable *in vivo* expression even in the absence of antibiotic selection. The main drawback to this strategy is that production levels of recombinant protein are often lower than can be achieved with multicopy plasmids. To address this problem, strong chromosomal promoters were identified by random integration of the M6 encoding gene (*emm6*) into the *Strep. gordonii* chromosome. These strains then formed the basis for the development of a series of specially engineered recipient hosts that could serve for chromosomal recombination with DNA fragments carrying *emm6* based gene fusions (Pozzi et al., 1997). In nearly all cases the M protein itself acted both as a fusion partner and to display the recombinant proteins on the cell surface. The signal sequence of M6 is able to direct the recombinant protein into the secretion pathway and the C terminal domain of M6 provides a cell wall anchoring signal that results in attachment of the protein to the peptidoglycan (Pozzi et al., 1997). Removal of the C-terminal anchoring sequence leads to efficient secretion in the external milieu. The resulting integrants were shown to be totally stable *in vivo* and produced the heterologous molecule *in situ*, with no negative impact on their colonization capacity (Beninati et al., 2000). Nevertheless, these recombinant strains still carry genes encoding for antibiotic resistance markers.

Several antigens and epitopes have been displayed on the surface of *Strep. gordonii* using the chromosomal expression systems described above at levels of up to 10,000 molecules per cell (Pozzi et al., 1997; Pozzi, University of Sienna, personal communication). Polypeptide antigens ranging in size from 15 to 441 amino acids in length of viral, bacterial, and eukaryotic origin have been produced using this system. Two different chromosomal expression sites have been used to concomitantly express two different antigens on the cell surface of *Strep. gordonii* (Pozzi et al., 1997).

Recently, the construction of a GFP-tagged *Strep. gordonii* strain has been reported but this fluorescent strain has been used to study biofilm formation *in vitro* and not yet for *in vivo* experiments (Aspiras et al., 2000).

Vaccine Delivery Using Lactic Acid Bacteria

Research aimed at developing LAB as vaccine delivery vehicles was initiated almost a decade ago in several laboratories throughout Europe and included work on both persisting and non-persisting species and strains, that is, *Lc. lactis, Lactobacillus* spp., and *Strep. gordonii*. Studies with other non-pathogenic Gram-positive bacteria (i.e., *Staphylococcus carnosus* or *xylosus*) and attenuated strains of *Listeria monocytogenes* were initiated as well (Nguyen et al., 1993; for reviews, see Stahl et al., 1997; Guzman et al., 1997). LAB research has been supported, among other sources, through two successive research networks funded by the European Commission (contracts BIO2-CT94-3055 and BIO4-CT96-0542) which focused on the use of common antigens (namely, tetanus toxin fragment C and the gp50 protein of Aujeszky's disease virus) and common biological reagents and methods of analysis of immune responses, in order to perform a controlled comparison of the three LAB systems under study (for a review, see Mercenier et al., 2000). The present state of knowledge is summarized below in sections dealing with each delivery system in turn.

Vaccine Delivery Using *Lc. lactis*

Oral administration of *Lc. lactis* to mice or humans results in only a transient passage of the bacteria through the intestinal tract (Klijn et al., 1995). The strategy has therefore been to use the bacteria as self-loading microparticles.

Iwaki et al. (1990) were the first to use the recombinant lactococci as vaccine delivery vehicles. In this report, oral immunization with killed recombinant lactococci expressing surface protein antigens from *Streptococcus mutans* was shown to elevate systemic and local immune responses to the antigen.

To date most immunological studies have been carried out with *Lc. lactis* producing tetanus toxin fragment C (TTFC) as the model antigen. TTFC is a 47 KDa non-toxic polypeptide carrying the ganglioside binding domain of the holotoxin that has been shown to be immunogenic in mice and guinea pigs (Fairweather et al., 1987). Initially, strains of *Lc. lactis* expressing TTFC were shown to be immunogenic by immunizing mice subcutaneously with live bacteria and measuring levels of the TTFC-specific serum antibody (Wells et al., 1993b). These studies were extended to include comparative studies of immunogenicity with strains of *Lc. lactis* expressing TTFC intra-cellularly or on the surface using the cell wall anchoring domain of lactococcal proteinase PrtP as a fusion partner with TTFC (Norton et al., 1995, 1996). Immunization with different numbers of bacteria indicated that the levels of serum antibody elicited to TTFC were dependent on the dose of antigen. Interestingly, the cell surface associated form of TTFC was apparently 10- to 20-fold more immunogenic than alternative forms of the antigen (Norton et al., 1996). Unfortunately, these systems for antigen expression have not yet been compared using the mucosal route of immunization.

Nasal administration of lactococci synthesizing high cytoplasmic levels of TTFC (using pLET1 vector and lactococcal T7 system described above) elicited significant levels of IgG antibody response in the serum (Norton et al., 1997). Mice were inoculated with either 5×10^8 or 5×10^9 c.f.u of expressor or control strains of lactococci on days 1, 7, and 29 with and without 10 μg of cholera toxin as an adjuvant. The mean antibody response elicited by 5×10^8 c.f.u of the TTFC expressor strain of *Lc. lactis* (containing an estimated 6 μg of TTFC) was greater than those induced by inoculation with 10-fold higher amounts (60 μg) of purified recombinant TTFC. The use of cholera toxin (CT) as a mucosal adjuvant significantly enhanced responses to purified recombinant TTFC but not to TTFC delivered in lactococci. The serum antibodies elicited by 5×10^8 or 5×10^9 c.f.u of lactococci were capable of protecting mice from subcutaneous (s.c.) challenge with $20 \times LD_{50}$ of tetanus toxin. The induction of a local mucosal antibody response to TTFC was investigated by the ELISPOT assay that is used to enumerate antigen-specific antibody producing lymphocytes. Nasal inoculation of 5×10^9 c.f.u of TTFC expressing lactococci induced anti-TTFC IgA producing lymphocytes in the lung and nasal mucosa. Interestingly co-administration of CT markedly increased the number of lymphocytes producing IgA antibody to TTFC whereas this had no effect on the level of serum antibody responses to TTFC (Norton et al., 1997).

Further studies were conducted with lactococci constitutively producing TTFC in the cytoplasm at relatively moderate levels (estimated at 1% of total protein; using the pTREX1 vector; Robinson et al., 1997). These strains were shown to elicit protective level serum antibody responses to TTFC by both intra-nasal (i.n.) and oral (intra-gastric) routes of administration. It was also established for the i.n. route of administration that the antibody titers were similar whether the bacteria were given live or killed prior to inoculation with mitomycin C or formalin. A comparison of live versus killed bacteria has not yet been reported for the oral route of immunization. The anti-TTFC specific antibody isotypes comprised both IgG1 and IgG2a subclasses as previously shown for the i.n. route (Norton et al., 1997). Mucosal anti-TTFC specific antibodies were also detected in the feces of the immunized mice. Following i.n. inoculation the fecal IgA response to TTFC increased to high levels on day 35 and 41 post-immunization. In mice orally vaccinated with TTFC expressing lactococci the IgA antibody response was already at a high level by day 15 post-vaccination but fell to the same level as the control groups by day 38. Further studies will be required in order to more accurately determine the magnitude and kinetics of IgA responses induced by recombinant *Lc. lactis*.

Antibody responses to antigens of *Lc. lactis* have also been detected in the serum of mice immunized intra-nasally and orally with recombinant lactococci (Robinson et al., 1997). Anti-lactococcal antibody responses were about 10-fold lower than the TTFC specific responses but nevertheless indicated that a response to the bacterial vector is elicited in immunized mice. T cell proliferation assays with splenocytes from mice immunized with recombinant lactococci have also demonstrated the presence of a cellular response to lactococcal antigens (Dr K. Robinson; University of Cambridge, personal communication). Similar immunization studies with the glutathione S-transferase (P28) antigen of *Schistosoma mansoni* have been described. This antigen was expressed at good levels (estimated 5–10% of total protein) in *Lc. lactis* using the lactococcal T7 system but was found to be less immunogenic than TTFC by both systemic and mucosal routes of immunization (Chamberlain et al., 1997).

The second model antigen studied by the EC LABVAC network was gp50 of Aujesky's Disease Virus (ADV). This virus infects swine through the respiratory tract with young piglets being most susceptible. It had already been shown that the stimulation of mucosal immune responses against the virus was an effective strategy to inhibit virus replication at the primary site of infection and that gp50 was a protective vaccine antigen (Ishii et al., 1988; Mukamoto et al., 1991; Takada et al., 1994). Thus, the LAB were considered potentially good vaccine delivery vehicles for a gp50 subunit vaccine.

The gp50 antigen expressed in *Lc. lactis* lacked the eukaryotic secretion leader and C-terminal transmembrane domain as these were considered likely to interfere with expression in LAB. However, no expression of gp50 was obtained in *Lc. lactis* or *E. coli* and the plasmids constructs were prone to structural instability in both hosts (J. Wells, University of Cambridge, unpublished results). It was hypothesized that the lack of expression or instability of the plasmids constructs might be due to the high G + C content (>70%) of the gp50 gene. Therefore, a synthetic gene with a codon usage adapted for expression in *Lc. lactis* was assembled using a PCR based method of gene synthesis (Stemmer et al., 1995). This antigen was finally expressed at high levels (5%) in *Lc. lactis* (Rush, C. and Wells, J. M., 1998, University of Cambridge, unpublished results) and at moderate levels in *Lb. plantarum* NCIMB8826 (Chagnaud, P., Reveneau, N., and Mercenier, A., Institut Pasteur de Lille, 1999, unpublished results). Both recombinant strains were immunogenic by the systemic route. Moreover, i.n. immunization of mice with gp50 expressing lactococci elicited serum antibodies to gp50 and cellular responses to the native antigen (Rush, C. and Wells, J., University of Cambridge, 2000, unpublished data).

Lc. lactis has also been used to express a type 3 capsular polysaccharide (CPS) from *Strep. pneumoniae* (Gilbert et al., 2000). Only three of the four type 3 CPS biosynthetic genes present in *Strep. pneumoniae* were found to be necessary for the production of 120 mg/L of an extracellular polysaccharide. The type 3 CPS produced by *Lc. lactis* was shown to be structurally identical to that of *Strep. pneumoniae* by nuclear magnetic resonance spectroscopy and immunological analysis. Immunization of mice intraperitoneally with *Lc. lactis* expressing CPS or comparable amounts of purified type 3 CPS from *Strep. pneumoniae* elicited identical immune responses to the capsule. These encouraging results indicate that further investigations into the delivery of recombinant capsule antigens via mucosal routes of administration are warranted.

Vaccine Delivery Using *Lactobacillus* spp.

As compared to *Lc. lactis* and *Strep. gordonii*, the initial choice of a candidate *Lactobacillus* vaccine strain is more complex due to the existence of a diversity of strains which may vary in their persistence, ability to survive *in vivo*, and their intrinsic immunomodulatory properties (Pouwels et al., 1998; Mercenier et al., 2000). As mentioned above, the *Lactobacillus* genus is very broad, including isolates from different origins that probably adapted themselves to specific ecological niches (e.g., fermented foods, silage, humans, animals, etc.). It is generally accepted that the persistence or colonization capacity is host- and tissue- or site-specific. So it might be anticipated that "optimal" vector strains will have to be selected to target different hosts or different mucosal areas in the same host. However, the experiments conducted so far with lactobacilli as antigen delivery systems have been restricted to mice, in which strains of different origins (see Table 9.2) all perform well. The differences observed so far in terms of immunogenicity (see below) seemed to be related mainly to the antigen production level in the recombinant strain and to the capacity of the strain to survive passage through the stomach and/or to reside temporarily in the GI tract. In principle, depending on the characteristics of the candidate vaccine strains, lactobacilli may lead to the development of different delivery systems. The use of a "non-commensal" food starter strain unable to establish itself in a body cavity, would generate an approach similar to *Lc. lactis* (i.e., "live microparticles" pre-loaded with antigen). In contrast, strains belonging to (or similar to) the endogenous microflora and able to "colonize" or persist in a mucosal niche would be very close to the *Strep. gordonii* system (i.e., colonizing "cell factory" able to synthesize the antigen *in situ*). In theory, it might be speculated that both types of lactobacilli would be perceived differently by the MALT, thus leading to different immune responses. However, to the best of our knowledge, there is no direct evidence supporting this hypothesis as yet.

Table 9.2. *Lactobacillus* Strains Used as Antigen Expression Host

Species	Strain	Origin	Persistence in Mice (days)[a]	Survival Rate (human)
Lb. paracasei	LbTGS1.4	Murine vagina	4–6	ND[b]
Lb. casei (zeae)	ATCC393	dairy	3–5	ND
Lb. plantarum	256	silage	3–5	ND
	NCIMB 8826	human	4–6	7%
Lb. fermentum	KLD	human	4–6	1%
Lc. lactis	MG1363	dairy	<1	0.5%

Adapted from Mercenier et al., 1996; Vesa et al., 2000.
[a]Persistence levels evaluated as CFU/mg feces vary between individual strains.
[b]Not determined.

Because of the species- (and strain-) dependence of most genetic tools, a limited number of strains have been evaluated so far for their local delivery capacity. Very few strains of *Lactobacillus* have been described as expression hosts for model antigens (see Table 9.2, reviewed in Wells et al., 1996; Rush et al., 1997; Mercenier et al., 2000).

As in the case of *Lc. lactis*, the most detailed immunization studies have been performed, using TTFC as a model antigen. Three main *Lactobacillus* strains were studied and compared to *Lc. lactis* and *Strep. gordonii*, that is, *Lb. casei (zeae)* ATCC393, *Lb. plantarum* 256 and *Lb. plantarum* NCIMB8826. A fourth strain, *Lb. fermentum* KLD has been evaluated as well, but progress with this host has been hampered by the difficulty in constructing recombinant strains producing high amounts of the antigen (L. Plant and P. Conway, University of New South Wales, personal communication). This typically reflects upon the difficulty to adapt genetic tools to the strain under study, a situation that has delayed the first reports of successful local immunizations with lactobacilli (see Mercenier et al., 2000). However, once optimized strains are constructed they perform equally well as *Lc. lactis* (see text below).

TTFC was produced intra-cellularly or at the cell surface in both *Lb. casei* 393 and *Lb. plantarum* 256. The latter species turned out to be a better expression host in terms of antigen expression levels, as had also been found for another antigen by Hols et al. (1997). Replicative plasmids were constructed that carried the TTFC encoding gene under the control of an inducible (α-amylase from *Lb. amylovorus*) or a constitutive (lactate dehygrogenase from *Lb. casei*) promoter. Cell wall anchoring was achieved using the targeting signal of the *Lb. casei* major protease (PrtP) leading to exposure of 10^3–10^4 molecules/cell as estimated by flow cytometry (Maassen et al., 1999; Shaw et al., 2000). In this series of plasmids, all expression signals and most vector sequences were of *Lactobacillus* origin.

In the case of *Lb. plantarum* NCIMB 8826, immunization protocols were optimized mainly with recombinant cells producing TTFC in the cytoplasm. However, this bacterium was also engineered to secrete TTFC or produce it at the cell surface as a fusion with the M6 carrier (see section on *Strep. gordonii*). Subcutaneous, i.n., and intra-gastric immunizations of C57bl/6 mice demonstrated that the three recombinant strains were able to elicit antigen specific serum IgG and local IgA responses (Reveneau, N. et al., 2002). As for *Lc. lactis*, but in contrast to the results obtained by Shaw et al. (2000), cell surface presentation of the antigen seemed to be more immunogenic when relative production levels were taken into account. However, the corresponding *Lactobacillus* strains turned out to be rather unstable, exhibiting structural rearrangements of the plasmid during propagation (Reveneau, N., Chagnaud, P., and Mercenier, A., Institut Pasteur de Lille, 2000, unpublished).

An elegant chromosomal integration system was thus developed for *Lb. plantarum* (Hols, P. and Delcour, J., Université Catholique de Louvain-La-Neuve, personal communication) which leads to either non-disruptive integration of the suicide plasmid in the tRNAser locus or to single copy integration in the *L-ldh* gene. In the latter case, upon a spontaneous second recombination event, excisants were isolated that carried the TTFC encoding gene as an unique heterologous sequence (see Mercenier et al., 2000). Even though the integrants and excisants produced less antigen than strains harbouring multi-copy plasmids, they were shown to be immunogenic by both the s.c. and i.n. routes (Grangette, C., Geoffroy, M.-C., Chagnaud, P., Müller-Alouf, H., and Mercenier, A., Institut Pasteur de Lille, 1999; unpublished). Importantly the L-LDH deficient *Lb. plantarum* strain is not impaired as compared to the wild type strain, regarding its viability or persistence in mice (Favier, C., Hols, P., Goudercourt, D., Müller-Alouf, H., Grangette, C., and Vaughan, H., University of Wageningen, Université Catholique de Louvain-La-Neuve and Institut Pasteur de Lille, 2000, unpublished). Expression signals developed for the strain NCIMB 8826 included both constitutive (lactate deyhydrogenase, pLDH; lactococcal promoter 32) and the lactococcal nisin-inducible (pNis) promoters. The latter permitted dose–response curves (Pavan et al., 2000) to be performed, and demonstrated that the level of intra-cellularly produced antigens is a key factor governing the immune response.

As *Lb. casei* turned out to be a less effective antigen delivery system than *Lb. plantarum* (Shaw et al., 2000), only immunization results with the latter host are summarized below. Even though no head-to-head comparison of the two *Lb. plantarum* strains studied so far has been performed, the results obtained with both carriers are comparable. Using recombinant *Lb. plantarum* 256 and 8826 strains synthesizing TTFC intra-cellularly, high serum IgG responses were generated after i.n. or intra-gastric administration to mice. Immunization with *Lb. plantarum* 256/TTFC was significantly more effective through the nasal than the intra-gastric route, leading to serum IgG titers of approximately 10^4 and 10^2, respectively. The i.n. immunization schedule, which included administration of $2–5 \times 10^9$ live cells at three consecutive days for both priming and boosting, led to a detectable IgA antibody response in bronchoalveolar lavage (BAL) fluids and to the presence of high TT-specific antibody secreting cells in cervical lymph nodes and spleen. High serum IgG titers against TTFC were also measured in response to a single-dose immunization protocol. Intra-nasal immunization with *Lb. plantarum* 256 expressing TTFC on the cell surface only elicited a weak serum IgG response and were non-immunogenic by the oral route despite the fact that this strain was producing only 5- to 10-fold less amounts of antigen than the highly immunogenic strains that expressed the antigen intra-cellularly (Shaw et al., 2000).

Local immunizations with *Lb. plantarum* 8826/TTFC were performed using similar bacterial doses and a slightly different regime, that is, a single- or double-dose of lactobacilli for priming and two booster immunizations all given at 3 week intervals. The single-dose protocol led to anti-TTFC serum IgG levels that correlated to the actual dose of antigen delivered. Strains producing TTFC at up to 10% total protein content (8826/pMEC46; Pavan et al., 2000) elicited a strong immune response even after priming (end point titer of 10^4), which then increased 10 to 100 fold after boosting. Similar titers were obtained with a strain producing 5–10 times less TTFC (8826/pMEC4; Grangette, C., Müller-Alouf, H., Geoffroy, M.-C., Chagnaud, P., and Mercenier, A., Institut Pasteur de Lille, 1999, unpublished) at the end of a single-dose protocol, underlining again that absolute levels of antigen expressed in lactobacilli particularly impact on immunogenicity (Shaw et al., 2000; Grangette et al., 2001).

The IgG response to TTFC was found to be quite long-lasting as it decreased only by one order of magnitude 7 months after the last boost (Müller-Alouf, H., Grangette, C., Goudercourt, D., and Mercenier, A., Institut Pasteur de Lille, 2000, unpublished). Both types of recombinant strains led to specific IgA responses in BAL fluids and to antigen-specific T cell proliferation in cervical lymph nodes. However, no response was detectable when stimulation was performed with *Lb. plantarum* in the latter assay, in contrast to the results reported for *Lc. lactis* (see above). This difference in intrinsic immunogenicity between lactic acid bacterial vectors was observed in two independent laboratories (Rush, C. and Wells, J. M., University of Cambridge, 1999, unpublished; Grangette, C., Müller-Alouf, H., Goudercourt, D., and Mercenier, A., Institut Pasteur de Lille, 1999, unpublished). Interestingly, as in the case of *Lc. Lactis*, serum antibody titers did not differ substantially whether live or killed (mytomycin C or UV treated) strains were used to immunize mice. However, in the case of *Lb. plantarum* 8826 at least, protection studies including both direct lethal challenge and sero-neutralization assays, demonstrated that live bacteria induced a better protection than inactivated ones (Grangette et al., 2001). This was also the case after intra-gastric immunization, where end-point titers as high as 10^{5-6} (serum IgG) were obtained with the best *Lb. plantarum* 8826 recombinant strains (Grangette, C. et al., 2002). The immunization route did not seem to impact on the isotypic responses as in both cases IgG1, IgG2b, and, to a lesser extent, IgG2a subclasses were measured.

Ongoing work linked to the development of *Lactobacillus* based vehicles includes selection of strains with different intrinsic immunological properties, identification and transfer or inactivation of adhesion factors (Pouwels et al., 1998; Roos, 1999), and construction of biologically contained strains (Hols, P. and Delcour, J., Université Catholique de Louvain-La-Neuve, personal communication).

Important questions that remain to be addressed in the case of lactobacilli, include the following:

1. Is persistence of the strain in the body more important than its survival or viability?
2. Is adhesion of *Lactobacillus* to the mucus or to the epithelial cells influencing the immune response and does bacteria–host signalling play an important role?
3. Should the intrinsic immunomodulation or adjuvant property of the strain be "tailored" to the final target (e.g., Th1/Th2 balance, pro- or anti-inflammatory effect)?
4. Can the system be manipulated to induce either active immunization or oral tolerance (i.e., a combination of appropriate antigen location, colonization and immunomodulation capacity of the strain)?
5. Should a *Lactobacillus* vaccine strain be selected on the basis of specific probiotic traits?

Vaccine Delivery Using *Streptococcus gordonii*

The first evidence that a recombinant commensal bacterium can be used as a live vector to deliver antigens at mucosal surfaces was obtained with *Strep. gordonii* (Medaglini et al., 1995). Several papers and reviews describe the results obtained with this delivery system (see Pozzi et al., 1997; Medaglini et al., 1997a). Therefore, only key features are summarized below. Antigens have almost exclusively been expressed in this host on the cell surface as genetic fusions to the M6 protein of *Strep. pyogenes*, using the chromosomal expression system described above. Nevertheless, the model antigen TTFC has been synthesized both on the cell surface and in the cytoplasm of *Strep. gordonii* in order to investigate the effects of antigen location on immunogenicity (G. Pozzi, personal communication). Subcutaneous and i.n. immunization of mice with recombinant strains of *S. gordonii* displaying TTFC at the cell surface elicited serum IgG responses that conferred good to partial protection against a lethal challenge with TT (i.e., 82% of s.c. immunized mice and 38% of i.n. immunized mice were protected). In addition i.n. immunization elicited IgA to TTFC in lung washes. Notably, the IgG1/IgG2a ratio varied from ~6 to 1 depending on the route (s.c. vs. i.n.) of administration (Medaglini et al., 2001).

Immunization studies in mice with recombinant strains of *Strep. gordonii* have shown that a single oro-nasal dose (in the range 10^7 to 10^9 c.f.u) results in high rates of nasopharangeal colonization, which are comparable to the results obtained with wild type strains

(Oggioni et al., 1995; Medaglini et al., 1995). Recently, Lee et al. showed that oral colonization of mice with *Strep. gordonii* expressing a pertussis toxin S1 subunit (PTS1) elicited sIgA antibodies but not serum antibodies to PTS1 (Lee et al., 2002).

Recombinant strains of *Strep. gordonii* have also been shown to colonize the vaginal mucosa of mice following intra-vaginal administration of a single dose of bacteria (Pozzi et al., 1997). This opens up the possibility of utilizing recombinant *Strep. gordonii* to vaccinate against sexually transmitted pathogens (Medaglini et al., 1997b, 1998).

Strep. gordonii expressing M6 fusions to the E7 epitope of human papilloma virus or Ag5.2, a bee venom allergen, have been used for i.n. and vaginal immunization of mice (Medaglini et al., 1997a). In both cases, antigen-specific local (sIgA) and serum antibodies (predominantly IgG1 and IgG2a) were elicited (Medaglini et al., 1997a,b; Pozzi et al., 1997). In the studies with E7 expressing *Strep. gordonii*, antigen-specific IgA antibodies were detected in the vaginal washes up to 10 weeks after administration of the strains. It was also shown that the immune response depended on effective colonization since killed recombinant bacteria did not induce a local response (Medaglini et al., 1997a,b, 1998; Pozzi et al., 1997).

Very few intra-gastric immunizations were reported for this delivery system. However, recombinant strains producing LTB at the cell surface were shown to be able to induce both serum IgG and fecal IgA, even though *Strep. gordonii* does not colonize the intestinal mucosa of mice (Ricci et al., 2000).

These initial studies have been extended to immunization of cynomologous monkeys using strains of *Strep. gordonii* expressing the E7 or HIV1-V3 epitopes. In this primate, no vaginal colonization was observed but repeated administrations of the recombinant bacteria led to the induction of antigen specific local (IgA) and serum antibody (Medaglini et al., 1998). Both the E7 and HIV1-V3 polypeptide antigens were known to contain T cell epitopes and T cell proliferative responses were measured *in vitro* to the E7 and HIV1-V3 antigens after immunization of monkeys with the corresponding antigen expressor strains of *Strep. gordonii* (Di Fabio et al., 1998; Oggioni et al., 1999).

Recent studies have also shown that mouse dendritic cells (DCs) are activated following phagocytosis of *Strep. gordonii*, indicating that they are likely to be efficient at presenting antigens of this bacterium and promoting primary T cell responses. Ovalbumin (OVA) expressed on the surface of recombinant *Strep. gordonii* was indeed processed and presented on MHC class I molecules 10^6 times more efficiently than soluble OVA (Rescigno et al., 1998). These data were extended to human DCs generated from peripheral blood monocytes. Corinti et al. (1999) used recombinant *Strep. gordonii* strains expressing TTFC on the cell surface to deliver this MHCII-restricted antigen into DCs. The authors demonstrated that, upon phagocytosis by the DCs, the recombinant strain induced DC maturation and stimulated the synthesis of chemokines very active in attracting T cells. These effects were much more pronounced than those induced with soluble TTFC or TTFC conjugated to inert particles, and required less antigen (Corinti et al., 1999, 2000). These are important observations as DCs play a key role as sentinels that recognize invading organisms in tissues facing the external environment.

Induction of Oral Tolerance

In general, humans and animals have low level or undetectable immune responses to food antigens and commensal bacteria. However, this may vary depending on the nature of the antigen, especially in diseased states that lead to inflammation at mucosal surfaces (Strobel and Mowat, 1998). The precise mechanisms by which the homeostatic state of the intestinal ecosystem is established and maintained are still not completely understood but it is, presumably, crucial in preventing deleterious immune responses, such as allergy, against food antigens. It also plays an important role in maintaining the integrity of the mucosal barrier.

It has long been recognized that feeding of soluble proteins can result in a lack of immunological response to subsequent systemic injections of the same antigen (Mowat, 1985; Husby et al., 1995; Metzler and Wraith, 1995). This phenomenon, commonly referred to as "oral tolerance", has been experimentally investigated as a method of treatment for autoimmune diseases (Weiner et al., 1995). It has been proposed that intestinal epithelial cells may be involved in the induction of oral tolerance on the basis that they have the ability to express MHCII molecules but lack molecules on the cell surface that provide a second vital stimulus to T cells (Sanderson et al., 1993). Recent data indicate that the second signal required for activation of T cells besides the antigen–MHC interaction with the T cell receptor is mediated through interaction of B7.1 and B7.2 molecules, found on professional APCs, with the CD28 receptor on T cells (Freeman et al., 1993). Thus, epithelial cells may actively tolerize T cells in the mucosal tissue by failing to provide the second signal of T cell activation. There is also evidence from studies in animal models that the mucosal immune system may generate specific cells that suppress systemic immune responses, while a mucosal IgA response is still present (James, 1997). Several tolerization and treatment studies in animal models of autoimmune disease have involved feeding of large quantities of autoantigens. It has been proposed that in these circumstances tolerance may result from T cell anergy caused by high doses of antigen (see MacDonald, 1994; Yoshida et al., 1997). In addition to active suppression and clonal anergy, deletion of antigen-reactive T cells has also been reported (Chen et al., 1995). Evidently there are different possible mechanisms of tolerance and these may vary depending on the form of the antigen, the dose of antigen, and frequency of administration (Yoshida et al., 1997; Strobel and Mowat, 1998).

The mechanism of tolerance to commensal bacteria is unknown but may involve differences in the capacity of commensal and pathogenic bacteria to activate the immune system (see Wold et al., 1989). Routes of entry into the body and specific interactions with dendritic cells could, for example, play a key role in activating a positive immune response, but the initial steps leading to either immunogenic or tolerogenic responses remain the subject of active investigation (Strobel and Mowat, 1998; Autenrieth and Schmidt, 2000; Hayday and Viney, 2000; MacPherson et al., 2000).

It is evident from the experiments described here that, contrary to what might have been expected, the non-pathogenic non-invasive LAB are able to induce a positive immune response that is dependent on the dose of bacteria, the nature and the amount of antigen, as well as the location of the antigen in the bacterial cells. Moreover, it has been proposed that these carriers might also be used to induce oral tolerance by secreting soluble antigens into the intestinal tract. Maassen et al. (1999) have recently described the construction of strains of *Lb. casei* that secrete human myelin basic protein (hMBP) or hMBP as a fusion to β-glucuronidase, with the prospect of evaluating these strains in a rat model of experimental autoimmune encephalomyelitis (EAE). In this model oral administration of myelin basic protein was shown to inhibit autoimmune damage of the myelin sheath surrounding nerve axons (Bitar and Whitacre, 1988; Higgins and Weiner, 1988). So far, no studies describing treatment of EAE with recombinant *Lactobacillus* secreting MBP have been reported. The authors, however, confirmed efficient secretion of hMBP by the recombinant

Lactobacillus strain by performing efficient parenteral immunization with the bacterial culture broth (Maassen et al., 1999).

Prevention and Treatment of Allergy

Several dietary and clinical studies have suggested that consumption of LAB can reduce the symptoms of allergy and inhibit IgE production (Halpern et al., 1991; Trapp et al., 1993; Alm et al., 1999; van de Water, 1999; Yasu et al., 1999; Cross et al., 2001). Allergy is mediated by a dominant T-helper 2 lymphocyte (Th2) response to an allergenic molecule leading to high levels of IL4, IL5, and production of IgE. It has been proposed that LAB might reduce allergy by hydrolytically degrading allergens in the GI tract (Sutas et al., 1996) and by exerting an immunoregulatory effect on the immune system. Several clinical studies involving the consumption of foods containing LAB indicate increased production of type I and type II interferons that might modulate the development of Th2 responses to allergenic molecules (reviewed in detail by Cross et al., 2001). Experimental evidence is also accumulating for an immunoregulatory role of LAB that is mediated directly through the induction of pro-T-helper 1 lymphocyte responses via stimulation of IL-12 and IL-18 and TNFα production by macrophages and dendritic cells. However some studies have shown that not all LAB promote Th1 responses and that cytokine induction by LAB is clearly a strain dependent property (D'Andrea et al., 1993; Marin et al., 1997; Hessle et al., 1999; Miettinen et al., 1999). Furthermore, some LAB have been shown to suppress autoimmune disorders that are mediated by Th1 cells producing high levels of IFNγ (Kato et al., 1998; Madsen et al., 1999).

In a recent study by Kruisselbrink et al. (2001) the immunomodulatory effect of *Lb. plantarum* was evaluated in a model of dust mite allergy. Mice were sensitized to dust mite peptide (Der p1) that induces a dominant Th2 response and then treated intranasally with *Lb. plantarum* expressing the Der p1 peptide fused to a carrier protein β-glucuoronidase or a control strain in which the Der p1 peptide was replaced with a peptide from ovalbumin. Immunization of the mice led to a strong T cell response to the allergenic peptide resulting in high levels of IFNγ and IL-5 production. In the mice treated with *Lb. plantarum*, there was a significant decrease in the IFNγ production for both the control strain and the strain producing Der p1 whereas a decrease in IL-5 production was only measured in mice treated with *Lb. plantarum* expressing of the Der p1 peptide. These findings contrast with reports of specific Th1 promoting properties of LAB discussed above since antigen specific Th1 (IFNγ) responses were decreased by intra-nasal administration with *Lb. plantarum*. There was, however, a specific down-regulation of the Th2 (IL-5) component of the response to the antigen in mice treated with the strain expressing Der p1. Taken together these findings indicate that LAB expressing allergens may be good candidates for the treatment and possibly also the prevention of allergic disorders. However, it is clear that more research is needed to unravel the mechanisms that lie behind the immunomodulatory effects observed in humans and experimental animal models.

Delivery of Therapeutic Proteins via the Mucosal Surface

The development of high level inducible expression systems for *Lc. lactis* promoted interest in the use of these bacteria as production hosts for recombinant proteins.

Vectors including signal secretion leaders of lactococcal origin were developed to secrete heterologous proteins into the growth medium (see Wells et al., 1993c; Corthier and Renault, 1999; de Vos, 1999; Langella and Leloir, 1999). Recent improvements include the design of a series of vectors that allowed secretion and cell wall anchoring of the staphylococcal nuclease in *Lc. lactis* and lactobacilli (Dieye et al., 2001). Proteolysis of secreted proteins does not seem to be a problem in *Lc. lactis* strains lacking the PrtP protease and very few proteins are naturally secreted by *Lc. lactis*, indicating that this might be a useful approach to obtain an initial high level of purity of an expressed protein.

The first report of cytokine expression in *Lc. lactis* was for murine IL-2 using the lactococcal T7 system to secrete a fully biologically active IL-2 protein in the growth medium (Steidler et al., 1995). The cytokine was easily purified in yields of approximately 3 mg/L. N-terminal sequencing of purified IL-2 showed that the recombinant protein was properly processed and indistinguishable from native IL-2. More recently, a number of other cytokines and biologically active proteins have been expressed and secreted in *Lc. lactis* including IL-10 (Steidler et al., 2000).

The possibility of using recombinant *Lc. lactis* to orally deliver cytokines to the immune system was investigated by measuring immune responses in mice intra-nasally immunized with either *Lc. lactis* expressing TTFC or with strains of *Lc. lactis* that co-expressed TTFC intra-cellularly and secreted murine IL-2 or murine IL-6. All three strains were shown to produce approximately the same level of TTFC. The IL-2 and IL-6 producing strains were shown to secrete fully biologically active cytokines at levels of approximately 0.9 μg/ml in normal culture medium. The peak level of serum antibody responses to TTFC were 10- to 15-fold higher in mice immunized with the cytokine expressing strains than in the strains producing antigen alone. The effect of the cytokines was only observed when live cells were used, suggesting that the lactococci were producing cytokine *in vivo*. Notably, co-expression of IL-6 also led to increased serum IgA reponses to TTFC. Moreover, it is interesting to note that, while immune responses to the heterologous protein were enhanced in the double recombinant strains, this did not impact on the intensity of the immune response against the bacterial vector itself (Steidler et al., 1998).

A recent study by Steidler et al., has shown that intra-gastric administration of IL-10 secreting *Lc. lactis* has a preventive or therapeutic effect in two different mouse models of colitis (Shanahan, 2000; Steidler et al., 2000). The rationale for this approach is based on the role of IL-10 as a modulator of the regulatory T cells that control inflammatory responses to intestinal antigens and its activity in the restoration of T cell tolerance to the intestinal microflora (Duchmann et al., 1996; Asseman et al., 1999). A 50% reduction in inflammatory symptoms was observed after repeated administration of recombinant lactococci producing murine IL10 (mIL10), which is comparable in efficacy to alternative anti-inflammatory treatments. This positive effect required local *de novo* synthesis of mIL10, as UV-killed recombinant lactococci did not improve histological inflammation scores. The local delivery of this cytokine by lactococci avoids possible adverse effects from systemic exposure to the cytokine and provides a therapeutic effect at much lower doses. This exciting new approach to the treatment of inflammatory bowel disease (IBD) highlights the benefits of manipulating the enteric bacteria. As stressed by the authors, live recombinant lactococci might be useful for intestinal delivery of therapeutic proteins that are unstable or difficult to produce in large quantities.

Recently, Drouault et al. described the construction of recombinant *Lc. lactis* strains secreting a staphylococcal lipase (Drouault et al., 2000). In a further study by the same group the therapeutic effect of *Lc. lactis* expressing *Staphylococcus hyicus* lipase were evaluated in a porcine model of pancreatic insufficiency (Drouault, 2002). In this model, pancreatic insufficiency was induced by ligation of the pancreatic duct and coefficient of fat absorption measured after feeding of high fat diets (containing 15% lipids) mixed with control and lipase expressing strains of *Lc. lactis*. In this study the lipase was expressed intra-cellulary as higher amounts could be produced and it was previously shown that *Lc. lactis* lose viability in the upper jejuno–ileum and release their cellular contents (Drouault et al., 1999). The coefficient of fat absorption was higher (91.9% ± 3.7%) after consumption of food mixed with the lipase expressing *Lc. lactis* strain than after consumption of food mixed with the inactive control strain (78.4% ± 2.4%). The final diet (two daily meals of 300 g) contained a substantial dose of lactococci, that is, approximately 1×10^{10} *Lc. lactis* cells/g but nevertheless indicated the potential for using this approach to treat pancreatic insufficiency in humans.

A very elegant demonstration of the use of recombinant *Strep. gordonii* expressing a microbicidal single chain antibody (ScFv H6) to treat experimental vaginitis caused by *Candida albicans* was achieved by Beninati et al. (2000). These authors have engineered *Strep. gordonii* either to secrete H6 ScFv into the culture medium or to express it as a fusion protein on the cell surface. Both types of recombinant strains were able to stably colonize the rat vagina, which led to an efficient curing of the infection in 75% and 37.5% of the rats, respectively. A post-challenge intra-vaginal administration of a single dose of the H6-secreting strain was as efficacious as the current chemical treatment by fluconazole. This work indicates that commensal bacteria can be engineered to deliver an anti-infective agent *in vivo* without having to give repeated doses (Beninati et al., 2000). Another recent study showed that oral administration of *Lb. casei* (*zeae*) producing single chain antibodies that recognize the streptococcal antigen I/II of *Streptococcus mutans*, a pathogen involved in dental caries, markedly reduced *S. mutans* bacterial counts and caries scores (Kruger et al., 2002).

Conclusions and Future Prospectives

To date mucosal immunization with harmless recombinant LAB has shown that these non-pathogenic and non-invasive bacterial vectors are capable of eliciting specific local and systemic immune responses to the foreign antigen they synthesize. Using *Lc. lactis, Strep. gordonii*, or *Lactobacillus* spp. as a delivery vehicle it was shown that immune responses to TTFC are elicited when the antigen is expressed intra-cellularly or on the cell surface. It is not yet clear which mode of expression is optimal because immunogenicity may depend on the level of antigen and the species (or possibly even the strain) of LAB used as the vaccine carrier. The studies described to date are therefore not directly comparable even though they point to the fact that, at equal antigen dose, the cell wall presentation might be more immunogenic. However, the metabolic burden imposed on the strain by efficient secretion/anchoring of heterologous molecules may hamper its stability or viability. An alternative to circumvent this drawback is to achieve high (e.g., a few percent of total protein content) intra-cellular production of the antigen, when possible. In this respect the genetic system recently developed for *Lc. Lactis* by Walker and Klaenhammer (2001) might prove to be of high value. These authors have engineered lactococcal strains to confer them the capacity to externalize intracellular proteins independently of the classical secretion and export pathways (Walker and Klaenhammer, 2001).

Although it might be speculated that, as in the case of *Strep. gordonii*, live persisting bacteria will be superior to non-persisting ones when immunizing by less sensitive routes, that is, oral or vaginal, solid data still have to be generated to support this hypothesis in the case of lactobacilli. Experiments to directly compare immune responses to antigens expressed in colonizing or non-colonizing species of LAB are underway.

Finally, it remains to be determined whether killed rather than live bacteria can be used for certain applications. In the case of cytokine delivery using *Lc. lactis* the enhancement of immune responses by co-expressed cytokine was dependent on the use of live bacteria (Steidler et al., 1998, 2000). This indicated that active cytokine was not associated with the bacterial cells and that it was secreted *de novo* by live bacteria after inoculation. Intra-nasal immunization with live and killed *Lc. lactis* and *Lb. plantarum* expressing antigens intra-cellularly elicited similar levels of serum antibody to TTFC (Robinson et al., 1997; Grangette et al., 2001) although live bacteria were reported to induce better levels of protection (Grangette et al., 2002). In contrast, immune responses to antigens expressed on the cell surface of *Strep. gordonii* were measured after vaginal immunization with live but not killed strains. However, in this case only a single dose was given and the antigen was surface located. Taken together, these findings suggest that LAB can be used as killed whole cells for vaccines but it will depend on other factors such as amount of antigen associated with the cell, number of doses, and the route of administration.

Evidence to date indicates that the LAB are themselves relatively poorly antigenic, most likely due to tolerance to antigens found on commensal LAB. These microorganisms might thus serve as ideal vaccine carriers if the mechanisms involved in tolerance to LAB were not conferred to heterologous antigens using appropriate immunization regimes. At the present time it not known to what extent the intrinsic immunomodulatory capacity of the LAB carrier might influence the nature of the induced immune response (e.g., bias towards Th1 or Th2 profile).

TTFC has served as a good model antigen for studies on vaccine delivery using LAB; a substantial amount of data has been accumulated for different bacterial delivery systems. Now, attention is being turned to additional disease targets and vaccine antigens including bovine rotavirus non-structural protein 4, *Brucella abortus* L7/L2 antigen, *Bacillus anthracis* toxin, human papilloma virus type 16 E7 protein, and bovine beta-lactoglobulin (Shaw et al., 2000; Chatel et al., 2001; Enouf et al., 2001; Bermudez-Humaran, 2002; Ribeiro et al., 2002). Hopefully, these ongoing studies will demonstrate that LAB vaccines have sufficient potency (i.e., give protective level immune responses using minimal doses) for use as commercial vaccines.

Our progress toward development of more effective oral vaccines is hampered by a lack of knowledge of the factors that lead to the induction of adaptive responses by pathogenic bacteria encountered at mucosal surfaces. However, there are still a number of factors that can be empirically investigated in relation to the use of LAB as vaccine carriers. It is possible that the LAB can be further manipulated to contain factors from pathogenic bacteria that are known to help stimulate adaptive immune responses without posing any risk of harm or disease. As already mentioned we also need to know more about the fate of mucosally administered LAB and the effects of persistence and adherence on immunogenicity and protection. Therefore, we need to unravel the mechanisms of antigen presentation by LAB carriers and to better understand how and with which immune cell types they interact. Both lines of research have just begun to be investigated.

It has been proposed that LAB manipulated to secrete antigen into the GI tract rather than producing it intra-cellularly or on the cell surface might induce tolerance to that immunogen instead of an adaptive immune response. Recent research with LAB secreting autoantigens or allergens in experimental models of autoimmune or allergic disease suggests that they may be suitable for the treatment of allergic and autoimmune disorders although much more work is needed to gain an understanding of the mechanisms involved.

Apart from their use as antigen delivery vehicles, the LAB might also be engineered in the future to deliver therapeutic antibodies, enzymes, immunomodulatory molecules, or peptides in the GI tract (e.g., Beninati et al., 2000; Steidler et al., 2000; Kruisselbrink et al., 2001; Drouault, 2002). Before LAB can indeed be used in humans it will be necessary to construct strains for human or animal use that will meet the safety requirements of the regulatory bodies. This implies that the existing food grade expression systems should be further developed for this purpose (see references in de Vos, 1999 and Pavan et al., 2000). As our knowledge of mucosal immunology and factors affecting the efficacy of LAB as delivery vehicles increases there will be considerable potential to improve the existing technology.

The results generated in an EU-funded project on LAB (LABVAC, 1997–2000) have consolidated the proof that different LAB species are able to efficiently present a foreign antigen to the MALT. Notably, both systemic and mucosal antibody responses were elicited after delivery of recombinant LAB producing the model antigen TTFC by the i.n. intra-gastric, or vaginal route. The anti-TTFC serum IgG responses were very high, that is, end-point titers up to 10^5–10^6. When tested in a lethal challenge or seroneutralization assay, these responses were shown to be protective. It should also be mentioned that comparative studies conducted in different laboratories of the LABVAC consortium demonstrated that the induced immune responses were highly reproducible, which is an important issue when developing local delivery systems. At present, it might be concluded that the three LAB species studied so far are equally promising, each of them being characterized by specific advantages and drawbacks. Whether there will be a need in the future to tailor the choice of the LAB vector to a specific application remains an open question. At present the LAB represent a promising mucosal delivery system for both vaccines and therapeutic molecules. The European Commission is continuing to support the development of LAB delivery systems to treat or prevent important medical diseases through the efforts of new RTD projects LABDEL (QLK3-2000-00340) and DEPROHEALTH (QLK1-2000-00146).

Acknowledgements

J. M. W. and A. M. are grateful for financial support from the European Commission for the LABDEL project (contract QLRT-2000-00340) and DEPROHEALTH project (contract QLK1-2000-00146) that are coordinated by J. M. W. and A. M., respectively. The authors thank Dr. Owen for providing figure 9.2.

References

Adams, M. R., and Marteau, P. (1995). On the safety of lactic acid bacteria from food. *International Journal of Food Microbiology* 27: 263–264.

Aguirre, M., and Collins, M. D. (1993). Lactic acid bacteria and human clinical infection. *Journal of Applied Bacteriology* 75: 95–109.

Allan, C. H., Mendrick, P. L., and Trier, J. S. (1993). Rat intestinal M cells contain acidic endosomal–lysomal compartments and express class II major histocompatability complex determinants. *Gastroenterology* 104: 698–708.

Alm, J. S., Swartz, J., Lilja, G., Scheynius, A., and Pershagen, G. (1999). Atopy in children of families with an anthroposophic lifestyle. *Lancet* 353:1485–1488.

Aspiras, M. B., Kazmerzak, K. M., Kolenbrander, P. E., McNab, R., Hardegen, N., and Jenkinson, H. F. (2000). Expression of green fluorescent protein in *Streptococcus gordonii* DL1 and its use as a species-specific marker in coadhesion with *Streptococcus oralis* 34 in saliva-conditioned biofilms. *In vitro, Applied and Environmental Microbiology* 66: 4074–4083.

Asseman, C., Mauze, S., Leach, M. W., Coffman, R. L., and Powrie, F. (1999). An essential role for interleukin 10 in the function of regulatory T cells that inhibit intestinal inflammation. *Journal of Experimental Medicine* 190: 995–1004.

Autenrieth, I. B., and Schmidt, M. A. (2000). Bacterial interplay at intestinal mucosal surfaces: Implications for vaccine development. *Trends in Microbiology* 8: 457–464.

Beninati, C., Oggioni, M. R., Boccanera, M., Spinoza, M. R., Maggi, T., Conti, S., Magliani, W., De Bernardis, F., Teti, G., Cassone, A., Pozzi, G., and Polonelli, L. (2000). Therapy of mucosal candidiasis by expression of an anti-idiotype in human commensal bacteria. *Nature Biotechnology* 18: 1060–1064.

Bergmann, K.-C., and Waldman, R. H. (1988). Stimulation of secretory antibody following oral administration of antigen. *Review of Infectious Diseases* 10: 939–950.

Bermudez-Humaran, L. G., Langella, P., Miyoshi, A., Gruss, A., Guerra, R. T., Montes de Oca-Luna, R., and Le Loir, Y. (2002). Production of human papillomavirus type 16 E7 protein in *Lactoccus lactis. Applied Environmental Microbiology* 68: 917–922.

Bitar, D. M., and Whitacre, C. C. (1988). Suppression of experimental auto-immune encephalomyelitis by the oral administration of myelin basic protein. *Cell Immunology* 112: 364–370.

Brandtzaeg, P., Backkevold, E. S., and Fardstad, I. N. (1999). Regional specialization in the mucosal immune system: What happens in the microcompartments? *Immunology Today* 20: 141–151.

Bumann, D., Hueck, C., Aebischer, T., and Meyer, T. F. (2000). Recombinant live *Salmonella* spp. for human vaccination against heterologous pathogens. *FEMS Immunology and Medical Microbiology* 27: 357–364.

Chamberlain, L., Wells, J. M., Robinson, K., Schofield, K., and Le Page, R. (1997). Mucosal immunization with recombinant *Lactococcus lactis*. In: G. Pozzi and J. M. Wells (Eds.), *Gram-positive bacteria as vaccine vehicles for mucosal immunization* (pp. 83–106). Berlin: Springer-Verlag.

Chen, Y., Inobe, J. I., Marks, R., Gonnella, P., Kuchroo, V. K., and Welner, H. L. (1995). Peripheral deletion of antigen-reactive T cells in oral tolerance. *Nature* 376: 177–180.

Chatel, J. M., Langella, P., Adel-Patient, K., Commissaire, J., Wal, J. M., and Corthier, G. (2001). Induction of mucosal immune response after intranasal or oral inoculation of mice with *Lactococcus lactis* producing bovine beta-lactoglobulin. *Clinical and Diagnostic Laboratory Immunology* 8: 545–551

Conley, M. E., and Delacroix, D. L. (1987). Intravascular and mucosal immunoglobulin A: Two separate but related systems of immune defence. *Annals of Internal Medicine* 106: 892.

Corinti, S., Medaglini, D., Cavani, A., Rescigno, M., Pozzi, G., Ricciardi-Castaglioni, P., and Girolomoni, G. (1999). Human dendritic cells very efficiently present a heterologous antigen expressed on the surface of recombinant Gram-positive bacteria to CD4+ T lymphocytes. *Journal of Immunology* 163: 3029–3036.

Corinti, S., Medaglini, D., Prezzi, C., Cavani, A., Pozzi, G., and Girolomoni, G. (2000). Human dendritic cells are superior to B cells at presenting a major histocompatibility complex class II-restricted heterologous antigen expressed on recombinant *Streptococcus gordonii. Infection and Immunity* 68: 1879–1883.

Corthier, G., and Renault, P. (1999). Future directions for research on biotherapeutic agents: Contribution of genetic approaches on lactic acid bacteria. In: G. W. Elmer (Ed.), *Biotherapeutic agents and infectious diseases* (pp. 269–304). Totowa, NJ: Humana Press Inc.

Cross, M. L., Stevenson, L. M., and Gill, H. S. (2001). Anti-allergy properties of fermented foods: An important immunoregulatory mechanism of lactic acid bacteria? *International Immunopharmacology* 1(5): 891–901.

D'Andrea, A., Aste-Amezaga, M., Valiante, N. M., Ma, X., Kubin, M., and Trinchieri, G. (1993). Interleukin 10 (IL-10) inhibits human lymphocyte interferon gamma-production by suppressing natural killer cell stimulatory factor/IL-12 synthesis in accessory cells. *Journal of Experimental Medicine* 178: 1041–1048.

de Vos, W. M. (1999). Gene expression systems for lactic acid bacteria. *Current Opinion in Microbiology* 2: 289–295.

Dieye, Y., Usai, S., Clier, F., Gruss, A., and Piard, J.-C. (2001). Design of a protein-targeting system for lactic acid bacteria. *Applied Environmental Microbiology* 183: 4157–4166.

Di Fabio, S., Medaglini, D., Rush, C. M., Corrias, F., Panzini, G. L., Pace, M., Verani, P., Pozzi, G., and Titti, F. (1998). Vaginal immunization of cynomolgus monkeys (*Macaca fascicularis*) with *Streptococcus gordonii* expressing HIV-1 and HPV-16 antigens. *Vaccine* 16: 485–492.

Drouault, S., Corthier, G., Ehrlich, S. D., and Renault, P. (1999). Survival, physiology, and lysis of *Lactococcus lactis* in the digestive tract. *Applied and Environmental Microbiology* 65: 4881–4886.

Drouault, S., Corthier, G., Ehrlich, S. D., and Renault, P. (2000). Expression of the *Staphylococcus hyicus* lipase in *Lactococcus lactis. Applied Environmental Microbiology* 66: 588–598.

Drouault, S., Juste, C., Marteau, P., Renault, P., and Corthier, G. (2002). Oral treatment with *Lactococcus lactis* expressing *Staphylococcus hyicus* lipase enhances lipid digestion in pigs with induced pancreatic insufficiency. *Applied Environmental Microbiology* 68: 3166–3168.

Duchmann, R., Schmitt, E., Knolle, P., Meyer zum Buschenfelde, K. H., and Neurath, M. (1996). Tolerance towards resident intestinal flora in mice is abrogated in experimental colitis and restored by treatment with interleukin-10 or antibodies to interleukin-12. *European Journal of Immunology* 26: 934–938.

Dupont, L., Boizet-Bonhoure, B., Coddeville, M., Auvray, F., and Ritzenthaler, P. (1995). Characterisation of genetic elements required for site-specific integration of *Lactobacillus delbrueckii* subsp. *bulgaricus* bacteriophage mv4 and construction of an integration-proficient vector for *Lactobacillus plantarum*. *Journal of Bacteriology* 177: 586–595.

Dutot, P. (1996). Evaluation des lactobacilles comme vecteurs vivants de vaccination, PhD thesis, Université Louis Pasteur, Strasbourg, France.

Enouf, V., Langella, P., Commissaire, J., Cohen, J., and Corthier, G. (2001). Bovine rotavirus non-structural protein 4 (NSP4) produced by *Lactococcus lactis* is antigenic and immunogenic. *Applied and Environmental Microbiology* 67: 1423–1428.

Fairweather, N. F., Lyness, V. A., and Maskell, D. J. (1987). Immunisation of mice against tetanus toxin with fragments of tetanus toxin synthesised in *Escherichia coli*. *Infection and Immunity* 55: 2541–2545.

Finzi, G., Carnaggia, M., and Copella, C. (1993). Cathepsin E in follicle-associated epithelium of intestine and tonsils: Localization to M cells and possible role in antigen processing. *Histochemistry* 99: 201–211.

Freeman, G. J., Gribben, J. G., and Boussiotis, V. A. (1993). Cloning of B7-2: A CTLA-4 counter-receptor that costimulates human T cell proliferation. *Science* 262: 909–911.

Geoffroy, M. C., Guyard, C., Quatannens, B., Pavan, S., Lange, M., and Mercenier, A. (2000). Use of green fluorescent protein to tag lactic acid bacterium strains under development as live vaccine vectors. *Applied and Environmental Microbiology* 66: 383–391.

Gicquel, B. (1995). BCG as a vector for the construction of multivalent recombinant vaccines. *Biologicals* 23: 113–118.

Gilbert, C., Robinson, K., Le Page, R. W. F., and Wells, J. M. (2000). Heterologous expression of an immunogenic pneumococcal type 3 capsular polysaccharide in *Lactococcus lactis*. *Infection and Immunity* 68: 3251–3260.

Grangette, C., Müller-Alouf, H., Goudercourt, D., Geoffroy, M.-C., Turneer, M., and Mercenier, A. (2001). Mucosal immune responses and protection against tetanus toxin after intranasal immunization with recombinant *Lactobacillus plantarum*. *Infection and Immunity* 69: 1547–1553.

Grangette, C., Muller-Alouf, H., Geoffroy, M., Goudercourt, D., Turneer, M., and Mercenier, A. (2002). Protection against tetanus toxin after intragastric administration of two recombinant lactic acid bacteria: Impact of strain viability and *in vivo* persistence. *Vaccine* 20(27–28): 3304–3309.

Gruzza, M., Duval-Iflah, Y., and Ducluzeau, R. (1992). Colonization of the digestive tract of germ-free mice by genetically engineered strains of *Lactococcus lactis*: Study of recombinant DNA stability. *Microbial Releases* 1: 165–171.

Gruzza, M., Fons, M., Ouriet, M. F., Dubal-Iflah, Y., and Ducluzeau, R. (1994). Study of gene transfer *in vitro* and in the digestive tract of gnotobiotic mice from *Lactococcus lactis* strains to various strains belonging to human intestinal flora. *Microbial Releases* 2: 183–189.

Guarner, F., and Schaafsma, G. J. (1998). Probiotics. *International Journal of Food Microbiology* 39: 237–238.

Guzman, C. A., Weiss, S., and Chakraborty, T. (1997). *Listeria monocytogenes*—A promising vaccine carrier to evoke cellular immune responses. In: G. Pozzi and J. M. Wells (Eds.), *Gram-positive bacteria as vaccine vehicles for mucosal immunisation* (pp. 145–173). Berlin: Springer-Verlag.

Halpern, G. M., Vruwink, K. G., Van de Water, J., Keen, C. L., and Gershwin, M. E. (1991). Influence of long-term yoghurt consumption in young adults. *International Journal of Immunotherapy* 7: 205–210.

Hathaway, L. J., and Kraehenbuhl, J. P. (2000). The role of M cells in mucosal immunity. *Cell Molecular Life Science* 57: 323–332.

Hayday, A., and Viney, J. L. (2000). The ins and outs of body surface immunology. *Science* 290: 97–100.

Hessle, C., Hanson, L. A., and Wold, A. E. (1999). Lactobacilli from human gastrointestinal mucosa are strong stimulators of IL-12 production. *Clinical Experimental Immunology* 116: 276–282.

Higgins, P. J., and Weiner, H. L. (1988). Suppression of experimental auto-immune encephalomyelitis by oral administration of myelin basic protein and its fragments. *Journal of Immunology* 140: 440–445.

Hols, P., Slos, P., Dutot, P., Reymund, J., Chabot, P., Delplace, B., Delcour, J., and Mercenier, A. (1997). Efficient secretion of the model antigen M6-gp41E in *Lactobacillus plantarum* NCIMB 8826. *Microbiology* 143: 2733–2741.

Ishii, H., Kobayashi, Y., Kuroki, M., and Kodama, Y. (1988). Protection of mice from lethal infection with Aujeszky's disease virus by immunization with purified gVI. *Journal of Genetic Virology* 69: 1411–1414.

Iwaki, M., Okahashi, N., Takahashi, I., Kanamoto, T., Sugita-Konishi, Y., Aibara, K., and Koga, T. (1990). Oral immunization with recombinant *Streptococcus lactis* carrying the *Streptococcus mutans* surface protein antigen gene. *Infection and Immunity* 58: 2929–2934.

James, S. P. (1997). The gastrointestinal mucosal immune system. In: M. M. Levine, G. C. Woodrow, J. B. Kaper, and G. C. Cobon (Eds.), *New generation vaccines* (pp. 151–171). New York: Marcel Dekker, Inc.

Jones, B. D., Ghori, N., and Falkow, S. (1994). *Salmonella typhimurium* initiates murine infection by penetrating and destroying the specialized epithelial M cells of the Peyer's patches. *Journal of Experimental Medicine* 180: 15–23.

Kantele, A., Hakkinen, M., Moldoveanu, Z., Lu, A., Savilahti, E., Alvarez, R. D., Michalek, S., and Mestecky, J. (1998). Differences in immune responses induced by oral and rectal immunizations with *Salmonella typhi* Ty21a: Evidence for compartmentalization within the common mucosal immune system in humans. *Infection and Immunity* 66: 5630–5635.

Kato, I., Endo-Tanaka, K., and Yokokura, T. (1998). Suppressive effects of the oral administration of *Lactobacillus casei* on type II collagen-induced arthritis in DBA/1 mice. *Life Sciences* 63(8): 635–644.

Klaenhammer, T. R. (1995). Genetics of intestinal lactobacilli. *International Dairy Journal* 5: 1019–1058.

Klijn, N., Weerkamp, A. H., and de Vos, W. M. (1995). Genetic marking of *Lactococcus lactis* shows its survival in the human gastrointestinal tract. *Applied and Environmental Microbiology* 61: 2771–2774.

Kruisselbrink, A., Heijne Den Bak-Glashouwer, M. J., Havenitch, C. E., Thule, J. E., and Janssen, R. (2001). Recombinant *Lactobacillus plantarum* inhibits house dust mite-specific T-cell responses. *Clinical Experimental Immunology* 126: 2–8.

Kullen, M. J., and Klaenhammer, T. R. (2000). Genetic modification of lactobacilli and bifidobacteria. *Current Issues in Molecualr Biology* 2: 41–50.

Krüger, C., Hu, Y., Pan, Q., Marcotte, H., Hultberg, A., Delwar, D., van Dalen, P. J., Pouwels, P. H., Leer, R. J., Kelly, C. G., van Dollenweerd, C., Ma, J. K., and Hammarström, L. (2002). *In situ* delivery of passive immunity by lactobacilli producing single-chain antibodies. *Nature Biotechnology* 20: 702–706

Lamm, M. E. (1997). Interaction of antigens and antibodies at mucosal surfaces. *Annual Review of Microbiology* 57: 311–340.

Langella, P., and Leloir, Y. (1999). Heterologous protein secretion in *Lactococcus lactis*: A novel antigen delivery system. *Brazilian Journal of Medical and Biological Research* 32: 191–198.

Lee, S. F., Halperin, S. A., Wang, H., and Mac Arthur, A. (2002). Oral colonization and immune responses to *Streptococcus gordonii* expressing a pertussis toxin S1 fragment in mice. *FEMS Microbiology Letters* 208: 175–178.

Levine, M. M., Galen, J., Barry, E., Noriega, F., Chatfield, S., Sztein, M., Dougan, G., and Tacket, C. (1996). Attenuated *Salmonella* as live oral vaccines against typhoid fever and as live vectors. *Journal of Biotechnology* 44: 193–196.

Locht, C. (2000). Live bacterial vectors for intranasal delivery of protective antigens. *Pharmaceutical Science and Technology Today* 3: 121–128.

Maassen, C. B. M., Laman, J. D., Heijne den Bak-Glashouwer, M. J., Tielen, F. J., van Holten-Neelen, J. C. P. A., Hoogteijling, L., Antonissen, C., Leer, R. J., Pouwels, P. H., Boersma, W. J. A., and Shaw, D. M. (1999). Instruments for oral disease-intervention strategies: Recombinant *Lactobacillus casei* expressing tetanus toxin fragment C for vaccination or myelin proteins for oral tolerance induction in multiple sclerosis. *Vaccine* 17: 2117–2128.

Maassen, C. B. M., van Holten-Neelen, J. C. P. A., Balk, F., den Bak-Glashouwer, M. J. F., Leer, R. J., Laman, J. D., Boersma, W. J. A., and Claassen, E. (2000). Strain-dependent induction of cytokine profiles in the gut by orally administered *Lactobacillus* strains. *Vaccine* 18: 2613–2623.

Madsen, K. L., Doyle, J. S., Jewell, L. D., Tavernini, M. M., and Fedorak, R. N. (1999). *Lactobacillus* species prevents colitis in interleukin 10 gene-deficient mice. *Gastroenterology* 116(5): 1107–1114.

MacDonald, T. T. (1994). Oral tolerance. Eating your way towards immunosuppression. *Current Biology* 4: 178–181.

MacPherson, A. J., Gatto, D., Sainsbury, E., Harriman, G. R., Heingartner, H., and Zinkernagel, R. M. (2000). A primitive T cell-independent mechanism of intestinal mucosal IgA responses to commensal bacteria. *Science* 288: 2222–2226.

Martin, M. C., Alonso, J. C., Suarez, J. E., and Alvarez, M. A. (2000). Generation of food-grade recombinant lactic acid bacterium strains by site-specific recombination. *Applied Environmental Microbiology* 66: 2599–2604.

Mazanec, M. B., Kaetzel, C. S., Lamm, M. E., Fletcher, D., and Nedrud, J. G. (1992). Intracellular neutralization of virus by immunoglobulin A antibodies. *Proceedings of the National Academy of Sciences, USA* 89: 6901–6905.

McGhee, J. R., Mestecky, J., Dertzbaugh, M. T., Eldridge, J. H., Hirasawa, M., and Kiyono, H. (1992). The mucosal immune system: From fundamental concepts to vaccine developments. *Vaccine* 10: 75–88.

Medaglini, D., Ciabattini, A., Spinosa, M. R., Maggi, T., Marcotte, H., Oggioni, M. R., and Pozzi, G. (2001). Immunization with recombinant *Streptococcus gordonii* expressing tetanus toxin fragment C confers protection from lethal challenge in mice. *Vaccine* 19: 1931–1939

Medaglini, D., Oggioni, M., and Pozzi, G. (1998). Vaginal immunisation with recombinant Gram-positive bacteria. *American Journal of Reproductive Immunology* 39: 199–208.

Medaglini, D., Pozzi, G., and King, T. P., and Fischetti, V. A. (1995). Mucosal and systemic immune responses to a recombinant protein expressed on the surface of the oral commensal bacterium *Streptococcus gordonii* after oral colonization. *Proceedings of the National Academy of Sciences USA* 92: 6868–6872.

Medaglini, D., Ricci, S., Maggi, T., Rush, C. M., Manganelli, R., Oggioni, M. R., and Pozzi, G. (1997a). Recombinant Gram-positive bacteria as vehicles of vaccine antigens. *Biotechnology Annual Review* 3: 297–312.

Medaglini, D., Rush, C. M., Sestini, P., and Pozzi, G. (1997b). Commensal bacteria as vectors for mucosal vaccines against sexually transmitted diseases: Vaginal colonisation with recombinant streptococci induces local and systemic antibodies in mice. *Vaccine* 15: 1330–1337.

Mercenier, A., Dutot, P., Kleinpeter, P., Aguirre, M., Paris, P., Reymund, J., and Slos, P. (1996). Development of lactic acid bacteria as live vectors for oral or local vaccines. *Advances in Food Science* 18: 73–77.

Mercenier, A., Müller-Alouf, H., and Grangette, C. (2000). Lactic acid bacteria as live vaccines. *Current Issues in Molecular Biology* 2: 17–25.

Mestecky, J., and McGhee, J. R. (1987). Immunoglobin A (IgA): Molecular and cellular interactions involved in IgA biosynthesis and immune response. *Advances in Immunology* 40: 153.

Michalek, S. M., Eldridge, J. H., Curtiss III, R., and Rosenthal, K. L. (1994). Antigen delivery systems: New approaches to mucosal immunization In: P. L. Ogra, M. D. Mestecky, M. E. Lamm, W. Strober, J. R. McGhee, and J. Bienenstock (Eds.), *Handbook of mucosal immunology* (pp. 373–390). San Diego: Academic Press Inc.

Michetti, P., Mahan, M. J., Slauch, J. M., Mekalanos, J. J., and Neutra, M. R. (1992). Monoclonal secretory immunoglobulin A protects mice against oral challenge with the invasive pathogen *Salmonella typhimurium. Infection and Immunity* 60: 1786.

Miettinen, M., Matikainen, S., Vuopio-Varkila, J., Pirhonen, J., Varkila, K., Kurimoto, M., and Julkunen, I. (1998). Lactobacilli and streptococci induce interleukin-12 (IL-12), IL-18, and gamma interferon production in human peripheral blood mononuclear cells. *Infection and Immunity* 66: 6058–6062.

Moore, W. E. C., and Holdeman, L. V. (1974). Human fecal flora: The normal flora of 20 Japanese-Hawaiians. *Applied Microbiology* 27: 961.

Mowat, A. M. (1985). The role of antigen recognition and suppressor cells in mice with oral tolerance to ovalbumin. *Immunology* 56: 253–260.

Mukamoto, M., Watanabe, I., Kobayashi, Y., Icatlo, F. C. J., Ishii, H., and Kodama, Y. (1991). Immunogenicity in Aujesky's disease virus structural glycoprotein gVI (gp50) in swine. *Veterinary Microbiology* 29: 109–121.

Müller-Alouf, H., Grangette, C., Goudercourt, D., Reveneau, N., and Mercenier, A. (1999). Comparative cytokine inducing pattern of lactic acid bacteria used for mucosal vaccine development. *Immunology Letters* 69: 33.

Nagler-Anderson, C. (2000). Tolerance and immunity in the intestinal immune system. *Critical Review of Immunology* 20: 103–120.

Nguyen, T. N., Hansson, M., Stahl, S., Bachi, T., Robert, A., Domzig, W., Binz, H., and Uhlen, M. (1993). Cell-surface display of heterologous epitopes on *Staphylococcus xylosus* as a potential delivery system for oral vaccination. *Gene* 128: 89–94.

Nicoletti, C. (2000). Unsolved mysteries of intestinal M cells. *Gut* 47: 735–739.

Norton, P. M., Brown, H. W. G., Wells, J. M., Macpherson, A. M., Wilson, P. W., and Le Page, R. W. F. (1996). Factors affecting the immunogenicity of tetanus toxin fragment C expressed in *Lactococcus lactis. FEMS Immunology and Medical Microbiology* 14: 167–177.

Norton, P. M., Le Page, R. W. F., and Wells, J. M. (1995). Progress in the development of *Lactococcus lactis* as a recombinant mucosal vaccine delivery system. *Folia Microbiologia* 40: 225–230.

Norton, P. M., Wells, J. W., Brown, H. W. G., Macpherson, A. M., and Le Page, R. W. F. (1997). Protection against tetanus toxin in mice nasally immunized with recombinant *Lactococcus lactis* expressing tetanus toxin fragment C. *Vaccine* 15: 616–619.

Oggioni, M. R., Manganelli, R., Contorni, M., Tommasino, M., and Pozzi, G. (1995). Immunization of mice by oral colonization with live recombinant commensal streptococci. *Vaccine* 13: 775–780.

Oggioni, M. R., Medaglini, D., Romano, L., Peruzzi, F., Maggi, T., Lozzi, L., Bracci, L., Zazzi, M., Wiesmuller, K. H., Manca, F., Valensin, P. E., and Pozzi, G. (1999). Immunogenicity and antigenicity of the V3 domain of HIV-1 gp120 expressed on the surface of *Streptococcus gordonii. AIDS Research Human Retroviruses* 15: 451–459.

O'Hagan, D. T. (1994). Oral immunization and the common mucosal immune system. In: D. T. O'Hagan (Ed.), *Novel delivery systems for oral vaccines* (pp. 1–24). Florida, USA: CRC Press, Inc.

Owen, R. L., Pierce, N. F., and Cray, W. C., Jr (1988). Effects of bacterial inactivation methods, toxin production, and oral immunization on uptake of *Vibrio cholerae* by Peyer's patch lymphoid follicles. In: S. Kuwahara, and N. F. Pierce (Eds.), *Advances in research on cholera and related diarrheas* (pp. 189–197). Tokyo: KTK Scientific Publishers.

Pappo, J., and Mahlman, R. T. (1993). Follicle epithelial M cells are a source of IL-1 in Peyer's patches. *Immunology* 78: 505–507.

Pavan, S., Hols, P., Delcour, J., Geoffroy, M. C., Grangette, C., Klerebezem, M., and Mercenier, A. (2000). Adaptation of the nisin-controlled expression system in *Lactobacillus plantarum*: A tool to study *in vivo* biological effects. *Applied and Environmental Microbiology* 66: 4427–4432.

Pouwels, P. H., Leer, R. J., Shaw, M., Heijne den Bak-Glashouwer, M.-J., Tielen, F. D., Smit, E., Martinez, B., Jore, J., and Conway, P. L. (1998). Lactic acid bacteria as antigen delivery vehicles for oral immunisation purposes. *International Journal of Food Microbiology* 41: 155–167.

Pouwels, P. H., Leer, R. J., and Boersma, W. J. A. (1996). The potential of *Lactobactillus* as a carrier for oral immunisation: Development and preliminary characterisation of vector systems for targeted delivery of antigens. *Journal of Biotechnology* 44: 183–192.

Pouwels, P. H., and Leer, R. J. (1993). Genetics of lactobacilli: plasmids and gene expression. *Antonie Van Leeuwenhoek* 64: 85–107.

Pozzi, G., and Oggioni, M. R. (1994). The human oral commensal *Streptococcus gordonii* as live vector for vaccines. In: A. Totolian (Ed.), *Pathogenic streptococci: present and future* (pp. 163–165). St Peterburg: Lancer Publications.

Pozzi, G., Oggioni, M. R., and Medaglini, D. (1997). Recombinant *Streptococcus gordonii* as a live vehicle for vaccine antigens. In: G. Pozzi and J. M. Wells (Eds.), *Gram-positive bacteria as vaccine vehicles for mucosal immunisation* (pp. 35–60). Berlin: Springer-Verlag.

Reid, G. (2000). Probiotic therapy and functional foods for prevention of urinary tract infections: state of the art and science. *Current Infectious Diseases Reports* 2: 518–522.

Rescigno, M., Citterio, C., Théry, M., Rittig, M., Medaglini, D., Pozzi, G., Amigorena, S., and Ricciardi-Castagnoli, P. (1998). Bacteria-induced neo-biosynthesis, stabilization, and surface expression of functional class I molecules in mouse dendritic cells. *Proceedings of the National Academy of Sciences USA* 95: 5229–5234.

Reveneau, N., Geoffroy, M.-C., Locht, C., Chagnaud, P., and Mercenier, A. (2002). Comparison of the immune responses induced by local immunizations with recombinant *Lactobacillus plantarum* producing tetanus toxin fragment C in different cellular locations. *Vaccine* 20: 1769–1777.

Ribeiro, L. A., Azevedo, V., Le Loir, Y., Oliveira, S. C., Dieye, Y., Piard, J. C., Gruss, A., and Langella, P. (2002). Production and targeting of the *Brucella abortus* antigen L7/L2 in *Lactococcus lactis*: A first step towards food-grade live vaccine against brucellosis. *Applied and Environmental Microbiology* 68: 910–916.

Ricci, S., Medaglini, D., Rush C. M., Marcello, A., Peppoloni, S., Manganelli, R., Palu, G., and Pozzi, G. (2000). Immunogenicity of the B monomer of *Escherichia coli* heat-labile toxin expressed on the surface of *Streptococcus gordonii*. *Infection and Immunity* 68: 760–776.

Roberts, M., Chatfield, S. N., and Dougan, G. (1994). *Salmonella* as carriers of heterologous antigens. In: D. T. O'Hagan (Ed.), *Novel delivery systems for oral vaccines* (pp. 27–58). Florida, USA: CRC Press Inc.

Robinson, K., Chamberlain, L. M., Schofield, K. M., Wells, J. M., and Le Page, R. W. F. (1997). Oral vaccination of mice against tetanus with recombinant *Lactococcus lactis*. *Nature Biotechnology* 15: 653–657.

Roos, S. (1999). Adhesion and autoaggregation of *Lactobacillus reuteri* and description of a new *Lactobacillus* species with mucus binding properties. PhD thesis, Swedish University of Agricultural Sciences, Uppsala, Sweden.

Rush, C. M., Mercenier, A., and Pozzi, G. (1997). Expression of vaccine antigens in *Lactobacillus*. In: G. Pozzi and J. M. Wells (Eds.), *Gram-positive bacteria as vaccine vehicles for mucosal immunisation* (pp. 107–144). Berlin: Springer-Verlag.

Sanderson, I. R., Ouellette, A. J., Carter, E. A., Walker, W. A., and Harmatz, P. R. (1993). Differential regulation of B7 mRNA in enterocytes and lymphoid cells. *Immunology* 79: 434–438.

Shanahan, F. (2000). Therapeutic Manipulation of Gut Flora. *Science* 289: 1311–1312.

Shaw, D. M., Gaerthé, B., Leer, R. J., Van der Stap, J. G. M. M., Smittenaar, C., Heijne den Bak-Glashouwer, M. J., Thole, J. E. R., Tielen, F. J., Pouwels, P. H., and Havenith, C. E. G. (2000). Engineering the micro-flora to vaccinate the mucosa: serum immunoglobulin G responses and activated draining cervical lymph nodes following mucosal application of tetanus toxin fragment C-expressing lactobacilli. *Immunology* 100: 510–518.

Sirard, J. C., Niedergang, F., and Kraehenbuhl, J. P. (1999). Live attenuated *Salmonella*: A paradigm of mucosal vaccines. *Immunology Review* 171: 5–26.

Stahl, S., Samuelson, P., Hansson, M., Andreoni, C., Goetsch, L., Libon, C., Liljeqvist, S., Gunneriusson, E., Binz, H., Nguyen, T. N., and Uhlen, M. (1997). Development of non-pathogenic staphylococci as vaccine delivery vehicles. In: G. Pozzi and J. M. Wells (Eds.), *Gram-positive bacteria as vaccine vehicles for mucosal immunisation* (pp. 61–81). Berlin: Springer-Verlag.

Steidler, L., Hans, W., Schotte, L., Neirynck, S., Obermeier, F., Falk, W., Fiers, W., and Remaut, E. (2000). Treatment of murine colitis by *Lactococcus lactis* secreting interleukin-10. *Science* 289: 1352–1355.

Steidler, L., Robinson, K., Chamberlain, L., Schofield, K. M., Remaut, E., Le Page, R. W. F., and Wells, J. M. (1998). Mucosal delivery of murine interkeukin-2 (IL-2) and IL-6 by recombinant strains of *Lactococcus lactis* coexpressing antigen and cytokine. *Infection and Immunity* 66: 3183–3189.

Stemmer, W. P., Crameri, A., Ha, K. D., Brennan, T. M., and Heyneker, H. L. (1995). Single-step assembly of a gene and entire plasmid from large numbers of oligodeoxyribonucleotides. *Gene* 164: 49–53.

Stoolman, L. M. (1989). Adhesion molecules controlling lymphocyte migration. *Cell* 56: 907.

Strobel, S., and Mowat, A. M. (1998). Immune responses to dietary antigens: oral tolerance. *Immunology Today* 19: 173–181.

Sutas, Y., Soppi, E., Korhonen, H., Syvaoja, E. L., Saxelin, M., Rokka, T., and Isolauri, E. (1996). Suppression of lymphocyte proliferation *in vitro* by bovine caseins hydrolyzed with *Lactobacillus casei* GG-derived enzymes. *Journal of Allergy and Clinical Immunology* 98: 216–224.

Takada, A., Shimizu, Y., and Kida, H. (1994). Protection of mice against Aujeszky's disease virus infection by intranasal vaccination with inactivated virus. *Journal of Veterinary Medical Science* 56: 633–637.

Taylor, H. P., and Dimmock, N. J. (1985). Mechanisms of neutralization of the influenza virus by secretory IgA is different from that of monomeric IgA or IgG. *Journal of Experimental Medicine* 161: 198.

Trapp, C. L., Chang, C. C., Halpern, G. M., Keen, C. L., and Gershwin, M. E. (1993). The influence of chronic yogurt consumption on populations of young and elderly adults. *International Journal of Immunotherapy* 9: 53–64.

Van de Water, J., Keen, C. L., and Gershwin, M. E. (1990). The influence of chronic yogurt consumption on immunity. *Journal of Nutrition* 129(7 Suppl): 1492S-5S.

Vesa, T., Pochart, P., and Marteau, P. (2000). Pharmacokinetics of *Lactobacillus plantarum* NCIMB 8826. *Lactobacillus fermentum* KLD, and *Lactococcus lactis* MG 1363 in the human gastrointestinal tract. *Alimentary Pharmacology Therapies* 14: 823–828.

Walker, S. A., and Klaenhammer, T. R. (2001). Leaky *Lactococcus* cultures that externalize enzymes and antigens independently of culture lysis and secretion and export pathways. *Applied Environmental Microbiology* 67: 251–259.

Weiner, H. L., Miller, A., and Khoury, S. J. (1995). Treatment of autoimmune diseases by oral tolerance to autoantigens. *Advanced Experimental Medical Biology* 371B: 1217–1223.

Wells, J. M., Norton, P. M., and Le Page, R. W. F. (1995). Progress in the development of mucosal vaccines based on *Lactococcus lactis*. *International Dairy Journal* 5: 1071–1079.

Wells, J. M., and Pozzi, G. (1997). An overview of Gram-positive bacteria as vaccine vehicles for musocal immunization. In: G. Pozzi and J. M. Wells (Eds.), *Gram-positive bacteria as vaccine vehicles for mucosal immunisation* (pp. 1–8). Berlin: Springer-Verlag.

Wells, J. M., Robinson, K., Chamberlain, L. M., Schofield, K. M., and Le Page, R. W. F. (1996). Lactic acid bacteria as vaccine delivery vehicles. *Anton van Leeuwenhoek* 70: 317–330.

Wells, J. M., and Schofield, K. M. (1996). Cloning and expression vectors for lactococci. In: T. F. Bozoglu and R. Bibek (Eds.), *Lactic acid bacteria: Current advances in metabolism, genetics, and applications* (pp. 37–62). NATO ASI Series Vol H 98. Heidelberg: Springer-Verlag.

Wells, J. M., Wilson, P. W., and Le Page, R. W. (1993a). Improved cloning vectors and transformation procedure for *Lactococcus*. *Journal of Applied Bacteriology* 74: 629–636.

Wells, J. M., Wilson, P. W., Norton, P. M., Gasson, M. J., and Le Page, R. W. F. (1993b). *Lactococcus lactis*: High-level expression of tetanus toxin fragment C and protection against lethal challenge. *Molecular Microbiology* 8: 1155–1162.

Wells, J. M., Wilson, P. W., Norton, P. M., and Le Page, R. W. (1993c). A model system for the investigation of heterologous protein secretion pathways in *Lactococcus lactis*. *Applied Environmental Microbiology* 59: 3954–3959.

Winner, L., Mack, J., Weltzin, R. A., Mekalanos, J. J., Kraehenbuhl, J. P., and Neutra, M. R. (1991). New model for analysis of mucosal immunity: Intestinal secretion of monoclonal immunoglobulin A from hybridoma tumors protects against *Vibrio cholerae* infection. *Infection and Immunity* 59: 977.

Wold, A. E., Dahlgren, U. I. H., Hanson, L. A., Mattsby-Baltzer, I., and Midvetdt, T. (1989). Difference between bacterial and food antigens in mucosal immunogenicity. *Infection and Immunity* 57: 2666–2673.

Yasui, H., Shida, K., Matsuzaki, T., and Yokokura, T. (1999). Immunomodulatory function of lactic acid bacteria. *Antonie Van Leeuwenhoek* 76: 383–389.

Yoshida, T., Hachimura, S., and Kaminogawa, S. (1997). The oral administration of low-dose antigen induces activation followed by tolerization, while high-dose antigen induces tolerance without activation. *Clinical Immunological Immunopathology* 82: 207–215.

10

The Genetics of Phage Resistance in *Lactococcus lactis*

Shirley A. Walker and Todd R. Klaenhammer

Summary

Because of the nature of the cheese fermentation process, bacteriophage problems continue to appear in the Cheddar cheese industry, resulting in slowed or failed fermentation tanks and substantial economic losses. Extensive research in this area has lead to a vast accumulation of genetic information on *Lactococcus lactis*, the mechanisms by which it protects itself from phage attack, the phages themselves, and the phage–host interactions. This body of information has not only yielded a greater understanding of the natural defense mechanisms of *Lc. lactis*, but has also allowed for the development of novel, genetically engineered defense strategies. This chapter will address important aspects of phage resistance in *Lc. lactis*, both natural and novel. The means by which phages overcome these mechanisms will also be highlighted to illustrate the dynamic nature of phage–host interactions in the cheese environment. In addition, the continuing need to elevate the platform of knowledge of these model phage–host relationships will be emphasized, in our efforts to stay one step ahead of the dynamic evolutionary and adaptive ability of bacteriophages in fermentation environments.

Introduction

Lactococcus lactis is an industrially important member of the lactic acid bacteria (LAB) used widely in the fermentation of dairy products, including sour cream, buttermilk, and various cheeses such as cheddar. In addition to its role in these important food fermentations, its long history of safe use in the food industry and generally recognized as safe (GRAS) status affords *Lc. lactis* the potential to play an even greater role in food biotechnology. The ever-expanding knowledge of the molecular genetics of *Lactococcus*,

Shirley A. Walker and Todd R. Klaenhammer • Department of Food Science, North Carolina State University, Campus Box 7624, Raleigh, North Carolina 27695-7624, USA; e-mail: klaenhammer@ncsu.edu

including the development of cloning vectors and efficient transformation procedures, chromosomal integration methods, and efficient, regulatable, expression systems, has opened the door to the creation of specialized lactococcal strains. One look at the chapters in this book illustrates the growing importance of this important microorgansim. A significant problem encountered with *Lactococcus* has been its susceptibility to bacteriophage, which can lead to slow acid development and decreased turnover of dairy product in the processing plant. In fact, phage infection remains a major cause of slow acid production in dairy fermentations (Sanders, 1987). Highly specialized strains developed for specific functions using biotechnology are especially vulnerable since repeated use can allow the accumulation of phages capable of attacking the strain, greatly limiting its long-term usefulness in industry. It is not surprising, then, that the current utilization of this important microorganism in the food industry, coupled with the extensive research being conducted on expanding its uses, has placed greater demands on starter culture manufacturers to find ways to protect their valuable lactococcal strains from phage attack.

This review is intended to overview current research dealing with the genetics of phage resistance mechanisms, both natural and genetically engineered, in *Lc. lactis*. In some cases, relevant research regarding phage resistance in *Streptococcus thermophilus* will also be addressed, since increasing use of this microorganism in thermophilic dairy fermentations, especially mozzarella cheese, has lead to increased bacteriophage problems. While significant advances have been made in the study of bacteriophage genetics and speciation, these issues will not be covered in this review unless pertinent to phage resistance. For detailed coverage on bacteriophage genetics, the reader is referred to Chapter 3.

Natural Host-Encoded Phage Resistance Mechanisms

In response to the diverse populations of phages present in mesophilic dairy fermentations, *Lactococcus* species have developed a number of defense mechanisms, many of them plasmid encoded, to inhibit the proliferation of bacteriophages. Some of these mechanisms are encoded on conjugative plasmids or are associated with insertion elements, which promotes their dissemination to other lactococcal strains. These natural host defense mechanisms fall into four major categories: bacteriophage adsorption inhibition, inhibition of phage DNA injection, restriction/modification (R/M), and abortive (Abi) mechanisms. These mechanisms have been extensively reviewed (Hill, 1993; Klaenhammer and Fitzgerald, 1994; Dinsmore and Klaenhammer, 1995; Garvey et al., 1995b; Daly et al., 1996; Allison and Klaenhammer, 1998). The following section will cover the major advances, with an emphasis on more recent studies, made in each of these areas and how they might be utilized in the rational design of phage-insensitive strains. Additionally, advances made in the understanding of how phages overcome these defense mechanisms will be discussed, since this will be a critical component of our continuing efforts to maximize phage resistance while minimizing the evolution of new phages.

Bacteriophage Adsorption Inhibition

Since phage adsorption is the first step in the phage infection cycle, adsorption inhibition represents one of the first natural lines of defense in lactococcal starter cultures, as well as one of the least characterized of the phage defense mechanisms. The isolation of bacteriophage insensitive mutants (BIMs), altered in their ability to adsorb different phages, remains an important strategy used by starter culture companies to maintain phage resistant derivatives of important lactococcal strains (reviewed by Klaenhammer and Fitzgerald, 1994; Daly et al., 1996). Many of these BIMs result from chromosomal mutations that alter or mask phage cell–surface receptors, and are often unstable due to reversion of the phenotype. However, the study of BIMs has offered some insight into this defense mechanism. For example, by studying a non-adsorbing *Lc. lactis* mutant, Valyasevi et al. (1990) found that a rhamnose component of the extracellular wall polysaccharide was important for the binding of phages kh and ml3 to *Lc. lactis* KH. In addition, they found that galactose was also important for binding of five phages. In another example, Gopal and Crow (1993) found that differences in the loosely associated material (LAM) of *Lc. lactis* subsp. *cremoris* E8 and its phage-resistant mutant 398 were responsible for the inability of the phage to adsorb to strain 398. The LAM of strain 398 was more abundant, contained five times more rhamnose, two times more galactose, and lacked a 21 kDa protein.

While the two examples cited above highlight the importance of cell wall components in phage adsorption, Geller et al. (1993) identified a cell membrane receptor for phage ϕc2 (c2 species). Using a complementation strategy in a mutant no longer able to adsorb ϕc2, they found that a 99.4 kDa membrane protein, encoded by *pip*, was responsible for the adsorption of ϕc2 and other members of the c2 species to *Lc. lactis* C2. Pip, which represents the only phage receptor to be characterized at the molecular level, contains four to six possible membrane spanning regions and a putative secretion signal in the amino terminus. Homologs to *pip* have also been identified in many other strains of *Lc. lactis* (Geller et al., 1993). In addition to Pip, Valyasevi et al. (1991) also identified a 32-kDa membrane protein important for the infectivity of both ϕc2 and sk1. The protein works as part of a 350-kDa membrane complex. In this case, however, phage adsorption is normal, but the efficiency of plaquing (EOP) is severely inhibited. Hill (1993) has suggested that the 32-kDa membrane protein might be involved in DNA injection. To date, the relationship between Pip and the 32 kDa proteins is unknown.

A number of plasmids which encode adsorption inhibition phenotypes have also been identified. The first such plasmid, pME0030, was identified by Sanders and Klaenhammer (1983) and was found to significantly reduce the adsorption efficiency of ϕ18 to its host. de Vos et al. (1984) found that pSK112 was responsible for the adsorption inhibition phenotype of the phage-resistant strain SK110. By comparing cell wall components of SK110 and the cured, phage-sensitive derivative SK112, they found that the lipotechoic acid (LTA) in the cell wall fraction of SK110 contained galactose, while the LTA in SK112 did not (Sijtsma et al., 1990). The galactosyl-containing component probably acts by steric hindrance, shielding the phage receptors so that attachment cannot occur. Plasmid pCI528 from *Lc. lactis* UC503 has been shown to give complete resistance to prolate and small isometric phages and is responsible for a "fluffy" phenotype when pelleted by centrifugation (Lucey et al., 1992). Analysis of the cell surface polysaccharides detected greater levels of galactose and rhamnose in the plasmid-containing strain than in the plasmid-cured derivative. Electron microscopy showed a thick, irregularly distributed extracellular substance, and mild alkali treatment of the plasmid-containing host restored phage adsorption and phage sensitivity, indicating that the polysaccharide extracellular substance probably acted by shielding the phage receptor. Recently, Forde et al. (1999) identified another plasmid in *Lc. lactis* subsp. *cremoris* HO2 which displayed an adsorption inhibition phenotype, providing complete protection against ϕ712 and partial protection against ϕc2. As with pCI528, this plasmid was also responsible for a "fluffy" phenotype upon centrifugation. Harrington and Hill (1992) identified a unique adsorption inhibition phenotype while studying a phage-insensitive mutant isolated after infection with ϕD1. While the strain was still able to adsorb ϕD1 at normal levels, it adsorbed phage c2 less efficiently than the parental strain. Characterization identified a 26.75-kb plasmid, pAH90, not present in the parent. The plasmid was found to be a cointegrate of the two parental plasmids, pAH82 and pAH33, neither of which displayed an adsorption inhibition phenotype. Cointegration therefore activated a silent adsorption inhibition phenotype. To date, the molecular mechanisms behind the adsorption inhibition phenotypes encoded on the plasmids described above have not been characterized.

While the above studies are an important start in the understanding of phage adsorption, further work is required to characterize this important phage defense strategy. Since phage adsorption is the initial step in the phage infection cycle, an understanding of its mechanisms and ways to prevent it will be important in the development of strains with resistance mechanisms that act at different points in the lytic cycle. While in many cases the adsorption inhibition phenotype is highly host–phage specific, some do act on a broader spectrum of phages and would be more widely applicable. For example, the extensive molecular characterization of Pip, the receptor for ϕc2 and other prolate phages, has lead to the development of a novel phage defense mechanism effective against members of the industrially significant c2 species (Garbutt et al., 1997). This mechanism, described in the section on novel mechanisms for phage defense, represents an important application of fundamental information regarding phage adsorption.

Inhibition of Phage DNA Injection

In a few instances, phage adsorption to the cell is normal, but phage DNA penetration is inhibited. The first example of this defense mechanism was described in *Lactobacillus casei* YIT9002, where electron microscopy showed that phage PL-1 adsorbed normally to the host, but DNA was not injected (Watanabe et al., 1984). More recently, Garvey et al. (1996) identified a third phage defense mechanism on the lactococcal plasmid pNP40 in addition to the two abortive infection mechanisms, AbiE and AbiF, described below. While AbiF alone reduced the EOP of phage ϕc2 to 10^{-4}, pNP40 completely blocked ϕc2 plaque formation (Garvey et al., 1996). In addition, pNP40 increased the survival rate of the lactococcal host to 90%, a feature not indicative of abortive infection alone. Further study showed that while pNP40+ cells adsorbed phage ϕc2 normally, no phage DNA could be detected in the cell until late into the infection cycle (30 min as opposed to 5 min for the control), indicating that DNA injection was impaired or delayed. Electroporation of phage ϕc2 DNA into pNP40+ cells, however, resulted in a significant increase in the number of successful infection centers. The authors concluded that pNP40 contained an early-acting phage defense mechanism that inhibited DNA injection (Garvey et al., 1996). Lastly, Akcelik (1998) recently reported that *Lc. lactis* subsp. *lactis* PLM-18 adsorbed phage la2 normally, but inhibited its DNA injection. The mechanism appeared to be chromosomally encoded. To date, none of these examples have been studied on a molecular level. However, Garvey et al. (1996) have speculated that a gene product of pNP40 may possibly interact with one of two membrane proteins, Pip or a 32-kDa protein, known to be involved in the interaction of ϕc2 with the host cell membrane. While further work is required to fully understand the molecular mechanism behind this natural phage-defense strategy, the inhibition of DNA injection represents another powerful weapon in the phage defense arsenal of *Lc. lactis*.

Restriction/Modification Mechanisms

Restriction/modification (R/M) mechanisms are widely distributed in *Lactococcus* and protect the cell from bacteriophage infection by restricting the foreign DNA. The majority of these R/M systems are plasmid encoded, and were identified in *Lc. lactis* using host-dependent replication of phages. R/M systems act early in the phage infection cycle and thus do not severely impact cell viability (reviewed by Klaenhammer and Fitzgerald, 1994). Therefore, restriction/modification can be a powerful phage defense mechanism, restricting the EOPs of sensitive phages anywhere from 10^{-1} to 10^{-6}. However, a small proportion of phages can escape restriction and become modified. These phages would thus be able to proliferate unrestricted, resulting in increased titers of phage in the environment. Phages may also be able to overcome an R/M system in other ways (reviewed by Klaenhammer and Fitzgerald, 1994). For example, the phage genome may possess a gene encoding for an antirestriction protein or for its own methylase. Alternatively, phages may escape restriction by reducing/eliminating the number of recognition sites in the phage genome. A novel escape mechanism was described by Hill et al. (1991a), who found that phage ϕ50 (P335 species) had acquired the amino domain of the *Lla*I methylase, along with its expression signals, by recombination with pTR2030. This phage was able to methylate its own genome and was no longer sensitive to the R/M mechanism present on this plasmid. The ability of phages to overcome R/M systems, along with the diversity of phages often present in the processing environment, is undoubtedly partly responsible for the wide distribution of R/M systems, alone or in combination with other R/M or phage defense systems, in the dairy lactococci.

Three main classes of R/M systems are recognized (reviewed by Bickle and Kruger, 1993). Type I systems require three subunits (*hsd*R, a restriction subunit; *hsd*M, a modification subunit; and *hsd*S, a specificity subunit) which, when complexed, cleave the DNA a far distance from an asymmetrical recognition site. Type II systems require a separate enzyme for restriction and modification, each capable of recognizing the restriction site. DNA cleavage occurs within a symmetrical recognition site. Type IIS systems are a subclass of Type II systems, except that cleavage occurs at a fixed distance from an assymetrical recognition site. Lastly, Type III systems also involve two genes, a restriction gene and a modification gene. Cleavage occurs only when the two enzymes are complexed at a fixed distance from an assymetrical recognition site. To date, examples of each R/M type have been identified in *Lc. lactis* strains.

By far, type II R/Ms represent the most commonly identified R/M systems in *Lactococcus*. To date, eight Type II systems have been characterized, either biochemically or genetically, in *Lc. lactis*. Basic characteristics are listed in Table 10.1. For more detailed information, the reader is referred to Table 4 in Allison and Klaenhammer (1998). In most cases, the R/M systems consist of two enzymes, a restriction endonuclease and a methylase. However, three of the R/M systems are unique in that they contain two methylases: *Lla*A1 (Nyengaard et al., 1995), *Lla*DCH1 (Moineau et al., 1995a), and *Scr*F1 (Davis et al., 1993). The reason behind this is not known. For *Scr*F1, Twomey et al. (1997) have suggested that two methylases might counteract the degeneracy of the recognition site in certain sequence contexts. For *Lla*DCH1 (Moineau et al., 1995a), the two methylases (M.*Lla*IIA and M.*Lla*IIB) show significant homology to the two methylases of the isoschizomer, *Dpn*II, of *Streptococcus pneumoniae* (M.*Dpn*II and M.*Dpn*A, respectively). While M.*Dpn*II modifies only double stranded DNA, M.*Dpn*A methylates both single- and double-stranded DNA, and may be involved in facilitating the natural transfer of plasmid DNA between two strains

Table 10.1. Restriction/Modification Systems of *Lactococcus lactis* and *Streptococcus thermophilus*

Designation (Identified on)	Type	Restriction Site[a]	Methylase Type	ϕ's affected	Reference
Lactococcus lactis					
*Scr*F1 chromosome	II	CC/NGG	Two m^5C	c2 species	Davis et al. (1993) Twomey et al. (1993) Twomey et al. (1997)
*Lla*I pTR2030	IIS	Unknown	N^6A	P335 species	Hill et al. (1989a) Hill et al. (1991a) O'Sullivan et al. (1995) O'Sullivan and Klaenhammer (1998)
*Lla*A1 pFW094	II	/GATC	m^6A		Nyengaard et al. (1993) Nyengaard et al. (1995)
*Lla*BI pJW563	II	C/TRYAG	m^6A	936 and c2 species	Nyengaard et al. (1993) Nyengaard et al. (1995) Nyengaard et al. (1996)
*Lla*DII pHW393	II	Unknown	Unknown	936 and c2 species	Madsen and Josephsen (1998)
*Lla*DCHI pSRQ700	II	/GATC	Two m^6A	936, c2, and P335 species	Moineau et al. (1995a) Moineau et al. (1995b)
*Lla*497I	II	CC/WGG	Unknown		Mayo et al. (1991)
*Lla*KR2I pKR223	II	/GATC	m^5c	936 species ϕsk1	Twomey et al. (1998) McKay et al. (1989)
*Lla*CI	II	A/AGCTT			Josephsen et al. (1998)
*Lla*1403I pIL26143	IC	Unknown	N^6A	ϕbIL170	Schouler et al. (1998a)
Lla chromosomal	IC	Unknown	N^6A	bIL67	Schouler et al. (1998b)
*S.Lla*W12I pAW122	IC	Unknown			Madsen et al. (2000)
S.Lla PCIS3	I	Unknown			Seegers et al. (2000)
S.Lla PCIS1	I	Unknown			Seegers et al. (2000)
S.Lla chromosomal	I	Unknown			Seegers et al. (2000)
*Lla*F1 pND801	III	Unknown		Isometric phage ϕ712	Su et al. (1999)
Streptococcus thermophilus					
*Sth*134I chromosomal	II	C/CGG	Unknown		Solaiman and Somkuti (1990)
*Sth*117I chromosomal	II	CC/WGG	Unknown		Solaiman and Somkuti (1991)
*Ssl*I chromosomal	II	CC/WGG	Unknown		Benbadis et al. (1991)
*Sth*455I chromosomal	II	CC/WGG	Unknown		Guimont et al. (1993)
*Sth*132I chromosomal	IIS	CCCG(N_4)/ GGGC(N_8)	Unknown		Poch et al. (1997)

With the exception of data for *Lla*C1, *Lla*KR2I, and *Lla*F1, the information in this table is condensed from Table 4 in Allison and Klaenhammer (1998).

[a]"/" site of cleavage; N = any nucleotide; W = A or T; R = G or A; Y = C or T; *S.Lla* represents a specificity subunit only.

by methylating the incoming single-stranded DNA (Lacks et al., 1991). Moineau et al. (1995a) speculated that M.*Lla*IIB may have a similar function in *Lc. lactis*.

Moineau et al. (1995a) also point out another interesting feature of the *Dpn*II system of *Streptococcus pneumoniae*. In contrast to *Dpn*II, some strains carry a complementary R/M system, *Dpn*I, which acts on methylated DNA (Lacks and Greenberg, 1977). Therefore, if phages escape the *Dpn*II system in one strain by becoming methylated, they will be restricted by the *Dpn*I system present in another strain. The authors speculate that a *Dpn*I-like system might be harbored by some lactococcal strains, but remains undetected by the use of unmodified phages in identifying R/M systems. They suggest that using modified phages to search for such a complementary system might be useful in increasing phage protection, since a major problem with R/M systems is the modification and subsequent proliferation of some of the infecting phages. *Lactococcus* has developed a number of ways to protect itself from this phenomenon, including the presence of multiple R/M systems or the presence of multiple phage resistance mechanisms in general. It is, therefore, not unlikely that a *Dpn*I-like system exists in certain cultures.

One Type IIS R/M system, *Lla*I, was identified on pTR2030 from the prototype *Lc. lactis* strain ME2 (Hill et al., 1989a). Although the methylase of *Lla*I (M.*Lla*I) shows considerable homology to the type IIS methylases of the *Fok*I and *Sts*I systems (Hill et al., 1991a), the *Lla*I R/M system is novel in that restriction requires three genes: *llaI.1, llaI.2*, and *llaI*.3, and therefore has similarities to the type I R/M systems (O'Sullivan et al., 1995). In addition to the genes encoding for restriction and modification, the *Lla*I operon also contains a gene, *llaI.C*, which encodes for a regulatory factor similar to other regulatory proteins involved in type II R/Ms (O'Sullivan and Klaenhammer, 1998). When provided *in trans*, C.*Lla*I enhances the restriction efficiency of *Lla*I. Subsequent study showed that C.*Lla*I did not increase transcription of the *Lla*I operon, but rather worked at the post-transcriptional level. Significant homology between C.*Lla*I and the Rop protein of *E. coli* suggests that C.*Lla*I might act by stabilizing the *llaI* mRNA (O'Sullivan and Klaenhammer, 1998). The presence of a helix-turn-helix motif, found in many proteins capable of binding nucleic acids, in C.*Lla*I strengthens this view. Interestingly, growth of cultures at 40°C completely abolished the enhancement of restriction by C.*Lla*I, thereby providing a possible molecular explanation for the increased phage sensitivity of many lactococcal strains at elevated temperatures.

Schouler et al. (1998a,b) recently described two type IC R/M systems in *Lc. lactis* IL1403: one encoded on plasmid pIL26143 (*lla1403I*; Schouler et al., 1998a) and a second one chromosomally encoded (Schouler et al., 1998b). In addition, they found that some plasmids encoded only the *hsd*S (specificity) subunit (Schouler et al., 1998b). These *hsdS* genes were able to interact with the host-encoded *hsdR* and *hsdM* genes to alter the specificity of restriction, a phenomenon they termed combinational variation. This combinational variation could enhance the resistance of *Lactococcus* to bacteriophages in the environment by allowing the acquistion of novel specificities. Schouler et al. (1998b) also suggested that the use of a single subunit to confer specificity on both restriction and modification functions would allow type I R/M systems to evolve more rapidly, possibly allowing *Lc. lactis* to adapt fairly quickly to evolving bacteriophage.

Two other recent studies appear to confirm the importance of combinational variation to enhanced phage resistance. Seegers et al. (2000) identified three *hsd*S genes in *Lc. lactis* UC509.9, two on separate plasmids and one on the chromosome. Madsen et al. (2000) identified an *hsd*S gene encoding the type 1C *S.Lla*W12I specificity subunit in *Lc. lactis* W12, which, together with the complete type I R/M system, conferred increased phage resistance to the host.

Another interesting feature of the plasmid-encoded type IC systems described above was their proximity to, and perhaps linkage within operons encoding for replication functions. Schouler et al. (1998b) suggested that this location could increase plasmid stability by post-segregational killing of plasmid-free cells. Such a function was recently shown for type II R/M systems (Kulakauskas et al., 1995; Naito et al., 1995). In addition, this localization near replication genes suggests that the plasmid-encoded, type IC R/M systems may be activated under stress conditions, possibly including phage infection (Schouler et al., 1998a).

The most recent addition to the lactococcal R/M family was *Lla*FI, the only type III R/M system to be identified in *Lc. lactis*, and in Gram-positive bacteria in general (Su et al., 1999). This review will not cover the details of this system in detail. However, its identification clearly illustrates the diversity of R/M systems harbored by *Lc. lactis* starter cultures in response to the diverse bacteriophage population encountered in the processing plants, since examples of all three R/M types have now been described in this microorganism. Continued study of R/M systems will be an important aspect of developing highly resistant lactococcal starter strains, since these systems can be systematically combined with each other and with other phage resistance mechanisms (see Stacking of Phage Defense Mechanisms below).

Although not much is known about the genetics of R/M systems in *Streptococcus thermophilus*, five R/M systems have been identified and partially characterized (Table 10.1). Four of these R/Ms are type II systems, including *Sth*134I (Solaiman and Somkuti, 1990), *Sth*117I (Solaiman and Somkuti, 1991), *Ssl*I (Benbadis et al., 1991), and *Sth*455I (Guimont et al., 1993). One type IIS system was also identified, *Sth*132I (Poch et al., 1997). In all cases, the R/M systems are chromosomally encoded, although the genetics have not been determined. In addition to these R/M systems, Moineau et al. (1995b) reported that the type II lactococcal R/M system *Lla*DCHI was functional when expressed from its own promoter in *Strep. thermophilus*, resulting in EOPs of 10^{-5}–10^{-8} when tested with several *Strep. thermophilus* phages isolated from cheese plants. A significant feature which allowed use of this enzyme in this thermophilic microorganism is that *Lla*DCHI, unlike many lactococcal R/M systems, is not sensitive to elevated temperatures of 42°C (Moineau et al., 1995b). The finding that a lactococcal R/M system could be used effectively in *Strep. thermophilus* was significant, because it offered a way to expand the phage resistance of this increasingly important fermentation bacterium. One drawback, however, was that the base lactococcal plasmid containing *llaDCHI* did not replicate in *Strep. thermophilus*. Therefore, the *llaDCHI* operon was subcloned into a cloning vector capable of replicating in this organism. Further work is needed to make the system food grade, and even then, regulatory issues must be addressed in order to utilize a lactococcal gene in *Strep. thermophilus*.

Abortive Infection

Abortive infection mechanisms operate after phage adsorption and DNA injection and are generally characterized by a decrease in the burst size of the phage, an increase in the latent period, a decrease in the number of centers of infection, and a high death rate for the host cell (reviewed by Klaenhammer and Fitzgerald, 1994; Allison and Klaenhammer, 1998). These characteristics make abortive mechanisms very powerful against phage proliferation, since the release of progeny phage is diminished or eliminated. It is unclear whether death of the cell results from the resistance mechanism itself or from irreversible effects of the phage infection cycle that redirect cell functions. Either way, cell death before the development or release of phage progeny can act as an effective trap to prevent the build up of phage in the culture medium.

To date, 16 genes encoding abortive mechanisms have been identified in *Lc. lactis*. The basic characteristics of each Abi mechanism are listed in Table 10.2. For more comprehensive information, consult the recent review by Allison and Klaenhammer (1998). In addition, an undesignated abortive mechanism has been identified on the plasmid pMRC01 (Ryan et al., 1996; Coakley et al., 1997). The majority of these genes are encoded on plasmids, and interestingly, with one exception (AbiN; Prevots et al., 1998), contain a lower GC content (23.9–29%) than the reported average GC content for *Lc. lactis* (37%) (Garvey et al., 1995b). The chromosomally encoded AbiN (34%) is interesting

Table 10.2 Abortive Infection (Abi) Mechanisms Identified in *Lactococcus lactis*

Designation	Phages Affected	Point of Action	Reference
AbiA pTR2030	936 species (sk1) P335 species (ϕ31) c2 species	At or before replication	Hill et al. (1989b) Hill et al. (1990b) Dinsmore and Klaenhammer (1997) Dinsmore et al. (1998)
AbiB pIL415	936 species (ϕbil70, ϕbil66)	Degradation of phage transcripts	Cluzel et al. (1991) Parreira et al. (1996)
AbiC pTN20	936 species P335 species	Unknown	Durmaz et al. (1992)
AbiD pBF61	936 species (sk1) c2 species	Unknown	McLandsborough et al. (1995)
AbiD1 pIL105	936 species (bIL66, bIL70) c2 species (c6A, bIL67)	Unknown	Bidnenko et al. (1995) Anba et al. (1995)
AbiE pNP40	936 species	No evidence of DNA packaging	Garvey et al. (1995a) Garvey et al. (1997)
AbiF pNP40	936 species (ϕ712) c2 species (c2)	Affects rate of DNA replication	Garvey et al. (1995a) Garvey et al. (1997)
AbiG pCI750	936 species (ϕ712) c2 species (c2)	Possibly phage transcription	O'Connor et al. (1996) O'Connor et al. (1999)
AbiH chromosomal	ϕ59 (isometric) ϕ53 (prolate)	Unknown	Prevots et al. (1996)
AbiI pND852	936 species (ϕ712) c2 species (c2)	No evidence of DNA packaging	Su et al. (1997)
AbiJ pND859	936 species (ϕ712)	Unknown	Deng et al. (1997)
AbiK	P335 species	Affects phage DNA replication	Emond et al. (1997)
PSRQ800	936 species c2 species	Affects phage DNA maturation	Boucher et al. (2000)
AbiL	936 species (ϕ712) c2 species (c2)	Unknown	Deng et al. (1999)
AbiN chromosomal	ϕ59 (sm. isometric) ϕ53 (prolate)	Unknown	Prevots et al. (1998)
AbiO pPF144	c2 species (ϕ53, c2) 936 species (ϕ59, ϕ712)	Unknown	Prevots and Ritzenthaler (1998)
AbiQ pSRQ900	936 species c2 species	No evidence of DNA packaging? Possibly head morphogenetic pathway	Emond et al. (1998)
AbiR PKR223	c2 species	Affects DNA replication	Twomey et al. (2000)

because it is present in an operon containing prophage genes (Prevots et al., 1998). In addition, most of the Abi mechanisms are encoded by a single gene. AbiE (Garvey et al., 1995a), AbiG (O'Connor et al., 1996), AbiL (Deng et al., 1999), and AbiR (Twomey et al., 2000) are exceptions, each requiring two genes usually arranged in an operon. AbiR is the first abortive system encoded by two separated genetic loci (Twomey et al., 2000). To date, none of the identified *abi* genes appear to be induced upon phage infection of the host. While AbiD, AbiD1, and AbiF share limited protein homology (26–47% identity), most Abi proteins show little to no homology to other proteins in the data bases, making deductions as to their mode of action somewhat difficult. Even protein homology may not reflect similar functions, however, as AbiF appears to affect phage DNA replication while AbiD and AbiD1 do not. In addition, Emond et al. (1997) found that while no protein homology was evident between AbiA and AbiK, amino acid composition analysis showed that they might belong to a similar family of proteins. Interestingly, AbiA and AbiK appear to act at similar points in the phage lytic cycle (see below).

Abortive mechanisms may act at a number of points in the phage infection cycle, including DNA replication, transcription, translation, regulation, or at some point in the morphogenetic pathway. While little is known about the exact molecular mechanism of action of the Abi proteins in *Lactococcus*, some information is available for a few of the Abi systems. Of the 17 Abi proteins studied to date, four are known to act at or before phage DNA replication: AbiA (Hill et al., 1991b), AbiF (Garvey et al., 1995a), AbiK (P335 phages; Emond et al., 1997), and AbiR (Twomey et al., 2000). In all cases, phage DNA replication was diminished or extremely retarded in the presence of these Abi proteins, although the exact mechanism of DNA replication inhibition is not known. However, Dinsmore and Klaenhammer (1997) have identified two regions on the phage ϕ31 (P335 species) genome responsible for the action of AbiA on this bacteriophage: an early expressed open reading frame (ORF245) and an intergenic region between two additional ORFs, ORF71 and ORF169, both of which lie upstream of ORF245. The study of two AbiA resistant (AbiA^R) phage ϕ31 derivatives, ϕ31A and ϕ31B, identified point mutations in each of these regions, respectively (Dinsmore and Klaenhammer, 1997). Furthermore, expression of the mutant ORF245 identified from ϕ31A *in trans* reduced the sensitivity of ϕ31 to AbiA. The presence of the 118 bp fragment containing the intergenic region between ORF71 and ORF169, either from the wildtype ϕ31 or from ϕ31B, *in trans* also severely decreased the sensitivity of ϕ31 to AbiA. This 118 bp fragment did not contain any complete ORFs, and it was found that the DNA fragment itself was responsible for the reduced effectiveness of AbiA, suggesting that AbiA, alone or in combination with a phage-encoded factor, binds this intergenic region. Since this 118 bp fragment did not reduce AbiA activity on phage ul36 (P335 species), sk1 (936 species), or c2 (c2 species, prolate), AbiA probably requires a phage-encoded protein to mediate its actions (Dinsmore and Klaenhammer, 1997). The exact mechanism involved in the interaction between AbiA and these two regions of ϕ31 remains to be determined. Dinsmore et al. (1998) have identified a leucine zipper and an adjacent basic region in AbiA, which were critical to its action against representative phages of all three industrially important species. The presence of a leucine zipper suggests that AbiA may act as a dimer or heterodimer, interacting with itself or with a phage-encoded protein. The fact that a basic region associated with a leucine zipper (B-zip) represents an important motif involved in DNA binding suggests that AbiA may act by binding phage DNA, possibly in the 118-bp intergenic region.

Bidnenko et al. (1995) also took advantage of spontaneously appearing phage bil66 mutants resistant to AbiD1 to study its mode of action. They found that a 1.33 kb DNA fragment from the mutant phages would allow the growth of AbiD1^S phages in AbiD1$^+$ cells when provided *in trans*. Molecular characterization of the fragment, which contained four ORFs, identified point mutations in ORF1 which were partly responsible for the observed phenotype. ORF3 was also found to be critical, since expression of ORF3 on a high-copy-number vector *in trans* was able to overcome the effects of AbiD1 on phage bil66. The current theory is that AbiD1 interacts with ORF1 to decrease the levels of ORF3 below that required for normal phage development. This repression of ORF3 levels was not at the level of transcription. AbiD1 may therefore act to prevent translation of ORF3 or to inactivate the ORF3 product. The presence of two helix-turn-helix motifs in AbiD1 points to a possible ability to bind DNA or RNA to exert its actions.

Lastly, Rince et al. (2000) identified a 324-bp fragment from the phage sk1(AbiF insensitive) genome which reduced the effectiveness of AbiF on sensitive phage 712. Molecular analysis of the region suggested that AbiF might act on the *cos* ends of sensitive small isometric phages.

Two other abortive mechanisms, AbiB (Parreira et al., 1996) and AbiG (O'Connor et al., 1999), have been found to affect the level of phage RNA transcripts. AbiB results in the decay of early, middle, and late sensitive phage transcripts within 10–15 min of infection, resulting in the accumulation of transcripts of about 200 bp (Parreira et al., 1996). The degradation products result from endonucleolytic cleavage preferentially at U/U, A/U, and U/A sites. The authors speculate that AbiB may act by having latent RNase activity, which is stimulated by a phage product, by interacting with an early phage product to activate a bacterial RNase, or by activating a phage-encoded RNase. AbiG, on the other hand, appears to act by inhibiting phage sk1 and late c2 RNA synthesis (O'Connor et al., 1999). However, it has not been fully determined whether or not transcription is the primary target of AbiG.

The point in the phage lytic cycle at which the remainder of the abortive systems act is currently unknown. However, since phage DNA accumulates in many of these Abi+ hosts at a normal rate, including AbiC (Durmaz et al., 1992; Moineau et al., 1993b), AbiE (Garvey et al., 1995a), AbiI (Su et al., 1997), and AbiQ (Emond et al., 1998), they must act at a point later than phage replication. In the case of AbiE, AbiI, AbiK (936 species; Boucher et al., 2000), and AbiQ, the replicated phage DNA does not appear to be packaged. While no evidence exists that AbiE and AbiI actually affect phage DNA packaging, some evidence does suggest that AbiQ may exhibit this mode of action. Emond et al. (1998) showed that AbiQ is active against members of the 936 and c2 phage species and results in the accumulation of immature, concatemeric phage DNA. AbiQ, therefore, appears to prevent the cleavage of the concatemers. Although the molecular mechanism was not determined, the authors speculate that AbiQ may target the head morphogenetic pathway of the phage. This argument was strengthened by an observed limited amino acid homology between the λ gpA (terminase) and gpB (head–tail connector) analogues of c2-like and 936-like phages, suggesting that AbiQ could interact with one of these phage products and have similar effects on both groups of phages (Emond et al., 1998). In addition, AbiK also appears to prevent DNA maturation in the 936-like phages, as only immature forms of phage DNA were found (Boucher et al., 2000). Interestingly, AbiK appears to impact the 936 and P335 phages differently.

Abortive mechanisms are a powerful weapon in the phage defense arsenal, since they can act at different points in the phage infection cycle and can inhibit the proliferation of phages which escape the earlier acting defense systems. However, as with most of the defense systems described in this chapter, phages are often able to overcome abortive systems used as the sole defense mechanism. Two examples of point mutations that resulted in a phage's loss of sensitivity to an abortive system were described above for AbiA (Dinsmore and Klaenhammer, 1997) and AbiD1 (Bidnenko et al., 1995). In addition, presentation of AbiA (Dinsmore and Klaenhammer, 1994), AbiC (Moineau et al., 1994), and AbiK (Bouchard and Moineau, 2000) on high-copy number vectors resulted in insensitive, recombinant phages which had recombined with the host genome. In the case of AbiA, the recombinant phages were also found to be resistant to *per31* (see below), suggesting that recombination leads to the replacement of the phage φ31 origin of replication (*ori*). With AbiK, recombination also resulted in a new *ori* in one of the mutant phages.

The continued study of abortive defense mechanisms will be an important component of the development of phage-resistant strains. The study of mutant and recombinant phages can lead to a better understanding of the molecular mechanisms behind the abortive phenotype, as well as elucidate the means phages use to circumvent their action. Increased information on the actual mechanism of defense will aid in the design of more effective phage defense strategies. In addition, study of the regulation of genes encoding abortive mechanisms could lead to effective ways to increase the efficiency of these systems. A few examples of increasing abortive activity already exist. For many of the systems, including AbiA (Dinsmore and Klaenhammer, 1994), AbiC (Durmaz and Klaenhammer, 1995), and AbiK (Emond et al., 1997), increasing copy number has lead to increased efficiency of the system. In other cases, such as AbiD1 (Anba et al., 1995) and AbiN (Prevots et al., 1998), high levels of expression may be toxic for *L. lactis*. Interestingly, AbiK also appeared toxic to *Lc. lactis* if expression was increased using both a high-copy number vector and a strong promoter (Emond et al., 1997). Combining certain Abi mechanisms has also been shown to increase their efficiency in some instances. For example, McLandsborough et al. (1998) recently enhanced phage resistance by combining Abi mechanisms from two different strains (AbiE/AbiD and AbiF/AbiD) on one plasmid. It should be noted, however, that not all combinations are additive, and some combinations can even lead to decreased efficiency of one of the Abi systems (Durmaz and Klaenhammer, 1995). Lastly, continuing efforts to identify new abortive systems provide greater opportunities for the design of strains which can stay one or more steps ahead of the ever-evolving bacteriophage.

Stacking of Phage Defense Mechanisms

While each of the mechanisms described above can be powerful defense strategies in and of themselves, few of them alone can inhibit the proliferation of phages over an extended period of time. Thus, an important strategy has been to develop strains which carry multiple phage-resistance mechanisms aimed at different parts of the phage lytic cycle and/or at different species of phages. This strategy developed in recognition of the fact that many phage-insensitive commercially available lactococcal strains harbor plasmids with multiple phage resistance mechanisms and/or multiple plasmids which encode for phage resistance. For comprehensive reviews on plasmids encoding for phage resistance, please see Klaenhammer and Fitzgerald (1994), Daly et al. (1996), Hill (1993), and Allison and Klaenhammer (1998). The first documented example was the prototype strain *Lc. lactis* subsp. *cremoris* ME2, which Sanders and Klaenhammer (1983) showed contained 13 plasmids. Three of these plasmids were involved in phage resistance. pME0030 encodes for adsorption inhibition (Sanders and Klaenhammer, 1983), pTR2030 encodes for *Lla*I and AbiA (Hill et al., 1989a), and pTN20 encodes for an R/M system and AbiC (Higgins et al., 1988; Durmaz et al., 1992). Most recently, Forde et al. (1999) identified at least four plasmids encoding different phage resistance mechanisms (adsorption inhibition, R/M, and abortive) in *Lc. lactis* subsp. *cremoris* HO2. This example illustrates the value of "stacking" complementary phage resistance mechanisms acting at different points in the lytic cycle in the design of phage-insensitive strains, since many of the strains described above have remained relatively phage-insensitive even after continued use in the cheese industry.

To mimic this natural stacking phenomenon, laboratories around the world have exploited the conjugative ability of many of these phage-resistance encoding plasmids to transfer them, alone or in combination, to other lactococcal starter cultures (Sing and Klaenhammer, 1986; Jarvis, 1988; Coffey et al., 1989; Kelly et al., 1990; Harrington and Hill, 1991; Klaenhammer, 1991; Coakley et al., 1997; O' Sullivan et al., 1998; Forde et al., 1999). Selection for transconjugants is aided by the presence of naturally encoded, food-grade selectable markers on many of these plasmids, including phage resistance itself, bacteriocin production or immunity, and lactose/sucrose utilization. The resulting phage-insensitive strains can be used without regulatory approval since conjugation is considered a natural means of genetic transfer. Many of these strains have been used successfully in starter culture rotation programs in the United States (Sanders, 1988; Klaenhammer, 1991) and in Ireland (Kelly et al., 1990; Klaenhammer and Fitzgerald, 1994).

While the above information has been extensively reviewed in the past, a recent report (O'Sullivan et al., 1998) demonstrated the success which can be achieved with this type of stacking strategy. In this study, three different phage resistance mechanisms, R/M (encoded by pAH82), Abi (encoded by pMRC01), and adsorption inhibition (encoded by pAH90), were introduced singly or in combinations of two and three, into a plasmid-free *Lc. lactis* strain, MG1614. A plasmid containing genes for lactose utilization (*lac*) and proteinase activity (*prt*), pLP712, was then introduced to yield a strain with desirable fermentation characteristics. By using an isogenic strain to test the various combinations of these mechanisms, the complementary effects of stacking were more clearly evident. The strain DPC5000, which contained all three phage defense mechanisms, exhibited high levels of resistance to all known phages lytic for the parental strain, including two members of the 936 phage species and four members of the c2 species. In addition, the strain possessed desirable fermentation characteristics and, on the basis of the Heap and Lawrence starter activity test, was predicted to withstand phage attack in a commercial setting for extended periods of time.

All of the above examples utilized natural conjugation strategies to stack complementary phage defense mechanisms. Many other examples have been described in which electroporation was used to introduce nonconjugative, lactococcal plasmids, as well as recombinant plasmids, encoding for phage resistance into *Lc. lactis*. Continued research into the development of food-grade vectors for *Lc. lactis*, as well as efforts to achieve regulatory approval for use of food-grade, recombinant mechanisms and electroporation, will increase the number of available strategies for the design of phage-insensitive strains.

Rotation and Replacement Strategies to Prevent Phage Proliferation

To maintain proper end-product consistency and quality despite stricter time schedules, many cheese factories have moved from mixed starter cultures to defined starter cultures, which can contain one, two, or more defined lactococcal strains known to possess desirable fermentation characteristics (reviewed by Daly et al., 1996). Ideally, at least two phage-unrelated strains are utilized, so that if one strain becomes susceptible to phage attack, the other(s) will carry on the fermentation. When phages against one of the strains are detected, the strain is then replaced with another phage-unrelated strain or with a BIM derived from the original strain. This type of replacement strategy prevents the build-up of any one type of phage in the plant, but requires monitoring of the plant environment on a regular basis. An alternative rotation strategy was proposed by Moineau et al. (1994). In this strategy, strains that are attacked by different species of phages would be rotated to prevent the build-up of particular phage species in the production environment. In addition, Moineau (1997) proposed a rotation in the production of cheese varieties as a way to prevent the accumulation of phages.

A problem with the current rotation strategies is the scarcity of phage-unrelated strains. In addition, BIMs for a particular strain may not be available, since in many cases the mutant derivatives lack the fermentative capability of the parent strain. One response to this problem was the development of the phage defense rotation strategy (Sing and Klaenhammer, 1993; Durmaz and Klaenhammer, 1995), in which an isogenic strain carrying different phage resistance mechanisms is rotated. Rotation of different phage resistance mechanisms ensures that phages which escape one line of defense will encounter a different defense targeting a different point in the phage lytic cycle. Their study, for example, rotated a strain carrying different R/M and Abi mechanisms (Sing and Klaenhammer, 1993) or a strain carrying different combinations of R/M and Abi mechanisms (Durmaz and Klaenhammer, 1995). The rotation strategy not only kept the number of phages in the population low, but also reduced the emergence and subsequent proliferation of mutant phages which can arise in response to many defense mechanisms (Durmaz and Klaenhammer, 1995). Several advantages exist for utilizing a single-strain rotation strategy (Sing and Klaenhammer, 1993). For instance, use of a single strain known to possess excellent fermentative characteristics would deliver end products of consistent quality. In addition, the diversity of phages present in a plant would be reduced by the use of a single propagating host, and screening procedures to monitor for phages would be greatly simplified as well. Lastly, and probably most important in this age of genetic engineering, strains developed for a very specific function can be protected, thus increasing their long-term usefulness to the industry.

One of the key features of any successful rotation strategy is monitoring of the production plant for the presence of disruptive phages. Most laboratories use starter activity tests or spot-sensitivity assays to detect phages against certain strains in their rotation schemes. With current advances in molecular biology, however, more rapid methods of detection, similar to ones being developed for the detection of food-borne pathogens, are being sought. One method utilized DNA probes to phages of the c2 and 936 species to detect the presence of 10^5–10^7 phages/ml in treated skimmed milk, whole milk, and whey samples (Moineau et al., 1992). Despite the ability to process many samples at once, the procedure still required 24 hr to complete. Some success has been achieved in using enzyme-linked immunosorbent assay (ELISA) to detect phages of different species. One system used polyclonal antibodies raised to native phages of the c2 and 936 species to detect 10^7 phages/ml (Lembke and Teuber, 1979). Two other methods have utilized monoclonal antibodies to the major capsid protein (MCP) of various phages. According to Azaiez et al. (1998), the MCP is an excellent target for detection for three reasons: (1) the MCP is the most abundant protein in the phage structure, (2) previous studies have shown that the MCP is expressed in excess, and (3) members of the same phage species have similar structural protein profiles. In the first study, monoclonal antibodies were raised against the denatured major capsid protein of phage ul36 (P335 species) and were used to detect 10^7 phages/ml of ul36 in partially denatured milk samples (Moineau et al., 1993a). In this example, the antibodies were less effective at detecting other phages of the P335 species, whose members tend to be more diverse than members of the 936 and c2 species (Alatossava and Klaenhammer, 1991; Moineau et al., 1993c). Recently, monoclonal antibodies were raised against the native MCPs of a c2-like phage and were used to detect 10^7–10^8 phages/ml of six different representatives of the c2 species (Azaiez et al., 1998). The ELISA methods have a distinct advantage in that they can be performed in less than half a day, thus providing fairly rapid information on the species of phages present so that action can be taken to include a strain which does not propagate that particular species of phage. However, further work is required to lower the detection limits and to ensure that antibodies used are adequate to detect most members of the important species attacking lactococcal starter cultures. Lastly, multiplex PCR was used to detect, in a single reaction, the presence of phages of the 936, P335 and c2 species (Labrie and Moineau, 2000). The detection limits were 10^4–10^7 PFU/ml whey sample or lysate, which could be improved to 10^3–10^5 PFU/ml when a concentration step was used. The primer sets for the c2- and 936-like phages were targeted to conserved regions on the *mcp* or major structural protein, respectively, while the primer set for the P335 species was targeted to a genomic region common to its diverse members. Clearly, PCR offers a very powerful method for detection of the three most common phage species affecting cheese production.

Novel Mechanisms for Phage Defense

Phage Encoded Resistance

Recent advances in the molecular biology of *Lc. lactis* and its bacteriophages has opened the door to the development of novel, recombinant phage defense mechanisms which can be added to the above arsenal. One fairly successful avenue for the development of these novel mechanisms has been the utilization of phage sequences to inhibit phage proliferation. A good example is represented by phage encoded resistance (Per) which provides a phage origin of replication (*ori*) *in trans* to compete with and inhibit phage replication (Hill et al., 1990a; O'Sullivan et al., 1993). This phage resistance mechanism works in an abortive infection manner and was first demonstrated with *ori*s isolated from two P335 phages, ϕ50 (*per50*; Hill et al., 1990a) and ϕ31 (*per31*; O'Sullivan et al., 1993). When present on a low-copy-number vector, *per50* and *per31* result in explosive amplification of the vector, with a concomitant reduction in phage efficiency of plaquing (EOP) (0.42 and 0.3, respectively) and plaque size (Hill et al., 1990a; O'Sullivan et al., 1993). On a high-copy-number vector, both cause a significant decrease in EOP (10^{-4} and 10^{-7}, respectively) (O'Sullivan et al., 1993), probably by titrating out critical replication proteins required for phage replication. While highly effective, one drawback to the use of *per50* and *per31* in high copy is the emergence of *per* resistant (*per*^{R}) mutant phages (O'Sullivan et al., 1993). Characterization of several *per31*^{R} phages showed that they had recombined with the *Lc. lactis* NCK203 chromosome to replace the phage ϕ31 origin of replication (O'Sullivan et al., 1993; Durmaz and Klaenhammer, 2000).

Another problem encountered with the Per defense mechanism is the narrow range of phages affected. While *per31* is specific for ϕ31, *per50* inhibits, to varying degrees, a number of ϕ50-related P335 phages, including ϕCS, ϕD1, ϕ48, ul36, ϕA1, and ϕB1 (Hill et al., 1990a). However, *per50* has no affect on ϕ31, and neither *per31* nor *per50* are effective against phages of other species, including the industrially significant c2 and 936 species. Although phage origins have been identified for three other lactococcal phages, Tuc2009 (McGrath et al., 1999), c2 (Waterfield et al., 1996), and sk1 (Chandry et al., 1997), only the origin from Tuc2009 has been shown to produce a negative effect on phage proliferation (EOP 0.1 when placed in a high copy number vector; McGrath et al., 1999). To date, therefore, the Per phage defense mechanism has demonstrated success only against a limited number of lactococcal phages. Further work will be required to determine the practicality of expanding this mechanism to inhibit a broader range of phages attacking *Lc. lactis*. In contrast, a 320 bp fragment containing the origin of replication from ϕSfi21, a bacteriophage which infects *Streptococcus thermophilus* Sfi1, has been shown to produce a Per-like phenotype when presented *in trans* on a high-copy-number vector during phage infection (EOP $<10^{-6}$ for 17/25 phages tested) (Foley et al., 1998). The origin was identified on a 5 kb DNA replication module which is conserved in >70% of *Strep. thermophilus* phages (Desiere et al., 1997), indicating that this phage-defense mechanism might find greater application in the protection of this bacterium.

Antisense RNA Technology

Antisense RNA technology offers another approach to utilize phage sequences in providing barriers to phage attack. Binding of antisense RNA to target mRNA is thought to prevent translation, either by preventing ribosome loading or by destabilizing the mRNA and making it more susceptible to RNase attack (Inouye, 1988). Naturally occurring antisense mechanisms have been described in several systems (for reviews, see Inouye, 1988; Simons, 1988). Additionally, antisense strategies have been used successfully to control gene expression in animals (Izant and Weintraub, 1984), plants (Ecker and Davis, 1986), and bacteria (Coleman et al., 1984).

Attempts to use antisense mechanisms to protect *Lc. lactis* from bacteriophage attack, however, have yielded variable and mostly marginal results. Using the major coat protein gene, *mcp*, of ϕF4-1, Chung et al. (1992) achieved a reduction in EOP to 0.77–0.5, depending on the extent of the *mcp* gene included in the antisense construct. In contrast, Moineau et al. (1993b) found that the major structural proteins of P335 phage ul36 were produced in excess, making them poor targets for antisense technology. Kim and Batt (1991a,b) cloned an entire ORF (*gp51C*) of unknown function from ϕ7–9 in an antisense orientation. When the entire coding region was used, this antisense construct resulted in a reduction in the EOP of ϕ7–9 to 10^{-2}. This same EOP reduction was observed upon infection with phages related to ϕ7–9, which also contained this ORF. In addition, resistance to phage ϕ7–9 was also achieved by antisense RNA directed against two ORFs immediately downstream of *gp51C* (*gp18C* and *gp24C*), although the resistance was far less efficient (EOP approximately 0.45) than that achieved with *gp51C* (Kim et al., 1992). More recently, Polzin et al. (1996) used an antisense strategy to target several ORFs from the early and late regions of the prolate phage c2. The ORFs included *e5*, a putative subunit of DNA polymerase; *e12*, a putative transcription factor; *l7*, a major tail protein, and *l12*, a terminase. Even though there was some evidence that the antisense constructs did lower the expression levels of some of the ORFs, no inhibition was observed at low or high copy for any of the constructs. Lastly, in our laboratory, an antisense strategy was used to target the transcriptional activator, *tac31A*, of the phage ϕ31 late promoter (Walker and Klaenhammer, 1998). Although the anti-*tac* construct in high copy was able to significantly reduce expression of β-galactosidase from the phage promoter, as determined from a $P_{\phi 31}$ :: *lacZ.st* fusion, it was not able to inhibit proliferation of φ31. In addition, high-copy antisense constructs of other putative ORFs (early/middle expressed ORF1, late expressed ORFs 3–6) identified near the phage φ31 late promoter (Walker et al., 1998) also had no effect on the ability of phage φ31 to plaque on its host (Walker and Klaenhammer, 2000).

One significant barrier to the successful use of an antisense strategy may be that the levels of antisense RNA product expressed by the cell have not been high enough to effectively compete with expression of sense RNA from the phage DNA. Recent work in our laboratory has centered on combining antisense technology with an explosive vector to increase the ratio of antisense RNA to target, phage mRNA at the appropriate point in the phage infection (Walker and Klaenhammer, 2000). To accomplish this objective, the antisense cassettes described above containing the first four φ31 late ORFs (ORF3–ORF6) were subcloned to pTRK360, a low-copy-number vector containing *per31*. Phage infection of the host would result in explosive amplification of the low-copy vector, thereby significantly increasing levels of antisense RNA transcripts later in the lytic cycle. In addition, the presence of *per31* also lowered the burst size of phage φ31 4-fold, resulting in fewer sense, target mRNAs expressed from the phage genome. The combination of *per31* and the antiORF4 cassette resulted in a 3-fold decrease in the EOP of phage φ31 when compared to *per31* alone (EOP 0.11 vs. 0.36) and a greater than 2-fold decrease in the efficiency of forming centers of infection (ECOI 0.75 vs. 0.35). The function of ORF4 in phage development is currently unknown.

While the success of the *ori31* + antiORF4 is an exciting step forward, there are still several serious challenges to overcome in the use of such an antisense strategy to protect *Lc. lactis* from phage infection. First, since this strategy requires both a phage φ31 origin and coding region, it would not be effective against the heterogeneous population of phages which attack *Lc. lactis*. Second, as stated above, few of the lactococcal phage origins identified by genome sequencing have been shown to result in explosive replication when present on a vector (Waterfield et al., 1996; Chandry et al., 1997). Lastly, more work is needed to identify appropriate phage targets for antisense development, especially targets that are conserved among a number of industrially important phages. Despite these drawbacks, however, this antisense strategy has the potential to play a significant role in the arsenal of phage defense mechanisms available for lactic acid bacteria. Besides phage origins, antisense constructs could possibly be combined with any other phage defense that affects phage replication and/or burst size to increase the ratio of antisense RNA to target phage mRNA. Also, the stacking of antisense constructs which target ORFs from different phases in the phage lytic cycle may prove more productive than a single antisense construct. Availability of sequencing data and the recent intense research into the molecular biology of the lactococcal bacteriophages will surely identify targets that are fairly conserved within a phage species, thereby making antisense strategies more broadly applicable.

Genetically Engineered Suicide System

Recently, a novel genetically engineered abortive defense system which utilized a phage-specific late promoter was designed to act as a genetic trap for phages (Djordjevic and Klaenhammer, 1997; Djordjevic et al., 1997). In this system, the phage-inducible late promoter from the lytic bacteriophage φ31 (φ31P: O'Sullivan et al., 1996; Walker, 2000; Klaenhammer, 1998) was linked to the lethal *Lla*IR restriction cassette (O'Sullivan et al., 1995) without the corresponding methylase gene (Djordjevic et al., 1997). Phage infection would transcriptionally activate the phage promoter to express the lethal gene, thereby killing the host and destroying the phage genome. The construct in high copy resulted in an EOP reduction of approximately 10^{-4} for φ31. In addition, only 15% of the infected cells released phage into the medium. However, as with other phage defense mechanisms, a low number of phages were able to overcome the suicide system (EOP of 0.4 vs. 10^{-4}) (Djordjevic and Klaenhammer, 1997). These phages were found to possess a mutation in the transcriptional activator of the phage φ31 late promoter which resulted in a 50% reduction in the strength at which the promoter was activated (Djordjevic and Klaenhammer, 1997). Subsequent improvements were made in the suicide system by replacing the phage φ31 late promoter with a stronger, mutated version (φ31P4X; Walker and Klaenhammer, 1998) or by including *Lla*IC, a regulatory protein which enhances restriction by the *Lla*IR cassette (O'Sullivan and Klaenhammer, 1998). These improvements resulted in a 2.2-fold and a 5-fold reduction in EOP, respectively, compared to the original φ31P :: *Lla*IR cassette (Djordjevic and Klaenhammer, 1997). The emergence of resistant phages against these improved suicide systems was not evaluated. Lastly, stacking of the suicide defense system with high copy versions of AbiA or *per31* resulted in a complete inability of phage φ31 to plaque on the recombinant host (Djordjevic and Klaenhammer, 1997).

The success of this suicide system offers exciting possibilities in genetically engineering abortive type phage defense mechanisms. In this instance, however, the defense mechanism is very specific for φ31 and φ31 derivatives. While the system could be designed for any bacteriophage if a phage-specific promoter were available, only the identification of a phage-inducible promoter conserved in a number of bacteriophages would make this system more broadly applicable. One exciting outgrowth of this work has been the identification of a phage-specific promoter from a bacteriophage which infects *Strep. thermophilus* (Jenny et al., 1997). Using Southern hybridization, this promoter element appeared to be conserved in a number of streptococcal bacteriophages isolated from cheese manufacturing plants, suggesting that a similar type of suicide system might have broader application for *Strep. thermophilus*. Initial work utilizing this promoter fused to the lactococcal *Lla*IR restriction cassette in low copy yielded encouraging results (EOP 0.2), but further work is needed to optimize the system for this important bacterium (Jenny et al., 1997).

Deletion or Replacement of Chromosomal Elements

Finally, two interesting examples of novel phage defense mechanisms involve the alteration or replacement of chromosomal elements to inhibit phage proliferation. In one case, site-specific integration was used to inactivate sequences in the NCK203 chromosome which contributed to the emergence of new phages insensitive to AbiC (Moineau et al., 1994) or *per31* (Durmaz and Klaenhammer, 2000). Inactivation prevented the evolution and subsequent proliferation of the recombinant lytic phages. In the second case, the gene for a bacteriophage receptor (*pip*), encoded by the *Lc. lactis* chromosome and involved in sensitivity to phages of the c2 species, was replaced with a mutated version (Garbutt et al., 1997). The replacement, which left no non-lactococcal DNA or antibiotic markers, resulted in a strain resistant to infection by c2 phages, but not to phages of the P335 (small isometric), 936 (small isometric), and 949 species (large isometric) (Kraus and Geller, 1998).

Novel phage defense mechanisms generated by recombinant DNA techniques offer an exciting way to increase our ability to inhibit phage proliferation and/or evolution. The accumulation of information on bacteriophage genetics and the molecular mechanisms behind natural phage defense mechanisms will provide new avenues for the continued development of these types of novel strategies.

Media Additives

So far, we have dealt with the genetic components harbored by or added to lactococcal starter cultures to protect them from phage infection. In the initial years of studying phage defense mechanisms, a good deal of work was put into developing bulk starter medium or media additives, such as chelating agents to tie up Ca^{+2} ions required for adsorption by most lactococcal bacteriophages, which could be used to prevent phage infection during preparation of the bulk starter (reviewed by Daly, 1983). In addition, the applicability of immunizing cows with phages and using the resultant whey as an additive in bulk starter tanks to neutralize phages before infection, has been evaluated. Unfortunately, the titer of phage-specific antibodies present in the whey was too low to be commercially effective, and very little work into this area has been accomplished in this age of genetics. Recently, however, Geller et al. (1998) were able to achieve sufficiently high titers of phage-specific antibodies in bovine colostrum to inhibit phage disruption of *Lc. lactis* in milk fermentations. While there was little to no cross-reaction of antibodies made to a phage of one species with phages of different species, antibodies prepared against one phage were able to cross react with at least one other phage of the same species. While this particular strategy cannot be used since colostrum is not a food-grade ingredient, the report illustrates that such a strategy could have potential for commercial use in bulk starter vats if antibodies could be economically prepared from high-titer colostrum samples (Geller et al., 1998).

Final Comments

The revolution in biotechnology has allowed the development of specialized *Lc. lactis* strains for use in the food industry, putting even greater pressure on researchers to develop highly effective phage defense mechanisms to protect their investment. Fortunately, these same biotechnological advances have also lead to an exponential increase in the information on bacteriophages and the systems *Lc. lactis* has developed to inhibit them. As our information increases, we will be in a position to strategically utilize these defense mechanisms, both natural and recombinant, to drastically reduce the negative impact of bacteriophage infection on milk fermentations. The lessons learned with *Lc. lactis* will also be invaluable in developing phage-defense mechanisms for other LAB members, since increased use of other genera in fermentations can be expected to result in the proliferation of phages capable of inhibiting their growth.

References

Akcelik, M. (1998). A phage DNA injection-blocking type resistance mechanism encoded by chromosomal DNA in *Lactococcus lactis* subsp. *lactis* PLM-18. *Milchwissenschaft Milk Science International* 53: 619–622.

Alatossava, T., and Klaenhammer, T. R. (1991). Molecular characterization of three small isometric-headed bacteriophages which vary in their sensitivity to the lactococcal phage resistance plasmid pTR2030. *Applied and Environmental Microbiology* 57: 1346–1353.

Allison, G. E., and Klaenhammer, T. R. (1998). Phage resistance mechanisms in lactic acid bacteria. *International Dairy Journal* 8: 207–226.

Anba, J., Bidnenko, E., Hillier, A., Ehrlich, D., and Chopin, M.-C. (1995). Characterization of the lactococcal *abiD1* gene coding for phage abortive infection. *Journal of Bacteriology* 177: 3818–3823.

Azaiez, S. R. C., Fliss, I., Simard, R. E., and Moineau, S. (1998). Monoclonal antibodies raised against native major capsid proteins of lactococcal c2-like bacteriophages. *Applied and Environmental Microbiology* 64: 4255–4259.

Benbadis, L., Barel, J.-R., and Hartley, D. L. (1991). Purification, properties, and sequence specificity of *SslI*, a new type II restriction endonuclease from *Streptococcus salivarius* subsp. *thermophilus*. *Applied and Environmental Microbiology* 57: 3677–3678.

Bickle, T. A., and Kruger, D. H. (1993). Biology of DNA restriction. *Microbiology Reviews* 57: 434–450.

Bidnenko, E., Ehrlich, D., and Chopin, M.-C. (1995). Phage operon involved in sensitivity to the *Lactococcus lactis* abortive infection mechanism AbiD1. *Journal of Bacteriology* 177: 3824–3829.

Bouchard, J. D., and Moineau, S. (2000). Homologous recombination between a lactococcal bacteriophage and the chromosome of its host strain. *Virology* 270: 65–75.

Boucher, I., Eomond, E., Dion, E., Montpetit, D., and Moineau, S. (2000). Microbiological and molecular impacts of AbiK on the lytic cycle of *Lactococcus lactis* phages of the 936 and P335 species. *Microbiology* 146: 445–453.

Chandry, P. S., Moore, S. C., Boyce, J. D., Davidson, B. E., and Hillier, A. J. (1997). Analysis of the DNA sequence, gene expression, origing of replication and modular structure of the *Lactococcus lactis* lytic bacteriophage sk1. *Molecular Microbiology* 26: 49–64.

Chung, D. K., Chung, S. K., and Batt, C. A. (1992). Antisense RNA directed against the major capsid protein of *Lactococcus lactis* subsp. *cremoris* bacteriophage F4-1 confers partial resistance to the host. *Applied Microbiology and Biotechnology* 37: 79–83.

Cluzel, P.-J., Chopin, A., Ehrlich, S. D., and Chopin, M.-C. (1991). Phage abortive infection mechanism from *Lactococcus lactis* subsp. *lactis*, expression of which is mediated by an Iso-IS*S1* element. *Applied and Environmental Microbiology* 57: 3547–3551.

Coakley, M., Fitzgerald, G. F., and Ross, R. P. (1997). Application and evaluation of the phage resistance- and bacteriocin-encoding plasmid pMRC01 for the improvement of dairy starter cultures. *Applied and Environmental Microbiology* 63: 1434–1440.

Coffey, A., Fitzgerald, G. F., and Daly, C. (1989). Identification and characterization of a plasmid encoding abortive infection from *Lactococcus lactis* ssp. *lactis* UC811. *Netherlands Milk Dairy Journal* 43: 229–244.

Coleman, J., Green, P. J., and Inouye, M. (1984). The use of RNAs complementary to specific mRNAs to regulate the expression of individual bacterial genes. *Cell* 37: 429–436.

Daly, C. (1983). The use of mesophilic cultures in the diary industry. *Antonie van Leeuwenhoek* 49: 297–312.

Daly, C., Fitzgerald, G. F., and Davis, R. (1996). Biotechnology of lactic acid bacteria with special reference to bacteriophage resistance. *Antonie van Leeuwenhoek* 70: 99–110.

Davis, R., van der Lelie, D., Mercenier, A., Daly, C., and Fitzgerald, G. F. (1993). *Scr*FI restriction-modification system of *Lactococcus lactis* subsp. *cremoris* UC503: Cloning and characterization of two *Scr*FI methylase genes. *Applied and Environmental Microbiology* 59: 777–785.

Deng, Y.-M., Liu, C.-Q., and Dunn, N. W. (1999). Genetic organization and functional analysis of a novel phage abortive infection system, AbiL, from *Lactococcus lactis*. *Journal of Biotechnology* 67: 135–149.

Deng, Y.-M., Harvey, M. L., Liu, C.-Q., and Dunn, N. W. (1997). A novel plasmid-encoded phage abortive infection system from *Lactococcus lactis* biovar. *diacetylactis*. *FEMS Microbiology Letters* 146: 149–154.

Desiere, F., Lucchini, S., Bruttin, A., Zwahlen, M.-C., and Brussow, H. (1997). A highly conserved Dna replication module from *Streptococcus thermophilus* phages is similar in sequence and topology to a module from *Lactococcus lactis* phages. *Virology* 234: 372–382.

de Vos, W. M., Underwood, H. M., and Davies, F. L. (1984). Plasmid encoded bacteriophage resistance in *Streptococcus cremoris* SK11. *FEMS Microbiology Letters* 23: 175–178.

Dinsmore, P. K., and Klaenhammer, T. R. (1994). Phenotypic consequences of altering the copy number of *abiA*, a gene responsible for aborting bacteriophage infections in *Lactococcus lactis*. *Applied and Environmental Microbiology* 60: 1129–1136.

Dinsmore, P. K., and Klaenhammer, T. R. (1995). Bacteriophage resistance in *Lactococcus*. *Molecular Biotechnology* 4: 297–314.

Dinsmore, P. K., and Klaenhammer, T. R. (1997). Molecular characterization of a genomic region in a *Lactococcus* bacteriophage that is involved in its sensitivity to the phage defense mechanism AbiA. *Journal of Bacteriology* 179: 2949–2957.

Dinsmore, P. K., O'sullivan, D. J., and Klaenhammer, T. R. (1998). A leucine repeat motif in AbiA is required for resistance of *Lactococcus lactis* to phages representing three species. *Gene* 212: 5–11.

Djordjevic, G. M., and Klaenhammer, T. R. (1997). Bacteriophage-triggered defense systems: Phage adaptation and design improvements. *Applied and Environmental Microbiology* 63: 4370–4376.

Djordjevic, G. M., O'Sullivan, D. J., Walker, S. A., Conkling, M. A., and Klaenhammer, T. R. (1997). Triggered-suicide system designed for bacteriophage defense of *Lactococcus lactis*. *Journal of Bacteriology* 179: 6741–6748.

Durmaz, E., and Klaenhammer, T. R. (1995). A starter culture rotation strategy incorporating paired restriction/modification and abortive infection bacteriophage defenses in a single *Lactococcus lactis* strain. *Applied and Environmental Microbiology* 61: 1266–1273.

Durmaz, E., and Klaenhammer, T. R. (2000). Genetic analysis of chromosomal regions of *Lactococcus lactis* acquired by recombinant lytic phages. *Applied and Environmental Microbiology* 66: 895–903.

Durmaz, E., Higgins, D. L., and Klaenhammer, T. R. (1992). Molecular characterization of a second abortive phage resistance gene present in *Lactococcus lactis* subsp. *lactis* ME2. *Journal of Bacteriology* 174: 7463–7469.

Ecker, J., and Davis, R. (1986). Inhibition of gene expression in plant cells by expression of antisense RNA. *Proceedings of the National Academy of Science USA* 83: 5372–5376.

Emond, E., Dion, E., Walker, S. A., Vedamuthu, E. R., Kondo, J. K., and Moineau, S. (1998). AbiQ, an abortive infection mechanism from *Lactococcus lactis*. *Applied and Environmental Microbiology* 64: 4748–4756.

Emond, E., Holler, B. J., Boucher, I., Vandenbergh, P. A., Vedamuthu, E. R., Kondo, J. K., and Moineau, S. (1997). Phenotypic and genetic characterization of the bacteriophage abortive infection mechanism AbiK from *Lactococcus lactis*. *Applied and Environmental Microbiology* 63: 1274–1283.

Foley, S., Lucchini, S., Zwahlen, M.-C., and Brussow, H. (1998). A short noncoding viral DNA element showing characteristics of a replication origin confers bacteriophage resistance to *Streptococcus thermophilus*. *Virology* 250: 377–387.

Forde, A., Daly, C., and Fitzgerald, G. F. (1999). Identification of four phage resistance plasmids from *Lactococcus lactis* subsp. *cremoris* HO2. *Applied and Environmental Microbiology* 65: 1540–1547.

Garbutt, K. C., Kraus, J., and Geller, B. L. (1997). Bacteriophage resistance in *Lactococcus lactis* engineered by replacement of a gene for a bacteriophage receptor. *Journal of Dairy Science* 80: 1512–1519.

Garvey, P., Rince, A., Hill, C., and Fitzgerald, G. F. (1997). Identification of a RecA homolog ($RecA_{LP}$) on the conjugative lactococcal phage resistance plasmid pNP40: Evidence of a role for chromosomally encoded $RecA_{L}$ in abortive infection. *Applied and Environmental Microbiology* 63: 1244–1251.

Garvey, P., Hill, C., and Fitzgerald, G. F. (1996). The lactococcal plasmid pNP40 encodes a third bacteriophage resistance mechanism, one which affects phage DNA penetration. *Applied and Environmental Microbiology* 62: 676–679.

Garvey, P., Fitzgerald, G. F., and Hill, C. (1995a). Cloning and DNA sequence analysis of two abortive infection phage resistance determinants from the lactococcal plasmid pNP40. *Applied and Environmental Microbiology* 61: 4321–4328.

Garvey, P., van Sinderen, D., Twomey, D. P., Hill, C., and Fitzgerald, G. (1995b). Molecular genetics of bacteriophage and natural defense systems in the genus *Lactococcus*. *International Dairy Journal* 5: 905–949.

Geller, B. L., Ivey, R. G., Trempy, J. E., and Hettinger-Smith, B. (1993). Cloning of a chromosomal gene required for phage infection of *Lactococcus lactis* subsp. *lactis* C2. *Journal of Bacteriology* 175: 5510–5519.

Geller, B. L., Kraus, J., Schell, M. D., Hornsby, M. J., Neal, J. J., and Ruch, F. E. (1998). High titer, phage-neutralizing antibodies in bovine colostrum that prevent lytic infection of *Lactococcus lactis* in fermentations of phage-contaminated milk. *Journal of Dairy Science* 81: 895–900.

Gopal, P. K., and Crow, V. L. (1993). Characterization of loosely associated material from the cell surface of *Lactococcus lactis* supbsp. *cremoris* E8 and its phage-resistant variant strain 398. *Applied Environmental Microbiology* 59: 3177–3182.

Guimont, C., Henry, P., and Linden, G. (1993). Restriction/modification in *Streptococcus thermophilus*. Isolation and characterisation of a type II restriction endonuclease *Sth*455I. *Journal of Applied Microbiology and Biotechnology* 39: 216–220.

Harrington, A., and Hill, C. (1991). Construction of a bacteriophage-resistant derivative of *Lactococcus lactis* subsp. *lactis* 425A by using the conjugal plasmid pNP40. *Applied and Environmental Microbiology* 57: 3405–3409.

Harrington, A., and Hill, C. (1992). Plasmid involvement in the formation of a spontaneous bacteriophage insensitive mutant of *Lactococcus lactis*. *FEMS Microbiology Letters* 75: 135–141.

Higgins, D. L., Sanozky-Dawes, R. B., and Klaenhammer, T. R. (1988). Restriction and modification activities from *Streptococcus lactis* ME2 are encoded by a self-transmissable plasmid, pTN20, that forms cointegrates during mobilization of lactose-fermenting ability. *Journal of Bacteriology* 179: 3435–3442.

Hill, C. (1993). Bacteriophage and bacteriophage resistance in lactic acid bacteria. *FEMS Microbiology Reviews* 12: 87–108.

Hill, C., Miller, L. A., and Klaenhammer, T. R. (1990a). Cloning, expression, and sequence determination of a bacteriophage fragment encoding bacteriophage resistance in *Lactococcus lactis*. *Journal of Bacteriology* 172: 6419–6426.

Hill, C., Miller, L. A., and Klaenhammer, T. R. (1990b). Nucleotide sequence and distribution of the pTR2030 resistance determinant (*hsp*) which aborts bacteriophage infection in lactococci. *Applied and Environmental Microbiology* 56: 2255–2258.

Hill, C., Miller, L. A., and Klaenhammer, T. R. (1991a). *In vivo* genetic exchange of a functional domain from a type II A methylase between lactococcal plasmid pTR2030 and a virulent bacteriophage. *Journal of Bacteriology* 173: 4363–4370.

Hill, C., Massey, I. J., and Klaenhammer, T. R. (1991b). Rapid method to characterize lactococcal bacteriophage genomes. *Applied and Environmental Microbiology* 57: 283–288.

Hill, C., Pierce, K., and Klaenhammer, T. R. (1989a). The conjugative plasmid pTR2030 encodes two bacteriophage defense mechanisms in lactococci, restriction/modification (R+/M+) and abortive infection (Hsp+). *Applied and Environmental Microbiology* 55: 2416–2419.

Hill, C., Romero, D. A., McKenney, S., Finer, K. R., and Klaenhammer, T. R. (1989b). Localization, cloning, and expression of genetic determinants for bacteriophage resistance (Hsp) from the conjugative plasmid pTR2030. *Applied and Environmental Microbiology* 55: 1684–1689.

Inouye, M. (1988). Antisense RNA: Its functions and applications in gene regulation—a review. *Gene* 72: 25–34.

Izant, J., and Weintraub, H. (1984). Inhibition of thymidine kinase gene expression by anti-sense RNA: A molecular approach to genetic analysis. *Cell* 36: 1007–1115.

Jarvis, A. W. (1988). Conjugal transfer in lactic streptococci of plasmid-encoded insensitivity to prolate- and small isometric-headed bacteriophages. *Applied and Environmental Microbiology* 54:777–784.

Jenny, P. A., Djordjevic, G. M., and Klaenhammer, T. R. (1997). Designing a phage-triggered suicide system for thermophilic dairy starter culture *Streptococcus thermophilus*. Presented at the American Society for Microbiologists local meeting, October 24, 1997, Raleigh, NC.

Josephsen, J., Jorgen-Jensen, B., and Nyengaard, N. R. (1998). Determination of the recognition sequence of the type II restriction endonuclease, *Lla*CI, from *Lactococcus lactis* W15. *FEMS Microbiology Letters* 163: 25–29.

Kelly, W., Dobson, J., Jorck-Ramberg, D., Fitzgerald, G., and Daly, C. (1990). Introduction of bacteriophage resistance plasmids into commercial *Lactococcus* starter strains. *FEMS Microbiology Reviews* 87: P63 (Abstract).

Kim, J. H., and Batt, C. A. (1991a). Antisense RNA mediated bacteriophage resistance in *Lactococcus lactis*. *Applied and Environmental Microbiology* 57: 1039–1045.

Kim, J. H., and Batt, C. A. (1991b). Identification of a nucleotide sequence conserved in *Lactococcus lactis* bacteriophages. *Gene* 98: 95–100.

Kim, S. G., Bor, Y.-C., and Batt, C. A. (1992). Bacteriophage resistance in *Lactococcus lactis* ssp. *lactis* using antisense ribonucleic acid. *Journal of Dairy Science* 75: 1761–1767.

Klaenhammer, T. R. (1991). Development of bacteriophage-resistant strains of lactic acid bacteria. *Biochemical Society Transactions* 19: 675–681.

Klaenhammer, T. R., and Fitzgerald, G. F. (1994). Bacteriophage and bacteriophage resistance. In: M. J. Gasson and W. M. de Vos (Eds.), *Genetics and biotechnology of lactic acid bacteria* (pp. 106–168). Glasgow, UK: Blackie Academic and Professional.

Kraus, J., and Geller, B. L. (1998). Membrane receptor for prolate phages is not required for infection of *Lactococcus lactis* by small or large isometric phages. *Journal of Dairy Science* 81: 2329–2335.

Kulakauskas, S., Lubys, A., and Ehrlich, S. D. (1995). DNA restriction-modification systems mediate plasmid maintenance. *Journal of Bacteriology* 177: 3451–3154.

Labrie, S., and Moineau, S. (2000). Multiplex PCR for detection and identification of lactococcal bacteriophages. *Applied and Environmental Microbiology* 66: 987–994.

Lacks, S. A., Springhorn, S. S., and Cerritelli, S. (1991). Restriction/modification systems of pneumoncocci: Why two methylases in the *Dpn*II system? In: G. M. Dunny, P. P. Cleary, and L. L. Mckay (Eds.), *Genetics and molecular biology of streptococci, lactococci and enterococci* (pp. 71–76). Washington, DC: American Society for Microbiology.

Lacks, S. A., and Greenberg, B. (1977). Complementary specificity of restriction endonucleases of *Diplococcus pneumoniae* with respect to DNA methylation. *Journal of Molecular Biology* 114: 153–168.

Lembke, J., and Teuber, M. (1979). Detection of bacteriophages in whey by an enzyme-linked immunosorbent assay. *Milchwissenschaft* 34: 457–458.

Lucey, M., Daly, C., and Fitzgerald, G. F. (1992). Cell surface characteristics of *Lactococcus lactis* harbouring pCI528, a 46 kb plasmid encoding inhibition of bacteriophage adsorption. *Journal of General Microbiology* 138: 2137–2143.

Madsen, A., and Josephsen, J. (1998). Cloning and characterization of the lactococcal plasmid-encoded type II restriction/modification system, *Lla*DII. *Applied and Environmental Microbiology* 64: 2424–2431.

Madsen, S., Westphal, C., and Josephsen, J. (2000). Characterization of a novel plasmid-encoded HsdS subunit, *S.Lla*W12I, from *Lactococcus lactis* W12. *Plasmid* 44: 196–200.

Mayo, B., Hardisson, C., and Brana, A. F. (1991). Nucleolytic activities in *Lactococcus lactis* subsp. *lactis* NCDO 497. *FEMS Microbiology Letters* 79: 195–198.

McGrath, S., Seegers, J. F. M. L., Fitzgerald, G. F., and van Sinderen, D. (1999). Molecular characterization of a phage-encoded resistance system in *Lactococcus lactis*. *Applied and Environmental Microbiology* 65: 1891–1899.

McKay, L. L., Bohanon, M. J., Polzin, L. M., Rule, P. L., and Baldwin, K. A. (1989). Localization of separate genetic loci for reduced sensitivity towards small isometric-headed bacteriophage sk1 and the prolate-headed phage c2 on pGBK17 from *Lactococcus lactis* subsp. *lactis* KR2. *Applied and Environmental Microbiology* 55: 2702–2709.

McLandsborough, L. A., Sechaud, L., and McKay, L. L. (1998). Synergistic effects of *abiE* or *abiF* from pNP40 when cloned in combination with *abiD* from pBF61. *Journal of Dairy Science* 81: 362–368.

McLandsborough, L. A., Kolaetis, K. M., Requena, T., and McKay, L. L. (1995). Cloning and characterization of the abortive infection genetic determinant *abiD* isolated from pBF61 of *Lactococcus lactis* subsp. *lactis* KR5. *Applied and Environmental Microbiology* 61: 2023–2026.

Moineau, S. (1997). Bacteriophages and phage resistance in *Streptococcus thermophilus*: An update. *Proceedings from the 34th Marschall Italian & Specialty Cheeses* (pp. 9–17). Madison, WI.

Moineau, S., Walker, S. A., Vedamuthu, E. R., and Vandenbergh, P. A. (1995a). Cloning and sequencing of *Lla*II restriction/modification genes from *Lactococcus lactis* and relatedness of this system to the *Streptococcus pneumoniae Dpn*II system. *Applied and Environmental Microbiology* 61: 2193–2202.

Moineau, S., Walker, S. A., Holler, B. J., Vedamuthu, E. R., and Vandenbergh, P. A. (1995b). Expression of a Lactococcus lactis phage resistance mechanism by *Streptococcus thermophilus*. *Applied and Environmental Microbiology* 61: 2461–2466.

Moineau, S., Pandian, S., and Klaenhammer, T. R. (1994). Evolution of a lytic bacteriophage via DNA acquisition from the *Lactococcus lactis* chromosome. *Applied and Environmental Microbiology* 60: 1832–1841.

Moineau, S., Bernier, D., Jobin, M., Hebert, J., Klaenhammer, T. R., and Pandian, S. (1993a). Production of monoclonal antibodies against the major capsid protein of the *Lactococcus* bacteriophage ul36 and development of an enzyme-linked immunosorbent assay for direct phage detection in whey and milk. *Applied and Environmental Microbiology* 59: 2034–2040.

Moineau, S., Durmaz, E., Pandian, S., and Klaenhammer, T. R. (1993b). Differentiation of two abortive mechanisms by using monoclonal antibodies directed toward lactococcal bacteriophage capsid proteins. *Applied and Environmental Microbiology* 59: 208–212.

Moineau, S., Pandian, S., and Klaenhammer, T. R. (1993c). Restriction/modification systems and restriction endonucleases are more effective on lactococcal bacteriophages that have emerged recently in the dairy industry. *Applied and Environmental Microbiology* 59: 197–202.

Moineau, S., Fortier, J., and Pandian, S. (1992). Direct detection of lactococcal bacteriophages in cheese whey using DNA probes. *FEMS Microbiology Letters* 92: 169–174.

Naito, T., Kusano, K., and Kobayashi, J. (1995). Selfish behavior of restriction-modification systems. *Science* 267: 897–899.

Nyengaard, N. R., Falkenberg Klok, J., and Josephsen, J. (1996). Cloning and analysis of the restriction-modification system *Lla*BI, a bacteriophage resistance system from *Lactococcus lactis* subsp. *cremoris* W56. *Applied and Environmental Microbiology* 62: 3494–3498.

Nyengaard, N., Vogensen, F. K., and Josephsen, J. (1995). Restriction-modification systems in *Lactococcus lactis*. *Gene* 157: 13–18.

Nyengaard, N., Vogensem, F. K., and Josephsen, J. (1993). *Lla*AI and *Lla*BI, two type-II retriction endonucleases from *Lactococcus lactis* subsp *cremoris* W9 and W56 recognizing, respectively, 5′-/GATC-3′ and 5′-C/TRYAG-3′. *Gene* 136: 371–372.

O'Connor, L., Tangney, M., and Fitzgerald, G. F. (1999). Expression, regulation, and mode of action of the AbiG abortive infection system of *Lactococcus lactis* subsp. *cremoris* UC653. *Applied and Environmental Microbiology* 65: 330–335.

O'Connor, L., Coffey, A., Daly, C., and Fitzgerald, G. F. (1996). AbiG, a genotypically novel abortive infection mechanism encoded by plasmid pCI750 of *Lactococcus lactis* subsp. *cremoris* UC653. *Applied and Environmental Microbiology* 62: 3075–3082.

O'Sullivan, D., Coffey, A., Fitzgerald, G. F., Hill, C., and Ross, R. P. (1998). Design of a phage-insensitive dairy starter via sequential transfer of naturally occurring conjugative plasmids. *Applied and Environmental Microbiology* 64: 4618–4622.

O'Sullivan, D. J., Hill, C., and Klaenhammer, T. R. (1993). Effect of increasing the copy number of bacteriophage origins of replication, *in trans*, on incoming-phage proliferation. *Applied and Environmental Microbiology* 59: 2449–2456.

O'Sullivan, D. J., and Klaenhammer, T. R. (1998). Control of expression of *Lla*I restriction in *Lactococcus lactis*. *Molecular Microbiology* 27: 1009–1020.

O'Sullivan, D. J., Walker, S. A., West, S. G., and Klaenhammer, T. R. (1996). Development of an expression strategy using a lytic phage to trigger explosive plasmid amplification and gene expression. *Bio/Technology* 14: 82–87.

O'Sullivan, D. J., Zagula, K., and Klaenhammer, T. R. (1995). *In vivo* restriction by *Lla*I is encoded by three genes, arranged in an operon with *llaIM*, on the conjugative *Lactococcus* plasmid pTR2030. *Journal of Bacteriology* 177: 134–143.

Parreira, R., Ehrlich, S. D., and Chopin, M.-C. (1996). Dramatic decay of phage transcripts in lactococcal cells carrying the abortive infection determinant AbiB. *Molecular Microbiology* 19: 221–230.

Poch, M. T., Somkuti, G. A., and Solaiman, D. K. Y. (1997). *Sth*132I, a novel class-IIS restriction endonuclease of *Streptococcus thermophilus* ST132. *Gene* 195: 201–206.

Polzin, K. M., Collins, L. J., Lubbers, M. W., and Jarvis, A. W. (1996). Effect of various mRNA's on bacteriophage c2 replication. Abstr. F2. Fifth Symposium on Lactic Acid Bacteria. Veldhoven, The Netherlands.

Prevots, F., and Ritzenthaler, P. (1998). Complete sequence of the new lactococcal abortive phage resistance gene *abiO*. *Journal of Dairy Science* 81: 1483–1485.

Prevots, F., Tolou, S., Delpech, B., Kaghad, M., and Daloyau, M. (1998). Nucleotide sequence and analysis of the new chromosomal abortive infection gene *abiN* of *Lactococcus lactis* subsp. *cremoris* S114. *FEMS Microbiology Letters* 159: 331–336.

Prevots, F., Daloyau, M., Bonin, O., Dumont, X., and Tolou, S. (1996). Cloning and sequencing of the novel abortive infection gene *abiH* of *Lactococcus lactis* ssp. *lactis* biovar. *diacetylactis* S94. *FEMS Microbiology Letters* 142: 295–299.

Rince, A., Tangney, M., and Fitzgerald, G. F. (2000). Identification of a DNA region from lactococcal phage sk1 protecting phage 712 from the abortive infection mechanism of AbiF. *FEMS Microbiology Letters* 182: 185–191.

Ryan, M. P., Rea, M. C., Hill, C., and Ross, R. P. (1996). An application in cheddar cheese manufacture for a strain of *Lactococcus lactis* producing a novel broad-spectrum bacteriocin, lacticin 3147. *Applied and Environmental Microbiology* 62: 612–619.

Sanders, M. E. (1988). Phage resistance in lactic acid bacteria. *Biochimie* 70: 411–421.

Sanders, M. E. (1987). Bacteriophages of industrial importance. In: S. M. Goyal, C. P. Gerba, and G. Bitton (Eds.), *Phage ecology* (pp. 211–244). NY: Wiley Interscience.

Sanders, M. E., and Klaenhammer, T. R. (1983). Characterization of phage-sensitive mutants from a phage-insensitive strain of *Streptococcus lactis*; evidence for a plasmid determinant that prevents phage adsorption. *Applied and Environmental Microbiology* 46: 1125–1133.

Schouler, C., Clier, F., Lerayer, A. L., Ehrlich, S. D., and Chopin, M.-C. (1998a). A type 1C restriction-modification system in *Lactococcus lactis*. *Journal of Bacteriology* 180: 407–411.

Schouler, C., Gautier, M., Ehrlich, S. D., and Chopin, M.-C. (1998b). Combinatorial variation of restriction modification specificities in *Lactococcus lactis*. *Molecular Microbiology* 28: 169–178.

Seegers, J. F., van Sinderen, D., and Fitzgerald, G. F. (2000). Molecular characterization of the lactococcal plasmid pCIS3: Natural stacking of specificity subunits of a type I restriction/modification system in a single lactococcal strain. *Microbiology* 146: 435–443.

Sijtsma, L., Wouters, J. T. M., and Hellingwerf, K. J. (1990). Isolation and characterization of lipoteichoic acid, a cell envelope component involved in preventing phage adsorption, from *Lactococcus lactis* subsp. *cremoris* SK110. *Journal of Bacteriology* 172: 7126–7130.

Simons, R. W. (1988). Naturally occurring antisense RNA control—a brief review. *Gene* 72: 35–44.

Sing, W. D., and Klaenhammer, T. R. (1993). A strategy for rotation of different bacteriophage defenses in a lactococcal single-strain starter culture system. *Applied and Environmental Microbiology* 59: 365–372.

Sing, W. D., and Klaenhammer, T. R. (1986). Conjugal transfer of bacteriophage resistance determinants on pTR2030 into *Streptococcus cremoris* strains. *Applied and Environmental Microbiology* 51: 1264–1271.

Solaiman, D. K. Y., and Somkuti, G. A. (1991). A type II restriction endonuclease of *Streptococcus thermophilus* ST117. *FEMS Microbiology Letters* 80: 75–80.

Solaiman, D. K. Y., and Somkuti, G. A. (1990). Isolation and characterization of a type II restriction endonuclease from *Streptococcus thermophilus*. *FEMS Microbiology Letters* 67: 261–267.

Su, P., Im, H., Hsieh, H., Kang, A. S., and Dunn, N. W. (1999). *Lla*FI, a type III restriction and modification system in *Lactococcus lactis*. *Applied and Environmental Microbiology* 65: 686–693.

Su, P., Harvey, M., Im, H. J., and Dunn, N. W. (1997). Isolation, cloning and characterization of the *abiI* gene from *Lactococcus lactis* subsp. *lactis* M138 encoding abortive phage infection. *Journal of Biotechnology* 54: 95–104.

Twomey, D. P., Daly, G. N., and Fitzgerald, G. F. (1997). Molecular characterization of the restriction endonuclease gene (*scrFIR*) associated with the ScrFI restriction/modification system from *Lactococcus lactis* subsp. *cremoris* UC503. *Microbiology* 143: 2277–2286.

Twomey, D. P., Davis, R., Daly, C., and Fitzgerald, G. F. (1993). Sequence of the gene encoding a second *Scr*FI m^5C methyltransferase of *Lactococcus lactis*. *Gene* 136: 205–209.

Twomey, D. P., DeUrraza, P. J., McKay, L. L., and O'Sullivan, D. J. (2000). Characterization of AbiR, a novel multicomponent abortive infection mechanism encoded by plasmid pKR223 of *Lactococcus lactis* subsp. *lactis* KR2. *Applied and Environmental Microbiology* 66: 2647–2651.

Twomey, D. P., McKay, L. L., and O'Sullivan, D. J. (1998). Molecular characterization of the *Lactococcus lactis* *Lla*KR2I restriction–modification system and effect of an IS982 element positioned between the restriction and modification genes. *Journal of Bacteriology* 180: 5844–5854.

Valyasevi, R., Sandine, W. E., and Geller, B. L. (1990). The bacteriophage kh receptor of *Lactococcus lactis* subsp. *cremoris* KH is the rhamnose of the extracellular wall polysaccharide. *Applied and Environmental Microbiology* 56: 1882–1889.

Valyasevi, R., Sandine, W. E., and Geller, B. L. (1991). A membrane protein is required for bacteriophage c2 infection of *Lactococcus lactis* subsp. *lactis* C2. *Journal of Bacteriology* 173: 6095–6100.

Walker, S. A., and Klaenhammer, T. R. (1998). Molecular characterization of a phage-inducible middle promoter and its transcriptional activator from the lactococcal bacteriophage ϕ31. *Journal of Bacteriology* 180: 921–931.

Walker, S. A., and Klaenhammer, T. R. (2000). An explosive antisense strategy to prevent the proliferation of a lytic, lactococcal bacteriophage. *Applied and Environmental Microbiology* 66: 310–319.

Walker, S. A., Dombroski, C. S., and Klaenhammer, T. R. (1998). Common elements regulating gene expression in temperate and lytic bacteriophages of *Lactococcus* species. *Applied and Environmental Microbiology* 64: 1147–1152.

Watanabe, K., Ishibashi, K., Nadashima, Y., and Sakurai, T. (1984). A phage-resistant mutant of *Lactobacillus casei* which permits phage adsorption but not genome injection. *Journal of General Virology* 65: 981–986.

Waterfield, N. R., Lubbers, M. W., Polzin, K. M., Le Page, R. W. F., and Jarvis, A. W. (1996). An origin of DNA replication from *Lactococcus lactis* bacteriophage c2. *Applied and Environmental Microbiology* 62: 1452–1453.

11

Antibiotic Resistance and Transfer in Lactic Acid Bacteria

Michael Teuber, Franziska Schwarz, and Leo Meile

Summary

Acquired antibiotic resistance, that is, resistance genes located on conjugative or mobilizable plasmids and transposons can be found in species of lactic acid bacteria (LAB) living in habitats (e.g., human and animal intestines) that are regularly challenged with antibiotics. Most data are available for pathogenic streptococci, enterococci, and enteric lactobacilli. However, conjugative genetic elements with antibiotic resistance traits detected in LAB from animals and food are very similar to elements characterized in pathogenic streptococci and enterococci, for example, θ-type replicating plasmids of the pAMβ1/pIP501 family, and transposons of the Tn*916* type. Observed resistance genes include *tetM, ermAM, cat, sat*, and *vanA*.

A composite 29,871 bp resistance plasmid detected in *Lactococcus lactis* subsp. *lactis* isolated from a raw milk soft cheese contains *tetS* previously described in *Listeria monocytogenes* and *Enterococcus faecalis, cat* and *str* from *Staphylococcus aureus*, and a new efflux protein for macrolide antibiotics. Three of its five IS elements are almost or completely identical with IS*1216* present in the *vanA* resistance transposon Tn*1546*. In streptococci (e.g., *Strep. pneumoniae*), transformation and homologous recombination have been proposed to lead to a mosaic gene structure of penicillin binding proteins, which provides protection against β-lactam antibiotics.

These data support the view that in antibiotic-challenged habitats LAB, like other bacteria, participate in the communication systems which transfer resistance traits over species and genus borders. The prevalence of such bacteria with acquired resistances, like enterococci, is high in animals (and humans) that are regularly treated with antibiotics. Antibiotic resistance traits as selectable markers in genetic modification of LAB for different purposes are presently being replaced, for example, by metabolic traits to generate food-grade vectors.

Michael Teuber, Franziska Schwarz, and Leo Meile • Laboratory of Food Microbiology, Swiss Federal Institute of Technology, ETH-Zentrum, CH-8092 Zurich, Switzerland

Ecological Aspects of Lactic Acid Bacteria Important for Antibiotic Resistance Development

The broad biochemical definition associates LAB of different phylogenetic branches of bacterial evolution: the "low GC taxa", for example, *Enterococcus, Lactobacillus, Lactococcus, Leuconostoc, Pediococcus*, and *Streptococcus* and the "high GC" genus *Bifidobacterium* (Schleifer and Ludwig, 1995). LAB are numerous in parts of the human and animal body (intestine, nasopharyngal, and vaginal mucosa), and the environments (mainly plants) where LAB are prominent in spontaneous fermentations, which developed into important food fermentations of plant material (sour dough, sauerkraut, etc.) and animal products (sausages, cheeses, and sour milk from meat and milk) (Teuber, 1993). Such food is an efficient vehicle for living bacteria from animal and plant sources into the human body. At cell densities of 10^8–10^9 viable bacteria per gram, one portion (100 g) of fermented product delivers 10^{10}–10^{11} viable microorganisms. In addition, some LAB from animal or human intestinal microflora have been adopted as "probiotic" food supplements including *Ent. faecium, Lactobacillus plantarum, Lb. acidophilus, Lb. casei* subsp. *rhamnosus*, and several *Bifidobacterium* and *Propionibacterium* species (Tannock, 1998). The existence of LAB in large numbers in habitats that are regularly challenged with antibiotics (diseased animals, humans, and plants) disposes these bacteria to a selective pressure resulting in resistance development.

It is the aim of this chapter to outline the state of resistance levels and mechanisms of action and transfer in LAB in the human/animal environments.

Antibiotic Resistance Phenomena and Transfer Mechanisms

Extensive recent reviews of the application of antibiotics in human and veterinary medicine (Levy, 1997; WHO, 1997), agriculture (National Research Council & Insitute of Medicine US, 1998; MAFF, 1998; Falkiner, 1998), and aquaculture (Reilly and Käferstein, 1997) have documented the evolution and enrichment of antibiotic-resistant bacteria: the phenomenon is regularly observed upon the introduction of a new antibiotic (Levy, 1997). The evolution of antibiotic resistance in microbial communities is enhanced by horizontal transfer of resistance genes over species and genus borders with the aid of conjugative plasmids, transposons, the possession of integrons, and insertion elements, as well as lytic and temperate bacteriophages (Davies, 1994). Within 50 years of large scale antibiotic application, which released an estimated amount of one million tons of antibiotics into the environment (Mazel and Davies, 1999), more than one mechanism of resistance against a particular antibiotic may have evolved including enzymatic inactivation of antibiotics (e.g., by β-lactamases, aminoglycoside actyl-, nucleotidyl-, and phosphoryl-transferases), restricted import of antibiotics (e.g., penicillin binding proteins), active export of antibiotics (e.g., by membrane inserted ATP-dependent efflux systems), and target modification (e.g., methylation of 23S rRNA, mutation of aminoacid sequence of topoisomerase IV) (Davies, 1997). For certain pathogenic and potentially pathogenic bacteria like staphylococci and enterococci, the evolution of highly resistant clones has inaugurated a crisis in antibiotic resistance (Neu, 1992). In the case of some vancomycin-resistant enterococci, there remains no clinically useful antibiotic for a successful treatment (Jett et al., 1994; McDonald et al., 1997).

The basic hypotheses governing antibiotic resistance evolution of bacteria have been accentuated by Levy (1997) in a number of drug resistance equations and rules:

1. Antibiotic application plus resistance traits/genes generate a resistance problem.
2. The severity and speed of resistance development are dependent on the selection density, that is, the amount of antibiotic per treated individual (human or animal) per geographic area.
3. Reversal of resistance levels in a biotope is more dependent on the survival of susceptible bacteria, and a re-colonization by them, than on the loss of resistance traits.
4. Resistance reservoirs are provided by pathogenic and commensal bacteria that have come into contact with antibiotics for a prolonged time.
5. Low level (chromosomal) resistance acquired by spontaneous mutation enhances the evolution of high level resistance by horizontal gene transfer (Baquero et al., 1997).

Antibiotic Resistance Profiles of Lactic Acid Bacteria

The knowledge of intrinsic chromosomally coded resistance of LAB to common antibiotics is necessary to recognize acquired resistance traits.

The resistance spectrum of *Bifidobacterium* was recently described by Charteris et al. (1998). The investigated (probiotic) bifidobacteria are susceptible to ampicillin, penicillin G, cephalosporin, bacitracin, chloramphenicol, erythromycin, clindamycin, nitrofurantoin, and tetracycline. Resistances—some being most likely intrinsic—exist towards vancomycin, gentamicin, kanamycin, streptomycin, fusidic acid, trimethoprim, norfloxacin, nalidixic acid, metronidazol, polymyxin B, and colistin. The mechanisms of resistances are unknown.

The resistance profiles of enterococci (*Ent. faecalis* and *Ent. faecium*) isolated from food or patients are widely varying, containing many acquired traits (see below). A possible baseline is provided by *Ent. faecium* strain 68, which is used as probiotic for man and animals and as a silage inoculant. This strain was isolated around 1920 in the pre-antibiotic era. It is susceptible to erythromycin (15 μg disc), framycetin (100 μg), streptomycin/penicillin (streptopen 35 μg), gentamicin (10 μg), penicillin G, tetracycline (30 μg), and chloramphenicol (30 μg). It is intrinsically resistant to kanamycin (30 μg), streptomycin (10 μg), and oxacillin (5 μg) (Teuber, unpublished data for an *Ent. faecium* strain 68 isolated from a pharmaceutical preparation in 1985 and 1997).

Investigated strains of *Lc. lactis* were sensitive to amikacin, ampicillin, first generation cephalosporin, chloramphenicol, erythromycin, gentamicin, imipenem, oxacillin, penicillin, piperacillin, sulfonamide, tetracycline, trimethoprim/sulfomethoxazol, and vancomycin (de Fabrizio et al., 1994). A slighty lowered susceptibility was observed towards carbenicillin, ciprofloxacin, dicloxacillin, and norfloxacin. Resistances were recorded towards colistin, fosfomycin, pipemidic acid, and rifamycin. Recently, multiple drug efflux proteins were discovered in *Lc. lactis* (van Veen and Konings, 1998), one being an ABC transporter (lmrA), the other a proton motive force dependent drug transporter (lmrP). A similar transporter (horA) was described in *Lb. brevis* ABBC45 (Sami et al., 1997): it is encoded on a high copy number plasmid and is responsible for a resistance to the bitter tasting hop resins humulone and isohumulone which are membrane active compounds (Teuber and Schmalreck, 1973; Schmalreck et al., 1975).

Twenty-six strains of *Lc. lactis* subsp. *cremoris* and subsp. *lactis* were all resistant to trimethoprim and almost all to sulfathiazole. Resistances to gentamicin, kanamycin, lincomycin, nafcillin, neomycin, nisin, rifampin, and streptomycin varied (Orberg and Sandine, 1985).

The industrially important lactobacilli for the food industry include the thermophilic *Lb. delbrueckii* subsp. *bulgaricus* and subsp. *lactis, Lb. helveticus* and *Lb. acidophilus* (as probiotic), the mesophilic *Lb. plantarum, Lb. casei* subsp. *rhamnosus, Lb. sake, Lb. curvatus*, and the heterofermentative *Lb. brevis, Lb. kefir, Lb. fermentum*, and *Lb. sanfranciscensis* (Teuber, 1993). Data on antibiotic resistance are scarce.

Thirty-one strains of *Lb. delbrueckii* subsp. *bulgaricus* as components of yogurt cultures showed obviously intrinsic resistance toward mycostatin, nalidixic acid, neomycin, polymyxin B, trimethoprim, colimycin, sulfamethoxazol, and sulfonamides. Susceptibilities to cloxacillin, dihydrostreptomycin, doxycyclin, furadantin, novobiocin, oleandomycin, oxacillin, and streptomycin were prominent, but kanamycin and streptomycin susceptibilities varied (Sozzi and Smiley, 1980). Many strains *of Lb. plantarum, Lb. casei, Lb. salivarius, Lb. leichmannii, Lb. acidophilus* carry intrinsic resistance toward vancomycin, which is due to the presence of D-alanin:D-alanine ligase-related enzymes (Elisha and Courvalin, 1995). The intrinsic vancomycin resistance of *Lactobacillus, Leuconostoc, and Pediococcus* species has been used to separate them from other Gram-positive bacteria on vancomycin-supplemented selective media (Simpson et al., 1988). An important observation is the high chromosomal mutation rate (10^{-4}) to nitrofurazone, kanamycin, and streptomycin resistance as compared to erythromycin and tetracycline resistance (10^{-9}) (Curragh and Collins, 1992). Fifteen strains of *Streptococcus thermophilus* from yogurt cultures showed varying resistance levels to colimycin, gentamicin, kanamycin, mycostatin, nalidixic acid, neomycin, polymyxin B., trimethoprim/sulfamethoxazol, streptomycin, and sulfonamides (Sozzi and Smiley, 1980).

The resistance situation within the pathogenic hemolytic and oral streptococci has been greatly influenced by the antibiotics used to treat streptococcal infections of the throat, ear, and lung by *Strep. pyogenes, Strep. pneumoniae* and related species. Whereas *Strep. pneumoniae* shows a high prevalence of resistance towards β-lactam antibiotics, *Strep. pyogenes* may have a substantial resistance towards macrolides like erythromycin (Hakenbeck, 1999; Kernodle, 2000; Weisblum, 2000).

A compilation of antibiotic resistance traits and genes of LAB is presented in Table 11.1 which assembles the most recent data on the occurrence of such defined resistances in the different commensal and pathogenic species of LAB.

Natural Transfer Tools of Lactic Acid Bacteria

Horizontal gene transfer in bacteria in natural environments (i.e., outside the microbiological laboratory) is by conjugation (Clewell, 1993) and most probably bacteriophages (e.g., Schmieger and Schicklmaier, 1999). Transformation may be a specific mechanism prevalent in oral and hemolytic streptococci within the human nasopharyngal cavity (Hakenbeck, 1999; Majewski, et al., 2000).

Conjugative plasmids contribute to the dissemination of antibotic resistance traits between bacteria in natural biotopes (humans, animals, plants, and their environments). Some of the conjugative antibiotic resistance plasmids from Gram-positive bacteria became the basis of the construction of vectors bearing selectable resistance traits (see below).

Conjugative transposons are characterized by transposase genes which induce excision of themselves and—after conjugative transfer—incorporation into the genomes

Table 11.1. Distribution of Antibiotic Resistance Determinants in Lactic Acid Bacteria

Genotype	Phenotype	Host Organisms	Location	Regulation	Reference
Glycopeptides					
*van*A	Van >256 Tei >32	*Ent. faecium* *Ent. faecalis* *Ent. hirae* *Ent. avium* *Ent. durans* *Ent. mundtii*	Plasmids, transposon *Tn*1546	Inducible	Fraimow and Courvallin, 2000
*van*B	Van 4 to 1000 Tei <1	*Ent. faecium* *Ent. faecalis* *Strep. bovis*	Chomosome, plasmid *Tn*1547 *Tn*5382	Inducible	ditto
*van*C1	Van 2 to 32 Tein <1	*Ent. gallinarum*	Chromosome	Constitutive or inducible	ditto
*van*C2	Van 2 to 32 Tei <1	*Ent. casseliflavius*	Chromosome	Constitutive or inducible	ditto
*van*C3	Van 2 to 32	*Ent. flavescens*	Chromosome	Constitutive or inducible	ditto
*van*D	Van 64 to 256 Tei 4 to 32	*Ent. faecium*	Chromosome	Constitutive or inducible	ditto
*van*E	Van 16 Tei 0.5	*Ent. faecalis*	Chromosome	?	ditto
Aminoglycosides					
1. Adenylyl-transferases					
ant(6)-1a	Strep	*Ent. faecalis*	Plasmid		Shaw and Wright, 2000
ant(9)-1b	Spec	*Ent. faecalis*	Plasmid		ditto
2. Phospho-transferases					
aph(3′)-IIIa	Kan, Amik, Isep, Neo, But, Ribos, Livid	*Ent. faecalis* *Strep. pneumoniae*	Plasmid *Tn*1545		ditto
aph(2″)-Ic	Gent, Net, Kan, Tob	*Ent. gallinarum*	Plasmid		ditto
aph(2″)-Id	Gent, Net, Kan, Tob	*Ent. casseliflavus*	Chromosome		ditto
3. Acetyl-transferases					
aac(6′)-1e	Kan, Tob, Amik, Neo, Fort	*Ent. faecalis*	Plasmid		ditto
aac(6′)-Ii	Kan, Tob, Amik, Neo	*Ent. faecium*	Chromosome		ditto

(*continued*)

Table 11.1. (*continued*)

Genotype	Phenotype	Host Organisms	Location	Regulation	Reference
4. Bifunctional enzyme					
aac(6′)-*aph*(2″)	Gent, Net, Siso, Kan, Tob, Amik, Isep, Neo, But Ribos, Livid	*Ent. faecalis*	Plasmid		ditto
Tetracyclines					
1. Efflux proteins					
tet(K)		*Bifidobacterium* *Enterococcus* *Streptococcus*			McMurry and Levy, 2000
tet(L)		*Enterococcus* *Streptococcus*			ditto
2. Ribosome protection					
tet(M)		*Ent. faecalis*	Plasmid chromosome *Tn*916	Inducible	ditto
tet(O)		*Strep. mutans*	Chromosome	Constitutive	ditto
tet(S)		*Ent. faecalis* *Lc. lactis*	Plasmid	?	ditto
tet(T)		*Strep. pyogenes*	Chromosome		
Chloramphenicol					
1. Multifunctional efflux proteins					
?		*Ent. faecalis* *Ent. faecium*	?	?	Lynch et al., 1999
2. Chloramphenicol-acetyl transferases	*cat*	*Enterococcus* *Lactobacillus* *Lc. lactis* *Strep. pyogenes*	Plasmids	Inducible?	Murray, 2000

Fluoroquinolones					
1. Topoisomerase IV					
*par*C		*Ent. faecalis* *Strep. pneumoniae*	Chromosome	Target mutation	Hooper, 2000
2. DNA gyrase					
*gyr*A		*Ent. faecalis* *Strep. pneumoniae*	Chromosome	Target mutation	ditto
*gyr*B		*Strep. pneumoniae*	Chromosome	Target mutation	ditto
3. Efflux Transporters					
?		*Ent. faecalis* *Strep. pneumoniae*	?	Decreased accumulation	ditto
Macrolide-lincosamide-streptogramins (MLS)					
1. Methyl-transferases					
*erm*AM	MLS	*Strep. sanguis*	Plasmid		Weisblum, 2000
*erm*AMR	MLS	*Ent. faecalis*	Plasmid		ditto
*erm*B-like	MLS	*Ent. faecalis*	Plasmid		ditto
*erm*GT	MLS	*Lb. reuteri*	Plasmid		ditto
*erm*TR	MLS	*Strep. pyogenes*			ditto
2. Acetylase					
*sat*A	streptogramin A	*Ent. faecium*	Plasmid		ditto
3. Efflux transporter (pmf)					
*mef*A	Macrolide	*Strep. pyogenes*			ditto
*mef*E	Macrolide	*Strep. pneumoniae*			ditto
*mef*214	Macrolide	*Lc. lactis*	Plasmid		Perreten et al., 2000
*mre*A	Macrolide	*Strep. agalactiae*			
β-***lactam antibiotics***					
1. β-lactamase					
blaZ		*Ent. faecalis*	Plasmid	Constitutive	Kernodle, 2000
2. Penicillin-binding proteins (PBP)					
pbp 5		*Ent. faecalis* *Ent. faecium* *Ent. raffinosus* *Ent. gallinarum* *Ent. hirae*	Chromosome		ditto

(continued)

Table 11.1. (*continued*)

Genotype	Phenotype	Host Organisms	Location	Regulation	Reference
1a, 1b, 2x, 2a, 2b, 3		*Strep. pneumoniae* *Strep. oralis* *Strep. mitis* *Strep. sanguis*	Chromosome: horizontal transfer by transformation	Leading to mosaic gene structures	ditto
Multidrug transporters					
lmrA (ABC)	MLS, Tet	*Lc. lactis*	Chromosome		van Veen et al., 1999
lmrP (pmf)	MLS	*Lc. lactis*	Chromosome		ditto
horA	Isohumulone, ethidium bromide	*Lb. brevis*	Plasmid		Sami et al., 1997

of recipient Gram-negative and Gram-positive bacteria. A well known example is the tetracycline resistance transposon Tn*916* from *Ent. faecalis* (Flannagan et al., 1994). Transposons are located on the chromosome or on plasmids, and sometimes on both, in one and the same bacterial strain.

To acquire antibiotic resistance genes LAB communicate actively and passively with other bacteria with the aid of conjugative plasmids and transposons. Indeed, plasmids are common in enterococci, lactococci, leuconostocs, pediococci, and streptococci and are present in some strains of *Strep. thermophilus*, lactobacilli, and bifidobacteria (Janzen et al., 1992; Mercenier et al., 1994; Dellaglio et al., 1995; Devriese and Pot, 1995; Sgorbati et al., 1995; Simpson and Taguchi, 1995; Teuber, 1995). Conjugative transposons (broad and narrow host range) have been described in enterococci, lactococci, and streptococci (Clewell, 1993).

Transfer of antibiotic resistance genes within LAB by bacteriophages and prophages seems theoretically possible, but has not been studied to any extent. In addition, the host range of such transfers would be rather limited to closely related strains within one species.

Antibiotic Resistance Transfer by Conjugative Plasmids in Lactic Acid Bacteria

Enterococci (*E. faecalis* and *E. faecium*) and some (oral) streptococci clearly represent the most promiscuous bacterial species discovered within the Gram-positive bacteria. Enterococci are part of the human and animal intestinal microflora. They have developed into important human pathogens, especially in immuno-compromised patients (Jett et al., 1994; Hancock and Gilmore, 2000). Infection is from the patients' own microflora or from other patients, hospital personnel, or possibly food. In food, enterococci are common in raw meat and milk (due to fecal contamination during production) and products made from these raw materials without pasteurization (raw milk cheeses and raw fermented sausages and ham) (Teuber et al., 1996; Giraffa et al., 1997).

A well characterized broad host range conjugative plasmid is pAMβ1 which was isolated from *Ent. faecalis* (see Figure 11.1). It carries a constitutive MLS resistance (to macrolides, lincosamides, and streptogramin B, see Table 11.1). Self-transfer at frequencies of about 10^{-4} per donor (and lower) has been observed in filter mating experiments to enterococci, staphylococci, *Clostridium, Lactobacillus, Lactococcus*, and *Bacillus* species (Macrina and Archer, 1993). Elaborate studies have shown that pAMβ1 could move from *Ent. faecalis* into the plasmid-free strain Bu2-60 of *Lc. lactis* subsp. *lactis* biovar *diacetylactis* during filter mating. From there it conjugated to 8 out of 18 commercial isolates of *Strep. thermophilus* with frequencies of 3.5×10^{-5}–7.6×10^{-9} per recipient: *Strep. thermophilus* transconjugants conjugated pAMβ1 into other *Strep. thermophilus* strains at 10^{-4}–10^{-7} per recipient. Back-transfer into *Lactococcus* Bu2-60 occurred at higher frequencies of about 10^{-4} (Kleinschmidt et al., 1993). pAMβ1 was quite stably maintained in *Strep. thermophilus* at 37°C, but lost within 90 generations of growth at 42°C.

Out of 13 *Lb. debrueckii* subsp. *bulgaricus*, 23 *Lb. delbrueckii* subsp. *lactis*, 44 *Lb. acidophilus*, 1 *Lb. helveticus*, 1 *Lb. brevis*, 5 *Lb. plantarum*, 6 *Lb. casei* subsp. *casei, 4 Lb. casei* subsp. *rhamnosus, 1 Lb. fermentum*, and *1 Lb. salivarius* subsp. *salicinius* strains only two strains—*Lb. brevis* 3030/62 and *Lb. helveticus* 3048b—accepted pAMβ1 during filter mating at about a frequency of 10^{-7}. In skimmed milk at 37°C, pAMβ1 was lost from *Lb. brevis* within 10 generations, at 30°C within 100 generations (Soeding et al., 1993). In cabbage juice or tomato juice, pAMβ1 stability was 80% within 77 generations at 30°C.

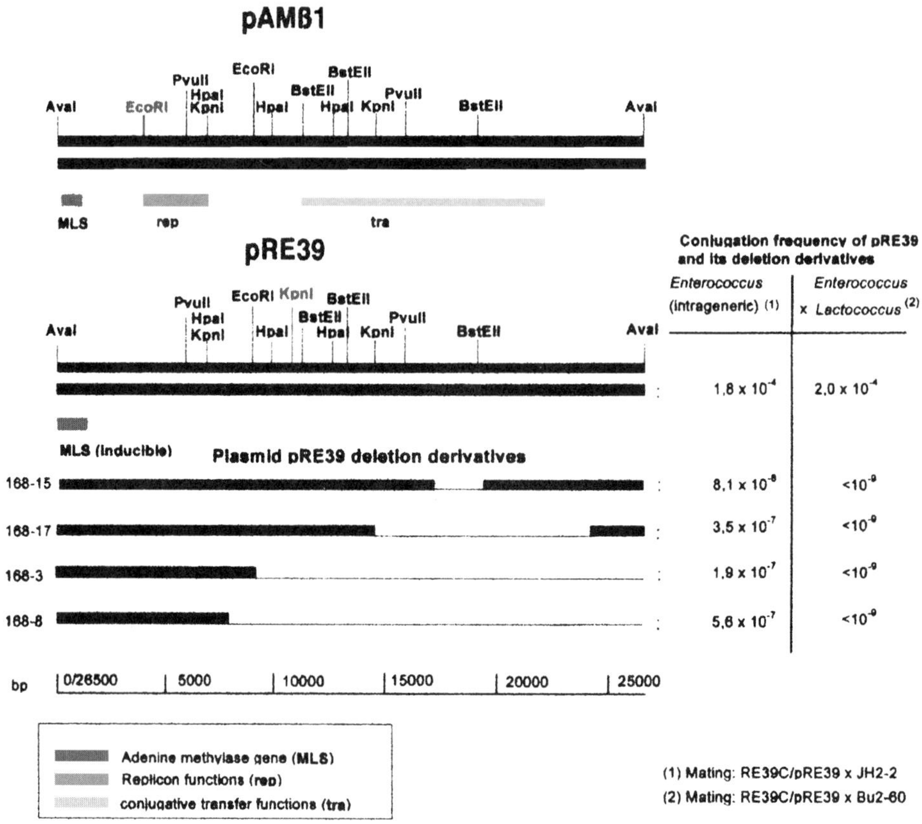

Figure 11.1. Physical map of the conjugative MLS-resistance plasmid pAMβ1 from *Ent. faecalis* (Macrina and Archer, 1993). Its restriction endonuclease profile is very similar to the conjugative MLS-resistance plasmid pRE39 from *Enterococcus* sp. RE39 isolated from raw minced beef (Teuber et al., 1996). The differences are one additional EcoRI site in pAMβ1 and one additional KpnI site in pRE39. The MLS methylase genes are identical, but constitutively expressed in pAMβ1 and erythromycin-inducible in pRE39. The replication and conjugative transfer functions seem to be in identical positions as indicated by the insert conjugation frequencies of deletion derivatives isolated from *Bacillus subtilis* after conjugative transfer (from Teuber et al., 1996).

Obviously many lactobacilli in contrast to lactococci (Gasson and Davies, 1980) cannot act as recipients of the broad host range resistance plasmid pAMβ1. Another broad host range plasmid, pIP501, originally isolated from *Strep. agalactiae* can be conjugated into *Streptococcus, Staphylococcus, Clostridium, Listeria*, and *Pediococcus* species. Like pAMβ1, pIP501 replicates by the θ-type mechanism, carries a MLS resistance gene, a region responsible for conjugative transfer, and a gene for a chloramphenicol acetyltransferase (Macrina and Archer, 1993). Although the conjugal transfer of pIP501 to other LAB has not been studied in greater detail, the replicon and resistance genes of this plasmid and some derivatives have been extensively used for the construction of cloning vectors for lactococci (de Vos and Simons, 1994). Indigenous conjugation systems in lacotococci are very common, reflecting the abundance of plasmid DNA (Gasson and Fitzgerald, 1994; Neve et al., 1987). Transferrable antibiotic resistance plasmids, however, have normally not been observed in starter cultures, most of which stem from the pre-antibiotic era. In contrast, reports of native conjugation systems *in Lactobacillus* are few: one plasmid associated transfer of lactose fermenting ability in *Lb. casei*, and bacteriocin production and immunity in *Lb. johnsonii* (Kullen and Klaenhammer, 1999). Likewise, conjugative plasmids have not been discovered in *Bifidobacterium* (Kullen and Klaenhammer, 1999). A similar situation is evident in *Leuconostoc* and *Pediococcus* which, however, can accept broad host range antibiotic resistance plasmids like pAMβ1, pVA797 :: Tn*917*, and pIP501 by high-frequency conjugation from *Lactococcus* harbouring these plasmids (Dessart and Steenson, 1991). Another efficient transfer system (10^{-2} in broth) is the sex pheromone induced conjugation by rolling-circle-replicating large plasmids of the pAD1 type (Clewell, 1993). Recently, it was demonstrated that clumping of donor and recipient cells (a prerequisite for conjugation) is induced by subinhibitory levels of chloramphenicol, erythromycin, or tetracyline even in the absence of pheromone production in the recipient (Wu et al., 1999).

Conjugative Transposons in LAB

Conjugative transposons are a main vehicle of antibiotic resistance transport in Gram-positive bacteria. They have been discovered in *Ent. faecalis* (Tn*916*, Tn*918*, Tn*920*, Tn*925*, Tn*2702*), *Ent. faecium* (Tn*5233*), *Strep. pyogenes* (Tn*3701*), *Strep. agalactiae* (Tn*93951*), and *Lc. lactis* (Tn*5276*, Tn*5301*). In enterococci and streptococci, they determine resistances to tetracycline (*tetM*), erythromycin (*ermAM, erm*), chloramphenicol (*cat*), and kanamycin (*aphA-3*). In lactococci, they code for nisin (*nis*) production and sucrose fermentativion (*sac*). They vary in size between 16 and 70 kb. They may be inserted into plasmids or the chromosome in one or multiple copies (inserts). Immunity and entry exclusion are absent. They may mobilize plasmids or chromosomal genes. The most remarkable observation, however, is the extreme host range which is a property of the Tn*916*/Tn*1545* family. It includes Gram-positive and Gram-negative bacteria of the following genera: *Acetobacterium, Acholeplasma, Actinobacillus, Alcaligenes, Bacillus, Butyrivibrio, Citrobater, Clostridium, Enterococcus, Escherichia, Eubacterium, Fusobacterium, Haemophilus, Lactobacillus, Lactococcus, Leuconostoc, Listeria, Mycoplasma, Neisseria, Peptostreptococcus, Staphylococcus, Streptococcus, Thermus*, and *Veillonella*, and probably more which have not yet been investigated (Clewell et al., 1995). Tn*916* has been completey sequenced (Flannagan et al., 1994). Resistance transfer rates are in the order of 10^{-9}–10^{-6} per donor in filter matings.

Despite the known nucleotide sequence and physical structure of Tn916 (see Figure 11.2), the actual molecular, ultrastructural, and biochemical mechanisms of conjugative transfer of this transposon remain unknown. However, a circular, single strand

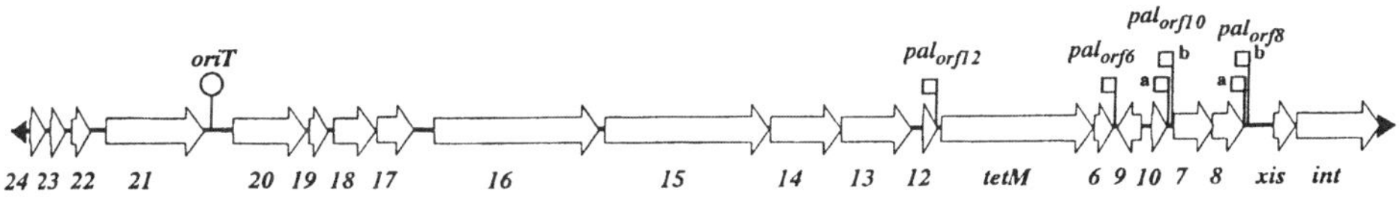

Figure 11.2. Physical map of the conjugative transposon Tn*916* (Flannagan et al., 1994). *TetM, xis*, and *int* are the transposon genes encoding tetracycline resistance protein TETM (ribosome protection), the excisionase and the integrase, resp. The main *orfs* of Tn*916* whose functions are still unknown are labelled according to Flannagan et al. (1994). The black arrows at the extremities of Tn*916* represent the terminal inverted repeats necessary for the formation of circular intermediates, replication, and conjugative transfer. The location of the origin of transfer (*ori* T) and of several relevant palindromes are indicated (from Celli and Trieu-Cuot, 1998; permission of publisher and authors applied for, pending).

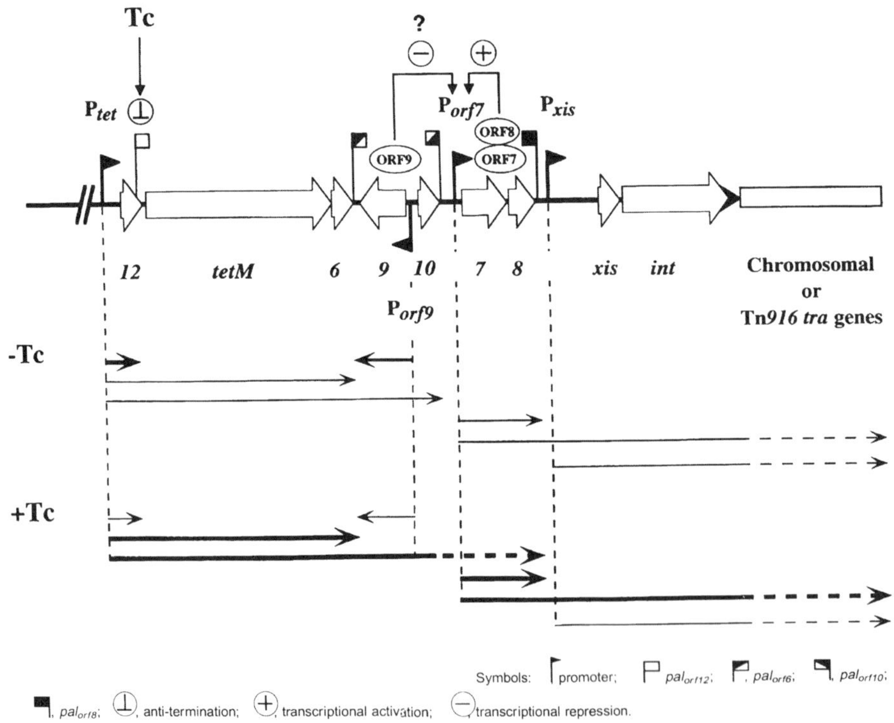

Figure 11.3. Regulation of expression of the transfer functions of Tn*916* by tetracycline. For explanation, see the text (from Celli and Trieu-Cuot, 1998; permission of publisher and authors applied for; pending).

DNA intermediate is a prerequisite of conjugal transfer. The role of tetracycline as regulator of induction of circularization of Tn*916* and expression of the transfer functions has been elucidated by Celli and Trieux-Cuot (1998) in elegant investigations, which are summarized in Figure 11.3. In the absence of tetracycline (Tc), most of the transcripts initiated at the promotor of *tetM* (P_{tet}) end at the palindrome of open reading frame 12 (pal_{orf12}). P_{orf9} transcribes *orf9* efficiently, whereas P_{orf7} directs a low level of transciption of *orf7* and *orf8*. Under these conditions, P_{orf7} and P_{xis} direct a low level of transcription of the transposition and downstream genes (i.e., the transfer of chromosomal genes, depending on whether a circularized or integrated element is considered). In the presence of tetracycline, the transcripts initiated at P_{tet} read through pal_{orf12}, pal_{orf6}, and pal_{orf10}, which leads to a decreased transcription of *orf9* but to an increased transcription of *orf7* and *orf8*. The resulting overexpression of ORF7 and ORF8 stimulates the activity of P_{orf7}, which leads to an increased transcription of the downstream genes (*orf7, orf8, xis, int*, and either the transfer genes of Tn*916* or the adjacent chromosomal genes). Increased transcription of *xis* and *int* is not supposed to result in an increase in excision, as this would not modify the ratio of the corresponding proteins. ORF9 could repress the activity of P_{orf7}. In this hypothesis, the presence of tetracycline in the medium would lead to a decreased expression of *orf9* and thus to an increased expression of *orf7* plus *orf8*. Absence or removal of tetracycline from the medium would lead to a decreased expression of *orf9* and thus to the opposite regulation. In plasmid pK214 from *Lc. lactis* (see below) the tetracycline resistance gene *tetS* is associated with an *orf9*-like and a truncated *orf7*-like sequence. The genetic

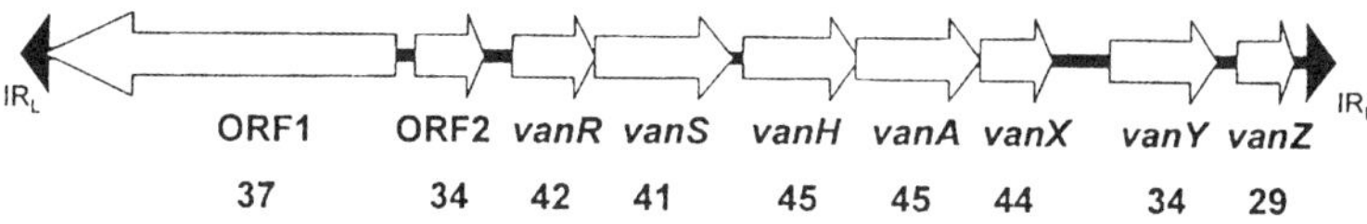

Figure 11.4. Structure of Tn*1546* (10,851 bp) carrying the *vanA* vancomycin-resistance gene cluster. The nine ORFs are delineated by 38 bp imperfect inverted repeats and include genes with resolvase and transposase activity (ORF1 and ORF2) as well as genes involved in regulation (*vanR* and *vanS*), synthesis of D-Ala-D-Lac (*vanH* and *vanA*), and hydrolysis of D-Ala-A-Ala precursors (*vanX* and *vanY*). The G + C content of each gene is shown. For a detailed model of peptidoglycan synthesis in glycopeptide-resistant enterococci see Fraimow and Courvalin (2000). (from Fraimow and Courvalin, 2000; permission of publisher and authors applied for, pending).

organization of this DNA in pK214 is similar to that of Tn*916*. Pairwise comparison of the homologous proteins revealed a high level of identity (ORF9 = 54%, ORF7 = 60%). This is interpreted as indicating that these tetracycline resistance genes and the associated regulatory proteins have evolved from a common ancestral regulon (Celli and Trieu-Cuot, 1998).

More complex transposons like Tn5253 (65.5 kb) may have an internal Tn*916*-like region that is capable of independent conjugative transposition. Another important, though not conjugative transposon, is Tn*1546*, which carries the vanA gene cluster responsible for vancomycin resistance in enterococci (see Figure 11.4). This transposon is easily mobilized, however, by conjugative plasmids (Arthur and Courvallin, 1993).

Transformation and Homologous Recombination

This mechanism of horizontal gene transfer seems to occur in nature in the streptococcal family of species, which inhabit the human and animal oral cavities and other parts of the body. Clear epidemiological evidence comes from the observation of the mosaic gene structures of penicillin binding proteins that are responsible for penicillin resistance in *Strep. pneumoniae* (Hakenbeck, 1999). The frequency of such an interspecies genetic exchange, however, decreases sharply with the extent of DNA sequence divergence between the donor and the recipient and follows an exponential relationship. Despite these divergences, measurable transformation rates were experimentally determined with *Strep. pneumoniae* as recipient and donor DNA from other streptococci like *Strep. mitis, Strep. oralis, Strep. parasanguis, Strep. crista, Strep. sanguis, Strep. anginosus, Strep. constellatus*, and *Strep. intermedius* (frequencies log 10 transformed between −2.6 and −6.8). No transformation of *Strep. pneumoniae* was obtained with DNA from *Strep. adjacens* (Majewski et al., 2000). Nevertheless, these transformation frequencies are obviously high enough to lead to interspecies transformation and homologous recombination in penicllin binding genes providing protection against β-lactam antibiotics.

LAB with Acquired and Transferable Antibiotic Resistances in Food

This topic is of importance since LAB are used as starter cultures for the production of fermented food. In addition, many types of food are still produced (in Europe) with unpasteurized raw material (meat and milk) which includes the endogenous microflora of the raw material.

Enterococci

Enterococci are commonly found in the intestines of farm animals and humans (Teuber, 1993). In food microbiology, they have been—like *E. coli*—regarded as indicators of fecal contamination. Because enterococci are widely dispersed with feces and manure in the environment and are able to multiply in a variety of organic material (milk, meat, vegetables) or in fermented food made from meat and milk (e.g., sausages and cheeses) they have been looked at as index organisms for unhygienic food processing if pasteurized substrates were used (Devriese and Pot, 1995). Food substances that consist of raw meat or milk, or that are made from these substrates by fermentation are almost always contaminated with enterococci. For some artisanal products, enterococci isolated from traditional raw milk cheeses are used as starter cultures (Giraffa et al., 1997). Certain *Ent. faecium* strains are applied as probiotics in farm animals and humans, and may be a component of silage inoculants (Elmer et al., 1996). Although enterococci were for a long time considered to be medically unimportant, within the last 20 years they have developed into serious pathogens specifically in nosocomial infections, where they cause abdominal abscesses, urinary tract infections, endocarditis, and bacteremia (Jett et al., 1994; Hancock and Gilmore, 2000).

The high level of antibiotic resistance observed in these bacteria (Table 11.1) has made them feared infectious agents in intensive care wards. Possible pathogenicity factors like hemolysins and cytolysins have been described. The most important species are *Ent. faecalis* and *Ent. faecium*, the first being more common in human illnesses; the second (though less common in human infections) may pose a larger resistance threat (Huycke et al., 1998).

In both species, the evolutionary development of resistance has been attributed to the possession of broad host range and extremely mobile genetic elements like conjugative plasmids and transposons (e.g., pAMβ1, or Tn*916*, Clewell et al., 1995). The molecular details of the structures and functions of these elements are fairly well studied and becoming understood (Clewell et al., 1995; Marra and Scott, 1999). It is noteworthy that transcription of the transfer functions of Tn*916* requiring excision of the element is dramatically increased in the presence of tetracycline (Celli and Trieu-Cuot, 1998).

An efficient genetic exchange between enterococci and staphylococci is evident from the recently described enterococcal transposon Tn5384 which evolved as a composite transposon through cointegration of enterococcal and staphylococcal plasmids (Bonafede et al., 1997).

Enterococci in Farm Animals and Meat

It has been shown that raw meat, raw milk, and products made from them without proper heat treatment frequently contain resistant enterococci (Rollins et al., 1985; Batish and Ranganathan, 1986; Knudtson and Hartman, 1993; Teuber et al., 1996; Giraffa et al., 1997; Aarestrup et al., 1998; Klein et al., 1998; Quednau et al., 1998). Data for meat (chicken, turkey, pigs, beef) were recently reviewed by Teuber et al. (1999). Not only are the tested isolates resistant to antimicrobial feed additives used at the time of testing (avoparcin, virginiamycin, tylosin, and bacitracin) but also to a battery of medically important antibiotics like penicillins, cephalosporins, vancomycin, streptomycin, erythromycin, fluoroquinolones, chloramphenicol, tetracyclines, neomycine, sulfonamides and trimetoprim, rifampicin, and clindamycin. The prevalence of multiply drug resistant strains is high (Klare et al., 1995a,b; Klein et al., 1998).

In epidemiological terms, this information provides important facts regarding the antibiotic resistance situation in enterococci from animals and their meat compared to clinical strains from humans. Resistance levels to tetracyclines (20–97%) and erythromycin (9–100%) are very high similar to recently investigated clinical isolates, for example, from the UK, Holland, and Switzerland (Guiney and Urwin, 1993; Liassine et al., 1998; van den Braak et al., 1998; Wüst et al., 1998). In contrast, ampicillin resistance is low, but penicillin and methicillin resistances are high, as is resistance to fluoroquinolones. Trimethoprim and sulfonamides range in antibiotic efficiency between 0% and 100%, indicating the dependence on the use of these antibiotics in these animals. Clear evidence that feeding antibiotics to chicken induces the selection of resistant enterococci, is provided in the case of bacitracin, a substance legally available in Europe as feed additive. If bacitracin is used resistance levels are between 28% and 100% (Teuber et al., 1999). In enterococci from cattle and pigs where bacitracin has not been employed, resistance levels are zero. Likewise, if tylosin is not used for feeding chicken or pigs, cross resistance to erythromycin is low (Ministry of Agriculture and Forestry Finland, 1997). Although the incidence of resistance to gentamicin is low in Europe, some strains isolated in our laboratory from chicken meat exported from China to Europe showed a high level gentamicin resistance (MIC > 1024 mg/L) coupled with a high level streptomycin resistance (MIC > 1024 mg/L). Gentamicin-resistant enterococci have also been reported in veterinary samples (e.g., from horses) and chicken meat in the USA (Thal et al., 1995). The gentamicin-resistant *Ent. faecalis* investigated in our laboratory contained the 6′-aminoglycoside acetyltransferase-2″-aminoglycoside phosphotransferase gene (AAC-APH, see Table 11.1) as detected by hybridization with a specific nucleotide probe derived from the nucleotide sequence of the AAC-APH from human isolates. This gene was not seen in the American isolates from chicken (reviewed by Teuber et al., 1999).

Multiple drug resistance (i.e., to more than one antibiotic) was between 63% and 100% of the resistant isolates. A frightening observation comes from the reports that vancomycin-resistant enterococci isolated from chicken meat and pork after enrichment in the presence of vancomycin reveal 100% multiple drug resistance; for example, an *Ent. faecium* isolate from minced pork was resistant to vancomycin, teicoplanin, avoparcin, penicillin, ampicillin (intermediate resistance), streptomycin, erythromycin, tetracycline, chloramphenicol, and ciprofloxacin (Klein et al., 1998).

The problem of vancomycin resistance in enterococci (VRE) has been reviewed in great detail (McDonald et al., 1997; Willems et al., 1999). If VRE from farm animals and food are to be a threat to the human population, colonization of a predisposed person has to precede infection. A wound infection of a chicken farm worker reported from the UK was obviously caused by a vancomycin-resistant enterococcus (Bates et al., 1993). The ban of avoparcin as a feed additive in Europe has resulted in a sharp drop in vancomycin-resistant enterococci between 1995 and 1996 in farm animals as shown in the Danish surveillance study (Aarestrup et al., 1998). A preliminary report from Germany has described a similar phenomenon in enterococci from human intestinal microflora obtained from healthy persons of the community (Witte, 1998). VRE has been reported in chicken meat from Sweden (Quedneau et al., 1998), a country where antibiotic feeds have been banned since 1986 (Ministry of Agriculture, Sweden, 1997). Vancomycin resistance was transferrable by conjugation to other enterococci *in vitro*. Whether Tn1546 was involved has not yet been investigated.

However, a detailed study on the molecular diversity and evolutionary relationships of Tn1546-like elements in vancomycin-resistant enterococci from humans and animals provided convincing evidence for the close relationship of these resistance determinants in human and animal isolates (Willems et al., 1999). Restriction length polymorphism (RFLP) analysis and sequencing of several complete VanA transposons of 13 VRE isolates representing 7 RFLP types identified 22 different Tn1546 derivatives within a body of 97 VRE. Differences included point mutations in *orf1, van*S, *van*A, *van*X, and *van*Y. In addition, insertions of IS1216V-IS3-like elements in *orf1*, of IS1251 in the vanS–vanH intergenic region, and of IS1216V in the vanX–vanY intergenic region were discovered. Presence of IS elements was often associated with deletions in Tn1546. Identical Tn1546 types were found among human and farm animal VRE in The Netherlands, suggesting a common resistance gene pool. VRE isolates from hospitals in Oxford (UK) and Chicago (USA) included in this molecular analysis suggested the possibility of horizontal transmission of the vancomycin resistance transposon. On the basis of the DNA polymorphism of Tn1546 (presented in Figure 11.5) the tracing of the routes of transmission of vancomycin resistance can be successfully exploited.

The ban on avoparcin use as being a contributor to vancomycin resistance was politically achieved because molecular methods proved unequivocally that the resistance genes involved (*van*A) were identical with the genes characterized in human clinical isolates (Klare et al., 1995a,b). In addition, avoparcin-induced vancomycin resistance was shown in the laboratory to be capable of transfer by conjugation to other enterococci and staphylococci (Noble et al., 1992; Klare et al., 1995a). A comparison of VRE from poultry (79% of 305 isolates including 58% high-level-vancomycin resistant *Ent. faecium*) with VRE from humans by genome-typing with pulsed-field gel electrophoresis did not reveal genetic overlap. Nucleotide-sequencing of the intergenic vanC–vanY region, however, showed full sequence conservation in more than 50% of the strains, suggesting that dissemination (by conjugation) of the resistance genes carried on transposable elements may be of greater importance than clonal dissemination of resistant strains (van den Braak et al., 1998).

Enterococci in Fermented Food

The numbers of viable enterococci in contaminated raw milk, poultry, pork, and beef are usually in the range of 10^2–10^4 per gram (Teuber et al., 1996). If these products are properly heat treated during cooking or processing (calculating with a D_{65} value of 2 min and a z value of 7–8) viable enterococci will be eliminated. If fermented products are made from the raw substrates of meat and milk, like sausages and cheeses, the contaminating enterococci (in addition to staphylococci, and eventually enterobacteria) may multiply to high numbers, for example, more than 10^7 CFU per gram in soft cheeses (Teuber et al., 1996). Based on the high prevalence of antibiotic-resistant enterococci in meat and milk, antibiotic-resistant enterococci should occur in fermented products from raw milk and meat.

In 1980, a preliminary study of 67 European cheeses made from raw and pasteurized milk yielded 27 (40%) samples containing enterococci (10^3–10^7 CFU per gram) (Sievers et al., 1993). In 15 (55%) of these cheeses, *Ent. faecalis, Ent. faecium*, and *Ent. durans* strains were isolated showing resistance to one or more of the following antibiotics: penicillin, cefalotin, furadoin, fucidin, erythromycin, tetracycline, and chloramphenicol. The multiple drug resistance level was 68% (Teuber et al., 1996); 25% of pasteurized and 67% of raw milk cheeses contained enterococci. The presence of enterococci in pasteurized cheeses is due to recontamination after pasteurization. A follow-up study in 1991 and 1995 investigating 53 hard, semi-hard, and soft cheeses presumably made from raw milk yielded 39 antibiotic-resistant *Ent. faecalis*, 12 *Ent. faecium*, 3 *Ent. casseliflavius*, 2 *Ent. durans*,

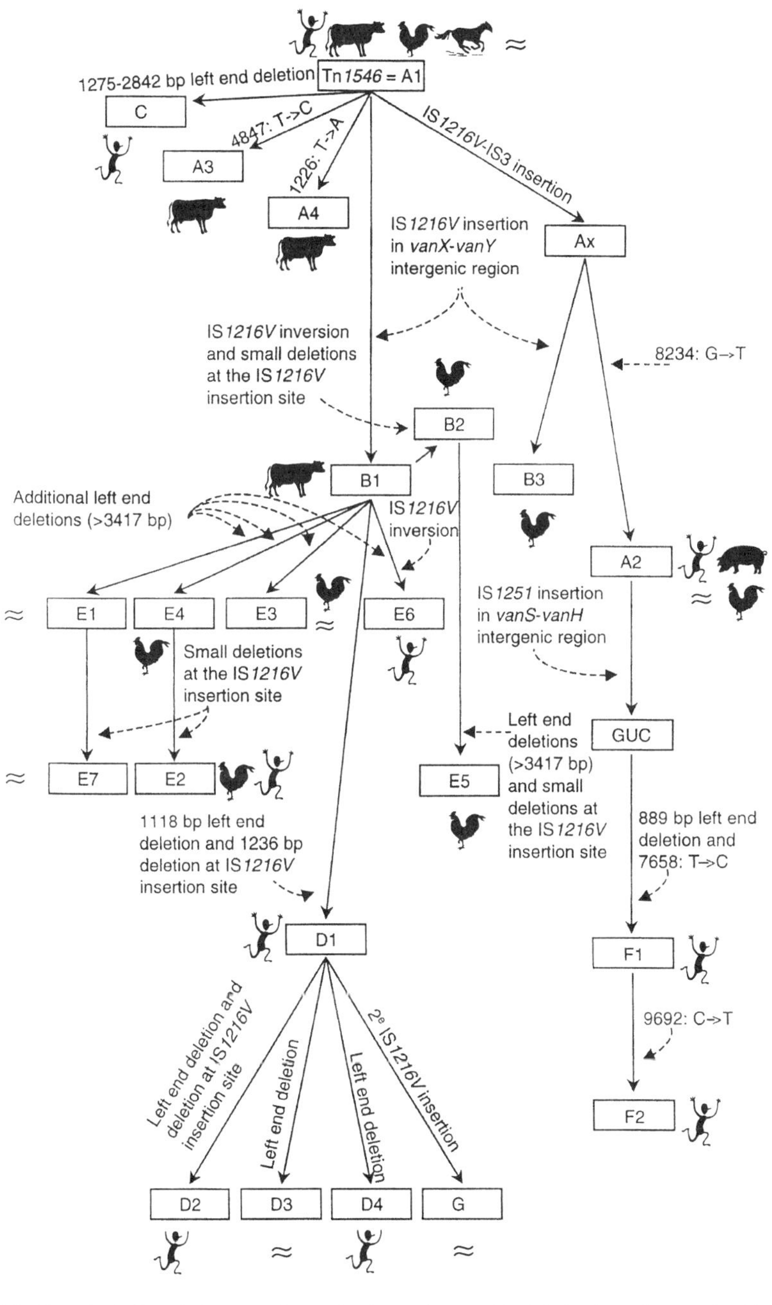

Figure 11.5. Hypothetical evolutionary scheme for the various Tn*1546* derivatives characterized by Willems et al. (1999) for the archetypal vancomycin-resistance transposon Tn*1546* (type A1, see Figure 11.4). Boxes represent the different Tn*1546* types. Filled arrows indicate transition of Tn*1546* type A1 to the other Tn*1546* types. The signets indicate the sources of the investigated strains (human, pig, calf, chicken, sewage (≈)). Investigated strains originated from different parts of Europe and the United States of America. The original figure is taken from Willems et al., 1999 (copy-right owners: ASM and authors have been asked for permission, answer pending).

and 3 undefined enterococcal strains. Resistance to penicillin (18%), erythromycin (48%), gentamicin (80%), tetracycline (59%), rifampicin (7%), chloramphenicol (32%), fusidic acid (14%), and vancomycin (4%) was detected. Prevalence of multiple drug resistance was 51%. A common multiple drug resistance type included resistance to tetracycline, chloramphenicol, erythromycin, and gentamicin. The vancomycin-resistant isolates have not yet been characterized.

Seventeen samples of minced meat, raw meat sausages, and ham yielded 8 *Ent. faecalis*, 6 *Ent. faecium*, 3 *Ent. casseliflavius*, 3 *Entt. durans*, and 26 undefined enterococcal strains (between 10^2 and 10^5 CFU per gram) which were resistant to one or more antibiotics including streptomycin, erythromycin, penicillin, tetracycline, rifampicin, gentamicin, and chloramphenicol. The incidence was 100% for streptomycin, 26% each for tetracycline and chloramphenicol, 13% for gentamicin, 8% for rifampicin, 6% for chloramphenicol, and 4% for penicillin. Using erythromycin and tetracycline as markers, 15% of the enterococcal isolates from cheese and sausage could transfer resistances to plasmid-free *Ent. faecalis* JH2-2 or *Lc. lactis* Bu2-60 by conjugation in filter mating experiments (see Table 11.2). Probably, conjugative plasmids like pRE39 and transposons like Tn*FO1* are involved since resistance genes can be located to chromosomal and/or plasmid DNA (see below).

Molecular Characterization of Antibiotic Resistance of Food-Borne Enterococci Compared to Clinical Specimens

The first studies of food-borne enterococci at a molecular level (Rollins et al., 1985) have clearly shown that the erythromycin resistance genes responsible were very similar in enterococci isolated from humans, chicken, and pigs. In addition, they were encoded on Tn*917*-like conjugative transposons. Recently, 88% of the enterococci isolated from broilers, cattle, pigs, and humans in the Danish surveillance studies (Aarestrup et al., 1998) were reported to carry erythromycin resistance genes identified by specific nucleotide probes as *ermB* (Jensen et al., 1999).

Following a similar line of experimentation, three of the conjugative enterococcal strains from our investigations were further characterized at a molecular level.

Enterococcus sp. RE39 from minced beef contained a conjugative 26 kb plasmid pRE39 similar to pAMβ1; however, its MLS resistance was inducible. pRE39 encoded an rRNA methylase with an amino acid sequence identical to the enzyme encoded on pAMβ1 (Teuber et al., 1996; see Figure 11.1). This gene was identified in an additional 18 of the enterococcal strains investigated from sausages and cheese by hybridization with a specific nucleotide probe and PCR, thus corroborating the Danish observations (Jensen et al., 1999). The host range of conjugative transfer by filter mating of pRE39 includes *Ent. faecalis* JH2-2, *Lc. lactis* Bu2-60, *List. innocua, Leuc. mesenteroides*, and *Bacillus subtilis*. Transfer frequencies on a receptor basis were high, having a value of 10^{-3}–10^{-6}.

The chloramphenicol and erythromycin resistances in *Ent. faecalis* RE25 are encoded on a 49 kb conjugative plasmid pRE25, which transfers these resistances to *List. innocua, Ent. faecalis* JH2-2, and *Lc. lactis* BU2-60 at frequencies of 10^{-5}–10^{-6}. The nucleotide sequence of the cloned chloramphenicol acetyltransferase is 100% identical with that of the *Strep. agalactiae* pIP501 gene (Perreten, Moschetti and Teuber GeneBank Acc. No. X92945). The erythromycin resistance region of this plasmid hybridized with the specific *erm* nucleotide probe from pAMβ1. The complete nucleotide sequence of this plasmid is currently being investigated. A completed coherent sequence of 26.000 kbp of pRE25 shows it to contain a substantial part of the known plasmid pIP501 (see Figure 11.6; Schwarz et al., 1999).

Table 11.2. **Conjugal Transfer of Tetracycline, Erythromycin and Chloramphenicol Resistances from *Enterococcus* Strains Isolated from Food (Teuber et al., 1996) to Plasmid-Free *Enterococcus faecalis* JH2-2 and *Lc. lactis* subsp. *lactis* Biovar. *Diacetylactis* Bu2-60 During Filter Mating**[a]

Product	Donor	Resistances	Selection	Recipients with Transfer Frequency: *Ent. faecalis* JH2-2	Recipients with Transfer Frequency: *Lc. lactis lactis* Bu2-60	Resistance Gene (hybridization)	Localization in the Donor Strains
Cheese							
Bösbachli	*Ent. faecalis* FO1	Tet Lm Erm Cm Gm	Tet5	10^{-5}	10^{-6}	*tetM*	Chromosome
							Plasmid (ca 30 kb)
			Erm5 Cm20	10^{-8}	—	ermAM (*cat*pIP501)	Plasmid (ca 27 kb)
Bösbachli	*Ent. faecalis* FO5	Tet Lm Erm Cm Gm	Tet5	ne	10^{-6}	*tetM*	Chromosome
							Plasmid (ca 30 kb)
			Erm5 Cm20	10^{-8}	—	*ermAM* (*cat*pIP501)	Plasmid (ca 30 kb)
Crottin	*Ent. faecalis* FE1	Tet Lm Gm	Tet5	ne	10^{-8}	*tetM*	Chromosome
Brie de Meaux	*Ent. faecalis* FF4	Lm Erm Gm Pen	Erm5	10^{-2}	—	*ermAM*	Plasmid (ca 30 kb)
Appenzeller 2	*Ent. faecalis* AP21	Tet Lm Erm Cm Gm	Erm5	10^{-5}	—	*ermAM*	Plasmid (ca 30 kb)
Appenzeller 5	*Ent. faecalis* AP51	Tet Lm Erm Gm	Erm5	10^{-6}	—	*ermAM*	Plasmid (ca 27 kb)
	Ent. faecalis AP53	Tet Cm Gm Pen	Tet5	10^{-5}	—	*tetM*	Chromosome
Appenzeller 6	*Ent. faecalis* AP62	Tet Lm Erm Cm Gm	Erm5	10^{-5}	—	*ermAM*	Plasmid (ca 30 kb)
Tête de Moine 1	*Ent. faecalis* TM11	Tet Lm Erm Cm Gm	Erm5	10^{-6}	—	*ermAM*	Plasmid (ca 27 kb)
San Carlo TI	*Ent. faecalis* 216	Lm Erm Cm Gm	Erm5	10^{-5}	—	*ermAM*	Plasmid (>50 kb)
Appenzeller 3	*Ent. faecium* AP34	Tet Gm	Tet5	10^{-5}	—	nh	Plasmid (>50 kb)
Meat products							
Salami 6	*Enterococcus* sp. RE45	Lm Tet	Tet5	ne	10^{-9}	*tetM*	Chromosome
							Plasmid (>50 kb)
Salami 3	*Ent. faecium* RE14	Tet Lm Erm	Tet5	ne	10^{-9}	*tetM*	Chromosome
							Plasmid (>50 kb)
			Erm5	10^{-6}	—	*ermAM*	Plasmid (ca 30 kb)
Salami 2	*Ent. faecium* RE1	Lm Erm Pen	Erm5	10^{-5}	—	*ermAM*	Plasmid (ca 30 kb)
Landjaeger 3	*Ent. hirae* RE22	Lm Erm	Erm5	10^{-7}	—	*ermAM*	Plasmid (ca 30 kb)

(continued)

Table 11.2. ***(continued)***

				Recipients with Transfer Frequency			
Product	Donor	Resistances	Selection	*Ent. faecalis* JH2-2	*Lc. lactis lactis* Bu2-60	Resistance Gene (hybridization)	Localization in the Donor Strains
Landjaeger 5	*Ent. faecalis* RE25	Tet Lm Erm Cm	Erm5	10^{-5}	10^{-6}	*ermAM* (*cat*pIP501)	Plasmid (49 kb)
			Cm20	10^{-5}	10^{-6}		
Landjaeger 5	*Ent. faecium* RE27	Lm Erm	Erm5	10^{-6}	—	*ermAM*	Plasmid (ca 30 kb)
Salami 5	*Ent. casseliflavus* RE37	Tet Lm Pen		10^{-6}	—	*ermAM*	Plasmid (ca 30 kb)
Minced meat	*Enterococcus* sp. RE39		Erm5	10^{-4}	10^{-3}	*ermAM*	Plasmid (26.5 kb)
Pancetta	*Ent. faecalis* RE52	Tet Lm Erm	Erm5	10^{-4}	—	*ermAM*	Plasmid (>50 kb)

[a] Erm5, erythromycin [5 μg/ml]; Cm20, chloramphenicol [20 μg/ml]; Tet5, tetracycline [5 μg/ml]; Gm, gentamicin; Lm, lincomycin; Pen, penicillin; ne, not examined; —, no transfer; nh, no hybridization with *tetM* gene probe. Conjugative transfer and allocation of resistance genes to transferred plasmids or the chromosome was investigated by Southern hybridization of total DNA extracts of resistant transconjugants after gel electrophoresis according to Perreten et al. (1997).

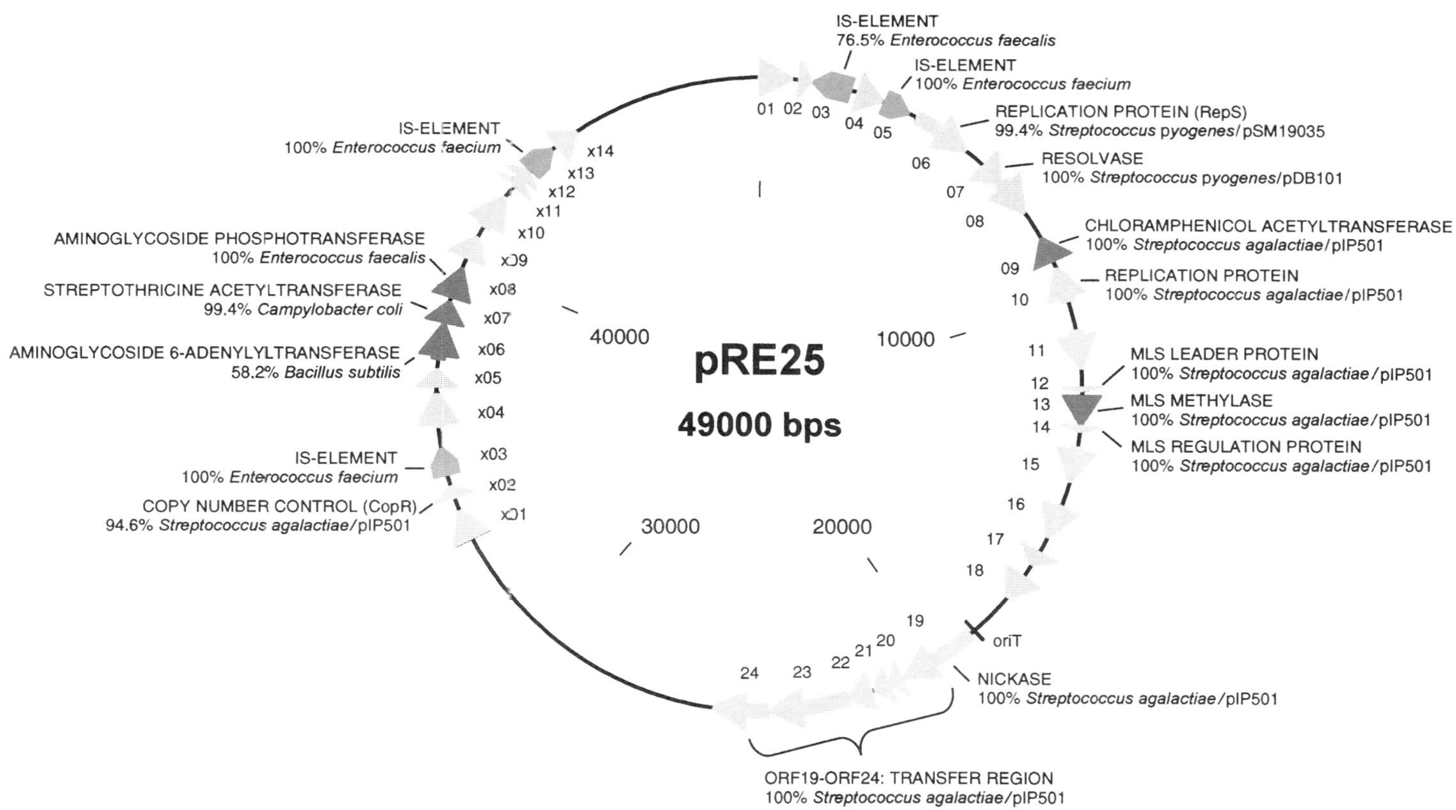

Figure 11.6. Partial structure of the conjugative multi-resistance plasmid pRE25 (49,000 bp) detected in *Ent. faecalis* strain RE25 isolated from a raw fermented sausage (Teuber et al., 1996, 1999; see also Table 11.2). The nucleotide sequences of all drawn out genes have been determined in our laboratory (Schwarz et al., 1999). Resistance genes are indicated in blue, IS-elements in green, all other ORFs in red. In addition, the homologies to known genes are given in percent amino acid identities. The *Ent. faecium* IS elements are identical with IS*1216* and IS*1216V*, resp., also present in Tn*1546* (ORF2 in Figure 11.4). The right arm of the plasmid is, in many parts, identical with published sequences of pIP501 from *Strep. agalactiae* (*orf09* to *orf24*; Macrina and Archer, 1993). The left arm of the plasmid contains two IS elements (*orfx03* and *orfx13*) of the IS*1216* type. Orientation of the direction of transcription is still arbitrary. *Orf05* is also identical to IS*1216*, *orf03* is a new IS element. Orfx07 representing streptothricin acetyltransferase of Gram-negative origin is noteworthy.

Transfer of the tetracycline resistance gene (at the nucleotide level 99.8% identical to *tetM* of transposon Tn*916*) from *Ent. faecalis* FO1 isolated from a raw milk mountain cheese (about 10^4 CFU per gram), to *Staph. aureus* (10^{-9}), *Ent. faecalis* JH2-2, *List. innocua* (10^{-6}), *Leuc. mesenteroides* (10^{-7}), and *Lc. lactis* Bu2-60 (10^{-6}) was achieved by filter mating. The mobile genetic element was identified as the Tn*916*-type transposon Tn*FO1*. It resides on the chromosome and on a 30 kb plasmid in this strain (Perreten et al., 1997a).

It must be concluded that antibiotic-resistant enterococci are present in some of our daily food supply. This explains their presence in the intestinal microflora of people who have not been treated with antibiotics but provide a community reservoir (Bates et al., 1993; Corpet, 1988; Liassine et al., 1998; van den Braak et al., 1998). The consumption of raw sausages or cheeses containing 10^5 to 10^7 multiple-drug-resistant enterococci per gram leads to the ingestion of 10^9 resistant bacteria in a meal containing 100 g of product. When these enterococci reach the intestine, at least a transient colonization is most likely to occur as has been shown in the case of intestinal "probiotic" bacteria including lactobacilli, bifidobacteria, and enterococci (Elmer et al., 1996; Tannock, 1998). Transfer of resistance genes into the endogenous intestinal microflora of the consumer is highly probable (Corpet, 1988; van den Braak et al., 1998; Witte, 1998). If the *Enterococcus*-contaminated food is carefully cooked or heat-treated, the spread of resistance would be blocked. However, as stated recently (MacDonald et al., 1997), a paucity of information exists on enterococcal colonization of the intestinal tract and the development of infection in humans. Nonetheless, colonization of germ-free animals and conjugative transfer of plasmids and transposons in this biotope has been reported in several instances (Doucet-Populaire et al., 1991; Brockmann et al., 1998). Fortunately, the clinical relevance of vancomycin-resistant enterococci in Europe still seems to be low (Grüneberg and Hryniewicz, 1998).

Lactobacillus

For bacteria to survive in an antibiotic containing habitat they must be expected to pick up antibiotic resistance genes from other bacteria. This has been observed (albeit in a small number of studies) for lactobacilli in habitats such as the bovine udder surface, the intestinal, vaginal, and nasopharyngal mucosae of man and animals (see Table 11.3). Strains of lactobacilli resistant to vancomycin (intrinsic), cefazolin, penicillin, tetracyclin, trimethoprim-sulfamethoxazole, and ciprofloxacin have been occasionally identified in cases of human *Lactobacillus*-bacteremia (Antony et al., 1996). As with food-borne pathogens, LAB contaminate milk and meat obtained from animals treated with antibiotics and carrying populations of resistant bacteria. Recently, tetracycline-resistant lactobacilli have been observed in raw salami type sausages in Belgium corroborating our previous results in Switzerland (Gevers et al., 2000).

Indeed, tetracycline-resistant *Lb. plantarum* has been found in several raw milk soft cheeses (G. Dasen, ETH Zurich, unpublished). Plasmid-borne erythromycin resistance (MLS type) was identified in a poultry isolate of *Lb. reuteri* (Tannock et al., 1994). Another poultry isolate of *Lb. reuteri* contained a 7 kb plasmid pTC82 harboring a gene for a chloramphenicol acetyltransferase homologous to that on the *Staph. aureus* plasmid pC194 (Lin et al., 1996). A *Lb. fermentum* isolated from pig feces ($>10^8$ CFU/gram) carried a 5.7 kb plasmid with an *erm* gene conferring high level erythromycin resistance (MIC $>$ 1 mg/ml), which was 98.2% identical to the gene of the enterococcal conjugative transposon Tn*1545* (Fons et al., 1997). As mentioned previously, the conjugative plasmid pAMβ1 can move from *Lactococcus* and *Enterococcus* species into *Lb. reuteri* and back

Table 11.3. Antibiotic Resistances and Resistance Plasmids in Enteric *Lactobacillus* Species from Animals

Species	Source	Plasmid Name and Size	Observed Resistances or Resistance Genes	Reference
Lb. acidophilus strain PA3	Pig		Tetracycline Erythromycin Oleandomycin Kanamycin Neomycin Gentamicin	Klaenhammer and Sutherland, 1980
Lb. acidophilus (20 strains)	Pig and calf feces	Several	Penicillin (1) Ampicillin (1) Cloxacillin (7) Aminoglycosides (20) Tetracycline (15) Erythromycin (10) Chloramphenicol (1) Bacitracin (6)	Vescovo et al., 1982
Lb. reuteri (16 strains)	Pig and calf feces	Several	Cloxacillin (16) Aminglycosides (16) Tetracycline (16) Erythromycin (13) Chloramphenicol (3) Rifamycin (3) Bacitracin (10)	Vescovo et al., 1982
Lb. reuteri	Poultry	pET 633 9.8 kb	*ermGT* (similar to *ermC* of pE 194)	Tannock et al., 1989
Lb. reuteri	Poultry	pLUL631	*erm* (similar to *ermB* of pIP501)	Connell and Tannock, 1989
Lb. reuteri G4	Chicken	pTC82	*catTC* (81% identity to *cat*PC 194)	Lin et al., 1996
Lb. fermentum	Pig	pLEM3 5.7 kb	*erm* (98.2% identity to Tn*1545 erm*)	Fons et al., 1997
Lb. plantarum	Raw pork	pCAT 8.5 kb	*cat*	Ahn et al., 1992

again (Tannock, 1987). Clearly, enteric lactobacilli participate in promiscuous gene transfer in their natural biotopes and in the laboratory. It is not surprising in the light of the experiences with enterococci that lactobacilli (e.g., *Lb. plantarum, Lb. acidophlus, Lb. brevis, Lb. casei*) isolated from "home-made" Spanish cheese (Serena, Gamonedo, Cabrales) did show resistance toward penicillin G, cloxacillin, streptomycin, gentamicin, tetracycline, erythromycin, and chloramphenicol (Herrero et al., 1996). Also, antibiotic-resistant lactococci and leuconostocs were isolated from the same material.

Of 14 *Lactobacillus* strains isolated from the crops of broiler chicken (*Lb. acidophilus, Lb. fermentum, Lb. crispatus, Lb. casei* subsp. *casei*, and *Lb. salivarius*) 12 strains were resistant to ciprofloxacin, 11 to gentamicin, 11 to streptomycin, 14 to trimethoprim/sulfamethoxazole, 8 to tetracycline, 2 to erythromycin, 5 to vancomycin (intrinsic), 14 to metronidazole (intrinsic), and all 14 to bacitracin, an antibiotic used as feed additive for the parent animals, but none to chloramphenicol, ampicillin, penicillin G, and rifampicin. All strains showed multiple drug resistance (three- to sixfold), but the question of intrinsic resistances has not been finally cleared; however, intrinsic resistances to tetracyline and erythromycin have not been reported for these bacteria in the literature.

Lactococcus

It has been known for some time that lactococci can accept antibiotic resitance genes like pAMβ1 by conjugation (Gasson and Davies, 1980). However, they should be sensitive to most clinically important antibiotics as summarized above in paragraph 3. Antibiotic resistant lactococci might develop in biotopes where they come into constant contact with antibiotics. Such a biotope is the dairy cow which is commonly treated with antibiotics to cure or prevent mastitis (National Research Council and Institute of Medicine, 1998; Teuber, 1999). From raw milk the bacteria are transferred into raw milk cheeses (Teuber, 1999b). We have isolated a multiply drug resistant *Lc. lactis* subsp. *lactis* pK214 from a raw milk soft cheese. The strain carries a resistance plasmid that was completely sequenced (Perreten et al., 1997b).

Genomics of the 29,871 bp Multiresistance Plasmid pK214 from Lactococcus lactis

Plasmid pK214 is resident in a *Lc. lactis* strain K214 which is streptomycin-, tetracycline-, and chloramphenicol-resistant (Perreten et al., 1997b). Genes encoding these three antibiotic resistances (*str, tet*, and *cat*) are found on this plasmid (see Table 11.4 and Figure 11.7). Since we have no cured strains of the original host *Lc. lactis* K214, further genes encoding the three resistances could be present in its genome or the other three plasmids.

Organization of pK214

A map describing the genetic organisation of pK214 is shown in Figure 11.2. The 29871-nucleotide sequence contains 29 open reading frames (ORFs), which may represent functionally translated or truncated genes. The deduced products and the most homologous proteins from the databanks are listed in Table 11.4. The average G + C content of pK214 is 32.4 mol% which is significantly lower than that of the *Lc. lactis* genomic DNA (36–38%; Kilpper-Bälz et al., 1982). It supports the idea that horizontal DNA transfer from other organisms with a lower G + C content has occurred. Comparative sequence analysis of the entire plasmid DNA and its putative ORFs demonstrates that the plasmid is composed of distinct DNA segments which originate in species like *Staphyloccoccus aureus* (32–36 mol % G + C), *Listeria monocytogenes* (37–39 mol% G + C), and *Ent. faecalis* or *Ent. faecium* (34–39 mol % G + C).

The DNA segment containing nucleotides 1–9000 is assumed to be the basic backbone of the *Lactococcus* plasmid into which DNA segments from other organisms have been integrated. Part of this *Lactococcus* segment is a *repB* gene encoding a RepB protein with high homology (around 80%) to Rep proteins typically found in *Lactococcus* plasmids like pWV02, pCI305, pCI528, pSL2, and pVS40. The RepB protein of pVS40 (von Wright and Räty, 1993) from *Lc. lactis* subsp. *lactis* biovar *diacetylatis* has a homology of 82.3% and that of pMRC01, a 60 kb conjugative plasmid from *Lc. lactis* DPC3147 strain, of 80.0% to pK214 (Dougherty et al., 1998). Interestingly, the pK214 region from ORF04 to ORF08 (positions 1824 to 6185) has an overall identity of 91.3% at the nucleotide level

Table 11.4. Genomics of the 29,871 bp Plasmid pK214 from *Lc. lactis* subsp. *lactis* Isolated from a Raw Milk Soft Cheese. ORFs Are Deduced from the Nucleotide Sequence and Compared to Known Amino Acid Sequences from Databanks

ORF No.	5′end pos. #	3′end pos. #	Known Protein with Highest Homology {organismsymbol 125 \f "Symbol" \s 9	% aa-Identity	% G/C-content	Accession No.
ORF01	21	593	DNA invertase of pMRC01 {*Lactococcus lactis*symbol 125 \f "Symbol" \s 9	71.0	29.1	AE001272
ORF02	681	1,448	*soj* protein {*Mycoplasma pneumoniae*symbol 125 \f "Symbol" \s 9	26.7	27.9	U34816
ORF03	1,451	1,750	Hypothetical protein	—	27.7	—
ORF04	1,824	2,189	orf59 gene product of pMRC01 {*Lactococcus lactis*symbol 125 \f "Symbol" \s 9	96.4	28.7	AE001272
ORF05	2,204	2,584	orf60 gene product of pMRC01 {*Lactococcus lactis*symbol 125 \f "Symbol" \s 9	99.0	30.4	AE001272
ORF06	2,610	3,554	orf61 gene product of pMRC01 {*Lactococcus lactis*symbol 125 \f "Symbol" \s 9	99.4	28.9	AE001272
ORF07	4,236	5,390	*repB* protein of pVS40 {*Lactococcus lactis*symbol 125 \f "Symbol" \s 9	82.3	35.5	L02920
ORF08	5,868	6,185	orf63 gene product of pMRC01 {*Lactococcus lactis*symbol 125 \f "Symbol" \s 9	95.9	31.1	AE001272
ORF09	7,231	8,925	*nel* protein (*traA* protein in *S. aureus*) of pMRC01 {*Lactococcus lactis*symbol 125 \f "Symbol" \s 9	97.3	29.6	AE001272
ORF10	9,592	10,353	IS*904* transposase {*Lactococcus lactis*symbol 125 \f "Symbol" \s 9	99.6	39.1	D00696
ORF11	10,534	11,790	*mef214* protein (*mefA*) {*Streptococcus pyogenes*symbol 125 \f "Symbol" \s 9	34.6	41.9	U70055
ORF12	11,879	12,331	*phnB* protein {*Eschericia coli*symbol 125 \f "Symbol" \s 9	29.9	37.7	J05260
ORF13	12,458	12,991	*p35* protein {*Eschericia coli*symbol 125 \f "Symbol" \s 9	38.0	44.4	X13270
ORF14	13,008	13,382	IS*904* truncated transposase {*Lactococcus lactis*symbol 125 \f "Symbol" \s 9	100.0	37.9	D00696
ORF15	14,256	13,438	IS*861* transposase {*Streptococcus agalactiae*symbol 125 \f "Symbol" \s 9	43.0	34.6	M22449
ORF16	15,678	15,127	*binL* protein (resolvase) {*Staphylococcus aureus*symbol 125 \f "Symbol" \s 9	79.2	37.7	X52734
ORF17	16,998	16,153	*rob* protein {*Eschericia coli*symbol 125 \f "Symbol" \s 9	32.7	37.9	M97495

(*continued*)

Table 11.4. (*continued*)

ORF No.	5′end pos. #	3′end pos. #	Known Protein with Highest Homology {organismsymbol 125 \f "Symbol" \s 9	% aa-Identity	% G/C-content	Accession No.
ORF18	17,155	17,841	Transposase of Tn*1546* {*Enterococcus faecium*symbol 125 \f "Symbol" \s 9	99.1	37.4	U49512
ORF19	18,908	18,060	Streptomycin adenylase of pS194 {*Staphylococcus aureus*symbol 125 \f "Symbol" \s 9	98.8	24.7	X06627
ORF20	19,755	18,916	*repD* protein of pC221 {*Staphylococcus aureus*symbol 125 \f "Symbol" \s 9	89.1	31.2	X02529
ORF21	21,663	20,452	*mob* protein (*repC*) {*Lactobacillus plantarum*symbol 125 \f "Symbol" \s 9	46.3	34.8	M33531
ORF22	22,563	21,916	Chloramphenicol acetyltransferase of pSBK203 {*Staphylococcus aureus*symbol 125 \f "Symbol" \s 9	99.5	24.1	M90091
ORF23	23,036	22,698	Truncated replication initator {*Listeria monocytogenes*symbol 125 \f "Symbol" \s 9	95.1	24.8	X68412
ORF24	23,201	23,887	Transposase of Tn*1546* {*Enterococcus faecium*symbol 125 \f "Symbol" \s 9	99.1	37.4	U49512
ORF25	24,429	24,199	orf7 gene product of Tn*916* {*Enterococcus faecalis*symbol 125 \f "Symbol" \s 9	56.2	37.7	L15633
ORF26	24,906	25,265	orf9 gene product of Tn*916* {*Enterococcus faecalis*symbol 125 \f "Symbol" \s 9	53.6	36.1	L15633
ORF27	25,946	25,779	Hypothetical protein of pIP811 {*Listeria monocytogenes*symbol 125 \f "Symbol" \s 9	100	35.1	L09756
ORF28	27,974	26,034	*tetS* protein of pIP811 {*Listeria monocytogenes*symbol 125 \f "Symbol" \s 9	99.8	33.3	L09756
ORF29	29,084	29,770	Transposase of Tn*1546* {*Enterococcus faecium*symbol 125 \f "Symbol" \s 9	100.0	37.4	U49512

with a segment of pMRC01 and up to 99.4% identity to selected ORFs (Table 11.4). As in the proven theta-type replicon of plasmid pCI305, the putative *repB* gene in pK214 is preceded by an AT-rich sequence (iteron) of 22-bp (5′-CCGAAAAAAACTGTGTATATG-3′) which is tandemly repeated three and one-half times (Foley et al., 1996). Therefore, in analogy to plasmid pCIP305, it is concluded that the region between positions 3970 and 4220 has to be regarded as containing the origin of replication (*oriV*) of pK214.

Other putative functions within the designated *Lactococcus* moiety could be assigned to another replication-associated protein (ORF02), a DNA nickase (ORF09), and a resolvase (ORF01), which is 92% identical with a corresponding sequence in the *Lc. lactis* plasmid pKR223 (Twomey et al., 2000). We detected 97.3% identity of ORF09 to the

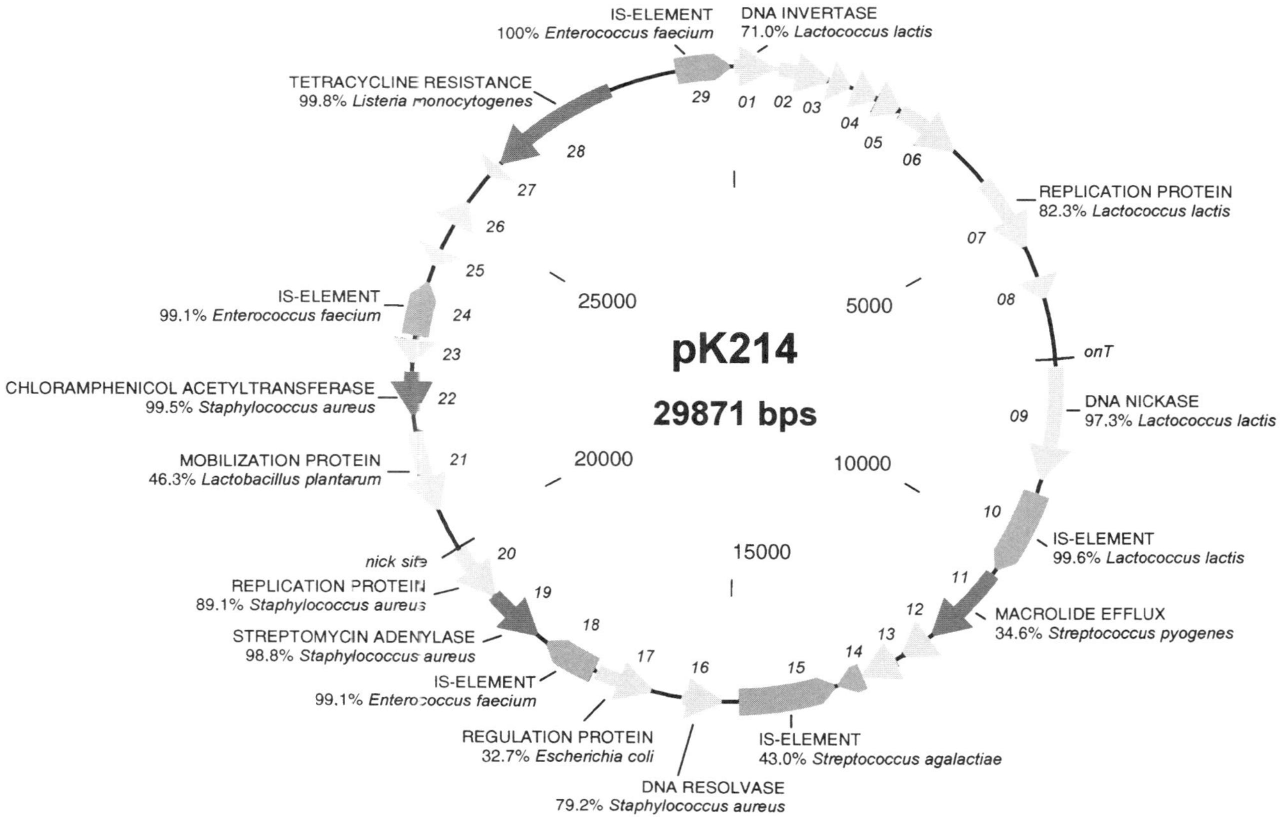

Figure 11.7. Structure of the multi-resistance plasmid pK214 from *Lactococcus lactis* subsp. *lactis* K214 which was isolated from a raw milk soft cheese (Brie de Meaux; Teuber et al., 1996). The complete nucleotide sequence revealed that the resistance genes are almost identical with genes previously reported in pathogenic bacteria like *Listeria monocytogenes* (tetracycline resistance) and *Staphylococcus aureus* (chloramphenicol and streptomycin resistance). The composite plasmid has obviously been assembled with the aid of insertion elements, like in pRE25 (see Figure 11.6), derived from IS element IS1216 (*orf18, orf24, orf29*). Orf15 is a new IS element also present in several copies in the completely sequenced genome of *Lc.lactis* IL1403 (Bolotin et al., 1999). Figure modified from Teuber (1999) based on Perreten et al. (1997b).

traA protein of pMRC01. The nickase gene of pK214, named *nel*, is not preceded by a nicking site (*oriT*) typically found upstream of nickase genes in conjugative plasmids of both Gram-positive and Gram-negative bacteria (Climo et al., 1996). Furthermore, other conjugative transfer functions seem to be absent from pK214. It would also explain why we failed to demonstrate conjugation-mediated plasmid transfer but succeeded in electroporation (Perreten et al., 1997b). Surprisingly, the G + C mol% values of the potential genes in the "*Lactococcus*" segment are lower than those of *Lactococcus* genomes.

Due to high sequence homologies of predicted gene products, we propose that segments from *Staphylococcus, Listeria, and Enteroccoccus* have been inserted into pK214 during its evolution. Since pK214 harbors five complete insertion sequence (IS) elements (three of them almost identical to the IS*1216* elements from *Ent. faecium* (Arthur and Courvalin, 1994), the heterologous segment acquisition may have been driven by these elements.

Insertion Sequence Elements of pK214

Two IS*904* elements (Dodd et al., 1990) obviously from *Lc. lactis* were found adjacent to the *Lactococcus* segment (described above) on the physical map of pK214 (Figure 11.3). One of these elements, however, is truncated. It seems to be interrupted by another IS element, named IS*215*. This new IS element contains two hypothetical proteins, two perfect inverted repeats of 14 nucleotides and two direct repeats of 5 bases. It belongs to the IS*3* family since its hypothetical transposase sequence has the characteristic D(35)E motif (Khan et al., 1990). Both invariant residues (Asp [D] at positions 13722–13720, and Glu [E] at positions 13614–13612, respectively) are surrounded by highly conserved residues of the motif. IS215 is identical with IS1077 present in seven copies in the genome of *Lc. lactis* IL1403, which was recently sequenced in its entirety (Bolotin et al., 1999).

Distinct segments resembling sequences from organisms other than *Lactococcus* are flanked by *Ent. faecium* IS-like elements. Three IS*1216*-like elements (IS*214*-I, IS*214*-II, IS*214*-III) are unidirectionally dispersed on pK214 (Figure 11.3). The observed high sequence homologies of these elements prove that they originate from *Ent. faecium*, where they have been shown to be be involved in high level vancomycin-resistant elements like Tn*1546* (Handwerger and Skoble, 1995; Rice and Carias, 1997; Jensen, 1998). Such mobile units (e.g., Tn*5385* or Tn*1546*-like transposons) were found to be intersected by one or several IS*1216*-like IS elements. Their roles in transposition of these huge mobile elements are still not clearly defined. In pK214, the pair IS*214*-I/IS*214*-II contains a segment probably originating from *Listeria*, whereas the pair IS*214*-II/IS*214*-III could represent the frame for a *Staph. aureus* derived segment (see below).

Antibiotic Resistance Genes of pK214

The segment containing ORF 16, 19, 20, and 22 seem to be derived from *Staphylococcus* since these ORFs show high homologies (78.8–99.5% identity) to proteins encoded on plasmids found in *Staphylococcus aureus*. Two hypothetical proteins represent antibiotic resistance determinants, namely ORF19 with 98.8% identity to a streptomycin-inactivating adenylase from the *Staphylococcus aureus* plasmid pS194 and ORF22 with 99.5% identity to the chloramphenicol acetyltransferase (Cat) from the *Staphylococcus aureus* plasmid pSBK203 (Table 11.4). Moreover, a homologous Cat protein was also identified on the multiresistant plasmid pWDB100 from *Listeria monocytogenes* (Hadorn et al., 1994). An alignment of the *cat* gene products belonging to the cat_{pC223} class (Trieu-Cuot et al., 1993) convincingly demonstrates their close evolutionary relationship (Figure 11.3). In addition, the regulatory region preceding the *cat* gene of pK214 is 100% identical to that of pWDB100 and pS194, respectively. A third antibiotic resistance gene, named *tetS*, corresponding to ORF28 resides on a pK214 segment, probably derived from *Listeria monocytogenes* (Figure 11.3). Its encoded gene product has a 99.8% identity with the tetracyline resistance protein found on plasmid pIP811 of *Listeria monocytogenes* BM4210 (Charpentier et al., 1994). A fourth antibiotic resistance protein is probably encoded by *mef214* (ORF 11) which is expressed and confers resistance to erythromycin in *E. coli*, but not in the original host *Lc. lactis*. It has the molecular characteristic of an efflux protein with 12 membrane spanning domains (Perreten et al., 2000). It is related to proton drug antiporters MefA and MefE of *Strep. pyogenes* and *Strep. pneumoniae*, respectively (Ainsa et al., 1998). No homology to the previously characterized lactococcal proton motive force-dependent drug transporter LmrP is present (Bolhuis et al., 1995).

Acquired Antibiotic Resistances in the Genetic Modification of Lactic Acid Bacteria

Molecular biology of LAB started when Gasson and Davies (1980) demonstrated conjugal transfer of the drug resistance plasmid pAMβ into lactic streptococci and when McKay's and other laboratories discovered a wealth of metabolic plasmids in commercial starter cultures of *Lc. lactis* and its subspecies (McKay, 1983; Pechmann and Teuber, 1980).

Vectors designed for pathogenic streptococci were the first to be applied in lactococcal gene cloning experments: derivatives of the 4.2 kb cryptic plasmid VA 380-I from *Strep. ferus*, of the 30 kb plamsid pIP501 from *Strep. agalactiae*, and of the 26.5 kb plasmid pAMβ1 from *Ent. faecalis* (for a review see de Vos and Simons, 1994) together with their original resistance genes if present. Lactococcal vectors were constructed from small cryptic plasmids such as pWV01 and pSH71. Antibiotic resistance genes as selectable markers were chosen on the basis of known experiences in other Gram-positive and Gram-negative bacteria: the chloramphenicol acetyltransferase gene from pC194, the erythromycin resistance gene from pE194, and the kanamycin nucleotidyl transferase (*knt-110*) gene from pUB110, all originating in *Staphylococcus aureus*. Very clearly, molecular biologists have used the natural principles of gene transfer and antibiotic resistance genes found in humans, animals, and food which are regarded as acquired antibiotic resistances. Recently, food-grade markers and vectors have been developed for LAB to avoid release of antibiotic-resistant, genetically modified LAB with food if they should be applied one day (for further literature see de Vos and Simons, 1994; Leenhouts et al., 1998).

Discussion and Conclusions

From a human point of view LAB have several important properties (Teuber, 1993):

1. Some species are serious human and animal pathogens (e.g., *Strep. pneumoniae, Strep. pyogenes, Strep. agalactiae*). However, these species are phylogenetically well separated from commensal and starter culture LAB (Stackebrandt and Teuber, 1988).

2. Some may be opportunistic pathogens in immunocompromised persons (e.g., *Ent. faecalis, Ent. faecium, Lb. rhamnosus*).
3. Most are commensal bacteria in human and animal habitats (mucosae, intestine) including "low and high GC" species (e.g., bifidobacteria, lactobacilli, lactococci, streptococci, enterococci).
4. They are responsible for economically important spontaneous fermentations of plant materials (e.g., lactobacilli, leuconostocs, pediococci, oenococci for sour dough, sauerkraut, silage, soy sauce, and wine).
5. Specific strains are applied as probiotic cultures to produce food with health claims (e.g., bifidobacteria, lactobacilli, enterococci).
6. They are the main components of starter cultures for the fermentation of more than 150 million tons of milk per year into yogurt, sour milk, and cheese (e.g., lactobacilli, lactococci, leuconostocs, and *Strep. thermophilus*). Such bacteria are generally recognized as safe (GRAS) for human consumption.
7. They are parts of starter cultures for fermented sausages and ham (e.g., *Lb. sake, Lb. curvatus*).
8. They are consumed in live form with the fermented products (up to 10^9 per gram product).
9. Finally, they are involved in the antibiotic resistance transfer cycles within the global biotopes as shown in this chapter.

All these functions are executed by LAB when living in association with other microbes in heavily crowded environments (e.g., 10^{10}–10^{11} bacteria per g of feces). This close contact with other bacteria is an excellent pre-condition for horizontal gene transfer be it by conjugation or transformation.

For example, it has been proposed that the excision and conjugative transfer of the broad host range transposon *Tn*916 is triggered by cell to cell contact (Scott, 1992). This transposon originating from *Ent. faecalis* has been shown to conjugate into many other species of the human nasopharyngal and intestinal microflora. This efficiency is explained by the observation that Tn*916* is not attacked by restriction enzymes in a new host. In addition, it can be accepted in more than one copy on the chromosome, or on a plasmid, or on both. Since excision and integration are often mutagenic leading to base substitutions or, sometimes, to shifts in the reading frame, conjugative transposons are important in creating and maintaining genome plasticity (Scott, 1992). Transposons are common in LAB (Clewell et al., 1995). Tn*916* contains the *tetM* gene (see Table 11.1). A similar transposon is TnFO1 from *Ent. faecalis* FO1, an isolate from a mountain raw milk cheese (Perreten et al., 1997a). This transposon, in contrast to Tn916, is able to excise from the *Lactococcus* chromosome and conjugate from there into *List. innocua*.

The presence of IS elements necessary for DNA excision and transposition has been demonstrated in LAB (Schaefer et al., 1991; Gasson and Fitzgerald, 1994). The detection of IS1181 in *Strep. thermophilus, Strep. salivarius, Lc. lactis*, and *Lb. delbrueckii* subsp. *bulgaricus* has been taken as evidence for horizontal gene transfer during dairy fermentations (Guedon et al., 1995). Horizontal gene transfer between pathogenic (*List. monocytogenes*), potentially pathogenic (*Ent. faecalis*), and starter culture bacteria (*Lc. lactis*) is supported by the occurrence of identical *tet*(S) genes in these species (Poyart-Salmeron et al., 1990; Francois et al., 1997; Perreten et al., 1997b).

Other tools for horizontal gene transfer are the many described conjugative and mobilizable plasmids in LAB (Gasson and Fitzgerald, 1994; Teuber, 1995; Chapter 2 by

Gasson). In lactococci, conjugative plasmids are carriers for vital technological functions including lactose transport and metabolism, citrate transport, casein degradation, oligopeptide transport, bacteriophage resistance, restriction/modification, extracellular polysaccharide synthesis, and bacteriocin production. Metabolic functions have also been shown to be located on transposons, for example, sucrose fermentation on the *Lc. lactis* conjugative nisin transposons Tn5276, Tn5301, Tn5306, and Tn5307 (Gasson and Fitzgerald, 1994).

A further horizontal gene transfer route that needs more scientific attention is transformation in streptococci in their natural environments (saliva, nasopharyngal cavity, and mucosae). It has been conclusively demonstrated that free DNA was able to transform *S. gordonii* DL1 in human saliva (Mercer et al., 1999). Using plasmid pVACMC1, erythromycin resistance was transformed into naturally competent *Strep. gordonii*. The half-life of the transformation capacity in human saliva was 50 s, enough to produce erythromycin-resistant transformants. These findings indicate that DNA released from bacteria or food sources within the mouth has the potential to transform naturally competent oral bacteria. It also corroborates the proposal that the mosaic structures of penicillin binding proteins in *Strep. pneumoniae* have arisen by transformation (Hakenbeck, 1999).

Horizontal gene transfer is obviously an essential mechanism for LAB to adapt to metabolic and antibiotic challenges and thereby survive in a specific environment. If necessary, antibiotic resistance genes take advantage of the existing horizontal tranfer routes also used for metabolic, regulatory, and phage resistance purposes. This is exemplified by the observation that LAB if living in a biotope challenged regularly with antibiotics (human intestine, animal intestine) acquire antibiotic resistance genes. The dependence of acquired resistance on the application of antibiotics can be clearly demonstrated with vancomycin-resistant enterococci in chicken fed with avoparcin (Aarestrup, 1995; van den Braak et al., 1998; Witte, 1998), virginiamycin (Hammerum et al., 1998), or bacitracin (Goldenberger, ETH Zürich, unpublished). Likewise, fermented food made from raw milk and meat may contain a certain proportion of LAB from the originating animals including enterococci, lactobacilli, and lactococci.

Another important observation relates to the fact that there is no barrier between pathogenic (e.g., streptococci), potentially pathogenic (e.g., enterococci), and commensal LAB (e.g., enteric lactobacilli, lactococci) regarding acquired resistances. Identical genes responsible for resistance are found, for example, for tetracycline (e.g., *tetM*), erythromycin (*ermAM*), chloramphenicol (*cat*), streptomyin (*str*), streptogramin (*sat*) in all three cohorts (see Table 11.1). Natural resistance transfer mechanisms identified in these LAB are also very similar and center around conjugative plasmids (e.g., pAMβ1, pAD1, or pIP501 type) and conjugative transposons (e.g., Tn*916* type). Communication of LAB with neighboring bacteria in a natural environment has been supported by *in vitro* and *in vivo* experiments (Brockmann et al., 1996; Doucet-Populaire et al., 1991; Witte, 1998; van den Braak et al., 1998) and the detection of conjugative and non-conjugative antibiotic resistance plasmids in commensal LAB (Teuber et al., 1996; Perreten et al., 1997b; Kullen and Klaenhammer, 1999). For the human population, recent work in Holland has shown that it is not the enterococcal clones coming from farm animals that spread permanently into the human intestinal microflora. It is rather a dispersal of antibiotic (e.g., vancomycin) resistance genes placed on conjugative transposons (e.g., Tn*1546*) or plasmids (van den Braak et al., 1998; Willems et al., 1999).

Molecular biology has used antibiotic resistance genes found in pathogenic bacteria (*cat, ery, nt* from *Staph. aureus*) to construct cloning vectors for LAB. These vectors are now being replaced by food-grade cloning and expression systems (see Leenhouts et al., 1998 for further references).

Like all other bacteria, LAB are prone to genetic exchange to enhance their survival in antibiotic-containing environments. For the food microbiologist, there is no question that it is necessary to avoid the distribution of bacteria with mobilizable antibiotic resistances (see WHO, 1997). Measures include the use of proper starter cultures and of proper substrates (e.g., pasteurized milk) for food fermentations (Teuber et al., 1996). In addition, generation of antibiotic-resistant bacteria in food animals and plants has to be minimized by a prudent use of antibiotics (Levy, 1997; Mazel and Davies, 1999).

References

Ahn, C., Collins-Thompson, D., Duncan, C., and Stiles, M. E. (1992). Mobilization and location of the genetic determinant of chloramphenicol resistance from *Lactobacillus plantarum* caTC2R. *Plasmid* 27: 169–176.

Ahrne, S., Moli, G., and Axelsson, L. (1999). Transformation of *Lactobacillus reuteri* with electroporation—studies on the erythromycin resistance plasmid pLUL631. *Current Microbiology* 24: 199–205.

Ainsa, J. A., Blokpoel, M. C. J., Otal, I., Young, D. B., de Smet, K. A. L., and Martin C. (1998). Molecular cloning and characterization of tap, a putative multidrug efflux pump present in *Mycobacterium fortuitum* and *Mycobacterium tuberculosis*. *Journal of Bacteriology* 180: 5836–5843.

Antony, S. J., Stratton, C. W., and Dummer, J. S. (1996). *Lactobacillus* bacteremia: Description of the clinical course in adult patients without endocarditis. *Clinical Infectious Diseases* 23: 773–778.

Aarestrup, F. M., Bager, F., Jensen, N. E., Madsen, M., Meyling, A., and Wegener, H. C. (1998). Resistance to antimicrobial agents used for animal therapy in pathogenic-, zoonotic-, and indicator bacteria isolated from different food animals in Denmark: A baseline study for the Danish Integrated Antimicrobial Resistance Monitoring Programme (DANMAP). *APMIS* 106: 745–770.

Arthur, M., and Courvalin, P. (1994). Genetics and mechanisms of glycopeptide resistance in enterococci. *Antimicrobial Agents and Chemotherapy* 37: 1563–1571.

Baquero, F., Negir, M. C., Morosini, M. I., and Blazquez, J. (1997). The antibiotic selection process: concentration-specific amplification of low-level resistant populations. In: D. J. Chadwick, and J. Goode (Eds.), *Antibiotic resistance. Origins, evolution, selection and spread* (pp. 87–105). Chichester: John Wiley & Sons.

Bates, J., Jordens, Z., and Selkon, J. B. (1993). Evidence for an animal origin of vancomycin-resistant enterococci. *The Lancet* 342: 490–491.

Batish, V. K., and Ranganathan, B. (1986). Antibiotic susceptibility of deoxyribonuclease-positive enterococci isolated from milk and milk products and their epidemiological significance. *International Journal of Food and Microbiology* 16: 203–206.

Berg, T., Firth, N., Apisiridej, S., Hettiaratchi, A., Leelaporn, A., and Skurray, R. A. (1998). Complete nucleotide sequence of pSK41: Evolution of staphylococcal conjugative multiresistance plasmids. *Journal of Bacteriology* 180: 4350–4359.

Bolhuis, H., Poelarends, G., van Veen, H. W., Poolman, B., Driessen, A. J. M., and Konings, W. N. (1995). The lactococcal lmrP gene encodes a proton motive force-dependent drug transporter. *Journal of Biological Chemistry* 270: 26092–26098.

Bolotin, A., Mauger, S., Malarme, K., Ehrlich, S. D., and Sorokin, A. (1999). Low-reduncancy sequencing of the entire *Lactococcus lactis* IL1403 genome. *Antonie van Leeuwenhoek* 76: 27–76.

Bonafede, M. E., Carias, L. L., and Rice, L. B. (1997). Enterococcal transposon Tn*5384*: Evolution of composite transposon through cointegration of enterococcal and staphylococcal plasmids. *Antimicrobial Agents and Chemotherapy* 41: 1854–1858.

Brockmann, E., Jacobsen, B. L., Hertel, C., Ludwig, W., and Schleifer, K. H. (1996). Monitoring of genetically modified *Lactococcus lactis* in gnotobiotic and conventional rats by using antibiotic resistance markers and specific probe or primer based methods. *Systematic and Applied Microbiology* 19: 203–212.

Celli, J., and Trieu-Cuot, P. (1998). Circularization of Tn*916* is required for expression of the transposon-encoded transfer functions: Characterization of long tetracycline-inducible transcripts reading through the attachment site. *Molecular Microbiology* 28: 103–117.

Charpentier, E., Gerbaud, G., and Courvalin, P. (1994). Presence of the *Listeria* tetracycline resistance gene *tet(S)* in *Enterococcus faecalis*. *Antimicrobial Agents and Chemotherapy* 38: 2330–2335.

Charpentier, E., Gerbaud, G., Jacquet, C., Rocourt, J., and Courvalin, P. (1995). Incidence of antibiotic resistance in *Listeria* species. *Journal of Infections Diseases* 172: 277–281.
Charteris, W. P., Kelly, P. M., Morelli, L., and Collins, J. K. (1998). Antibiotic susceptibility of potentially probiotic *Bifidobacterium* isolates from the human gastrointestinal tract. *Letters in Applied Microbiology* 26: 333–337.
Clewell, D. B. (1993). In: D. B. Clewell (Ed.), *Bacterial conjugation*. New York: Plenum Press.
Clewell, D. B., and Flannagan, S. E. (1993). The conjugative transposons of Gram-positive bacteria. In: D. B. Clewell (Ed.), *Bacterial Conjugation* (pp. 369–393). New York: Plenum Press.
Clewell, D. B., Flannagan, S. E., and Jaworsky, D. D. (1995). Unconstrained bacterial promiscuity: The Tn*916*–Tn*1545* family of conjugative transposons. *Trends in Microbiology* 3: 229–236.
Climo, M., Sharma, V. K., and Archer, G. L. (1996). Identification and characterization of the origin of conjugative transfer (*ori*T) and gene (*nes*) encoding a single-stranded endonuclease on the staphylococcal plasmid pGO1. *Journal of Bacteriology* 178: 4975–4983.
Corpet, E. E. (1988). Antibiotic resistance from food. *New England Journal of Medicine* 318: 1206–1207.
Curragh, H. J., and Collins, M. A. (1992). High levels of spontaneous drug resistance in *Lactobacillus*. *Journal of Applied Bacteriology* 73: 31–36.
Davies, J. E. (1994). Inactivation of antibiotics and the dissemination of resistance genes. *Science* 264: 375–382.
Davies, J. E. (1997). Origins, acquisition and dissemination of antibiotic resistance determinants. In: D. J. Chadwick and J. Goode (Eds.), *Antibiotic Resistance. Origins, evolution, selection and spread* (pp. 15–27). Chichester: John Wiley & Sons.
De Fabrizio, S. V., Parada, J. L., and Ledford, R. A. (1994). Antibiotic resistance of *Lactococcus lactis*—an approach of genetic determinants location through a model system. *Microbiologie—Aliments—Nutritions* 12: 307–315.
Dellaglio, F., Dicks, L. M. T., and Torriani, S. (1995). The genus *Leuconostoc*. In: B. J. B. Wood and W. H. Holzapfel (Eds.), *The genera of lactic acid bacteria* (pp. 235–278). London: Blackie Academic & Professional.
Dessart, S. R., and Steenson, L. R. (1991). High frequency intergeneric and intrageneric conjugal transfer of drug resistance plasmids in *Leuconostoc mesenteroides* ssp. *cremoris*. *Journal of Dairy Science* 74: 2912–2919.
Devriese, L. A., and Pot, B. (1995). The genus *Enterococcus*. In: B. J. B. Wood and W. H. Holzapfel (Eds.), *The genera of lactic acid bacteria* (pp. 327–367). London: Blackie Academic & Professional.
De Vos, W. M., and Simons, G. F. M. (1994). Gene cloning and expression systems in Lactococci. In: M. J. Gasson and W. M. de Vos (Eds.), *Genetics and biotechnology of lactic acid bacteria* (pp. 52–105). London: Blackie Academic & Professional.
Dodd, H. M., Horn, N., and Gasson, M. J. (1990). Analysis of the genetic determinant for production of the peptide antibiotic nisin. *Journal of General Microbiology* 136: 555–566.
Doucet-Populaire, F., Trieu-Cuot, P., Dosbaa, I., Andremont, A., and Courvalin, P. (1991). Inducible transfer of conjugative Transposon Tn*1545* from *Enterococcus faecalis* to *Listeria monocytogenes* in the digestive tracts of gnotobiotic mice. *Antimicrobial Agents and Chemotherapy* 35: 185–187.
Dougherty, B. A., Hill, C., Weidman, J. F., Richardson, D. R., Venter, J. C., and Ross, R. P. (1998). Sequence and analysis of the 60 kb conjugative, bacteriocin-producing plasmid pMRC01 from *Lactococcus lactis* DPC3147. *Molecular Microbiology* 29: 1029–1038.
Elisha, B. G., and Courvalin, P. (1995). Analysis of genes encoding D-alanine: D-alanine ligase-related enzymes in *Leuconostoc mesenteroides* and *Lactobacillus* spp. *Gene* 152: 79–83.
Elmer, G. W., Surawics, C. M., and McFarland, L. V. (1996). Biotherapeutic agents. A neglected modality for the treatment and prevention of selected intestinal and vaginal infections. *Journal of the American Medical Association* 275: 870–876.
Falkiner, F. R. (1998). The consequences of antibiotic use in horticulture. *Journal of Antimicrobial Chemotherapy* 41: 429–431.
Flannagan, S. E., Zitzow, L. A., Su, Y. A., and Clewell, D. B. (1994). Complete nucleotide sequence of the 18-kb conjugative transposon Tn*916* from *Enterococcus faecalis*. *Plasmid* 32: 350–354.
Foley, S., Bron, S., Venema, G., Daly, C., and Fitzgerald, G. F. (1996). Molecular analysis of the replication origin of the *Lactococcus lactis* plasmid pCI305. *Plasmid* 36: 125–141.
Fons, M., Hégé, T., Ladiré, M., Raibaud, P., Ducluzeau, R., and Maguin, E. (1997). Isolation and characterization of a plasmid from *Lactobacillus fermentum* conferring erythromycin resistance. *Plasmid* 37: 199–203.
Fraimow, H. S., and Courvallin, P. (2000). Resistance to glycopeptides in Gram-positive pathogens. In: V. A. Fischetti, R. P. Novick, J. J. Ferretti, D. A. Portnoy, and J. I. Rood (Eds.), *Gram-Positive pathogens* (pp. 621–634). Washington: ASM Press.

Gasson, M. J., and Davies, F. L. (1980). Conjugal transfer of the drug resistance plasmid pAMβ1 in the lactic streptococci. *FEMS Microbiology Letters* 7: 51–53.
Gasson, M. J., and Fitzgerald, G. F. (1994). Gene transfer systems and transposition. In: M. J. Gasson and W. M. de Vos (Eds.), *Genetics and biotechnology of lactic acid bacteria* (pp. 1–51). London: Blackie Academic & Professional.
Gevers, D., Huys, G., Devlieghere, F., Uyttendaele, M., Debevere, J., and Swings, J. (2000). Isolation and identification of tetracycline resistant lactic acid bacteria from pre-packed sliced meat products. *Systematic and Applied Microbiology* 23: 279–284.
Giraffa, G., Carminati, D., and Neviani, E. (1997). Enterococci isolated from dairy products: a review of risks and potential technological use. *Journal of Food Protection* 60: 732–738.
Grüneberg, R. N., and Hryniewicz, W. (1998). Clinical relevance of a European collaborative study on comparative susceptibility of Gram-positive clinical isolates to teichoplanin and vancomycin. *International Journal of Antimicrobial Agents* 10: 271–277.
Guedon, G., Bourgoin, F., Pebay, M., Roussel, Y., Colmin, C., Simonet, J. M., and Decaris, B. (1995). Characterization and distribution of two insertion sequences, IS1191 and iso-IS981, in *Streptococcus thermophilus*: Does intergeneric transfer of insertion sequences occur in lactic acid bacteria co-cultures? *Molecular Microbiology* 16: 69–78.
Guiney, M., and Urwin, G. (1993). Frequency and antimicrobial susceptibility of clinical isolates of enterococci. *European Journal of Clinical Microbiology and Infections Diseases* 12: 362–366.
Hakenbeck, R. (1999). β-Lactam-resistant *Streptococcus pneumoniae*: epidemiology and evolutionary mechanism. *Chemotherapy* 45: 83–94.
Hadorn, K., Kayser, F. H., and Hächler, H. (1994). Miniplasmid derived from *Listeria monocytogenes* multiresistance plasmid pWDB100 upon conjugal transfer into *Staphylococcus epidermidis* carries chloramphenicol resistance gene identical with staphylococcal gene. *Systematic and Applied Microbiology* 17: 492–500.
Hadorn, K., Hächler, H., Schaffner, A., and Kayser, F. H. (1993). Genetic characterization of plasmid-encoded multiple antibiotic resistance in a strain of *Listeria monocytogenes* causing endocarditis. *European Journal of Clinical Microbiology and Infections Diseases* 12: 928–937.
Hammerum, A. M., Jensen, L. B., and Aarestrup, F. M. (1998). Detection of the *satA* gene and transferability of virginiamycin resistance in *Enterococcus faecium* from food-animals. *FEMS Microbiology Letters* 168: 145–151.
Hancock, L. E., and Gilmore, M. S. (2000). Pathogenicicty of enterococci. In: V. A. Fischetti, R. P. Novick, J. J. Ferretti, D. A. Portnoy, and J. I. Rood (Eds.), *Gram-positive pathogens* (pp. 251–258). Washington: ASM Press.
Handwerger, S., and Skoble, J. (1995). Identification of chromosomal mobile element conferring high-level vancomycin resistance in *Enterococcus faecium*. *Antimicrobial Agents and Chemotherapy* 39: 2446–2453.
Herrero, M., Mayo, B., Gonzales, B., and Suarez, J. E. (1996). Evaluation of technologically important traits in lactic acid bacteria isolated from spontaneous fermentations. *Journal of Applied Bacteriology* 81: 565–570.
Hooper, D. C. (2000). Mechanisms of fluoroquinolone resistance. In: V. A. Fischetti, R. P. Novick, J. J. Ferretti, D. A. Portnoy, and J. I. Rood (Eds.), *Gram-positive pathogens* (pp. 685–693). Washington: ASM Press.
Huycke, M. M., Sahm, D. F., and Gilmore, M. S. (1998). Multiple-drug resistant enterococci: The nature of the problem and agenda for the future. *Emerging Infections Diseases* 4: 239–249.
Janzen, T., Kleinschmidt, J., Neve, H., and Geis, A. (1992). Sequencing and characterization of pST1, a cryptic plasmid from *Streptococcus thermophilus*. *FEMS Microbiology Letters* 95: 175–180.
Jensen, L. B., Fridmodt-Moller, N., and Aarestrup, F. M. (1999). Presence of *erm* gene classes in Gram-positive bacteria of animal and human origin in Denmark. *FEMS Microbiology Letters* 170: 151–158.
Jensen, L. B. (1998). Internal variations in Tn*1546*-like elements due to the presence of IS*1216V*. *FEMS Microbiology Letters* 169: 349–354.
Jett, B. D., Huycke, M., and Gilmore, M. S. (1994). Virulence of enterococci. *Clin. Microbiol. Rev.* 7: 462–478.
Kernodle, D. S. (2000). Mechanisms of resistance to β-lactam antibiotics. In: V. A. Fischetti, R. P. Novick, J. J. Ferretti, D. A. Portnoy, and J. I. Rood (Eds.), *Gram-Positive pathogens* (pp. 609–620). Washington: ASM Press.
Khan, E., Mack, J. P. G., Katz, R. A., Kulkosky, J., and Skalka, A. M. (1990). Retroviral integrase domain: DNA binding and the recognition of LTR sequences. *Nucleic Acids Research* 19: 851–861.
Kilpper-Bälz, R., Fischer, G., and Schleifer, K.-H. (1982). Nucleic acid hybridization of group D streptococci. *Current Microbiology* 7: 245–250.
Klaenhammer, T. R., and Sutherland, S. M. (1980). Detection of plasmid deoxyribonucleic acid in an isolate of *Lactobacillus acidophilus*. *Applied Environmental Microbiology* 39: 671–674.

Klare, I., Heier, H., Claus, H., Böhme, G., Marin, S., Seltmann, G., Hakenbeck, R., Altanassova, V., and Witte, W. (1995a). *Enterococcus faecium* strains with vanA-mediated high-level glycopeptide resistance isolated from animal foodstuffs and fecal samples of humans in the community. *Microbial Drug Resistance* 1: 265–272.

Klare, I., Heier, H., Claus, H., Reissbrodt, R., and Witte, W. (1995b). *vanA*-mediated high-level glycopeptide resistance in *Enterococcus faecium* from animal husbandry. *FEMS Microbiology Letters* 125: 165–172.

Klein, G., Pack, A., and Reuter, G. (1998). Antibiotic resistance patterns of enterococci and occurrence of vancomycin-resistant enterococci in raw minced beef and pork in Germany. *Applied Environmental Microbiology* 64: 1825–1830.

Kleinschmidt, J., Soeding, B., Teuber, M., and Neve, H. (1993). Evaluation of horizontal and vertical gene transfer and stability of heterologous DNA in *Streptococcus thermophilus* isolated from yogurt and yogurt starter cultures. *Systematic and Applied Microbiology* 16: 287–295.

Knudtson, L. M., and Hartman, P. A. (1993). Antibiotic resistance among enterococci isolates from environmental and clinical sources. *Journal of Food Protection* 56: 489–492.

Kullen, M. J., and Klaenhammer, T. R. (1999). Genetic modification of intestinal lactobacilli and bifidobacteria. In: G. W. Tannock (Ed.), *Probiotics, a critical review* (pp. 65–83). Wymondham: Horizon Scientific Press.

Leenhouts, K., Bolhuis, A., Venema, G., and Kok, J. (1998). Construction of a food-grade multiple-copy integration system for *Lactococcus lactis*. *Applied Microbiology and Biotechnology* 49: 417–423.

Levy, S. B. (1997). Antibiotic resistance: An ecological imbalance. In: D. J. Chadwick and J. Goode (Eds.), *Antibiotic Resistance. Origins, evolution, selection and spread* (pp. 1–14). Chichester: John Wiley & Sons.

Liassine, N., Frei, R., Jan, I., and Auckenthaler, R. (1998). Characterization of glycopeptide-resistant enterococci from a Swiss hospital. *Journal of Clinical Microbiology* 36: 1853–1858.

Lin, C. F., Fung, Z. F., Wu, C. L., and Chung, T. C. (1996). Molecular characterization of a plasmid-borne (pTC82) chloramphenicol resistance determinant (*cat*-TC) from *Lactobacillus reuteri* G4. *Plasmid* 36: 116–124.

Lynch, C., Courvalin, P., and Nikaido, H. (1997). Active efflux of antimicrobial agents in wild-type strains of enterococci. *Antimicrobial Agents and Chemotherapy* 41: 869–871.

Macrina, F. L., and Archer, G. L. (1993). Conjugation and broad host range plasmids in streptococci and staphylococci. In: D. B. Clewell (Ed.), *Bacterial conjugation* (pp. 313–368). New York: Plenum Press.

Majewski, J., Zawadzki, P., Pickerill, P., Cohan, F. M., and Dowson, C. G. (2000). Barriers to genetic exchange between bacterial species: *Streptococcus pneumoniae* transformation. *Journal of Bacteriology* 182: 1016–1023.

Marra, D., and Scott, J. R. (1999). Regulation of excision of the conjugative transposon Tn*916*. *Molecular Microbiology* 31: 609–621.

Mazel, D., and Davies, J. E. (1999). Antibiotic resistance in microbes. *CMLS, Cellular and Molecular Life Science* 56: 742–754.

McDonald, L. C., Kuehnert, M. J., Tenover, F. C., and Jarvis, W. R. (1997). Vancomycin-resistant enterococci outside the health-care setting: Prevalence, sources, and public health implications. *Emerging Infections Diseases* 3: 311–317.

McKay, L. L. (1983). Funcional properties of plasmids in lactic streptococci. *Antonie van Leeuwenhoek* 49: 259–274.

McMurry, L. M., and Levy, S. B. (2000). Tetracycline resistance in Gram-positive bacteria. In: V. A. Fischetti, R. P. Novick, J. J. Ferretti, D. A. Portnoy, and J. I. Rood (Eds.), *Gram-positive pathogens* (pp. 660–677). Washington: ASM Press.

Mercenier A., Pouwels, P. H., and Chassy, B. M. (1994). Genetic engineering of lactobacilli, leuconostocs and *Streptococcus thermophilus*. In: M. J. Gasson, and W. M. de Vos (Eds.), *Genetics and biotechnology of lactic acid bacteria* (pp. 252–293). London: Blackie Academic & Professional.

Mercer, D. K., Scott, K. P., Bruce-Johnson, W. A., Glover, L. A., and Flint, H. J. (1999). Fate of free DNA and transformation of the oral bacterium *Streptococcus gordonii* DL1 by plasmid DNA in human saliva. *Applied Environmental Microbiology* 65: 6–10.

Ministry of Agriculture and Forestry (Finland) (1997). Tylosin and spiramycin as feed additives—Influence on the efficacy of therapeutic macrolides. *Report from the Republic of Finland according to article 29 of the treaty between Member States of the European Union and the Republic of Finland on the scientific arguments for the adaptation to prohibit the use of tylosin and spiramycin as feed additives in animal nutrition by the National Veterinary and Food Research Institut (EELA)* E. Tast, T. Honkanen-Buzalski, and P. Mannerkop (Eds.), Helsinki: Publications of Ministry of Agriculture and Forestry 5/1997.

Ministry of Agriculture, Fisheries and Food (MAFF) (UK) (1998). *A review of antimicrobial resistance in the food chain*. July 1998. *A technical report for MAFF*. London: MAFF Publications.

Ministry of Agriculture (Sweden), Government Official Reports 132 (1997). *Antimicrobial feed additives*. Report from the Commission on Antimicrobial Feed Additives. Stockholm: Norsteedts Tryckeri AG.

Murray, I. A. (2000). Chloramphenicol resistance. In: V. A. Fischetti, R. P. Novick, J. J. Ferretti, D. A. Portnoy, and J. I. Rood (Eds.), *Gram-positive pathogens* (pp. 678–684). Washington: ASM Press.

National Research Council & Institute of Medicine (1998). *The use of drugs in food animals: benefits and risks*. Washington: National Academy Press.

Neu, H. C. (1992). The crisis in antibiotic resistance. *Science* 257: 1064–1973.

Neve, H., Geis, A., and Teuber, M. (1987). Conjugation, a common plasmid transfer mechanism in lactic acid streptococci of dairy starter cultures. *Systematic and Applied Microbiology* 9: 151–157.

Noble, W. C., Virani, Z., and Cree, R. G. A. (1992). Co-transfer of vancomycin and other resistance genes from *Enterococcus faecalis* NCTC 12201 to *Staphylococcus aureus*. *FEMS Microbiology Letters* 93: 195–198.

Orberg, P. K., and Sandine, W. E. (1985). Survey of antimicrobial resistance in lactic streptococci. *Applied Environmental Microbiology* 49: 538–542.

Pechmann, H., and Teuber, M. (1980). Plasmid pattern of group N (lactic) streptococci. *Zentralblatt für Bakteriologie C* 1: 133–136.

Perreten, V., Kollöffel, B., and Teuber, M. (1997a). Conjugal transfer of the Tn*916*-like transposon Tn*FO*1 from *Enterococcus faecalis* isolated from cheese to other Gram-positive bacteria. *Systematic and Applied Microbiology* 20: 27–38.

Perreten, V., Schwarz, F., Cresta, L., Boeglin, M., Dasen, G., and Teuber, M. (1997b). Antibiotic resistance spread in food. *Nature* 389: 801–802.

Perreten, V., Schwarz, F. V., Teuber, M., and Levy, S. B. (2000). Mef214, a new efflux protein conferring multiple antibiotic resistance in *Lactococcus lactis* subsp. *lactis* and in *Escherichia coli*. *Antimicrobial Agents and Chemotherapy* submitted.

Poyart-Salmeron, C., Carlier, C., Trieu-Cuot, P., Courtieu, A. L., and Courvalin, P. (1990). Transferable plasmid-mediated antibiotic resistance in *Listeria monocytogenes*. *The Lancet* 335: 1422–1426.

Quednau, M., Ahrne, S., Petersson, A. C., and Molin, G. (1998). Antibiotic-resistant strains of *Enterococcus* isolated from Swedish and Danish retailed chicken and pork. *Journal of Applied Microbiology* 84: 1163–1170.

Reilly, A., and Käferstein, F. (1997). Food safety hazards and the application of the principles of the hazard analysis and critical control point (HACCP) system for their control in aquaculture production. *Aquaculture Research* 28: 735–752.

Rice, L. B. (1998). Tn*916* family conjugative transposons and dissemination of antimicrobial resistance determinants. *Antimicrobial Agents and Chemotherapy* 42: 1871–1877.

Rice, L. B., and Carias, L. L. (1997). Transfer of Tn*5385*, a composite, multiresistance chromosomal element from *Enterococcus faecalis*. *Journal of Bacteriology* 180: 714–721.

Rinckel, L. A., and Savage, D. C. (1990). Characterization of plasmids and plasmid-borne macrolide resistance from *Lactobacillus* sp. strains. *Plasmid* 23: 100–133.

Rollins, L. R., Lee, L. N., and LeBlanc, D. J. (1985). Evidence for a disseminated erythromycin resistance determinant mediated by Tn*917*-like sequences among group D streptococci isolated from pigs, chickens, and humans. *Antimicrobial Agents and Chemotherapy* 27: 439–444.

Sami, M., Yamashita, H., Hirono, T., Kadokura, H., Kitamoto, K., Yoda, K., and Yamasaki, M. (1997). Hop-resistant *Lactobacillus brevis* contains novel plasmid harbouring a multidrug resistance-like gene. *Journal of Fermentation Bioengineering* 84: 1–6.

Schaefer, A., Jahns, A., Geis, A., and Teuber, M. (1991). Distribution of the IS elements ISS1 and IS904 in lactococci. *FEMS Microbiology Letters* 80: 311–318.

Schleifer, K.-H., and Ludwig, W. (1995). Phylogenetic relationships of lactic acid bacteria. In: B. J. B. Wood, and W. H. Holzapfel (Eds.), *The genera of lactic acid bacteria* (pp. 7–18). London: Blackie Academic & Professional.

Schmalreck, A. F., Teuber, M., and Hartl, A. (1975). Structural features determining the antibiotic potencies of natural and synthetic hop resins, their precursors and derivatives. *Canadian Journal of Microbiology*. 21: 205–212.

Schmieger, H., and Schicklmaier, P. (1999). Transduction of multiple drug resistance of *Salmonella enterica* serovar *thyphimurium* DT104. *FEMS Microbiology Letters* 170: 251–256.

Schwarz, F., Perreten, V., and Teuber, M. (1999). Characterization and partial sequence of a conjugative 49-kb antibiotic resistance plasmid from *Enterococcus faecalis* isolated from a dry sausage. Proc. 39th ICAAC, San Francisco, Poster No. 729a.

Scott, J. R. (1992). Sex and the single circle: conjugative transposition. *Journal of Bacteriology* 174: 6005–6010.

Sgorbati, B., Biavati, B., and Palenzona, D. (1995). The genus *Bifidobacterium*. In: B. J. B. Wood and W. H. Holzapfel (Eds.), *The genera of lactic acid bacteria* (pp. 279–306). London: Blackie Academic & Professional.

Shaw, K. J., and Wright, G. D. (2000). Aminoglycoside resistance in Gram-positive pathogens. In: V. A. Fischetti, R. P. Novick, J. J. Ferretti, D. A. Portnoy, and J. I. Rood (Eds.), *Gram-positive pathogens* (pp. 635–646). Washington: ASM Press.

Sievers, M., Teuber, M., Wirsching, F., Perreten, V., Eisenring, R., Fähndrich, P., Schlaepfer, S., Krusch, U., Simm, Ch., and Löhmer, A. (1993). Antibiotic resistance properties of enterococci and staphylococci from fermented food. *FoodMicro '93*, Book of Abstracts, p. 191.

Simpson, W. J., Hammond, J. R. M., and Miller, R. B. (1988). Avoparcin and vancomycin: Useful antibiotics for the isolation of brewery lactic acid bacteria. *Journal of Applied Bacteriology* 64: 299–310.

Simpson, W. J., and Taguchi, H. (1995). The genus *Pediococcus*, with notes on the genera *Tetratogenococcus* and *Aerococcus*. In: B. J. B. Wood, and W. H. Holzapfel (Eds.), *The genera of lactic acid bacteria* (pp. 125–172). London: Blackie Academic & Professional.

Soeding, B., Kleinschmidt, J., Teuber, M., and Neve, H. (1993). Assessment of abilities of conjugal transfer and stability of pAMβ1 in dairy lactobacilli with emphasis on thermophilic and nonstarter lactobacilli. *Systematic and Applied Microbiology* 16: 296–302.

Sozzi, T., and Smiley, M. B. (1980). Antibiotic resistances of yogurt starter cultures *Streptococcus thermophilus* and *Lactobacillus bulgaricus*. *Applied Environmental Microbiology* 40: 862–865.

Stackebrandt, E., and Teuber, M. (1988). Molecular taxonomy and phylogenetic position of lactic acid bacteria. *Biochimie* 70: 317–324.

Tannock, G. W. (1987). Conjugal transfer of plasmid pAMβ1 in *Lactobacillus reuteri* and between lactobacilli and *Enterococcus faecalis*. *Applied Environmental Microbiology* 53: 2693–2695.

Tannock, G. W. (Ed.) (1998). *Probiotics. A critical review*. Wymondham: Horizon Scientific Press.

Tannock, G. W., Luchansky, J. B., Miller, L., Connell, H., Thode-Andersen, S., Mercer, A. A., and Klaenhammer, T. R. (1994). Molecular characterization of a plasmid-borne (pGT633) erythromycin resistance determinant (*ermGT*) from *Lactobacilllus reuteri* 100–163. *Plasmid* 31: 60–71.

Teuber, M. (1993). Lactic acid bacteria. In: J. Rehm, G. Reed, A. Pühler, and P. Stadler (Eds.), *Biotechnology* (pp. 326–366, Vol. 1, 2nd ed.). Weinheim: Verlag Chemie.

Teuber, M. (1995). The genus *Lactococcus*. In: B. J. B. Wood and W. H. Holzapfel (Eds.), *The genera of lactic acid bacteria*. (pp. 173–234). London: Blackie Academic & Professional.

Teuber, M. (1999). Spread of antibiotic resistance with food-borne pathogens. *CMLS, Cellular and Molecular Life Science* 56: 755–763.

Teuber, M. (2000). Fermented milk products. In: B. M. Lund, T. C. Baird-Parker, and G. W. Gould (Eds.), *The microbiological safety and quality of food* (pp. 535–585, Vol. 1). Gaitherburg, MD: Aspen Publishers, Inc.

Teuber, M., and Perreten, V. (2000). Role of milk and meat products as vehicles for antibiotic-resistant bacteria. *ACTA Veterinaria Scandinavica Supplement* 93: 75–87.

Teuber, M., Perreten, V., and Wirsching, F. (1996). Antibiotikumresistente Bakterien: eine neue Dimension in der Lebensmittelmikrobiologie. *Lebensmittel-Technologie* 29: 182–199.

Teuber, M., Meile, L., and Schwarz, F. (1999). Acquired antibiotic resistance in lactic acid bacteria from food. *Antonie van Leeuwenhoek* 76: 115–137.

Teuber, M., and Schmalreck, A. F. (1973). Membrane leakage in *Bacillus subtilis* 168 induced by the hop constituents lupulone, humulone, isohumulone and lupulinic acid. *Archives of Microbiology* 94: 159–171.

Thal, L. A., Chow, J. W., Mahayni, R., Bonilla, H., Perri, M. B., Donabedia, S. A., Silverman, J., Taber, S., and Zervos, M. J. (1995). Characterization of antimicrobial resistance in enterococci of animal origin. *Antimicrobial Agents and Chemotherapy* 39: 2112–2115.

Twomey, D. P., DeUrraza, P. J., McKay, L. L., and O'Sullivan, D. J. (2000). Characterization of AbiR, a novel multicomponent abortive infection mechanism encoded by plasmid pKR223 of *Lactococcus lactis* subsp. *lactis* KR2. *Applied Environmental Microbiology* 66: 2647–2651.

Trieu-Cuot, P., de Cespédès, G., Bentorcha, F., Delbos, F., Gaspar, E., and Horaud, T. (1993). Study of heterogeneity of chloramphenicol acetyltransferase (CAT) genes in streptococci and enterococci by polymerase chain reaction: Characterization of a new CAT determinant. *Antimicrobial Agents and Chemotherapy* 37: 2593–2598.

Van den Braak, N., van Belkum, A., van Keulen, M., Vliegenthart, J., Verbrugh, H. A., and Endtz, H. P. (1998). Molecular characterization of vancomycin-resistant enterococci from hospitalized patients and poultry products in the Netherlands. *Journal of Clinical Microbiology* 36: 1927–1932.

Van Veen, H. W., and Konings, W. N. (1998). The ABC family of multidrug transporters in microorganisms. *Biochimica of Biophysica ACTA* 1365, 31–36.

Van Veen, H. W., Putnam, M., Margolles, A., Sakamoto, K., and Konings, W. N. (2000). Molecular pharmacological characterization of two multidrug transporters in *Lactococcus lactis*. *Pharmacology and Therapeutics* 85: 245–249.

Vescovo, M., Morelli, L., and Bottazzi, V. (1982). Drug resistance plasmids in *Lactobacillus acidophilus* and *Lactobacillus reuteri*. *Applied Environmental Microbiology* 43: 50–56.

Von Wright, A., and Räty, K. (1993). The nucleotide sequence for the replication region of pVS40, a lactococcal food grade cloning vector. *Letters in Applied Microbiology* 17: 25–28.

Weisblum, B. (2000). Resistance to the macrolide-lincosamide-streptogramin antibiotics. In: V. A. Fischetti, R. P. Novick, J. J. Ferretti, D. A. Portnoy, and J. I. Rood (Eds.), *Gram-positive pathogens* (pp. 694–710). Washington: ASM Press.

WHO (1997). *The medical impact of the use of antimicrobials in food animals*. Report of a WHO Meeting, Berlin, Germany, 13–17 October (1997). Geneva: WHO.

Willems, R. J. Ll, Top, J., van den Braak, N., van Belkum, A., Mevius, D. J., Hendriks, G., van Santen-Verheuvel, M., and van Embden, J. D. A. (1999). Molecular diversity and evolutionary relationships of Tn*1546*-like elements in enterococci from humans and animals. *Antimicrobial Agents and Chemotherapy* 43: 483–491.

Witte, W. (1998). Medical consequences of antibiotic use in agriculture. *Science* 279: 996–997.

Wu, K., An, F. Y., and Clewell, D. B. (1999). *Enterococcus faecalis* pheromone-responding plasmid pAD1 gives rise to an aggregation (clumping) response when cells are exposed to subinhibitory concentrations of chloramphenicol, erythromycin or tetracycline. *Plasmid* 41: 82–88.

Wüst, J., Zbinden, R., and Kayser, F. H. (1998). Die Empfindlichkeit von Bakterien gegen Chemotherapeutika (Zürich 1996). *Praxis* 87: 403–412.

12

The Ratio between Benefits and Risk of Fermented Foods Produced by Genetically Modified Lactic Acid Bacteria

Theo Verrips and Aat Ledeboer

Introduction

At present combinatorial (bio)chemistry combined with high throughput screening together with high throughput screening of natural compounds are, beside rDNA technology, the dominating technologies used by the pharmaceutical industry to find new solutions for the many diseases that are still not (well) cureable. Sometimes the high throughput screening and selection of natural compounds delivers remarkable and unexpected results. For instance a well designed screening for natural molecules that could replace insulin, did not result in the discovery of a molecule that fits on the binding site of the insulin receptor, but the natural compound (a non-peptidyl fungal compound) is able to penetrate the cell. There it recognizes the inner part of the receptor, subsequently changing its conformation in such a way that phosphorylation at the right site takes place. This phosphorylation induces down stream signal transduction cascades identical to those caused by insulin (Zhang et al., 1999).

It is fascinating to realize that Traditional Chinese Medicine is based on a process of screening enormous numbers of natural extracts and selecting the best ones (Needham et al., 1989). It is not known how many extracts have been screened and what exactly the selection methods were, but the results of the work of large numbers of Chinese scientists during many centuries are amazing, not at least because of the high standard of their data recording and management. Without knowing the molecular details, many books on medicine and plant extracts in China and India describe the beneficial effects of plant extracts,

Theo Verrips and Aat Ledeboer • Unilever Research, O. v. Noortlaan 120, 3133 AT Vlaardingen, The Netherlands; e-mail: theo.verrips@unilever.com

for example, (green) tea. Only recently several publications indicated that a certain component in tea, epigallocathechinegallate (EGCg), may have remarkable properties such as inhibiting urokinase, a protease involved in carcinogenesis, and blocking angiogenesis (Cao and Cao, 1999).

Most probably similar screening and selection processes have been practiced over thousands of years to develop the fermentation processes, that we know today (Reed, 1983). Again the selection criteria used are not known. However, it is very likely that keepability, tastefulness, and probable health benefits have been the selection criteria. Just as in modern high throughput screening and selection experiments, the ratio between negative and positive results was very much in favor of the negative results, but driven by the typical human curiosity and the necessity to answer the demands of the ever growing number of people, the screening and selection processes were continued, even after fatal events. The results of millennia of screening and selection, are at the tables of nearly all people every day, everywhere in the world. A summary of the main fermented foods and drinks in which lactic acid bacteria (LAB) play an important role is given in Table 12.1.

Although in the last 5,000 years undoubtedly the fermentation processes have improved, resulting in more standardized high quality fermentation products, no fundamental differences in the fermentation processes have developed over thousands of years. Of course the contributions of Louis Pasteur and others in the 19th century have increased our understanding of fermentation processes enormously and the fermentation processes could be better conducted then ever before, but their principles remain the same. Only now do we start to understand the mechanisms of improved keepability of fermented products or their health benefits, due to modern developments in biotechnology such as rDNA technology and high throughput screening.

However in contrast to some other areas, notably pharmaceutical rDNA products and rDNA enzymes in detergent products and to a certain extent enzymes in foods (Figure 12.1 and Table 12.2), new fermentation products based on rDNA technology are not on the market, in spite of the fact that rDNA technology has been applied frequently to microorganisms that are functional microorganisms in food fermentations, in particular lactic acid bacteria (Table 12.3). As shown in Figure 12.1, even transgenic plants, that were in 1983 (the year that rDNA insulin produced by a microorganism was introduced on the market) technically about 10 years behind microorganisms, have entered the market earlier than fermented products. This is caused by the lack of understanding of the Foods market by many molecular biologists. Whereas they were looking to what was technically feasible, they forgot that the question of clear benefit to the consumer versus (perceived) risk determines whether rDNA technology will become an important technology in fermented foods. This aspect was also neglected for transgenic plants and this is certainly one of the reasons that food products derived from transgenic plants are hardly accepted by consumers in Europe. However, in contrast to foods fermented with transgenic microorganisms, transgenic plants offer considerable benefits to farmers and the environment (Monsanto's Roundup herbicide resistant crops need less herbicides (about 10% less) and show increased yields (5–15%); Personal Communication Farmers Organization Argentina).

Just over a century ago Louis Pasteur (and others like Robert Koch) carried out revolutionary experiments in the many areas of biosciences and attacked many (scientific) dogmas. However he was supported enormously by his contemporaries, because he often used his scientific findings immediately to answer urgent and important unmet demands of consumers (Dubos, 1998). Provided that real (not the perceived) risks to consumers are

Table 12.1. Main Fermented Foods and Drinks in Which Lactic Acid Bacteria Are One of the Dominant Functional Microorganisms

Product Name	Substrate	Main Lactic Acid Bacteria (If Known)
Bakery products	Wheat	*Lactobacilli*
Banku	Maize, cassava	Lactic acid bacteria
Burukutu	Sorghum, cassava	Lactic acid bacteria
Busa	Rice, millet	*Lactobacilli*
Cheese	Milk	*Brevibacterium linens*
		Lactobacilli
		Lactococci
		Leuconostoc sp.
		Enterococci
		Pediococci
		Streptococci
Dawadawa	Locust bean	Lactic acid bacteria
Dosai	Black gram and rice	*Leuconostoc mesentoroides*
Hamanatto	Whole soybean, wheat flour	*Pediococci*
		Streptococci
Idli	Rice, black gram	*Leuconostic mesentoroides*
Kecap	Soybean, wheat	*Lactobacilli*
Kimchi	Vegetables	Lactic acid bacteria
Kishk	Wheat, milk	Lactic acid bacteria
Mahewu	Maize	*Lactobacillus delbrueckii*
Miso	Rice, soybean, wheat	*Lactobacilli*
Ogi	Maize	Lactic acid bacteria
Pickles	Cabbage, cucumbers	*Lactobacilli*
		Leuconostoc mesenteroides
		Pediococcus cerevisiae
Puto	Rice	Lactic acid bacteria
Sorghum beer	Sorghum, maize	Lactic acid bacteria
Soybean milk	Soybean	Lactic acid bacteria
Soy sauce	Soybean and wheat	*Lactobacilli*
		Pediococci
Sausages	Meat	*Lactobacilli*
		Pediococci
		Micrococcus caseolyticus
		Carnobacterium sps.
Tarhana	Wheat and milk	Lactic acid bacteria
Wine	Grape	*Lactobacilli*
		Leuconostoc sps.
		Pediococcus cerevisiae
Yogurt	Milk	*Lactobacillus delbrueckii*
		Streptococcus thermophilus

absent, or in the case of the environment within acceptable limits, Louis Pasteur's successes demonstrate that, if consumer demands are taken as the driving force, fermented foods using rDNA technology may become a success. That rDNA technology can be successful is demonstrated by the many new pharmaceutical products available on the market today.

In this chapter the supply chain (all the steps of a food product between breeding of plants to consumption of the product) of food products will be used to analyze how

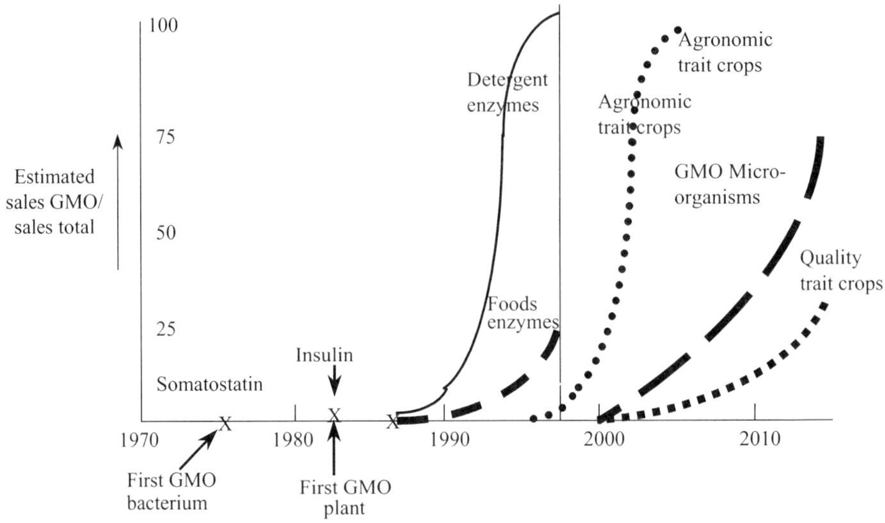

Figure 12.1. Penetration of GMO's and GMO derived products on the market (1998 data).

Table 12.2. Commercial Food Enzymes Made by rDNA Technology (as on the market at 1.5.1998; Source: Internal Unilever Competitors Analysis)

Enzyme	Commercial Name	Producer	Application
α-Galactosidase	α-galactosidase	NOVO N.	Animal feed
Xylanase	Bio-feed wheat	id	id
Lipase	Lipozym	id	Interesterification
ALDC	Maturex	id	Beer
Amylase	Novamyl	id	Bread
1,3 Lipase	Novozym 677	id	Bread
Xylanase	Peptopan	id	Bread
Amylase	Maltogene	id	Starch
Chymosin	Novoren	id	Cheese
Lipase	Novozym 398	id	Interesterification
Lipase	Novozym 435	id	id
Phytase	Pytan	id	Animal feed
Amylase	Termamyl	id	Starch
Transferase	Toryzym	id	Starch
Chymosine	Maxiran	DSM/Gb	Cheese
Phytase	Natuphos	id	Animal Feed
Chymosine	Chymogen	C. Hansen	Cheese
Chymosine	Chymax	Pfizer	Cheese
Xylanase	Biobake 710	Quest	Bread
Invertase		id	Chocolate
Glucanase		id	Beer
α-Galactosidase		id	Guar modification

fermented foods can be developed that may fulfill the demands of the consumers every day without imposing (unacceptable) risks to them. The supply chain analysis approach has been selected as the guide, because it is very likely that fermented foods in the future will contain various ingredients of transgenic origin, for example, transgenic plant material,

Table 12.3. Examples of Processes in Which Genetically Modified Lactic Acid Bacteria Are Used, that Potentially Can Be Brought to the Market

Process Description	Genetic Modification	Reference
α-Acetolactate decarboxylase mutants of *Lc. lactis* to enhance diacetylproduction in buttermilk	Use of an *ilv*-gene containing plasmid in the selection of a natural mutant; plasmid is eliminated later on	Curic et al. (1999)
Development of non-acidifying *L. bulgaricus* strains to produce mild, non-postacidifying yogurt	Transformation with a non-replicating plasmid, containing deleted lactose genes. Double cross-over with wild-type genes	Hottinger et al. (1992)
Development of a nisin resistant cheese starter culture. Nisin production prevents spoilage	Nisin resistance gene introduced in *Lc. lactis* starters by self-cloning	Hugenholtz and De Veer (1991)
Development of a cheese starter culture in which (auto)lysin genes are induced during ripening, to accelerate the ripening process	A phage lysin or autolysin gene is integrated by self-cloning behind a foodgrade inducible promoter	De Ruyter et al. (1997) Nauta et al. (1997)
Production of alanine overproducing strains to obtain sweet yogurt	Replacing the chromosomal *ldh* gene in *Lc. lactis* with the alanine dehydrogenase gene of *B. subtilis* converting pyruvate into L-alanine instead of lactate	Hols et al. (1999)
Acceleration of cheese ripening using a starter culture with an enhanced proteolytic activity	Replacing the *Lactococcus* protease gene by the neutral protease of *B. subtilis* var. *natto*	V. D. Guchte et al. (1990) McGarry et al. (1995)
Production of a yogurt containing a *Lactococcus* strain producing a vaccine for oral vaccination	Insertion of a gene encoding the tetanus toxin fragment C on a multi-copy plasmid and production in *Lc. lactis*	Robinson et al. (1997)

Table 12.4. Proven and Potential Positive Health Effects of Lactic Acid Bacteria

- Better intestinal lactose digestion
- Replacement of pathogenic bacteria and prevention of intestinal infections (e.g., reduction of *Helicobacter pylori*-induced ulcers)
- Positive effect on gut motility
- Improvement of the immune system, reducing virus infections and potentially resulting in reduced probability of colon cancer
- Decrease of enzymes involved in the synthesis of potential carcinogens (glucoronidase, nitro-, and azoreductase)
- Vehicle for passive immunization

enzymes produced by transgenic microorganisms or (living) transgenic microorganisms. As many potential benefits are described in other chapters of this volume, the risk aspects will receive most attention here. However some attention to potential benefits will be given as well (Table 12.4) to demonstrate the importance of the approach.

By analogy with microbial risk assessment (Verrips, 1989), risk is defined as the probability of a hazard occuring; hazard is defined as a harmful event to consumers or to the environment. This means that when a newly introduced gene encodes a protein that is intrinsically safe and does not provide a selection benefit for any receiving (micro)organism, the hazard is zero. Also for genes that are introduced for other reasons than to improve the functionality of the host, this analysis should be made. The consequence of zero hazard is that transgenic fermented food products containing genes encoding products with hazards equal to zero, are as safe as the untransformed products. If, on the other hand, the newly intoduced genes encode for proteins that pose no intrinsic hazard, but provide a receiving (micro)organism with a selection benefit, then the health hazard and the environmental hazard are not automatically zero. Consequently, the probability of transfer of the genes to receiver (micro)organisms has to be determined as well as the probability that such a transgenic (micro)organism has an advantage in its natural environment. Moreover in certain cases, for example, gut bacteria entering the sewage systems, they may benefit from newly acquired genetic information. It is remarkable that in the various regulations, health and environmental risks are not mentioned separately. Genes encoding proteins that pose a health hazard will not be considered in this chapter, as responsible companies will never start the development of such a food product; neither will authorities give permission for cloning such genes in plants and/or microorganisms that enter the food chain. On the other hand, genes encoding proteins that may provide the receiving (micro)organism with an ecological benefit, will be considered.

Potential Benefits of Genetically Modified Lactic Acid Bacteria

As stated in the Introduction, rDNA technology will only become a success if unmet consumer demands are fulfilled, because then the benefit:risk ratio (if there is any risk) will be very much in favor of the benefits. As is demonstrated by the large success of rDNA technology in the pharmaceutical area, that is what counts. Similarily rDNA enzymes in detergent products offer also clear performance and environmental benefits to consumers and the penetration of rDNA enzymes in these products is nearly 100%.

Clear consumer benefits of fermented foods will be:

(a) *Lactic acid bacteria with clear health benefits to consumers.* This will be a worldwide benefit. For the developing countries there are enormous opportunities to develop fermented foods that reduce infectious diseases (Tuomola et al., 1999), whereas for the developed countries the ever increasing health care costs will force governments to devote much more attention to disease prevention, and fermented products may play an important role in that scenario (Table 12.4);
(b) *Lactic acid bacteria that prolong the shelf life of fermented food products.* This is of particular importance to the developing countries that do not have the well controlled chilled distribution systems of the Western countries;
(c) *Lactic acid bacteria that upgrade the nutritional value of food products, by producing (micro)nutrients.* This is of particular importance for the developing countries, as some of the substrates of fermented products are "poor" in (micro)nutrients. A well-known example is cassava, used by millions of consumers, but very poor in proteins and consequently in essential amino acids;
(d) *Improvement of flavor of fermented products.* Flavor of food products are often consumer demand *number one* and with our increasing understanding of flavor

perception and the decay of the sensitivity of certain taste and odor perception systems as functions of age (Wysocki and Pelchat, 1993), it will be a challenge to develop feremented food products that answer the demands of ageing consumers as that may indirectly contribute to the well-being of these consumers.

Ad (a) During the last couple of years excellent programmes have started to determine potential health promoting aspects of LAB and to transfer the genetic information for these health effects to other LAB, thereby enlarging the number of fermented foods with clear and sustainable health benefits. Work is in progress to develop LAB as carriers for passive immunization (Pouwels et al., 1998). It is not yet certain whether this approach will be more efficient than other ways of passive or active immunization (Haq et al., 1995). However the consumer benefits, or better the benefits to humanity, of passive immunization are evident. For example, it is estimated that between 1 and 2 million young children die each year because of rotavirus infection in their gastrointestinal (GI) tract (Glass et al., 1994). It has been demonstrated that antibodies can neutralize these rotaviruses so well, that the infectious dose is not reached and consequently health problems are prevented (World Bank, 1993). Many other viruses and pathogenic microorganisms that exert their devastating activity in the GI tract of consumers may be neutralized by passive immunization as well. Consumer-friendly and affordable passive immunization can only be achieved using rDNA technology. It is very likely—although not all steps of the risk assessments proposed later in this chapter can be carried out on the basis of present knowledge—that the consumer benefits of passive immunization will outweigh the risks that may be related to the usage of genetically modified LAB. Replacement of (potentially) pathogenic bacteria by LAB in the GI tract is another realistic route to improve the health of consumers (Tuomola et al., 1999). There is an increasing amount of evidence that LAB can stimulate the mucosal immune system (Brassart and Schriffrin, 1997), which is of paramount importance to the health of consumers, as the immune system of the GI tract—which is larger than any other immune system in the human body—plays a crucial role in the elimination of transformed epithelial cells, food allergies, etc. Also a significant reduction of eczema and intestinal inflammation associated with food allergy in infants has been described (Kirjavainen et al., 1999). Moreover there is increasing evidence that with age the functionality of the (mucosal) immune systems decrease (Miller, 1996) and stopping or retarding this process, using fermented foods containing certain LAB, will be of great benefit. There are soft claims on the importance of LAB to prevent the conversion of potentially procarcinogens into carcinogens or to convert carcinogens (Hirayama and Rafter, 1999). Lowering of the cholesterol level by LAB is also claimed in the literature (Gilliland et al., 1985), but well-controlled experiments could show no assimilation of cholesterol or a benefit (Klaver and Van der Meer, 1993). These results—using the strains described in the literature as being beneficial (Gilliland et al., 1985) were confirmed in the laboratory of the authors. One of the potential beneficial aspects of genetically transformed LAB will be analyzed in the risk assessment later on in this chapter.

Ad (b) In the developing world, the amount of food products spoiled, before reaching the dish of the consumer, is still enormous (estimates indicate that up to 30% of all foods are spoiled). Although hard figures are lacking, for a considerable part this is due to microbial spoilage. There is excellent work done on antimicrobial compounds, such as nisin (Delves-Broughton, 1990), pediocin (Chikindas et al., 1993) and other bacteriocins (Van Kraaij, 1999) that are produced by LAB. Highly effective antimicrobial peptides from other organisms (Barra and Simmaco, 1995; Schonwetter et al., 1995) can be produced by transgenic LAB. These LAB, either as such, or in combination with cell wall degrading enzymes, provide a new and effective route to prevent microbial food spoilage, most likely consumer demand number one in developing countries.

Also the combination of transgenic plants producing insecticidal proteins (Jouanin et al., 1998) and increased and timely production of enzymes that lyse bacterial cell walls and cell walls of lower eukaryotes (already present in plants [Cornelissen et al., 1986]) and LAB that produce antimicrobial peptides, may contribute to an affordable food supply and consequently prevent malnutrition in the developing world. Improvement of the supply chain of food to the poorest of the world and not the absolute amount of food produced is the major problem (Conway and Toenniessen, 1999).

Ad (c) Lactic acid bacteria are often quite demanding with respect to their nutrients. In products like cheese this results in extensive degradation of milk proteins into amino acids and peptides which contribute significantly to the flavor of cheeses (Fox et al., 1996). However when LAB are grown on substrates relatively poor in proteins, like cassava, this is a clear disadvantage. However the biosynthetic pathways of amino acids in bacteria are quite well-known and especially *Brevibacteria* and *Corynebacteria* are excellent producers of amino acids (Jetten and Sinskey, 1995). Construction of LAB that can grow well on cassava and are able to convert carbohydrates and inorganic salts into amino acids may result in fermented cassava with better organoleptic properties and with a much higher nutritional value. Similarly, fermented products rich in folate, an important vitamin for pregnant women and often not present in sufficient amounts in the diet, should be a target. What is needed is a study of the nutritional requirements of African people now consuming cassava, and determination of their preferences for certain flavors, in order to develop in a rational way high quality fermentation products. Similarly, other indigenous food products may be upgraded in nutritional aspects.

Ad (d) As indicated before, in Western countries consumer demand number one is often optimal appearance and organoleptic properties of the food products. One of the attractive aspects of food fermentation processes is that diversity in organolept properties is created relatively late in the supply chain, for example, the steps in the supply chain of dairy products are equal for all types of fresh dairy products and cheeses up to the fermentation process (the few cheeses produced from unpasteurized milk excluded). Then, by using different starter cultures (and enzymes) and different process conditions in the actual fermentation process, an enormous diversity in products is created, offering the consumer the capacity to select products to their taste preferences. In this respect it is noteworthy that creating diversity at the final step in the supply chain is of economic importance. For the initial step, the economy of scale can be used to keep the price of such products low, whereas, during the fermentation process, with relatively small changes, enormous diversity can be created, as demonstrated in the production of beers, bread, cheeses, and wine. With age, taste perception decays, and some very nice products lose their attractiveness for the ageing consumers. With the enormous progress in understanding odor and taste perception (Buck and Axel, 1991; Shepherd, 1991; Vassar et al., 1993; Malnic et al., 1999) and its decay as a function of age (Wysocki and Pelchat, 1993), it will become possible to select different starter cultures (e.g., modified by genetic techniques) and process conditions to produce optimal products for the ever increasing market of wealthy consumers over 60 years of age.

The potential benefits to consumers, of food products fermented with LAB, is certainly not analyzed completely. In other parts of this book many other aspects will be discussed and the examples given above are just to illustrate that it is possible to get the balance between benefits and (theoretical) risks of fermented products right.

General Aspects of Risk Assessment of Genetically Modified Foods and Fermented Foods

It is important to define very precisely in which step of the supply chain a genetically modified ingredient or even raw material is used. A clear definition of what will be evaluated against which criteria is the only way to carry out risk assessments and to avoid those risk assessments that are mixed up with ethical debates. Provided that the newly introduced gene is encoding an intrinsically harmless protein, in general the risk assessments will provide the answers given in Figure 12.2a,b. The differences between these two figures are the presence, in the genetically modified organisms, of a gene encoding an antibiotic resistance marker. Although the evidence that antibiotic resistant genes are transferred from a genetically modified organism to another organism is still not quite clear, there are indications of such transfer (Lorenz and Wackernagel, 1994). As a result of many discussions with Consumer Organisations and environmentalists and their organizations, the author concluded that it is simply impossible to explain to a consumer why such a gene should be present in a genetically modified food product, even if there is neither a health nor an environmental risk. Moreover the presence of such a gene weakens the arguments of rDNA technologists that their method only adds useful information to the recipient organism in a well-defined way.

Figure 12.3/Table 12.5 shows the first of the decision schemes that will result finally in the decisions depicted in Figure 12.2a,b. For each raw material or ingredient used in the (fermented) food product the decision scheme should be used. Sometimes the first question will be answered with a "YES," followed by "STOP." This means that, when the ingredient or raw material originates from a transgenic animal, the evaluation process should be stopped. This is based on the view that a proper risk assessment of transgenic animals for usage as food cannot be carried out at present because there is a lack of knowledge in the area of safety of transgenic animals to consumers, and because the essential debate on the ethical aspects of foods from transgenic animals is not (yet) held.

From this decision scheme one is referred to either Figure 12.4 and Table 12.6 for raw materials or ingredients from plants, or to Figure 12.7 and Table 12.9 for a food ingredient derived from a transgenic microorganism, *but free from DNA of that microorganism*. For fermented food products manufactured with transgenic micro-organisms, that are still present and alive in the fermented product at the moment of consumption, Figures 12.5, 12.6 and Tables 12.7, 12.8 should be used to make a proper risk assessment.

All schemes result in clear answers as to whether the risk is acceptable or not. However it is a problem that certain probabilities, that are essential to carry out a proper risk assessment, are not available yet and are intrinsically difficult to determine. Therefore the better approach is to spend effort to determine whether there is an intrinsic health and/or environment hazard related to the introduction of the new genetic property.

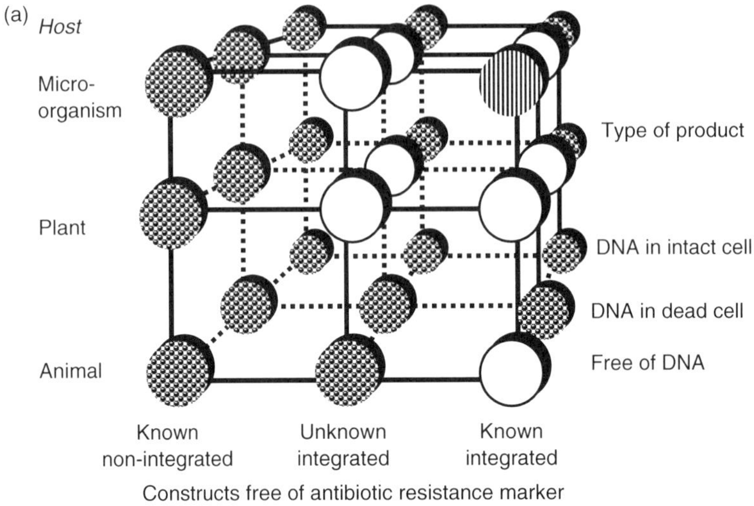

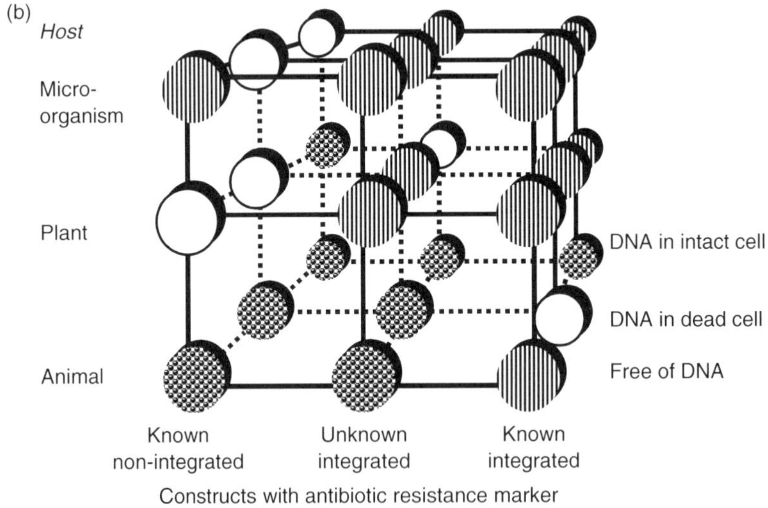

Figure 12.2. Risk cubes indicating health and environmental risks. (a) Products made by GMO's free of antibiotic resistance markers; (b) Products made by GMO's that contain antibiotic resistance markers. X-axis: Knowledge of new gene and how it is introduced in the Host; Y-axis: Nature of the Host; Z-axis: Nature of Product: *Free of rDNA*: for example, enzymes or antibodies made in approved fermentation processes; *DNA in dead cells*: the GMO is chemically or physically inactivated, for example, pasteurized products; DNA in intact cells: products containing active cells, for example, transgenic plants. Although always a complete Health and Environmental Assessment has to be carried out the results of such assessments will most probably be:

○ High Risk Concern;
● Risk Concern Low but still too many unknown factors;
◍ No Health or Environmental Risk expected.

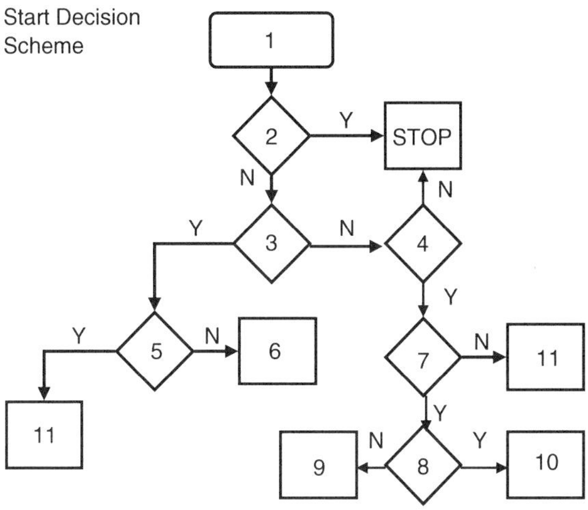

Figure 12.3. Introduction to risk assessment and to risk cubes.

Table 12.5. Decision Scheme to Determine the Nature of the Host Cell and Some Other Main Characteristics of the GMO

1(E).[a]	Recombinant DNA product
2(Q).	Is the host an Animal?
3(Q).	Is the host a commonly consumed Plant?
4(A).	Is the host a food grade microorganism?
5(Q).	Is the antibiotic resistance marker (used during construction) present in GMO?
6(A).	Go to Decision schemes for GM plants (Figure 12.4 and Table 12.6)
7 Q).	Is the antibiotic resistance marker eliminated?
8(Q).	Are living microorganisms present in the Food product?
9(A).	Go to Decision Scheme Food Ingredients (Figure 12.7 and Table 12.9)
10(A).	Go to Decision Scheme Fermented Foods (Figures 12.5, 12.6 and Tables 12.7, 12.8)
11(A).	Discuss with BT company why the antibiotic resistance marker is still present. This presence has an impact on the environment (horizontal transfer) and is a clear negative point in discussions with opinion makers and Consumer organizations.

[a] E = entry; A = action; Q = questions.

Supply Chain of Foods Prepared by Fermentation with Lactic Acid Bacteria

The hazard and risk aspects for fermented food products using rDNA technology in any step in the supply chain to be considered are:

1. is (are) the newly introduced gene(s) encoding a harmful product? If so stop the development of such systems;
2. can the newly introduced gene(s) provide the host with a benefit in its intended or "open" environment (this is a hazard factor!) and if so will that have consequences for other cells in the intended or "open" environment (risk assessment);

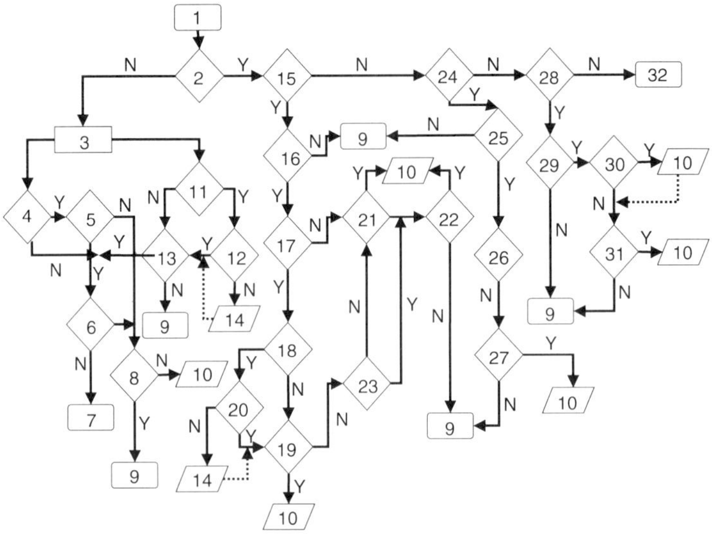

Figure 12.4. Foods derived from transgenic plants. Decision tree based on FDA statement of Policy May 1992 (Verrips, 1995).

3. can the newly introduced gene(s) be transferred to other (micro)organisms? If so (which means that the transfer occurs with a reasonable and quantifiable probability, e.g., a probability $<10^{-10}$) will this result in a benefit to the receiving (micro)organisms in its natural ecological system or in the "open" environment? If so will this have consequences on other cells operating in the natural ecological system or in the "open" environment?

A simplified model of a supply chain of a fermented food is given in Figure 12.8. This supply chain includes production of raw materials of animal and plant origin, harvesting (or collecting) these raw materials, pre-processing, addition of enzymes and/or microorganisms, fermentation, post-fermentation processes, distribution, and finally consumption. In principle all these steps have to be included for a proper risk assessment, although it will be clear that for fermented milk products, using non-GMO milk, the risk assessment can start at the point of addition of the recombinant enzyme and/or the genetically modified LAB.

As is shown in Table 12.1, beside milk (in Europe, United States), cassava (Africa), maize, sorghum, soybean, and rice (Asia) are the most important raw materials of foods fermented with LAB, and three of these raw materials (maize, soybean, and rice) are more and more of transgenic origin (Abelson and Hines, 1999; DellaPenna, 1999; Mazur et al., 1999; Moffat, 1999a,b; Serageldin, 1999; note that all these references are in one *Science* issue [Volume 285]). This means that a risk assessment of these raw materials has to be made as part of the total risk assessment of fermented foods in which one or several raw materials or ingredients are of transgenic origin. It is outside the scope of this chapter to go into detail of how a proper risk assessment of plant raw materials has to be made, but beside official guidelines, for example, of the FDA, the reader is referred to many earlier publications on this subject, also in relation to fermented foods (Verrips, 1995; Verrips and Van den Berg, 1996). Also the risk assessment of recombinant enzymes will not

Table 12.6. Food Derived from Transgenic Plants. Decision Tree Based on FDA Statement of Policy, May 1992 (Verrips, 1995)

1(E).[a]	Food derived from new (via rDNA technology modified) plant variety?
2(Q).	Will the modification result in nutritional effects?
3(A).	Assess the safety of the host plant and the donor of the DNA (gene)
4(Q).	Does the host species have a history of safe use?
5(Q).	Do characteristics of the host species, related species, or progenitor lines warrant analytical or toxicological tests?
6(Q).	Do test results provide evidence that toxicant levels in the new plant variety (GMO) do not present a safety concern?
7(A).	New variety (GMO) is not acceptable
8(Q).	Is the concentration and bio-availability of important nutrients in the GMO within the range ordinarily observed in the host species?
9(A).	No concern
10(A).	Consult FDA
11(Q).	Is food from the donor commonly allergenic?
12(Q).	Can it be demonstrated that the allergenic determinant has not been transferred to the GMO?
13(Q).	Do characteristics of the donor species, related species, or progenitor lines warrant analytical or toxicological tests?
14(A).	Consult FDA for additional or alternative testing
15(Q).	Will the modification result in the expression of proteins in the GMO?
16(Q).	Is the newly introduced protein present in food derived from the plant?
17(Q).	Is the protein derived from a food source substantially, or similar to, an edible protein?
18(Q).	Is food from the donor commonly allergenic?
19(Q).	Is the introduced protein reported to be toxic?
20(Q).	Can it be demonstrated that the allergenic determinant has not been transferred to the GMO?
21(Q).	Does the biological function of the introduced protein raise any safety concern, or is the introduced protein reported to be toxic?
22(Q).	Is the introduced protein likely to be a macro-nutrient of the human or animal diet?
23(Q).	Will the intake of the donor protein in the GMO be generally comparable to the intake of the same or similar protein in the donor or other food?
24(Q).	Will the modification result in the biosynthesis of new or modified carbohydrates in the GMO?
25(Q).	Has there been an intentional alteration in the structure, composition, or level of carbohydrate that does not normally occur in food carbohydrates?
26(Q).	Has any structural feature or functional group been introduced into the carbohydrate that does not normally occur in food carbohydrates?
27(Q).	Have there been any alterations that could affect digestibility or nutritional quality in a carbohydrate that is likely to be a macro-nutrient of the diet?
28(Q).	Will the modification result in the biosynthesis of new or modified fats or oils in the new variety?
29(Q).	Has there been an intentional alteration in the identity, structure, or composition of fats or oils in the GMO?
30(Q).	Has the intentional alteration been in a fat or oil that will be a macro-constituent of the diet?
31(Q).	Are any unusual or toxic fatty acids produced in the GMO?
32(E).	The product does not fit in this decision scheme

[a]E = entry; A = action; Q = questions.

be included, even though one of the most successful recombinant enzymes, chymosin, is solely used in the (milk) fermentation industry.

The risk assessment approach will be illustrated on two different fermentation products; one in which genetically modified LAB are used, but are not present in the end product (soy sauce), and one in which living lactic bacteria are present in the final product (yogurt).

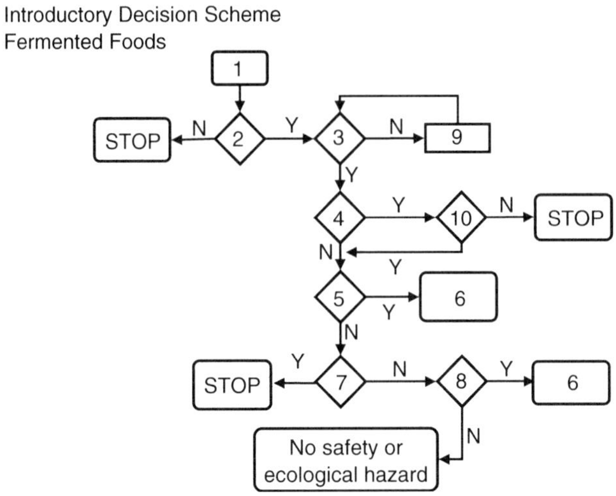

Figure 12.5. Introduction scheme to determine risk to consumers and environment of GMO fermented foods.

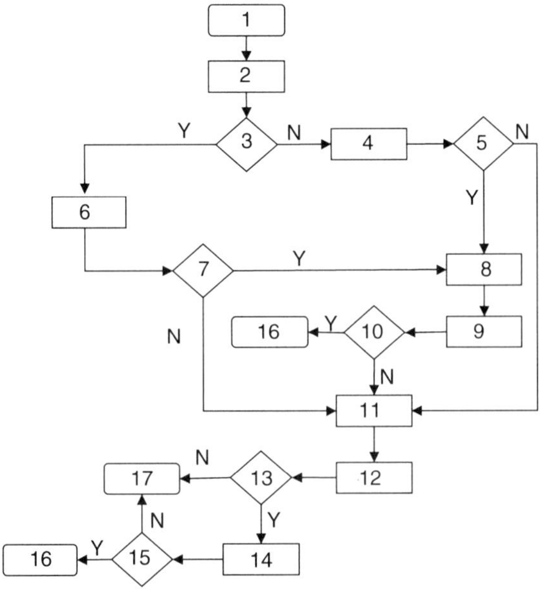

Figure 12.6. Structured assessment of risk related to with GMO fermented foods. (Note that the values for b, c, d, e, f, and g have to be determined experimentally and approved by governments (Verrips and Van den Berg, 1996).

Supply Chain of Soy Sauce

A simplified soy sauce process is depicted in Figure 12.9. It is assumed that a genetically modified lactic acid bacterium is used in this process, for example, a strain in which the resistance to salt is enhanced and that therefore is metabolically more active in the fermentation step in which salt is used to control undersirable microorganisms. Alternatively the lactic acid bacterium may contain genes encoding for enzymes to speed up the degradation of polysaccharides present in soy meal. Beside these newly introduced functional

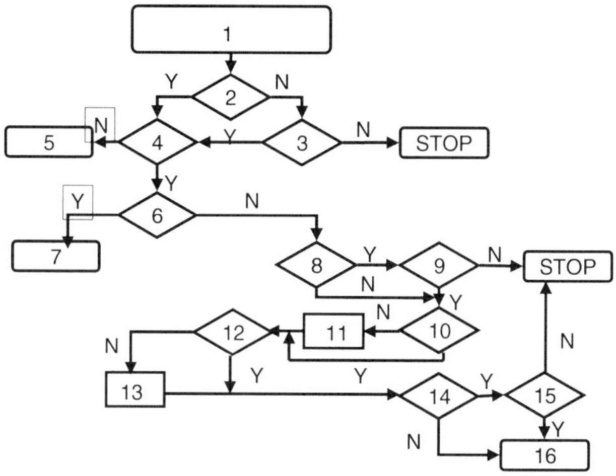

Figure 12.7. Structured assessment of cell free GMO derived Food components (e.g., enzymes) (Verrips, 1995).

Table 12.7. An Introduction Scheme to Determine Safety to Consumers and Some Environmental Consequences of Genetically Modified Microorganisms Used in Fermentation Processes

1(E).[a]	Generally Recognized As Safe genetically modified microorganism used in fermentations and still living in the final product
2(Q).	Encode the newly introduced gene for an intrinsically safe product?
3(Q).	Is the new gene stable integrated in the genome of the host cell?
4(Q).	Is an antibiotic resistance marker used during construction of the GMO?
5(Q).	Does the newly introduced gene encode for a protein that may result under certain conditions in an ecological advantage for the host cell?
6(A).	Carry out full risk assessment
7(Q).	Does the newly introduced gene encode for a protein that after transfer may result under certain conditions in an ecological advantage to recipient mammalian cells?
8(Q).	Does the newly introduced gene encode for a protein that after transfer may result under certain conditions in an ecological advantage to recipient microbial cells?
9(A).	Integrate new gene, preferably on pre-determined locus on the chromosome of the host
10(Q).	Is the antibiotic resistant marker gene eliminated?

[a]E = entry; A = action; Diamonds (Q = questions); Y = yes, N = no.

properties in one case it is assumed that either the lactic acid bacterium contains an antibiotic resistance marker (often used during transformation of micoorganisms as it provides a simple criterion to select transformed cells) or that an endogenous gene serves as a selection marker of the newly introduced genetic information (either an autonomous replicating plasmid or a plasmid that will integrate on the chromosome of the lactic acid bacterium). Another alternative is that the (antibiotic) resistance marker is eliminated (self cloning, De Vos and Simmons, 1994). So the first answers in the hazard analysis to be collected are:

1. are the genes used in the construct encoding proteins that are harmful to the consumer or to the environment?
2. are the genes used in the construct encoding proteins that will give recipient (micro)organisms a benefit in their ecological environment?

Table 12.8. A Structured Assessment of the Risk Related to the Introduction of Genetically Modified Lactic Acid Bacteria in (or as) Food Products (Verrips and Van den Berg, 1996)

1(E).[a]	Genetically modified lactic acid bacterium (GMO)
2(A).	Determine the distribution of the residence time of GMO in the GI tract of consumers. Take the time corresponding with 95 % of this distribution curve as $t(r)$
3(Q).	Will the GMO lyse with $P(b) > b$ in the GI tract within $t(r)$?
4(A).	Determine the probability $P(c)$ that intact cells of the GMO transfer genetic information to normal inhabitants of the GI tract. Use in these studies $t(r)$ as contact time and the conditions of the GI tract
5(Q).	Is $P(c) > c$?
6(A).	Determine the probability $P(f)$ that DNA originating from lysed GMO transform normal inhabitants of the GI tract (resulting in transformed inhabitants)
7(Q).	Is $P(f) > f$?
8(A).	Determine whether the transformed inhabitants obtain an advantage over untransformed inhabitants in the GI tract: $A(i)$. Define $A(i)$ in either faster growth rates $t'(g)$, better adhesion to epithelial cells h', or higher production of certain metabolites $\{p(x)', x = 1, \ldots\}$
9(A)	Determine the probability $P(e)$ that any of the events described under *action 8* will result in the formation of hazardous (= transformed inhabitant produce toxin or that will replace beneficial micro-organisms in the GI tract) microorganisms
10(Q).	Is $\{P(c) + P(f)\} * P(e) > e$?
11(A).	Determine also the probability $P(d)$ that the GMO will be transformed by genetic material originating from the common GI tract microorganisms (= modified GMO)
12(A).	Determine whether the modified GMO gains an advantage over untransformed GMO: $B(i)$. Define $B(i)$ in either faster growth rates $t''(g)$, better adhesion to epithelial cells h'', or higher production of certain metabolites $\{p(x)'', x = 1, \ldots\}$
13(Q).	Is $P(d) > d$?
14(A).	Determine the probability $P(g)$ that any of the events described under *action 12* will result in the formation of an hazardous GMO
15(Q).	Is $P(d) * P(g) > g$?
16(E).	This risk is unacceptable and the GMO should not be released
17(E).	This risk is acceptable and the GMO can be approved

[a] E = entry or end; A = action; Q = questions.

If, for either question one or two a positive answer is obtained, a complete risk assessment has to be carried out. It should be noticed that this is a hypothetical example, not providing any advantage to the consumer.

Supply Chain of Yogurt Produced with Genetically Modified Lactic Acid Bacteria

Yogurt manufacturing is a rather simple and short fermentation. Normally milk is collected (de-creamed) and pasteurized, after which a mixed culture of *Lactobacilli* and *Streptococci* (for certain varieties of yogurt *Bifidobacterium* is used as well) acidifies the milk to a pH between 4.3 and 4.6 within a couple of hours. It is assumed that the genetically modified *Lactobacillus* species contains new information, which provides this bacterium with the properties that ensure better survival in stomach and GI tracts of consumers, thereby reducing the probability that pathogenic bacteria will colonize the GI tract. Because of the increased survival this strain is also very suitable to produce antibody fragments that neutralize pathogenic bacteria or viruses present in the G/I tract. Although the authors are not aware if such a strain is already constructed, elsewhere in this book the ways to achieve this are outlined. Just as in the soy sauce case, it is assumed that the lactic acid bacterium contains either an antibiotic resistance marker or an endogenous

Table 12.9. Food Ingredient Produced with Recombinant Microorganisms, but Free of Any GMO or DNA Derived from that GMO (Verrips, 1995)

1(E).[a]	The food ingredient made by a recombinant microorganism (GMO)
2(Q).	Does the unmodified microorganism have a record of safe use in food products?
3(Q).	Can on the basis of feeding and/or toxicological studies the unmodified micro-organism be considered as safe in food products?
4(Q).	Is there sufficient knowledge and documentation that the newly introduced gene(s) encode(s) product(s) that is/are safe/acceptable in food products?
5(A).	Go to Novel Food guidelines
6(Q).	Does the GMO or an inherent part of it or the product(s) encoded by the newly introduced genetic material remain in the food product (criteria more than 1 GMO cell (or its equivalent in DNA)/ 25 ml)?
7(A).	Go to Decision Schemes Fermented Foods (Figures 12.5, 12.6 and Tables 12.7, 12.8)
8(Q).	May the consumption of the food containing the cell free product(s) encoded by the newly introduced gene(s), in the intended or expected consumed quantities result in any negative aspect on the health of the consumer?
9(Q).	Is it possible to reduce the quantities of the cell free product(s) encoded by the newly introduced gene(s) in food products to an acceptable level?
10(Q).	Are/is the newly introduced gene(s) stably integrated in the chromosome of the host cell?
11(A).	Integrate new genetic information stably on the host chromosome and/or ensure that during fermentation the GMO or its genes do not contaminate the environment
12(Q).	Is the GMO producing the food ingredient free of antibiotic resistance marker?
13(A).	Remove the antibiotic resistance gene (or ensure that during fermentation the GMO or its genes do not contaminate the environment)
14(Q).	Does the integration of the new genetic material disturb the metabolism of the GMO in such a way that hazardous products may be formed?
15(Q).	Does a 90 day feeding trial with the food product containing the cell free product(s) encoded by the newly introduced gene(s) show that the introduction of the new genetic material in the GMO does not have an effect on the metabolism of the GMO resulting in (a) hazardous compound(s)?
16(E).	Food products containing ingredients produced with this GMO can be approved

[a] E = entry; A = action; Q = questions.

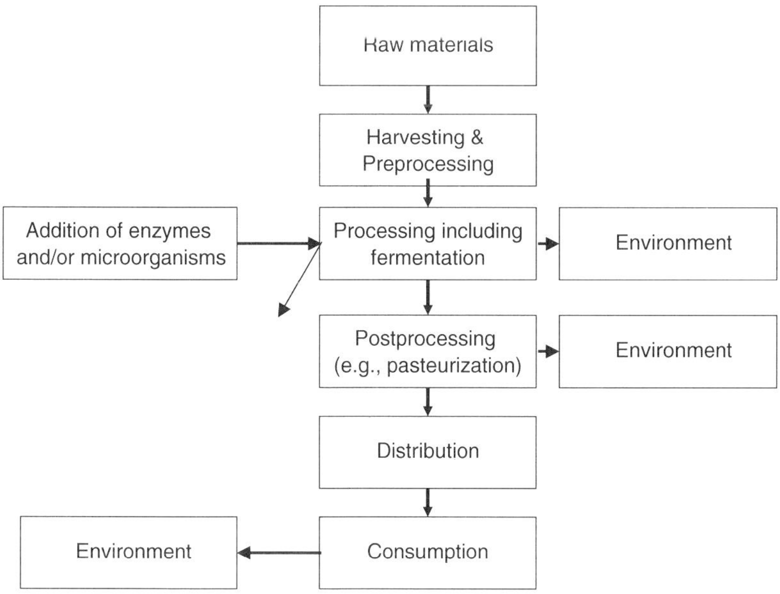

Figure 12.8. Simplified supply chain to show at which steps special care on the environmental risk has to be taken.

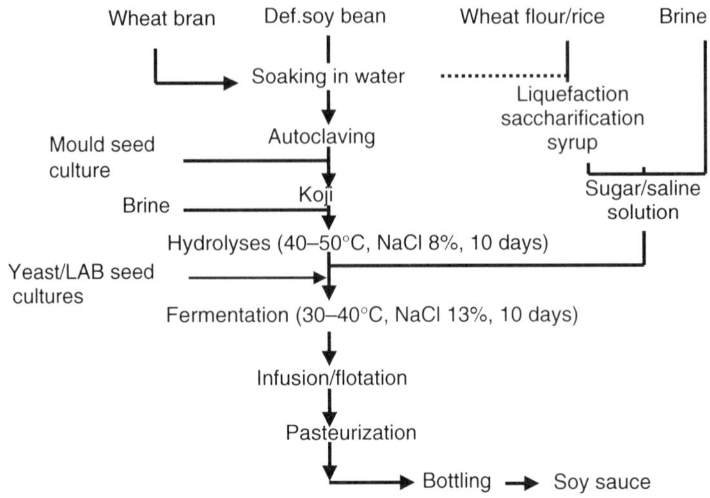

Figure 12.9. Simplified soya sauce fermentation process (in italics, possible introduction of transgenic material in the process).

gene as selection marker and that the modification is done either using an autonomous replicating plasmid or a plasmid that integrates on the chromosome of the lactic acid bacterium. The same schemes given in the example for soy sauce can be used, but the results will be quite different, and consequently in this example the risk assessment has to be completed up to the end of the supply chain (consumption of the products containing genetically modified LAB by consumers). Figures 12.5, 12.6 and Tables 12.7, 12.8 describe the questions in relation to the determination of the transfer of transgenic information from LAB either to eptithelial cells of the G/I tracts of consumers or to microorganisms present in the G/I tracts.

It is obvious that there are considerable advantages for the consumers of such a strain. However, because of the increased residence time, the probability of transfer of the genetic information to other residents of the G/I tract should be carefully studied, and in case of a probability $>10^{-10}$, the effects of this transfer on the properties of the modified micro-organisms should be studied in detail.

Conclusions

Making a risk assessment on fermented food product made by genetically modified microorganisms, or in the future, made from genetically modified plants, enzymes and microorganisms, without providing the benefits of the new food products to the consumer, is useless. Most likely no consumer will accept even the smallest risk, or even only a perceived risk, if there is no benefit for the consumer. Fermented foods in which LAB are (one of) the functional microorganisms, have a large number of proven or potential benefits, and these benefits can be increased by using rDNA technology and new screening and selection methods for the molecular structures providing these benefits. For quite some time there have been claims that LAB have a positive effect on gut motility, and experiments done within our company showed that indeed with a very high significance consumers (patients) with irritable bowel syndrome (IBS) could be cured by consuming milk fermented with *Enterococcus faecium* (Allen et al., 1992). However the mechanism of this benefit is still obscure. Modern screening techniques have resulted in the finding that a peptide can stimulate the motility of the gut system (Feighner et al., 1999) and soon the exact nature of the interaction of this peptide and its receptor will be known. Then it will be relatively simple to set up a system to study which LAB can interact with this receptor as well and when positive strains are found, whether this interaction can mimic the interaction of the peptide and this receptor and can cause the desirable effect. If in principle the effect is there but is quite weak, rDNA technology can either improve the interaction as such or it can provide more of the potential positive "epitopes" on the surface of the lactic acid bacterium. As IBS, or related problems with motility of the gut system, is quite a common problem of consumers (about one third of consumers have these problems to a certain degree), it is clear that the benefit can be considerable. Provided that the risk assessment, carried out by the authorities, shows that the health risk to the consumer is, even with the most sensitive methods available at present, not detectable, then the individual consumer should decide whether in this case the benefit outweighs the potential or proven environmental risk. Curing or prevention of IBS is certainly not the biggest benefit that fermented foods with genetically improved LAB can provide. Enormous (potential) benefits like the upgrading of nutritionally poor raw materials, passive immunization and stimulation of the immune system, thereby reducing the probability of colon cancer, should be studied in depth. When the expected benefits are proven beyond any doubt, the fact that in one or several steps rDNA technology will be used in the proper way, will certainly not be an obstacle for the consumer to buy these products.

References

Abelson, P. H., and Hines, P. J. (1999). The plant revolution. *Science* 285: 367–368.

Allen, W. D., Linggood, M., and Porter, P. (1992). Unilever Patent EPO508701.

Barra, D, and Simmaco, M. (1995). Amphibian skin: A promising resource for antimicrobial peptides. *TIBTECH* 13: 205–209.

Brassart, D., and Schriffrin, E. J. (1997). The use of probiotics to reinforce mucosal defence mechanisms. *Trends in Food Science and Technology* 8: 321–326.

Buck, L., and Axel, R. (1991). A novel multigene family may encode odorant receptors: A molecular basis for odor recognition. *Cell* 65: 175–187.

Cao, Y., and Cao, R. (1999). Angiogenesis inhibited by drinking tea. *Nature* 398: 381.

Chikindas, M. L., García-Garcerá, M. J., Driessen, A. J. M., Ledeboer, A. M., Nissen-Meyer. J., New, I. F., Abee, T., Konings, W. N., and Venema, G. (1993). PedeocinPA-1, a bacteriocin from *Pediococcus acidilactici* PAAC1.0, forms hydrophilic pores in the cytoplasmic membrane of target cells. *Applied and Environmental Microbiology* 59: 3577–3584.

Conway, G., and Toenniessen, G. (1999). Feeding the world in the twenty-first century. *Nature* 402S: C55–C58.

Cornelissen, B. J. C., Hooft van Huijsduijnen, R. A. M., and Bol, J. F. (1986). A tobacco mosaic virus-induced tobacco protein is homologous to the sweet-tasting protein thaumatin. *Nature* 321: 531–532.

Curic, M., Stuer-Lauridsen, B., Renault, P., and Nilsson, D. (1999). A general method for selection of α-acetolactate decarboxylase-deficient *Lactococcus lactis* mutants to improve diacetyl formation. *Applied and Environmental Microbiology* 65: 1202–1206.

DellaPanna, D. (1999). Nutritional genomics: Manipulating plant micronutrients to improve human health. *Science* 285: 375–379.

Delves-Broughton, J. (1990). Nisin and its application as a food preservative. *Journal of the Society of Dairy Technologists* 43: 73–76.

De Ruyter, P. G. A., Kuipers, O. P., Meijer, W. C., and de Vos, W. M. (1997). Food-grade controlled lysis of *Lactococcus lactis* for accelerated cheese ripening. *Nature Biotechnology* 15: 976–979.

de Vos, W. M., and Simmons, G. (1994). Gene cloning and expression systems in lactococci. In: M. J. Gasson, and W. M. de Vos (Eds.), *Genetics and biotechnology of lactic acid bacteria* (pp. 52–105). Glasgow: Blackie A. & P. Publishers.

Dubos, R. (1998). *Pasteur and modern science*. American Society for Microbiology Press.

Feighner, S. D. et al. (1999). Receptor for motilin identified in the human gastrointestinal system. *Science* 284: 2184–2188.

Fox, P. F., Wallace, J. M., Morgan, S., Lynch, C. M., Niland, E. J., and Tobin, J. (1996). Acceleration of cheese ripening. *Antonie van Leeuwenhoek* 70: 271–297.

Gilliland, S. E., Nelson, C. R., and Maxwell, C. (1985). Assimilation of Cholesterol by *Lactobacillus acidophilus*. *Applied and Environmental Microbiology* 49: 377–381.

Glass, R. I., Gentsch, J., and Smith, J. C. (1994). Rotavirus vaccines: Success by reassortment? *Science* 265: 1389–1390.

Haq, T. A., Mason, H. S., Clements, J. D., and Amtzenc, J. (1995). Oral immunization with a recombinant antigen produced in transgenic plants. *Science* 268: 714–715.

Hirayama, K., and Rafter, J. (1999). The role of lactic acid bacteria in colon cancer: Mechanistic considerations. *Antonie van Leeuwenhoek* 76: 391–394.

Hols, P., Kleerebezem, M., Schank, A. N., Ferain, T., Hugenholtz, J., Delcour, J., and de Vos, W. M. (1999). Conversion of *Lactococcus lactis* from homolactic to homoaniline fermentation through metabolic engineering. *Nature Biotechnology* 17: 588–592.

Hottinger, H., Mignot, O., and Mollet, B. (1992). Yogourt contenant des microorganismes vivants. European Patent Application 0518096.

Hugenholtz, J., and de Veer, G. J. C. M. (1991). Application of nisin A and nisin Z in dairy technology. In: G. Jung and H. G. Sahl (Eds.), *Nisin and novel lantibiotics* (pp. 440–447). The Netherlands: ESCOM, Leiden.

Jetten, M. S. M., and Sinskey, A. J. (1995). Recent advances in the physiology and genetics of amino acid producing bacteria. *Critical Reviews in Biotechnology* 15: 73–103.

Jouanin, L., Bonade-Bottino, M., Girard, C., and Gibaud, M. (1998). Transgenic plants for insect resistance. *Plant Science* 131: 1–11.

Kirjavainen, P. V., Apostolou, E., Salminen, S. J., and Isolauri, E. (1999). New aspects of probiotics—a novel approach to the management of food allergy. *Allergy* 54: 909–915.

Klaver, F. A. M., and van der Meer, R. (1993). The assimilation of cholesterol by lactobacilli and *Bifidobacterium* is due to their bile salt-deconjugating activity. *Applied and Environmental Microbiology* 59: 1120–1124.

Lorenz, M. G., and Wackernagal, W. (1994). Bacterial gene transfer by natural genetic transformation in the environment. *Microbiological Reviews* 58: 563–602.

Malnic, B., Hirono, J., Sato, T., and Buck, L. (1999). Combinatorial receptor codes for odors. *Cell* 96: 713–723.

Mazur, B., Krebbers, E., and Tingey, S. (1999). Gene discovery and product development for grain quality traits. *Science* 285: 371–375.

McGarry, A., Law, J., Coffey, A., Daly, C., Fox, P. F., and Fitzgerald, G. F. (1995). Effect of genetically modifying the lactococcal proteolytic system on ripening and flavor development in Cheddar cheese. *Applied and Environmental Microbiology* 60: 4226–4233.

Miller, R. A. (1996). The aging immune system: Primers and prospects. *Science* 273: 70–74.

Moffat, A. S. (1999a). Engineering plants to cope with metals. *Science* 285: 369–370.

Moffat, A. S. (1999b). Crop engineering goes south. *Science* 285: 370–371.

Nauta, A., van den Burg, B., Karsens, H., Venema, G., and Kok, J. (1997). Design of thermolabile bacteriophage repressor mutants by comparative molecular modelling. *Nature Biotechnology* 15: 980–983.

Needham, J., Gwei-Djen, L., and Hsing-Tsung, H. (1989). *Science and civilisation in China, Vol. 6, Biology and biological technology*. England: Cambridge University Press.

Pouwels, P. H., Leer, R. J., Shaw, M., Heijne-den Bok-Glaheuwer, M. J., Tielen, F. D., Smit, E., Martinez, B., Jore, J., and Conway, P. L. (1998). Lactic acid bacteria as antigen delivery vehicles for oral immunization purposes. *International Journal of Food Microbiology* 41: 155–167.

Reed, G. (1983). Foreword. In: H.-J. Rehm and G. Reed (Eds.), *Biotechnology, Vol. 5; Food and feed production with microorganisms*. Verlag Chemie.

Robinson, K., Chamberlain, L. M., Schoefield, K. M., Wells, J. M., and Le Page, R. W. F. (1997). Oral vaccination of mice against tetanus with recombinant *Lactococcus lactis*. *Nature Biotechnology* 15: 653–657.

Schonwetter, B. S., Stolzenvberg, E. D., and Zasloff, M. A. (1995). Epithelial antibiotics induced at sites of inflammation. *Science* 267: 1645–1648.

Serageldin, I. (1999). Biotechnology and food security in the 21st century. *Science* 285: 387–389.

Shepherd, G. M. (1991). Sensory transduction: Entering the mainstream of membrane signalling. *Cell* 67: 845–851.

Tuomola, E. M., Ouwehand, A. C., and Salminen, S. J. (1999). The effect of probiotic bacteria on the adhesion of pathigens to human intestinal mucus. *FEMS Immunology and Medical Microbiology* 26: 137–142.

Van de Guchte, M., Kodde, J., van der Vossen, J. M. B. M., Kok, J., and Venema, G. (1990). Heterologous gene expression in *Lactococcus lactis* subsp. *Lactis*: Synthesis, secretion and processing of the *Bacillus subtilis* neutral protease. *Applied and Environmental Microbiology* 56: 2606–2611.

Van Kraaij, C. M. J. (1999). *Probing the membrane activity of nisin by protein engineering* (pp. 5–26). Thesis, Utrecht University.

Vassar, R., Nigai, J., and Axel, R. (1993). Spatial segregation of odorant receptor expression in the mammalian olfactory epithelium. *Cell* 74: 309–318.

Verrips, C. T. (1989). Growth of microorganisms in compartmentalized products. In: G.W. Gould (Ed.), *Mechanism of action of food preservation procedures* (pp. 363–400). London: Elsevier Applied Science.

Verrips, C. T. (1995). Structured risk assessment of rDNA products and consumer acceptance of these products. In: H.-J. Rehm and G. Reed (Eds.), *Biotechnology (Vol. 12)*. VCH Publishers.

Verrips, C. T., and Van den Berg, D. J. C. (1996). Barriers to application of genetically modified lactic acid bacteria. *Antonie van Leeuwenhoek* 70: 299–316.

World Bank. (1993). *World Bank Development Report 1993: Investing in health*. New York: Oxford University Press.

Wysocki, C. J., and Pelchat, M. L. (1993). The effect of ageing on the human sense of smell, and its relationship to food choice. *Critical Reviews of Food Science and Nutrition* 33: 63–82.

Zhang, B., Salturo, G., Stalkowski, D., Li, Z. H., Zhang, Y., Roye, I., Vitella, D., Diez, M. T., Pelaez, F., Ruby, C., Kendall, R. L., Mao, X. Z., Griffin, P., Calaycay, J., Zierath, J. R., Heck, J. V., Smith, R. G., and Maller, D. L. (1999). Discovery of a small insulin mimetic with antidiabetic activity in mice. *Science* 284: 974–977.

Glossary of Terms

Abortive Infection: A broad collection of phage defense mechanisms which act at any number of points after phage adsorption and DNA injection to prevent proliferation and release of progeny phage. Abortive infection mechanisms usually result in death of the host, and are characterized by a reduced efficiency of plaquing (EOP), a decreased number of centers of infection, a reduced burst size, and reduced plaque size.

Adsorption Inhibition: The phage defense mechanism which blocks the first step in the phage infection cycle – attachment to the host. While current research suggests that certain carbohydrate or protein moieties play critical roles, these mechanisms remain largely unelucidated.

Antisense Technology: Antisense technology has been exploited to develop novel defense strategies which utilize the phage genome to inhibit proliferation of the phage. The antisense defense mechanism acts as an abortive inhibition mechanism in that, depending on the target gene, it acts at various stages in the phage lytic cycle and results in cell death. To utilize antisense technology, a phage gene, or other genetic sequence, is expressed in the antisense, or opposite, orientation to generate a mRNA complementary to the phage mRNA of interest. Interaction of the antisense mRNA with the phage target mRNA can inhibit translation, either by preventing ribosome loading, or destabalizing the target mRNA and making it more susceptible to RNase attack. If an appropriate target mRNA is selected, the antisense mRNA can inhibit the phage lytic cycle. In addition to the target, the appropriate ratio of antisense mRNA to target, sense mRNA is critical to the success of this mechanism.

Bacteriophage Insensitive Mutants (BIMs) are selected as survivors following high titer challenges with one or more phages. While varying mechanisms may be responsible, the predominant type of defense mechanism characterized in BIM's is one that interferes with phage adsorption via an alteration or masking of phage receptors. These mutations are often unstable, or may be accompanied by other undesirable traits such as slow acid development.

DNA Injection Inhibition: With this mechanism, phage adsorption takes place normally, but phage DNA is not detected until very late in the lytic cycle, if at all. While important, this mechanism is not well understood.

Efficiency of Plaquing (EOP): As used in this book, EOP is a measurement of the effectiveness of a phage defense strategy. EOP is calculated as follows: # plaques on strain containing defense mechanism / # plaques on sensitive, parent strain. As an example, an

EOP of 0.01 means that only 1 phage out of every 100 is capable of plaquing on the host carrying the defense mechanism of interest.

Phage Monitoring: Use of laboratory methods to detect phages in the cheese plant. If phages are detected, sensitive strains can be replaced with insensitive strains or derivatives to prevent the build up of the phage in the environment. While standard plaquing techniques can be used for phage detection, molecular methods including DNA hybridization, PCR, and ELISA, are currently under investigation.

Phage Encoded Resistance (*per*): A novel phage defense strategy which utilizes a portion of the phage genome to inhibit phage proliferation. In the examples descrubed, the phage origin of replication (*ori*) was presented on plasmids and resulted in inhibition of phage proliferation. Most likely, the *ori* on the plasmid acts as a false replication target, thereby titrating and depleting important replication proteins and decreasing the build-up of phage genomes. The *per* mechanism acts as an abortive inhibition mechanism in that cell death results after phage infection. For the most part, the *per* strategies described are very phage specific.

Restriction/modification: An early acting phage defense mechanism which utilizes two distinct enzymatic activities. First, presence of a restriction enzyme allows the strain to recognize and digest (restrict) foreign DNA, in this case phage DNA. Host DNA is protected by chemical modification using an encoded methylase. Since this mechanism acts early in the lytic cycle, immediately after DNA injection and cell viability is not typically affected, unless the phage escapes restriction. Restriction systems are inherently inefficient (EOP's @ 1/100 to 1/1000) and, therefore, modified phages inevitably appear in situations where R/M strains are used continuously. The types of restriction/modification systems are described in more detail within the text.

Rotation Strategies: Cheese manufacturers use rotation strategies to prevent the accumulation of phages in the dairy plant. Strains of varying phage sensitivities are used on a rotating basis so that phages capable of attacking one strain will encounter an insensitive strain and be prevented from further proliferation.

Stacking: Refers to the presence of multiple phage defense mechanisms in a single strain. Stacking occurs naturally in a number of prototype phage insensitive strains, and can protect them from a variety of phage types. In addition, stacking may also reduce the proliferation of mutant phages, since any phage capable of circumventing one mechanism may be inhibited by another acting at a different point in the lytic cycle. Stacking has also been accomplished by using conjugation or electroporation to introduce plasmids encoding varying phage defense mechanisms into strains of interest.

Index

936 phages 59, 73

A2 phage 66, 71, 84
ABC transporters *see* ATP-binding cassette (ABC) transporters
AbiA 300, 302
AbiB 301
AbiD1 300–1, 302
AbiE 294
AbiF 294
AbiG 301
AbiK 301, 302
AbiQ 301
abortive infection (Abi) 298–302
  genes 299–300
  of *Lc. lactis*, mechanisms of 299–300
  mode of action 300–1
  and phage infection cycle 300, 301
  phages overcoming 301–2
acetate kinase genes 175
acetyl transferases 321
acid resistance 266
acidification in milk fermentation 190
ackA gene 175
acmA gene 212
addressins 264
adenylyl transferases 321
adsorption inhibition, phage resistance by 292–4
aerotolerance 177
aggregation, cell 7, 32
aggregation-promoting factor 8
aggregation proteins 32
aldose sugar oxidization 171
alkaline shock protein 125
allergy prevention/treatment 280
amidases 55
amino acid biosynthesis 155, 158–9
amino acid degradation 159–60
amino acid uptake by lactococci 198
aminoglycoside resistance 321–2
aminopeptidases 189, 200–2
  aminopeptidase A 202
  aminopeptidase C 201
  aminopeptidase N 201, 209–11
aminopeptidases *contd.*
  aminopeptidase P 205
  of *Lc. lactis* proteolytic system 191
  narrow-specificity 202
  X-prolyl dipeptidyl aminopeptidase 203–4
animal gastro-intestinal tract 95
antibiotic feed additives 330, 331
antibiotic resistance 317–54
  acquired 317, 347
    in genetic modification 345, 347
    vs intrinsic 319
  avoiding distribution of 348
  distribution of determinants 321–4
  ecological aspects of LAB 318
  evolution hypotheses 319
  in farm animals 330–2
  in fermented food 332, 334
  highly resistant pathogens 318
  phenomena 318–19
  profiles of lactic acid bacteria 319–20
  transfer 320, 325
    by conjugative plasmids 320, 325–7
    from GMOs 363
    to intestinal microflora 338
    mechanisms 318–19
antibiotic resistance genes 5, 147, 196, 317, 318
antibiotic resistance markers 345, 369, 370
antigen-expressing *Lactobacillus* strains 147
antigens
  delivery to mucosa 261–5
  expression 147–8
  intracellular expression 267, 282
  M cell transported 264
  presentation 270
  secretion by LAB 283–4
antimicrobial activity
  lantibiotics 230
  transgenic LAB 362
antimicrobial peptides 225
antimicrobials 178
antisense RNA technology 4, 306–7
  barrier to successful use 307
  and phage resistance 82–3

antiterminator proteins 106, 107, 169, 170
arg genes 158–9
arginine biosynthesis 158–9
arginine deiminase (ADI) pathway 128–9, 159
Asa1 aggregation protein 32
Asc10 aggregation protein 32
AT drift 155
ATP-binding cassette (ABC) transporters 197, 199
  in antibiotic resistance 319
  in bacteriocin production 227, 244
  in lantibiotic export 233
  and producer self-protection 234
attB gene 53, 84
attenuation and immunogenicity 266
attP core 62
attP gene 53, 84
Aujesky's Disease Virus (ADV) 273
auto-induction 178
autolysin hydrolysis 212–13
autolysis 212
  and proteolysis 212–13
auxotrophy, amino acid 155, 158
avoparcin 330, 331, 332

B cells 264, 265
Bacillus spp.
  B. subtilis 7
    CR in 161–2, 163
    RNA polymerase 14
  bacteriocins against 226
  promoters 153
bacterial attachment site *see attP*
bacterial delivery systems *see* delivery vehicles
bacteriocin production 25, 132–4
  autoregulation 132
  instability 245
  in LAB 225–60
    Lactobacillus 178
  strength/timing of promotion 178
bacteriocinogenic strains 226
bacteriocins
  addition to starter cultures 212
  biosynthesis regulation 245
    HPK/RR system 245, 246
    induction 247–8
    pheremone 245–6
    quorum sensing model 247
    response regulators 247
    similar systems 246
    target promoters 247
  Class I *see* lantibiotics
  Class II 239–44
    biosynthesis regulation 239
    genes 237, 239–40, 243
    producer organisms 241–2
    regulatory circuit 243
  Class III producer organisms 242
  classification 226–7
bacteriocins *contd.*
  definition 225
  gene clusters 134, 240
  maturation 197
  pre-peptides 227, 228, 239
  producer self-protection 239
  sec-dependent 227, 239
  transporter genes 244
bacteriophage insensitive mutants (BIMs) 292–3
  scarcity of 304
bacteriophages *see* phages
benefits of GMOs 360–3, 372–3
betaine
  transport activity 127
  uptake systems 126
β-lactam antibiotic resistance 323
β-lactamase 323
Bifidobacterium 109
  antibiotic resistance 322, 323
  health-promoting 144
  resistance spectrum 319
bIL41 phage 70
bIL67 phage 56, 75, 77
bIL170 phage 59
biosynthetic pathways 130–5
  amino acid biosynthesis 130–1
  artificial promoters 134
  bacteriocin production 132–4
  carbon metabolism 132
  hybrid promoters 134
  nucleotide biosynthesis 131–2
  RNA stability 134–5
bitterness in cheese 209, 210, 213, 214
BK5-T phages 62, 65
blue/white selection of recombinants 5
bovine colostrum, antibodies in 309
bovine plasmin 211
Bradley phage classification 46
bronchial associated lymphoid tissue (BALT) 262
busA operon 126
butyrivibriocin 228

c2 phage 56, 73
  cell membrane receptor 293
  DNA replication 68
  early/late genes 56, 57, 58
  holins/lysins 75, 78
  origin of replication 67
  replication functions 67
carA gene 159
carB gene 131–2, 158
carbamoyl phosphate (CP) 158–9
carbohydrate metabolism 160
carbohydrate utilization genes 5
carbon catabolite repression (CR) 99–101
  CcpA-independent 107
  genetics 170
  glucose-mediated 173

carbon catabolite repression *contd.*
in *Lc. lactis* 100–1
in *Leuc. lactis* 106, 107
mechanisms in lactobacilli 160–1
see also CcpA-mediated CR
carbon metabolism 132
carbon starvation 130
carboxypeptidases 199, 200
carnobacteriocins 240, 244
immunity gene 243
producer organisms 241
carnosinase 203
casein degradation
in LAB 189–90
pathway, engineering of 208–9
proteinases 205
β-casein degradation 192–3
and proteinase classification 192–3
and temperature 196
caseinolytic pathway 189, 190, 207–8
casitone 207
casitone-dependent repression of proteolysis 215
cassettes
expression 148
plasmid-located DNA restriction 83
secretion 149
vectors comprised of 147
cat gene 317
catabolic control protein A *see* CcpA
catalase 177–8
CcpA 99–100, 103
in carbon metabolism 132
functions 100
homolog in lactobacilli 204
in *Leuc. lactis* 107
ccpA gene 162, 164–5
cluster, schematic representation of 164
location 163
mutation 167
ccpA-pepQ cluster/region 165, 204
CcpA-mediated CR 111, 161–5, 168
in phosphoketolase pathway 174
in sorbose metabolism 175
cell aggregation *see* aggregation, cell
cell membrane, permeabilization of 225–6, 230–1
wedge model of pore formation 231
cell wall anchor domain of PrtP 195
cell wall components in phage adsorption 293
cell wall hydrolases 212
cell wall weakening agents 12
Challis strain of *Strep. gordonii* 270–1
chaperones
heat-shock induced 196–7
protein 122
and stress responses 176
Cheddar cheese 291
cheese making
and antibiotic resistance 335, 341–2
cheese making *contd.*
bacterial contamination 332, 334, 338
experiments with Gouda 209
flavour development 212
flavour formation 213–14
organoleptic quality 209
phage problems 291
plant monitoring for phages 304
rennet action 208
ripening 83–4, 145
accelerated 213
bovine plasmin in *Lc. lactis* 211
rotation/replacement strategies 303–5
sensory evaluation 210
starter cultures 190
trials 189
chloramphenicol acetyl transferases 149, 322
chloramphenicol resistance 322, 334, 335–6
chromosomal integration
in *Lactobacillus plantarum* 275
plasmids 6–7
in *Strep. gordonii* 271
chromosome size/shape 2
chromosome walking strategy 31
CIRCE (controlling inverted repeat of chaperone expression) 123, 176
citrate fermentation, *Leuconostoc* 3
cloning heterologous genes 16
cloning systems, food-grade 209
cloning vectors 4–5
construction 347–8
for lactobacilli 269
and restriction-modification 14
Clostridium, bacteriocins against 226
Clp proteases 176, 196
ClpE function 123
ClpP function 123
clpP gene 123, 124
CluA amino acid sequence 32
cluA gene 32
co-integration 31
co-mobilization 10
codon frequencies in *Lactobacillus* 156–7
codon usage 155, 156, 157
rarity, species-specific 158
CodY 215
cold adaptation 125, 126
cold shock (CS) 113
proteins 177
colicin V 225
colitis models 281
commensal bacteria
immune response to 265
recombinant, as live antigen vector 277, 278
tolerance of 278–80
commercial importance *see* economic importance; industrial importance
comparative genomics 61–80, 109–10

competence
  in *Strep. gordonii* 271
  and transformation 8, 10–11, 347
composite resistance plasmids 317
computational methods 135
conjugal delivery systems 30
conjugation 7–8, 29–34
  frequencies 10
  as genetic tool 9–10, 146–7
    natural 320
  indigenous 30
conjugative plasmids 320, 325–7
  as genetic tool 346–7
conjugative transposons 35–9, 327–9
  in antibiotic resistance 320, 325
  host range 327
  Tn*916* transposon 327–8
constitutive-promoter library 134
consumer demands in science 356–7
Cop-binding operator 28
Cop protein 28
cos phages 49
cos sites 54
  lactococcal phages 70–1
  in P335 phages 60
  in phage synthesis 54
cotransfer (mobilization) 7
countertranscript RNA 4
covalently closed circular (CCC) DNA 30
Cp-1 phage holins 78
CR *see* carbon catabolite repression
cre elements/sequences 111, 162
cro early gene 52
Cro-like proteins 64–5, 67
Cro regulatory protein 52
csp genes 125, 126
CtsR stress regulator 124, 176
CylA 233
cytokines 261, 268–9, 281
cytolysin 229, 230, 234, 238

dairy fermentations 291, 292
dairy industry 95, 213, 291
  phages 45–6, 50
DEAD-box helicases 8
decision schemes 363
  food derived from GMOs 371
  food derived from transgenic plants 366, 367
  GMO main characteristics 365
  introductory, for fermented foods 368
    consumer safety/environmental consequences 369
  nature of host cells 365
dehydroalanine (Dha) 227, 232
dehydrobutyrine (Dhb) 227
deletion of chromosomal elements 308
delivery vehicles 265–71
  attenuating mutants 265
    LAB 266–71

delivery vehicles *contd.*
    Lactobacillus 178, 268–70
    Lactococcus lactis 267–8
    Strep. gordonii 270–1
  see also oral vaccines
dendritic cells 278
dental caries oral vaccine 282
dephosphorylation in inducer exclusion 166–7
Der p1 peptide 280
Dha 227, 232
Dha reductase 233
Dhb 232
di- and tripeptide transporter 206, 208
dipeptidases 202–3
dipeptide uptake 198
DNA
  AT rich 2
  autonomous molecules 2
  covalently closed circular (CCC) 30
  damage by oxidative stress 127–8
  E. coli chromosomal, replication of 53
  exogenous 8, 13
  inclusions for adaptability 2
  injection 293
  methylation 14
  packaging 49
    cos-site containing phage 70–1
    phage 54
  plasmid, segregational instability of 25
  single-stranded 27, 28
  see also phage DNA; rDNA products/technology
DNA gyrase 3, 7, 323
DNA homology
  P335 phages 81
  in phage classification 50–1
DNA-microarrays 135, 136
DNA topoisomerase 7
DnaK 123, 196–7
DT1 phage 1–2, 76, 77
DtpP 198
DtpT 198, 206, 208
dust mite allergy 280

early genes 52
  of 936 phages 59
  of bIL67 57
  of c2 56, 58
economic importance
  dairy industry 95
  fermentation 178
  lactic acid bacteria 143
  nisin 226
  stress response regulation 176
  see also industrial importance
EDTA inhibition of peptidases 204, 205
  aminopeptidases 200, 201, 205
  dipeptidases 202
  tripeptidases 203

efficiency of plaquing (EOP) 293, 294, 295
  reduction with antisense RNA technology 306
  reduction with Per 305
  reduction with suicide system 307–8
efflux proteins 322, 323
EII^{Man} complex 167–8, 173
electroporation 11, 12
  recovery of transformants 13
electrotransformation 10, 11
elements 31
Embden-Meyerhof pathway 95
endopeptidases 55
  of *Lc. lactis* proteolytic system 191, 199–200
  NisP 197
enterocin A 240, 241
enterocin B 241, 243
enterocin L50 243
enterococci
  antibiotic resistance 321, 322, 330–8
    community reservoir 338
    conjugal transfer of genes 335–6
    food-borne *vs* clinical 334, 338
    vancomycin 338
  distribution 325
  in food products 330–8
    farm animals/meat 330–2, 334, 335–6
    fermented food 332, 334
    as index organisms 330
  IS elements 37
  medical importance 330
  resistance spectrum 319
enterolysin A 227
environmental hazards 360
enzyme delivery systems 261
enzyme I (EI) 97, 100, 103
enzyme II (EII) 97
enzyme-linked immunosorbent assay (ELISA) 304
epicidin 228, 235
epidermin 228, 230, 231
epigallocathechinegallate (EGCg) 356
epilancin 232
EpiP leader peptidase 233
epithelial cells, induction of oral tolerance in 279
epithelial transport, M cell mediated 264
ericin 228
ermAM gene 317
erythromycin resistance 334, 338
  conjugal transfer of genes 335–6
Escherichia coli
  DNA replication 53
  expression vectors 17
  RNA polymerase 14–15
  Shine-Dalgarno sequence 15
European Commission support 284
evolution
  horizontal 81
  phages 80–1
    lytic *vs* lysogenic 64–5, 80–1

excisionase 64
exopeptidases 200–6
  aminopeptidases 200–2
  dipeptidases 202–3
  proline-specific peptidases 203–4
  tripeptidases 203
expanded major protein 54
experimental vaginitis model 282
expression signals, analysis of
  amino acid biosynthesis 155, 158
  codon usage 155, 156, 157
  promoters 150–5
expression vectors 17, 147–50, 179
  regulatable (NICE) 149
extrachromosomal elements 3

F4-1 phage 73
fermentation 95, 356
  failure, phage in 45–6
  homolactic-heterolactic shift 162
  importance of 143, 178
  milk 190
  of pentoses 174
  and stress responses 176
fermented food
  benefits:risks ratio of GMOs 355–75
  improvements with genetically modified LAB 360–2
  risk assessment 372
filter mating 338
flavour benefits with genetically modified LAB 360–1, 362
flavour generating enzymes 212, 213–14
fluorescence-activated cell sorter (FACS) analysis 147–8
fluoroquinolone resistance 323
FNR-like protein (FLP) 177
FNR protein 177
fOg44 phage 76, 78
follicle-associated epithelium (FAE) 262
food 357
  derived from transgenic plants 366, 367
  industry 160
  production 143
  spoilage 361
food allergens, tolerance of 278–80
food enzymes, rDNA-derived 358
food-grade expression vectors 317
fpg-recA operon 127
functional genomics, future of 135–6
functional module exchange 80
fusion plasmids 10

GadCB system, pH-regulating 129
gal genes 108
  regulators 99, 101–2
  silent 103–4

gal operon 98
galK 104
galK genes 105
galM genes 104
galP genes 99
galR genes 104
galactose
in *Lactococcus lactis* cell wall 293
metabolism 96, 99, 101
of *Lc. lactis* MG1363 98–9
in nisin regulation 236
uptake system 109
galactose permease 99
β-galactosidase
genes encoding 108
of *Leuc. lactis* 105
plasmid-encoded 170
GalE function 99
gallidermin 228
gastrointestinal associated lymphoid tissue (GALT) 262
gastrointestinal tract
Lc. lactis in 121
pathogens replaced by LAB 361
GC drift 155
gene cloning vectors 25
theta replicons 29
gene expression 14
Gram-negative species 17
heterologous 16–17
in lactobacilli 270
future of 179
genetic tools for 145–7
regulation studies 179
and Shine-Dalgarno sequences 15
gene modules 56
gene regulation 17, 96
gene transfer 7–13
conjugation 7–8
enterococci to staphylococci 330
horizontal 80, 346–7
natural 320
pathogens to starter culture bacteria 346
PepF1/PepF2 200
relevance to safety evaluation 25
transduction 8
transformation 8–9
transgenic information, risk of 372
transposition 9
genes
manipulation 2
organization in *Lc. lactis* 96
genetic arrangement 2
genetic engineering
caseinolytic pathway 189
phage-resistant mechanisms 82–3
strain improvement 4, 11
genetic switch *see* lysogenic-lytic decision
genetic tools 135
conjugation as 9–10
insertion sequences as 36
for lactobacilli 145–7, 269
natural 320, 325–9
phage-derived 82–4
expression systems 83
integration vectors, site-specific 84
lysin exploitation 83–4
phage resistance 82–3
transduction as 10
transformation as 10–13
genetically modified organisms *see* GMOs
genomics
functional, future of 135–6
power of 109–10
GFP-tagged *Strep. gordonii* 271
glucose, growth on 98
glycopeptide resistance 321
glycosidases 55
GMO-derived products 358
GMOs 2
acquired antibiotic resistance 345
benefits to farmers 356
in fermented food production 355–75
gene transfer in safety evaluation 25
lactic acid bacteria
potential benefits 360–3
potential commercial processes 359
penetration on market 358
probability of transfer of genes 360
safety assessment of 135
transgenic animals for food 363
gp50 antigen 273
GroEL/GroES 176
growth medium composition 208
growth phase and transformation frequencies 12
gut motility 372, 373

haemocin 225
hazards 360, 365–6
health benefits with genetically modified LAB 360, 361
health hazards 360
heat-shock gene regulation 125
heat-shock induced proteinases 196–7
heat-shock protease *see* HflB
heat-shock proteins (HSPs) 122, 175–6
encoding gene organization 123
gene regulation 124
induction 127
levels 123, 125
heat-shock response 122–3
heat-stable protein (HPr) 97, 165–7
in CcpA-mediated CR 161–2
effects of mutations 103–4
genes encoding 100, 103

heat tolerance of mutant genes 195, 196, 197
helicases 69–70
hematin and catalase 177
heterofermentative LAB 95
heterolactic pathway 160
HflB 123, 125, 127, 130
high temperature stress 122–5
his *operon* 130
histidine kinase 133
histidine protein kinase *see* HPK
HK022 phage repressor 66
holins 55–6, 74–8
  classification 56
  dual start motif 56
homing 32–3
homing lymphocytes 264
homofermentative LAB 95
homologous recombination 6, 146, 329
homoserine dehydrogenase 131
homoserine kinase 131
hop resin resistance 319
horizontal gene transfer 80
host recombination proteins 6
HPK 246
HPK/RR system 245
HPr protein *see* heat-stable protein (HPr)
hprK mutants 167
HpRK/P 167
HPr(SerP) 161–2, 165–7
HtrA 195–6
htrA insertion mutant 195, 196
human myelin basic protein (hMBP) 279
hydrolases, cell wall 212
hyperosmotic growth conditions 127

ICE*St1* 35
IL-2, murine 281
IL 10, murine 281
illegitimate recombination 6–7
immune response 280
immune system, mucosal, stimulation of 361, 373
immunity gene
  bacteriocins 243–4
  cloning/transfer 244
  lantibiotics 234–5
immunization
  of cows 309
  passive 361, 373
  studies
    cytokine delivery 281
    dust mite allergy 280
immunoglobulins
  IgA 262, 265, 275, 278
  IgE 280
  IgG 275
inducer control 166
inducer exclusion 100, 166
inducer expulsion 100
industrial applications 4
industrial importance 11
  of LAB 45, 291, 359
  of plasmids 3
  see also industrial importance
inhibitor target mechanism 4
insecticidal proteins from transgenic plants 362
insertion mutant *htrA* 195, 196
insertion sequence (IS)-mediated transposition events 31
insertion sequences 36
insertional inactivation mutants 35
integrase 61, 63, 64
integrase mRNA 53
integration
  sequences 9
  single-crossover 145
  site-specific 53, 145
  systems 270
integration vectors 6, 146
  site-specific, as genetic tools 84
integrative conjugative elements 35
integrative recombination 53, 146
intestinal ecosystem 262
intron maturase 32
introns 31, 32–3
irritable bowel syndrome 373
IS elements 37–8
isoprimeverose 171, 172
isoprimeverose transporter (XylP) 171
IS*SIS*/IS*SIT* elements 31, 36

katA gene 177

L10 phage 74
LAB *see* lactic acid bacteria
lac-gal genes 101–2
lac-gal operons 108
lac genes 97–8, 105, 106
lac operon 97, 98, 132
  of *L. casei* 168–9
  lacA genes 108
  lacF genes 210
  lacG genes 107–8
  lacL genes 108, 170
  lacLM genes 105, 108, 170–1
  lacM genes 108, 170
  lacS genes 102
  lacSZ genes 108
  in lactobacilli 169
  lacX gene 97
  lacZ genes 109
  in *Leuc. lactis* 106, 107
lac regulators 101–2, 132
LacR 97, 98
LacS 102
LacT 106, 107, 170
lactic acid 143

lactic acid bacteria 1–2, 45, 318
  and allergy treatment 280
  in antibiotic-challenged habitat 317
  antibiotic resistance 325, 329
  associated with food/beverages/feed 144
  economic importance 143
  fermentation 95
  in fermented food/drink 357
  "generally regarded as safe" (GRAS) status 266, 291
  genetically modified
    and fermented food 355–75
    potential benefits 360–3
    potential commercial processes 359
  importance 2, 345–6
  as mucosal delivery vehicles 261–90
  positive health effects 359
  and vaccine delivery 271–8
    Lactobacillus 274–7
    Lactococcus lactis 272–4
    Streptococcus gordonii 277–8
lacticin 229, 230, 232, 234, 235, 236, 238
Lactobacillus spp. 3
  antibiotic resistance 322, 323, 324, 338–40
    farm animals/meat 339–40
  CcpA-mediated CR in 162–5
  codon frequencies 156–7
  as commensal organisms 144
  conjugation in 8
  effect on cytokines 268–9
  fermentation 105–9
  gene expression 144–88
    genetic tools for 145–7
  gut survival/transit time 269
  health-promoting 144
  integration vectors 6
  L. bulgaricus 37, 38
  L. casei 37
  L. fermentum KLD-like cells 263
  L. helveticus 38
  L. johnsonii 38
  L. plantarum 109, 110
  L. sakei 150
  as mucosal delivery vehicle 268–70
  persistence in gut 268
  phage integration 63, 64
  phages 48, 51, 60–1, 74
    cos sites 71
    holins 78
    of known genomic sequence 56
    lysins 79–80
    pac sites 72
    replication functions 69–70
  plasmid transfer 325–6
  promoters
    lacking 151–2
    statistical analysis 153
Lactobacillus spp. *contd.*
    TG motif present 154
  resistance plasmids 339
  resistance spectrum 320
  sugar gene clusters/operons 112
  and vaccine delivery 274–7
lactocin 228
lactocin S 232, 236, 238
lactococcal sex factors *see* sex factors, lactococcal
lactococcins 242, 244
  972 227
Lactococcus spp.
  alternative sugar fermentation 101
  antibiotic resistance 340–5
    farm animals/meat 339
    fermented food 341–2
  conjugation in 7
  integration vectors 6
  IS elements 37, 38
  Lc. lactis
    712 30, 31
    antibiotic resistance 322, 323, 324, 335–6
    C2 31
    compared to *Bacillus subtilis* 121
    gene expression regulation 121–42
    "generally regarded as safe" (GRAS) status 291
    IL 1403 genome 215
    lactose metabolism 96–102
    localization in gut 267
    MG1363 30, 31, 34
    ML3 30
    model of gene organization/regulation 96
    as mucosal delivery vehicle 267–8
    persistence in gut 267
    phage integration 63
    phage resistance 291–315
    phage susceptibility 292
    plasmid-free strains 25, 30
    proteolysis in 189–223
    PTS genes 109, 110
    resistance spectrum 319–20
    stress responses *see* stress responses
    and vaccine delivery 272–4
  phages 48
    holins 77
    of known genomic sequence 57
    lysins 78–9
    pac sites 71
    protein composition 72–3
  plasmid function 3
  sugar gene clusters/operons 112
  transduction 8
lactose fermentation in *Leuconostoc* 3
lactose metabolism 95–6
  alternative system 101–2
  in lactobacilli and bifidobacteria 107

PEP-PTS 96–7, 105–7
PTS 97–8, 168, 169
lactose permease 102
lactose plasmid::sex factor co-integrates 36
lactose PTS genes 105–6
lactose repressor 108
lactose transport in *Leuc. lactis* 105
lactose transporter activity, control of 166
lambda phage
  gene organization 52
  lysogenic-lytic decision 51–2
  replication 53–4
  synthesis 54
Lan residues 232
LanP serine protease 233
LanT transporter 233
lanthionine 227
lantibiotics 226, 227–30
  bacteria synthesizing 227, 230
  biological activities 230–2
  biosynthesis 232–3
  biosynthesis regulation 235–7
    "leaky" terminators 236
    two-component system 235
  export/processing 233–4
  gene cluster organization 237, 238
  leader peptides 230
  pre-peptides 228–9, 232
  producer self-protection (immunity) 234–5
  two-peptide systems 230
LasN 232
LasP 234
late genes
  of 936 phages 59
  of bIL67 57
  of c2 57, 58
LcnC transporter 244
leader peptides 230
leading strand replication 27
Leloir pathway 96, 98, 101
Leuconostoc
  antibiotic resistance 339
  IS elements 38
  lac genes, plasmid encoded 105
  phages 48
linked trait curing 35
lipid II 231–2
lipoteichoic acid 7, 99, 293
Listeria, bacteriocins against 226
LL-H phage 74
  holins/lysins 76, 79–80
  origin of replication 69
loose tails 54
low pH stress 128–9
low temperature stress 125
ltnI gene 134
ltnR gene 134
luciferase reporter gene fusions 208
lymphocytes, homing 264
lymphoid follicles 262, 264
lysins 55, 74–6, 78–80, 83
lysis
  and flavour development 212
  phage 55–6
lysogenic-lytic decision/switch 51–2, 61, 64–5
lysogenic (temperate) phages 8, 10
  genetic organization 59
  as integration vectors 146
  life cycle 47
  lysogeny module 61
  superinfection exclusion functions 67
lysogenisation, resistance to 53
lysogeny modules 61–7
  LAB phages 62
  lysogenic phages 61
  site-specific integration 61–4
lytic (virulent) phages 8
  evolution from lysogenic 64–5
  genetic organization 59
  life cycle 46–7, 51, 52, 55

M cell mediated epithelial transport 264
M cells 262
macrolide-lincosamide-streptogramin (MLS) resistance 323, 325, 334
magnesium chloride in plasmid maintenance 13
major capsid protein (MCP) detection 304–5
manganese catalases 177
marker genes
  in plasmid vectors 5
  selectable 5, 9, 34
    antibiotic resistance 345
    movement away from antibiotic resistance 317
    and phage resistance 303
  in yoghurt production 372
marker proteins in *L. sakei* 150
matR/ltrB 32
meat products and antibiotic resistance 335–6, 338, 339–40
MeLan residues 232
metalloenzymes 200–1, 203
methyl-lanthionine 227
microbial risk assessment 360
microcins 225, 234
microfold cells *see* M cells
milk 165, 206
minus origin in rolling circle replication 27
misfolded proteins, sensor for 123
mob recombination site 7
mobA/ltrB 32
mobilization *see* cotransfer
mobilization protein gene (*mobA/ltrB*) 32
monoclonal antibodies 304–5
mozzarella cheese 292

mRNA 14, 16, 134, 135
mucin production 262
mucosal associated lymphoid tissue (MALT) 262, 264, 284
mucosal delivery vehicles 261–90
mucosal immune system stimulation 361
mucosal immunization *see* vaccines, mucosal
mucosal surfaces 261–5
mucosal transport of antigens 264
multidrug transporters 319, 324
multiple drug resistant organisms
  farm animals 330, 331
  fermented food 332, 334
mutacin 228, 229, 236, 238
mutagenesis of LacT, site-directed 170
mv1 phage 76
mv4 phage 84
Myoviridae 46

N early gene 52
NADH 162
NADP 162, 163
nasal vaccination 272–3, 277–8
nasopharyngeal associated lymphoid tissue (NALT) 262
nisin 197, 226, 230
  auto-inducible promoter 149–50
  bacteriocin production regulator 132, 133
  biosynthesis 232, 233
  biosynthetic gene clusters 133
  biosynthetic transfer of genes 35
  commercial importance 226
  and delivery vehicle 267–8
  gene cluster 132
  gene cluster organization 238
  gene expression 36
  pre-peptide sequences 228
  producer self-protection 234
  regulation 235–6
  sensor/regulator genes 270
  wedge model of pore formation 231
nisin-inducible gene expression system 211
NisP endopeptidase 197, 233
NisR response regulator 133
non-heme catalases 177
non-lantibiotics 226
nonconjugative plasmids 9
nucleotide biosynthesis 131–2
nukacin 229
nutritional benefits with genetically modified LAB 360, 362
nutritional requirements of LAB 155

Ø10MC phage 76, 78
Ø50 phage 82
Ø7201 phage 71, 73–4
Øadh phage 60–1
  holins 76, 78
  lysins 76, 79
Øadh phage *contd.*
  protein composition 74
  repressors 66
Øgle phage 60–1
  holins 76, 78
  lysins 76, 80
  protein composition 74
  repressors 66–7
ØLC3 phage 75, 77, 79
ØO1205 phage 60
  holins 75, 77
  lysins 75, 79
  protein composition 73
  repressor 66
ØUS3 phage 75, 78, 84
ØvML3 phage
  holins 75, 77
  lysins 75, 78, 83–4

Oenococcus oeni
  and arginine deaminase pathway 160
  extrachromosomal elements 3
  phage integration 63
  phages 48, 50, 51, 78, 80
oligopeptidases 189
oligopeptide permease (Opp) system 189, 198–9, 205–6
oligopeptide uptake in *Lc. lactis* 198–9, 205–6
open reading frames (ORFs)
  and antisense RNA technology 82
  involved in abortive infection 300–1
  in *Lactobacillus* phage 74
  in lactococcal phage 72, 77
  in lysogeny module 62
  in phage evolution 80
  in pK214 plasmid 341–2, 344
  in prolate-headed phage 56–7, 67
  in small isometric headed phage 59, 60, 68–9
  in *Strep. thermophilus* phage 73–4
  superinfection exclusion 67
  targeted by antisense RNA technology 306
  in Tn*916* 328
Opp system 213
oral tolerance 278–80, 283
oral vaccines *see* vaccines, oral
origin of replication
  c2 phage 67
  LL-H phage 69
  sk1 phage 68
  Tuc2009 phage 68
origin of transfer (*oriT*) 7, 33–4
ornithine biosynthesis 158
osmotic stress 126–7
oxidative pentose phosphate pathway 95
oxidative stress 127–8, 177

P001 phage 70, 75
P335 phages 59, 60, 62

P335 phages *contd.*
cos sites 70
DNA homology 81
protein composition 72
pac phages 49, 71–2
pac sites 54, 60
packaging
cos-site containing phage 70–1
phage DNA 54
pAMβ1/pIP501 plasmid family 4
pAMβ1 plasmid
in conjugal transfer 9, 29, 338–9
MLS resistance transfer 325
physical map 326
pancreatic insufficiency model 282
pC1528 plasmid 293
pCI305/pWV02 plasmid family 4
pCI2000 plasmid 29
pediocin family 227, 241, 244
Pediococcus 3, 38
P. pentosaceus 38
PEG *see* polyethylene glycol
penicillin-binding proteins 323, 329
pentose fermentation 174
PEP-PTS lactose fermentation 96–7, 105–7
Pep5 lantibiotic 230, 231, 232
pre-peptide sequences 228
producer self-protection 235
PepA 202
PepC 201–2
PepDA 215
PepF1/PepF2 200
PepM 215
PepN 201, 208
as debittering enzyme 209, 210, 214
overexpression vector 210
pepN gene 209, 211
PepO 199–200
PepO2 200
PepP 205, 234
PepQ 204
pepQ gene 164–5
PepR1 204
PepT 203
PepV 202–3
PepX 203–4, 208
peptidase genes as selectable markers 5
peptidase mutants, production of 206–7, 214
peptidases
function assessment 206
intracellular 212
of *Lc. lactis* proteolytic system 191, 199–205
non-essential nature in *Lc. lactis* 206, 213
physiological role in proteolysis 206–7
proline-specific 203–4
uptake of 207
see also endopeptidases; exopeptidases
peptide pheremone (Phe) 245–6, 247–8
peptide transport (PTR) family 198
peptide transport system expression 208
peptide uptake systems 197–9, 205–6
persistence of bacteria in gut 267, 268, 270, 282
Peye'r patches 262, 263
pFGI food-grade plasmid 210–11
pH, external *vs* internal 128
pH homeostasis 128
pH-inducible promoters 128
pH-regulating GadCB system 129
phage adsorption inhibition 292–4
phage attachment site *see attP*
phage defense mechanisms
antisense RNA technology 306–7
deletion/replacement of chromosomal elements 308
genetically engineered suicide system 307–8
novel mechanisms 305–8
phage encoded resistance (Per) 305–6
stacking of 302–3
phage defense rotation strategy 304
phage-derived expression systems 83
phage detection 304
phage DNA injection inhibition 294
phage-encoded repressor protein 47
phage encoded resistance (Per) 82, 305–6
phage resistance 67
combinational variation, importance of 297
host-encoded mechanisms 292–302
abortive infection 298–302
bacteriophage adsorption inhibition 292–4
phage DNA injection inhibition 294
restriction/modification mechanisms 295–8
in *Lactococcus lactis* 291–315
multiple mechanisms 302, 303
multiple plasmids 302
phage-resistant starter cultures 45
phage susceptibility of *Lc. lactis* 292
phages 78
biology 51–6
classification 46, 47–51
by DNA homology 50–1
by host range 48
by morphology 46, 48, 50
by serology 49
by structural protein profiles 49–50
conjugation mediated by 8
in dairy industry 45–6
escaping restriction 295
evolution 56, 80–1
in fermentation failure 45–6
gene order, conserved 56
of known genomic sequence 57
LAB 46, 56
biology of 56–61
comparative genomics 61–80

phages *contd.*
  lactococcal 62
    DNA packaging 70–1
    replication functions 67–9
    site-specific integration 61
  life cycle 46–7
    disruption 82
  lysis 74–80
  lytic/lysogenic cycles 8
  p355-type 51
  properties 45
  protein composition 54–5, 72–4
  replication 53–4, 67–70
    retarded by Abi 300
  resistance to abortive mechanisms 301–2
  see also specific types
pheremone (Phe) 245–6, 247–8
phospho-β-galactosidase genes 105, 107–8
phospho-transferases 321
phosphoenolpyruvate *see* PEP
phosphoketolase pathway 174–5
phosphorylation 100, 166–7
phosphotransferase system *see* PTS
Pip phage receptor 293
pIP501 plasmid
  conjugation 29
  MLS resistance transfer 326
  in mobilization 9
pK214 plasmid
  antibiotic resistance genes 344–5
  genetic organization 340, 342–4
  genomics 340, 341–2
  insertion sequence elements 344
  physical map 343
PL-1 phage 71, 76, 79
plantaricins
  gene cluster organization 240
  plantaricin-A 178
  pre-peptide sequences 229
  producer organisms 242
  response regulators 247
  transporter genes 244
plasmid-encoded traits 25–6, 30
plasmid incompatibility 13–14
plasmid-located DNA restriction cassette 83
plasmid vectors
  designed 29
  for lactobacilli 269
plasmids 2, 3, 5–6, 25–9
  chromosomal integration 6–7
  cloning vectors 4
  competing 13
  composite resistance 317
  conjugative, in antibiotic resistance 320, 325–7
  copy numbers 4
  encoding adsorption inhibition 293
plasmids *contd.*
  heterologous transmissible 29–30
  maintenance 13
  recombinant 6
  replication 3–4 *see* rolling circle replication; theta replication
  sequenced 27
  stability 5–6
pLS1 family 27
plus origin in rolling circle replication 27
Podoviridae 46, 48, 50
polyethylene glycol (PEG) 10, 12
portal protein 54
pRE25 plasmid 337
pRE39 plasmid 334
primosomes 53
pro-specific peptidases 191
probiotics 178, 318
proheads 54
prolate headed phages 56–7, 58, 73
prolidase 204
prolinase 205
proline 165
proline iminopeptidase (Pip) 205, 212
proline-specific peptidases 203–4
promoter-probe vector 17
promoters
  activity 16
  cloning 16
  comparative strengths 149
  induction 128
  for *Lc. lactis* 134
  in lysogenic-lytic switch 67
  sequencing 14, 150–5
  synthetic 16
prophage-encoded gene for phage resistance 83
prophages 47, 59
  integration/excision 146
proteases and stress responses 176
protection at mucosal surfaces 262
protein chaperones 122
protein composition 72–4
protein phosphorylation 161
protein profiles, structural 49–50
proteinases 205–6, 209
  in bacteriocin maturation 197
  functions 195
  heat-shock induced 196–7
  in *Lc. lactis* 194
    cell-wall located 189, 206
    classification by specificity 192–3
    Clp complex 196
    DnaK 196–7
    HtrA 195–6
  of *Lc. lactis* proteolytic system 191, 192–7

proteolysis
and autolysis 212–13
in *Lc. lactis* 189–223
components 191
dependence on 190
proteolytic systems 155, 158
Lc. lactis 205–7, 209–11, 214, 215
proton motive force-driven transport 198, 319
protoplast fusion, PEG induced 11
protoplast transformation 10
pRS01 plasmid 30–1, 32
PrtM maturation protein 193
prtM regulators 207, 208, 209, 215
PrtP proteinase 192, 199, 206, 213
in autolysis 212–13
with duplicated sell wall domain 215
genetics 193–4
as multi-domain enzyme 194–5
specificity 193
prtP regulators 207, 208, 209, 215
pseudocatalases 177
pSH71 plasmid replication 27
PTS 110, 165
dominant role in sugar transport 100
in galactose metabolism 99
genes 109–10
glucose/mannose 167–8
lactose metabolism 105–6
ribose metabolism regulation 174
sorbose metabolism 175
pts deficient mutants 166
PTS-mediated CR 175
ptsHI operon 166–7
purC(orf)QLF operon 131
purDEK operon 131
purine biosynthetic genes 131
PurR 131
pWC1 plasmid 28
pWV01 plasmid 27, 28
pWV01/pSH71 plasmid family 4
pWV02 plasmid 29
pyr operon 158
pyrimidine biosynthesis 131, 158
pyrKDbF operon 131
pyrrolidone carboxyl peptidase (Pcp) 202

quorum sensing model 247

rapid lactose fermentation by PEP-PTS 96–7
rbs gene cluster 174
rDNA products/technology 356, 358, 365–6, 373
RecA 130
recombinant proteins 17, 280
recombinants 6
blue/white selection of 5
identification of 5
recombinase, site specific 53
recombination
homologous *see* homologous recombination
site-specific 145
regulator genes of caseinolytic pathway 207
regulatory elements in lactobacilli 178–9
regulatory signal of the stringent response 130
Rep protein in rolling circle replication 27, 28
rep transcription 28
RepB protein 29, 340
replacement of chromosomal elements 308
replication
E. coli DNA 53
of phages *see* phages, replication
replication functions
lactococcal phages 67–9
S. thermophilus phages 69
sk1 phage 68
Tuc2009 phage 68
replication modules 69, 70
replication protein (REP) 3–4
replicons 4, 27
replisome organizer 69
reporter genes 36
repressor-encoding gene 65
repressors 4, 47, 61
class I 64–6
class II 65, 66–7
classification 64–5
co-operative binding 65
XylR 173
resistance plasmids, composite 317
resolvase-like protein 63
response regulator 133
restriction-modification 13, 14
restriction cassette 83
restriction/modification mechanisms 295–8
complementary systems 297
escape mechanisms 295
rhamnose 293
ribonucleic antiterminator (RAT) sequences 106
ribose metabolism 174
ribosome-binding sequence (RBS) *see*
Shine-Dalgarno sequence
ribosome protection 322
risk assessment
antibiotic resistance markers 364
food containing GMOs 367
food derived from GMOs 367, 369
genetic modification in food 363–5
introduction of GM LAB in food 370
microbial 360
plant raw materials 366
recombinant enzymes 366–7
risk cubes 364
rlt phage 72, 75, 83
RNA polymerase 14
RNA polymerase holoenzymes 14

RNA stability 134–5
RNAase III 135
rolling circle replication (RCR) 3–4, 5–6, 27–8
Roundup 356
ruminococcin 229

S-protein encoding gene 153
sakacin-A 240, 241, 244
sakacin-P 178, 240, 241, 247
salivaricin 229
salt stress/tolerance 127
sat gene 317
screening procedures 355–6
secretion vectors 179
segregational instability 25, 27
selection procedures 355–6
serine protease 233
serology in phage classification 49
sex factors
 integration/excision 34
 labile 7
 lactococcal 30–4
sex pheremones 7, 327
Sfi9 phage 76
Sfi11 phage 73, 75
Sfi21 phage 76, 82, 84
shelf life prolongation with GM LAB 360, 361–2
Shine-Dalgarno sequences 15–16, 17
shuttle vectors 10, 147–8
 bifunctional 5
 instant, production of 25
sIgA production 262, 265
sigma factors 14, 128, 130, 150
sigma replication *see* rolling circle replication (RCR)
signal peptidases 191
silage inoculant 145, 330
silent *gal* genes 103–4
single-crossover integration 145
single-stranded binding proteins 53
single-stranded DNA
 conversion to double-stranded 27, 28
 generation 27
Siphoviridae 46, 48, 50, 51
site-specific integration 53, 145, 308
site-specific integration vectors 84
site-specific recombination 6, 145
sk1 phage
 cos site 70
 early/late genes 58
 genetic organization 68
 holins 75, 77
 lysins 75, 78
 origin of replication 68
slow lactose fermenters 101
small isometric headed phages 59–61
 early/late genes 58
 genomic sequence information 59–60
sor operon 175
sorbose metabolism 175
sorting experiments 148, 194
SOS response 52
 to DNA damage 127, 175
soy sauce
 fermentation process, simplified 372
 supply chain 368–70
spacer region 16
spore outgrowth and nisin 226
spot-sensitivity assays 304
sso (single stranded DNA origin) 4
staphylococcal lipase secretion 281–2
staphylococcin 229, 230, 232
starter activity tests 304
starter cultures
 antibiotic resistance 326
 bacteriocin addition 212
 change from mixed to defined 303–4
 cheese 190
 cold adaptation 125
 development 143–4
 engineering 209
 enterococci in 330
 genetically modified LAB 362
 LAB as 95
 lysis 83
 media additives 309
 and phage evolution 81
 phage-resistant 45
 proteinase-deficient 209
 proteolytic enzymes 208
stem-loop structures 53, 177
streptin 228
streptococcin 229, 236, 238
Streptococcus spp.
 antibiotic resistance 321, 322, 323, 324
 extrachromosomal elements 3
 resistance spectrum 320
 Strep. gordonii
  colonization rates/persistence 270
  as delivery vehicle 270–1
  expressing antibody ScFv H6 282
  and vaccine delivery 277–8
  intra-vaginal vaccination 278
 Strep. thermophilus
  IS elements 37, 38
  lactose-galactose exchange 102–3
  lactose metabolism 103–4
  pAMβ1 plasmid transfer 325
  silent *gal* genes 104
 and transformation 8
Strep. thermophilus phages 48, 50, 60
 classification 71, 73
 DNA packaging 71
 holins 77–8
 integration 63, 64
 lysins 79
 pac sites 71–2

Strep. thermophilus phages *contd.*
protein composition 73–4
replication functions 69
stress regulators 124
stress response genes 122–7
stress responses 122–7, 175–7
cross protection 129–30
genomic approach 135–6
global regulation 129–30
high temperature 122–5
low pH 128–9
low temperature 125–6
osmotic 126–7
oxidative 127–8, 177
sublancin 229
subtilases 193, 194
subtilin 230
biosynthesis 233
biosynthetic gene clusters 133
pre-peptide sequences 228
producer self-protection 234
regulation 235–6
sucrose catabolism 35
sugar accumulation, control of 166
sugar degradation genes 113
sugar gene clusters/operons 111
sugar metabolism 160
sugar-related genes 111, 113
suicide system, genetically engineered 307–8
suicide vectors 6, 28
as genetic tools 36, 270
sulfhydryl-group inhibitors 201
sulfhydryl-group reagents 203
superinfection exclusion (Sie) functions 67
superoxide dismutase 127, 177
supply chains
LAB-fermented food 365–72
containing GMOs 370, 372
derived from GMOs 368–70
in risk assessment of GMOs 363
simplified, showing environmental risks 371
suppressor gene replacement 211
survival after freezing 126

T cytotoxic cells 264
T helper cells 264, 280
tagatose phosphate pathway 96, 97, 99
temperate phages *see* lysogenic (temperate) phages
temperature sensitive *dnaK* mutants 197
temperature sensitive *htrA* insertion mutants 195, 196
temperature sensitive plasmids 28, 36
terminase 54
terminators, *rho*-independent 15
tetanus toxin fragment C (TTFC) 147
immunization studies 275–7
future work 283, 284
tetanus toxin fragment C (TTFC) *contd.*
nasal vaccination 272–3, 290
oral vaccination 272
subcutaneous vaccination 277
sorting experiments 148–9
tetM gene 317
tetracycline 330
tetracycline resistance
conjugal transfer of genes 335–6
in enterococci 322, 325, 338
in *Lactobacillus* 338
tetracycline resistance gene 34
Tetragenococcus 3
TG motif 150, 153, 155
Lactobacillus promoters lacking 151–2
Lactobacillus promoters with 154
therapeutic proteins
mucosal delivery 280–2
secretion by LAB 284
thermolysin 201
theta replication 3, 28–9
c2 phage 68
plasmid stability 5
theta replicons 29
thiolpeptidase inhibitors 201
threonine biosynthesis 131
Tn*916* transposon 35, 327–8
and gene transfer 346
physical map 327
and tetracycline 330
Tn*917*-like transposons 334
Tn*917* transposon 9, 36
Tn*919* transposon 35
Tn*1546*-like transposons 331
Tn*1546* transposon 329, 334
TNO expression vectors 147
tolerization 279
topoisomerases 68, 323
topological organization of genomes 81
toxic oxygen compounds 127
TP901–1 phage 62–3, 72
transcript profiling 136
transcription 14–15
in amino acid degradation 160
initiation
and promoter activity 16
sigma factors 150
transcription attenuation 4
transcription initiation 177
transcription start sequences 150
transcriptional activators 131, 306
transcriptional antiterminators 169
transcriptional regulation 146
transcriptional regulator (LacR) *see* LacR
transcriptional terminator proteins 106
transduction 8
as genetic tool 10
specialized 8

transfer (*tra*) genes 7
transformation 8–9
  competence 8, 10–11
  efficiencies 11–12
  frequencies 11–12
  as genetic tool 10–13
    natural 320, 329
  and horizontal gene transfer 346
  Lc. lactis as delivery vehicle 267–8
transgenic plants/microorganisms *see* genetically modified organisms
translation 14, 15
  restricted 16–17
transmissible plasmids 29–30
transporter genes 244
transporter proteins 99
  of *Lc. lactis* proteolytic system 191
transposable genetic elements 35–9
transposition 9
transposon/insertion sequences 2
transposons 9
  in lactic acid bacteria 346
  self-transmissible 9
  tetracycline resistance 325
  see also conjugative transposons
tripeptidases 203
tripeptide uptake in *Lc. lactis* 198
tRna encoding genes 53
trp operon 130
tryptophan biosynthesis 158
Tuc2009 phage
  holins 75, 77
  lysins 75, 79
  origin of replication 68

vaccination studies
  Aujeszky's Disease Virus 271
  tetanus toxin fragment C 272–3
vaccines
  delivery to mucosa 261–5
  delivery using LAB 271–8
    Lactobacillus 274–7
vaccines *contd.*
    Lactococcus lactis 272–4
    Streptococcus gordonii 277–8
  intravaginal 278, 282
  live *vs* killed bacteria 283
  mucosal 265, 268
    see also bacterial delivery systems
  oral 2, 121, 265
    dental caries 282
    future work 283
vanA gene 317
VanA transposons 332
vancomycin resistance 320
  in enterococci (VRE) 331–2, 338
  transposon evolution 334
variacin 229
vector development 25, 281
virulent phages *see* lytic (virulent) phages
volatile compounds 208

wedge model of pore formation 231
whole genome sequence analysis 109, 110, 135, 215
wine fermentation, malo-lactic 160

X-prolyl dipeptidyl aminopeptidase 203–4
xpkA gene 174
xyl genes 172–3
  and glucose-mediated CR 173
  of *L. pentosus* 172
*xyl*O sequences 173
xylose 173
xylose fermenting species 171
xylose metabolism 171–3
α-xylosidase 172
XylP 171
xylP gene 171
XylQ 172
xylQ gene 171
XylR repressor 173
xylT Lactobacillus-E. coli shuttle vector 148

yoghurt supply chain 370, 372